Role of MicroRNA in Cancer Development and Treatment

Role of MicroRNA in Cancer Development and Treatment

Editors

Alessandra Pulliero
Alberto Izzotti

MDPI • Basel • Beijing • Wuhan • Barcelona • Belgrade • Manchester • Tokyo • Cluj • Tianjin

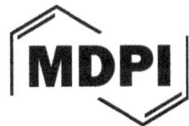

Editors
Alessandra Pulliero
Department of Health Sciences
University of Genoa
Genoa
Italy

Alberto Izzotti
Department of Experimental
Medicine
University of Genoa
Genova
Italy

Editorial Office
MDPI
St. Alban-Anlage 66
4052 Basel, Switzerland

This is a reprint of articles from the Special Issue published online in the open access journal *Journal of Personalized Medicine* (ISSN 2075-4426) (available at: www.mdpi.com/journal/jpm/special_issues/role_microRNA).

For citation purposes, cite each article independently as indicated on the article page online and as indicated below:

LastName, A.A.; LastName, B.B.; LastName, C.C. Article Title. *Journal Name* **Year**, *Volume Number*, Page Range.

ISBN 978-3-0365-3806-8 (Hbk)
ISBN 978-3-0365-3805-1 (PDF)

© 2022 by the authors. Articles in this book are Open Access and distributed under the Creative Commons Attribution (CC BY) license, which allows users to download, copy and build upon published articles, as long as the author and publisher are properly credited, which ensures maximum dissemination and a wider impact of our publications.

The book as a whole is distributed by MDPI under the terms and conditions of the Creative Commons license CC BY-NC-ND.

Contents

About the Editors vii

Alessandra Pulliero and Alberto Izzotti
Special Issue: "Role of MicroRNA in Cancer Development and Treatment"
Reprinted from: *J. Pers. Med.* **2022**, *12*, 503, doi:10.3390/jpm12030503 1

Giuseppe Valacchi, Erika Pambianchi, Simona Coco, Alessandra Pulliero and Alberto Izzotti
MicroRNA Alterations Induced in Human Skin by Diesel Fumes, Ozone, and UV Radiation
Reprinted from: *J. Pers. Med.* **2022**, *12*, 176, doi:10.3390/jpm12020176 5

Alessandra Pulliero, Deborah Traversi, Elena Franchitti, Martina Barchitta, Alberto Izzotti and Antonella Agodi
The Interaction among Microbiota, Epigenetic Regulation, and Air Pollutants in Disease Prevention
Reprinted from: *J. Pers. Med.* **2021**, *12*, 14, doi:10.3390/jpm12010014 37

Veronica Filetti, Carla Loreto, Luca Falzone, Claudia Lombardo, Emanuele Cannizzaro and Sergio Castorina et al.
Diagnostic and Prognostic Value of Three microRNAs in Environmental Asbestiform Fibers-Associated Malignant Mesothelioma
Reprinted from: *J. Pers. Med.* **2021**, *11*, 1205, doi:10.3390/jpm11111205 53

Katja Goričar, Marija Holcar, Nina Mavec, Viljem Kovač, Metka Lenassi and Vita Dolžan
Extracellular Vesicle Enriched miR-625-3p Is Associated with Survival of Malignant Mesothelioma Patients
Reprinted from: *J. Pers. Med.* **2021**, *11*, 1014, doi:10.3390/jpm11101014 67

Alberto Izzotti, Gabriela Coronel Vargas, Alessandra Pulliero, Simona Coco, Cristina Colarossi and Giuseppina Blanco et al.
Identification by MicroRNA Analysis of Environmental Risk Factors Bearing Pathogenic Relevance in Non-Smoker Lung Cancer
Reprinted from: *J. Pers. Med.* **2021**, *11*, 666, doi:10.3390/jpm11070666 85

Margherita Ferrante, Antonio Cristaldi and Gea Oliveri Conti
Oncogenic Role of miRNA in Environmental Exposure to Plasticizers: A Systematic Review
Reprinted from: *J. Pers. Med.* **2021**, *11*, 500, doi:10.3390/jpm11060500 101

Sara Tomei, Andrea Volontè, Shilpa Ravindran, Stefania Mazzoleni, Ena Wang and Rossella Galli et al.
MicroRNA Expression Profile Distinguishes Glioblastoma Stem Cells from Differentiated Tumor Cells
Reprinted from: *J. Pers. Med.* **2021**, *11*, 264, doi:10.3390/jpm11040264 117

Alberto Izzotti, Gabriela Coronel Vargas, Alessandra Pulliero, Simona Coco, Irene Vanni and Cristina Colarossi et al.
Relationship between the miRNA Profiles and Oncogene Mutations in Non-Smoker Lung Cancer. Relevance for Lung Cancer Personalized Screenings and Treatments
Reprinted from: *J. Pers. Med.* **2021**, *11*, 182, doi:10.3390/jpm11030182 131

Deborah Traversi, Alessandra Pulliero, Alberto Izzotti, Elena Franchitti, Licia Iacoviello and Francesco Gianfagna et al.
Precision Medicine and Public Health: New Challenges for Effective and Sustainable Health
Reprinted from: *J. Pers. Med.* **2021**, *11*, 135, doi:10.3390/jpm11020135 145

Barbara Marengo, Alessandra Pulliero, Maria Valeria Corrias, Riccardo Leardi, Emanuele Farinini and Gilberto Fronza et al.
Potential Role of miRNAs in the Acquisition of Chemoresistance in Neuroblastoma
Reprinted from: *J. Pers. Med.* **2021**, *11*, 107, doi:10.3390/jpm11020107 . . . . **175**

Maria Menini, Emanuele De Giovanni, Francesco Bagnasco, Francesca Delucchi, Francesco Pera and Domenico Baldi et al.
Salivary Micro-RNA and Oral Squamous Cell Carcinoma: A Systematic Review
Reprinted from: *J. Pers. Med.* **2021**, *11*, 101, doi:10.3390/jpm11020101 . . . . **193**

Rakhmetkazhy Bersimbaev, Olga Bulgakova, Akmaral Aripova, Assiya Kussainova and Oralbek Ilderbayev
Role of microRNAs in Lung Carcinogenesis Induced by Asbestos
Reprinted from: *J. Pers. Med.* **2021**, *11*, 97, doi:10.3390/jpm11020097 . . . . **207**

Michal Sima, Andrea Rossnerova, Zuzana Simova and Pavel Rossner
The Impact of Air Pollution Exposure on the MicroRNA Machinery and Lung Cancer Development
Reprinted from: *J. Pers. Med.* **2021**, *11*, 60, doi:10.3390/jpm11010060 . . . . **231**

Beatriz C. Lopes, Cristine Z. Braga, Fabrício V. Ventura, Jéssica G. de Oliveira, Edson M. Kato-Junior and Newton A. Bordin-Junior et al.
miR-210 and miR-152 as Biomarkers by Liquid Biopsy in Invasive Ductal Carcinoma
Reprinted from: *J. Pers. Med.* **2021**, *11*, 31, doi:10.3390/jpm11010031 . . . . **253**

About the Editors

Alessandra Pulliero

Alessandra Pulliero graduated with a BSc in Biology, Faculty of Mathematical, Physical and Natural Sciences, University of Padua, Italy. She received her doctorate in Environmental Medicine and Public Health, Faculty of Medicine, University of Padua Italy (2003–2006).

In 2001 she became Research fellow, for a research project funded by the MIUR entitled "Cross-talk between endoplasmic/sarcoplasmic reticulum and plasma membrane: interactions and functional relationships" at the University of Padua, Dept. of Biomedical Sciences Faculty of Medicine, University of Padua, Italy.

In 2007 she became Post Doc Researcher at the Dept. of Environmental Medicine and Public Health, University of Padua, Italy, for a research project (PRIN) entitled "Evaluation of exposure and individual susceptibility in subjects involved in the manipulation of antiblastic chemotherapy".

In 2008 she became Research assistant for a project on MicroRNA microarray and qPCR analyses and prevention of lung cancer. Setting up of microarray delivery systems. Analyzing microarray data. Involved in intracellular microRNA delivery by lipid nanoparticles. RNA interference and culture cells experiment at the Department of Health Sciences.

From 2013–2018 she was Research assistant at the University of Genoa on the project entitled "Development of preventive strategies of lung cancer by transfection with miRNA and modulation of DICER protein".

In 2017, Qualification of Associate in general and applied hygiene.

Alberto Izzotti

Prof. Izzotti has managed several research projects devoted to: (a) developing drugs for cancer prevention; (b) developing, in preclinical models, molecular tools applicable in the clinic; (c) shedding light on cancer ethio-pathogenesis; and (d) evaluating intermediate molecular biomarkers in clinical trials. Over the last ten years, he has mainly been involved in personalized medicine and postgenomic analyses using microarrays for evaluating the expression of genes and proteins. Since 2008, the research activity of Prof. Izzotti has been devoted to the study of microRNA, cancer chemopreventive agents, and gene transfer methods. Prof. Izzotti has managed several Grants for National and International projects.

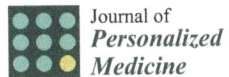

Editorial

Special Issue: "Role of MicroRNA in Cancer Development and Treatment"

Alessandra Pulliero [1,*] and Alberto Izzotti [2,3]

1 Department of Health Sciences, University of Genoa, Via Pastore 1, 16132 Genoa, Italy
2 Department of Experimental Medicine, University of Genova, 16132 Genova, Italy; izzotti@unige.it
3 UOC Mutagenesis and Cancer Prevention, IRCCS Ospedale Policlinico San Martino, 16132 Genova, Italy
* Correspondence: alessandra.pulliero@unige.it

Exposure to environmental contaminants may lead to changes in the expression of microRNAs (miRNAs), resulting in several health effects. miRNAs, small non-coding RNAs that regulate gene expression, have multiple transcript targets and thereby regulate several signaling molecules. Altered patterns of miRNAs can be responsible for changes linked to various health outcomes, suggesting that specific miRNAs are activated in pathophysiological processes. Genome-wide profiling demonstrates that miRNA expression signatures are associated with tumor type, tumor grade, and clinical outcomes, so miRNAs are potential candidates for diagnostic biomarkers, prognostic biomarkers, therapeutic targets, and preventive screening programs. Although miRNAs have multiple targets, their function in tumorigenesis is due to their regulation of a few specific targets. This Special Issue, entitled "Role of MicroRNA in Cancer Development and Treatment", focuses on the current state of pharmacogenomics and the extensive translational process required for clinical implementation, including the impact of environmental exposure on the MicroRNA machinery and cancer development. The present Special Issue provides a comprehensive overview of the current status of this interesting field of research. It comprises manuscripts reporting novel data as well as state-of-the-art reviews. The issue begins with five articles [1–4] focus on the role of microRNAs in environmental risk factors and lung cancer development.

Exposure to asbestos can cause cancer and other health conditions. A rare and aggressive cancer called mesothelioma is almost exclusively caused by asbestos exposure. Asbestos also causes a progressive lung disease called asbestosis. Environmental exposure to asbestos has been associated with a higher incidence of malignant mesothelioma. This study aimed to validate the predicted diagnostic significance of hsa-miR-323a-3p, hsa-miR-101-3p, and hsa-miR-20b-5p on a subset of mesothelioma patients exposed to asbestos and matched with healthy controls. PCR results showed that the three analyzed miRNAs were significantly down-regulated in cases vs. controls. In silico results showed a potential prognostic role of hsa-miR-101-3p due to a significant association of its higher expression and increased overall survival of mesothelioma patients [5]. Malignant mesothelioma is characterized by poor prognosis and short survival. Extracellular vesicles were isolated from serum samples obtained before and after treatment using ultracentrifugation on 20% sucrose cushion. Serum EV-enriched miR-103-3p, miR-126-3p and miR-625-3p were quantified using qPCR. After treatment, the expression of miR-625-3p and miR-126-3p significantly increased in mesothelioma patients with poor treatment outcome. Bioinformatics analysis showed enrichment of 33 miR-625-3p targets in eight biological pathways [6]. A review examines the role of microRNAs, the expression profile of which changes upon exposure to asbestos, in key processes of carcinogenesis, such as proliferation, cell survival, metastasis, neo-angiogenesis, and immune response avoidance [1]. As exposure to air pollution represents a dominant factor in the development of lung cancer and other respiratory system disorders, the authors identified the miRNAs commonly affected by

Citation: Pulliero, A.; Izzotti, A. Special Issue: "Role of MicroRNA in Cancer Development and Treatment". *J. Pers. Med.* **2022**, *12*, 503. https://doi.org/10.3390/jpm12030503

Received: 16 March 2022
Accepted: 18 March 2022
Published: 21 March 2022

Publisher's Note: MDPI stays neutral with regard to jurisdictional claims in published maps and institutional affiliations.

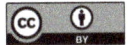

Copyright: © 2022 by the authors. Licensee MDPI, Basel, Switzerland. This article is an open access article distributed under the terms and conditions of the Creative Commons Attribution (CC BY) license (https://creativecommons.org/licenses/by/4.0/).

both conditions. Such molecules could serve as biomarkers of choice for identifying human populations at greater risk of lung cancer resulting from exposure to air pollution. The literature search identified a total of 25 miRNAs that meet such criteria. Among them, miR-222, miR-21, miR-126-3p, miR-155, and miR-425 may be considered the prominent molecules, as they were identified to be deregulated in multiple studies [3]. The knowledge of the mechanisms of action of environmental pollution now includes not only the alteration of the gut microbiota but also the interaction between different human microbiota niches such as the lung–gut axis. The epigenetic regulations can reprogram differentiated cells in response to environmental changes. In subjects at high risk of cancer, gut and lung microbiota are distinct from those of low-risk subjects, and disease progression is associated with microbiota alterations [4]. Next in this Special Issue are two contributions describing the relationship between miRNA profiles and oncogene mutations in non-smoker lung cancer and the identification, by microRNA analysis, of environmental risk factors using integrated DNA adducts and microRNAs analyses to retrospectively study the contribution of exposures to environmental carcinogens to lung cancer in 64 non-smokers living in Sicily and Catania city near to the Etna volcano [7]. MicroRNAs play a role in silencing mutated oncogenes, thus defending the cell against the adverse consequences of genotoxic damages induced by environmental pollutants. In addition, certain environmental compounds (i.e., diesel, ozone, and UV radiation) have been identified as persistent environmental pollutants due to their indestructible chemical and physical properties [8], in an experimental study, provide new information on the novel mechanisms on microRNA alteration in human skin biopsies exposed to diesel fumes, ozone, and UV light over 24 h of exposure. UV and ozone induced microRNA alteration immediately after exposure, whereas the peak of their deregulations induced by diesel fumes was reached only at the end of the 24 h. Diesel fumes mainly altered microRNAs involved in the carcinogenesis process, ozone in apoptosis, and UV in DNA repair. Epigenetics includes the study of the hypothesis that exposure to plasticizers causes changes in or the deregulation of a number of oncogenic miRNAs, and shows that the interaction of plasticizers with several redundant miRNAs, such as let-7f, let-7g, miR-125b, miR-134, miR-146a, miR-22, miR-192, miR-222, miR-26a, miR-26b, miR-27b, miR-296, miR-324, miR-335, miR-122, miR-23b, miR-200, miR-29a, and miR-21, might induce significant alterations. This systematic review points out the fact that the altered expression of microRNAs plays an important pathogenic role in exposure to plasticizers [9].

Consequently, human epigenetic studies have explored the identification and validation of miR-210 and miR-152 as non-invasive circulating biomarkers for the diagnosis and staging of breast cancer patients, confirming their involvement in tumor angiogenesis [10].

The expression of miRNAs was analyzed in primary tumors, metastases, and in bone marrow infiltrates of therapy-responsive and non-responsive neuroblastoma patients, in order to identify specific miRNAs involved in neuroblastoma metastasization and chemoresistance identifying miRNAs involved in the regulation of drug response and employed for therapeutic purposes [11]. Glioblastoma prognosis remains poor despite a remarkable amount of research programs; thus, this tumor remains a clinical challenge. The high level of inter- and intra-tumor heterogeneity is a major problem in the understanding of the physiopathology of the glioblastoma and requires a fine molecular analysis in order to lead to therapeutic solutions. The work of Tomei S. et al. [12] is part of this challenge. The authors investigated the microRNA profile of glioblastoma stem cells and their role in the progression of glioblastoma and patient outcome. Comparing the differential expression of miRNA in stem cells versus autologous differentiated cells might be of high interest. The authors found some new microRNAs correlated with the patient survival outcome. A review examines the role of the potential use of salivary microRNAs (miRNAs) as diagnostic and prognostic biomarkers for Oral squamous cell carcinoma patients aiding in the establishment of specific therapeutic strategies [13]. Precision and personalized medicine are useful tools for preventive strategies and could help with predicting morbidity and mortality and detecting chronic disease much earlier in the disease course, to improve the quality of care and quality of life of the patients and reduced healthcare time, efforts, and costs. Omics sciences offer a wide range of tools to improve public health including whole-genome and exosome sequencing. In future, disease prevention and treatment should be formulated at the individual level according to genomic features. Omics sciences have important implications for the prevention of both communicable and non-communicable diseases, especially because they can be used to assess health status during the whole course of life [14].

Funding: This research was partially funded by the University of Genoa, Italy PI Prof. Alberto Izzotti Grant '100008-2022-AI-FRA.

Acknowledgments: We would like to thank all the authors for providing excellent papers for this Special Issue of the *Journal of Personalised Medicine*, and for helping to further understanding and foster discussion within the field of the microRNA in cancer prevention. We would also like to thank the *Journal of Personalised Medicine* for the opportunity to edit this Special Issue. Finally, we would like to offer our sincere gratitude to the expert reviewers for offering fair and constructive criticism and oversight on the papers published in this issue.

Conflicts of Interest: The authors declare no conflict of interest.

References

1. Bersimbaev, R.; Bulgakova, O.; Aripova, A.; Kussainova, A.; Ilderbayev, O. Role of microRNAs in Lung Carcinogenesis Induced by Asbestos. *J. Pers. Med.* **2021**, *11*, 97. [CrossRef] [PubMed]
2. Izzotti, A.; Coronel Vargas, G.; Pulliero, A.; Coco, S.; Vanni, I.; Colarossi, C.; Blanco, G.; Agodi, A.; Barchitta, M.; Maugeri, A.; et al. Relationship between the miRNA Profiles and Oncogene Mutations in Non-Smoker Lung Cancer. Relevance for Lung Cancer Personalized Screenings and Treatments. *J. Pers. Med.* **2021**, *11*, 182. [CrossRef] [PubMed]
3. Sima, M.; Rossnerova, A.; Simova, Z.; Rossner, P. The Impact of Air Pollution Exposure on the MicroRNA Machinery and Lung Cancer Development. *J. Pers. Med.* **2021**, *11*, 60. [CrossRef] [PubMed]
4. Pulliero, A.; Traversi, D.; Franchitti, E.; Barchitta, M.; Izzotti, A.; Agodi, A. The Interaction among Microbiota, Epigenetic Regulation, and Air Pollutants in Disease Prevention. *J. Pers. Med.* **2021**, *12*, 14. [CrossRef] [PubMed]
5. Filetti, V.; Loreto, C.; Falzone, L.; Lombardo, C.; Cannizzaro, E.; Castorina, S.; Ledda, C.; Rapisarda, V. Diagnostic and Prognostic Value of Three microRNAs in Environmental Asbestiform Fibers-Associated Malignant Mesothelioma. *J. Pers. Med.* **2021**, *11*, 1205. [CrossRef] [PubMed]
6. Goričar, K.; Holcar, M.; Mavec, N.; Kovač, V.; Lenassi, M.; Dolžan, V. Extracellular Vesicle Enriched miR-625-3p Is Associated with Survival of Malignant Mesothelioma Patients. *J. Pers. Med.* **2021**, *11*, 1014. [CrossRef] [PubMed]
7. Izzotti, A.; Coronel Vargas, G.; Pulliero, A.; Coco, S.; Colarossi, C.; Blanco, G.; Agodi, A.; Barchitta, M.; Maugeri, A.; CT-ME-EN Cancer Registry Workers; et al. Identification by MicroRNA Analysis of Environmental Risk Factors Bearing Pathogenic Relevance in Non-Smoker Lung Cancer. *J. Pers. Med.* **2021**, *11*, 666. [CrossRef] [PubMed]
8. Valacchi, G.; Pambianchi, E.; Coco, S.; Pulliero, A.; Izzotti, A. MicroRNA Alterations Induced in Human Skin by Diesel Fumes, Ozone, and UV Radiation. *J. Pers. Med.* **2022**, *12*, 176. [CrossRef] [PubMed]
9. Ferrante, M.; Cristaldi, A.; Oliveri Conti, G. Oncogenic Role of miRNA in Environmental Exposure to Plasticizers: A Systematic Review. *J. Pers. Med.* **2021**, *11*, 500. [CrossRef] [PubMed]
10. Lopes, B.C.; Braga, C.Z.; Ventura, F.V.; de Oliveira, J.G.; Kato-Junior, E.M.; Bordin-Junior, N.A.; Zuccari, D.A. miR-210 and miR-152 as Biomarkers by Liquid Biopsy in Invasive Ductal Carcinoma. *J. Pers. Med.* **2021**, *11*, 31. [CrossRef] [PubMed]
11. Marengo, B.; Pulliero, A.; Corrias, M.V.; Leardi, R.; Farinini, E.; Fronza, G.; Menichini, P.; Monti, P.; Monteleone, L.; Elda Valenti, G.; et al. Potential Role of miRNAs in the Acquisition of Chemoresistance in Neuroblastoma. *J. Pers. Med.* **2021**, *11*, 107. [CrossRef] [PubMed]
12. Tomei, S.; Volontè, A.; Ravindran, S.; Mazzoleni, S.; Wang, E.; Galli, R.; Maccalli, C. MicroRNA Expression Profile Distinguishes Glioblastoma Stem Cells from Differentiated Tumor Cells. *J. Pers. Med.* **2021**, *11*, 264. [CrossRef] [PubMed]
13. Menini, M.; De Giovanni, E.; Bagnasco, F.; Delucchi, F.; Pera, F.; Baldi, D.; Pesce, P. Salivary Micro-RNA and Oral Squamous Cell Carcinoma: A Systematic Review. *J. Pers. Med.* **2021**, *11*, 101. [CrossRef] [PubMed]
14. Traversi, D.; Pulliero, A.; Izzotti, A.; Franchitti, E.; Iacoviello, L.; Gianfagna, F.; Gialluisi, A.; Izzi, B.; Agodi, A.; Barchitta, M.; et al. Precision Medicine and Public Health: New Challenges for Effective and Sustainable Health. *J. Pers. Med.* **2021**, *11*, 135. [CrossRef] [PubMed]

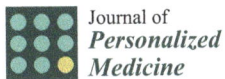

Article

MicroRNA Alterations Induced in Human Skin by Diesel Fumes, Ozone, and UV Radiation

Giuseppe Valacchi [1,2,3], Erika Pambianchi [1], Simona Coco [4], Alessandra Pulliero [5] and Alberto Izzotti [6,7,*]

1. Animal Science Department, Plants for Human Health Institute, North Carolina State University, Research Campus Kannapolis, Kannapolis, NC 28081, USA; gvalacc@ncsu.edu (G.V.); epambia@ncsu.edu (E.P.)
2. Department of Environmental Sciences and Prevention, University of Ferrara, 44121 Ferrara, Italy
3. Department of Food and Nutrition, Kyung Hee University, Seoul 130-701, Korea
4. Lung Cancer Unit, IRCCS Ospedale Policlinico San Martino, 16132 Genova, Italy; simona.coco@hsanmartino.it
5. Department of Health Sciences, University of Genova, 16132 Genova, Italy; alessandra.pulliero@unige.it
6. Department of Experimental Medicine, University of Genova, 16132 Genova, Italy
7. UOC Mutagenesis and Cancer Prevention, IRCCS San Martino Hospital, 16132 Genova, Italy
* Correspondence: izzotti@unige.it; Tel.: +39-010-3538522

Abstract: Epigenetic alterations are a driving force of the carcinogenesis process. MicroRNAs play a role in silencing mutated oncogenes, thus defending the cell against the adverse consequences of genotoxic damages induced by environmental pollutants. These processes have been well investigated in lungs; however, although skin is directly exposed to a great variety of environmental pollutants, more research is needed to better understand the effect on cutaneous tissue. Therefore, we investigated microRNA alteration in human skin biopsies exposed to diesel fumes, ozone, and UV light for over 24 h of exposure. UV and ozone-induced microRNA alteration right after exposure, while the peak of their deregulations induced by diesel fumes was reached only at the end of the 24 h. Diesel fumes mainly altered microRNAs involved in the carcinogenesis process, ozone in apoptosis, and UV in DNA repair. Accordingly, each tested pollutant induced a specific pattern of microRNA alteration in skin related to the intrinsic mechanisms activated by the specific pollutant. These alterations, over a short time basis, reflect adaptive events aimed at defending the tissue against damages. Conversely, whenever environmental exposure lasts for a long time, the irreversible alteration of the microRNA machinery results in epigenetic damage contributing to the pathogenesis of inflammation, dysplasia, and cancer induced by environmental pollutants.

Keywords: microRNAs; environmental risk factors; cutaneous tissues; ozone exposure

Citation: Valacchi, G.; Pambianchi, E.; Coco, S.; Pulliero, A.; Izzotti, A. MicroRNA Alterations Induced in Human Skin by Diesel Fumes, Ozone, and UV Radiation. *J. Pers. Med.* **2022**, *12*, 176. https://doi.org/10.3390/jpm12020176

Academic Editor: David Alan Rizzieri

Received: 6 October 2021
Accepted: 24 January 2022
Published: 28 January 2022

Publisher's Note: MDPI stays neutral with regard to jurisdictional claims in published maps and institutional affiliations.

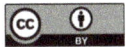

Copyright: © 2022 by the authors. Licensee MDPI, Basel, Switzerland. This article is an open access article distributed under the terms and conditions of the Creative Commons Attribution (CC BY) license (https://creativecommons.org/licenses/by/4.0/).

1. Introduction

The World Health Organization (WHO) estimated that circa 90% of the global urban population lives with pollutant levels exceeding WHO guideline limits. This has been linked to the premature death of seven million people each year [1]. The target organs of pollution include the lungs, gut, brain, and mainly the skin [2].

The skin is the largest sensory organ (approximately 2 m^2) in our body and is composed of two main layers: the epidermis and the dermis. The dermis is mainly formed of fibroblasts involved in the secretion of elastin and collagen fibers, embedded with nerve endings, sebaceous glands, hair follicles, and blood and lymphatic vessels. During the process of differentiation/keratinization, keratinocytes withdraw from the cell cycle and begin to express differentiation-dependent markers (i.e., keratins), eventually becoming anucleated densely keratinized corneocytes [3]. These cells are held together in the multilayered stratum corneum by a lipid-laden extracellular matrix (ECM), which performs the barrier function of the skin [4]. Recently, it has been demonstrated that the skin is not an impenetrable tissue, and it can even be a gateway for certain pollutants, even affecting internal organs [5].

The use of the word "pollution" can be misleading given that there are several different pollutants that can affect our health. Based on their chemical and physical properties as well as their sources, The United States Environmental Protection Agency (EPA) has identified the most common air pollutants, also known as "criteria air pollutants", as ozone (O_3), particulate matter (PM), carbon monoxide (CO), lead, sulfur dioxide (SO_2), and nitrogen dioxide (NO_2) [6]. Clear evidence of the correlation between each pollutant and skin disorder has not yet been established; however, the harmful effects of O_3, PM, and UV radiation have been well demonstrated. To date, only a few studies have compared the cutaneous effect of different pollutant exposure. Several skin diseases such as atopic dermatitis (AD), psoriasis, acne, and, in some cases, also skin cancer have been linked, either directly or indirectly, to pollution exposure, although the debate is still open. In particular, exposure to O_3 and PM have been demonstrated to be associated with skin aging, including wrinkle formation and dark spots, respectively [7]. In addition, the study by Xu et al. [8] demonstrated the association between ozone exposure and cutaneous conditions by analyzing the emergency room (ER) visits for skin conditions together with the levels of several air pollutants such as O_3, PM_{10}, SO_2, and NO_2. The authors were able to extrapolate that skin conditions such as urticaria, eczema, contact dermatitis, rash/other non-specific eruptions, and infected skin diseases were exacerbated by exposure to increased ozone levels. Another more recent publication has further examined the association of short-term changes in air quality with emergency department (ED) visits for urticaria in Canada. A total of 2905 ED visits were analyzed, and a positive and significant correlation was observed between air quality levels and ED visits for urticaria, confirming that air pollution can affect skin physiology [9,10].

O_3 and PM have quite different mechanisms of action, while O_3 is not able to penetrate the skin and reacts directly with the lipids present in the stratum corneum, PM can possibly enter the skin via the hair follicles or enable the skin to absorb components present in the PM (such as polycyclic aromatic hydrocarbons—PAH) and lead to an epidermal OxInflammatory reaction [11,12].

Indeed, it is now well established that ozone and diesel particles, together with UV radiation, can induce a proinflammatory response in parallel to an altered tissue redox homeostasis [13].

In addition to the ability of pollution to produce oxidative and inflammatory mediators, recent studies have indicated that DNA methylation patterns can be greatly influenced by environmental factors such as ambient air pollution, and these epigenetic changes are linked with diverse diseases [14–16].

In fact, several reports have shown that epigenetic alterations could be an important pathway through which environmental factors exert their effects [14,17]. Epigenetic refers to the alterations in gene expression levels that occur without changes in the underlying DNA sequence (such as DNA methylation, histone modification, miRNA, and noncoding RNA expression [18,19]). It should be mentioned that several pathologies, including cancers, have been associated with epigenetic modifications [18]. Exposure to environmental stimuli may result in epigenetic changes, which can impact gene expression and predisposition to developing pathological conditions. [20]. Understanding epigenetic alterations due to exposure to specific pollutants may lead to the development of biomarkers to assess the disease risk associated with air pollution. Micro-RNAs and noncoding RNAs (ncRNAs) play critical roles in gene expression and contribute to epigenetic control in the process [21]. For this reason, the present study aimed to evaluate the different miRNA epigenetic patterns related to the specific exposure of cutaneous tissues to pollutants such as ozone, diesel exhaust, and to the stressor UV radiation, which is the most toxic and most present in urban areas.

2. Materials and Methods

2.1. Ex Vivo Human Skin Explants Preparation

Human skin biopsies (12 mm diameter) were obtained from three healthy Caucasian donors (40–45 years old) who underwent elective abdominoplasties at Hunstad/Kortesis/Bharti Cosmetic Surgery clinic. In total, 24 punch biopsies were taken from the abdominal skin of each donor, and subcutaneous fat was removed with sterile scissors and a scalpel.

The biopsies, comprising dermal and epidermal layers, were rapidly rinsed with Phosphate-Buffered Saline (PBS, Gibco, New York, NY, USA). The biopsies were then moved into 6-well dishes containing 2 mL of complete Dulbecco's Modified Eagle Medium (DMEM) with 10% Fetal Bovine Serum (FBS) and 1% of antibiotics and antimycotics (100 U/mL penicillin and 100 µg/mL, Gibco, New York, NY, USA) added; then, they were incubated at 37 °C in 5% CO_2 for overnight recovery.

The following day the medium was replaced with a fresh one, and the biopsies were exposed to the different pollutants as discussed below.

The experiment was performed at least in triplicate for each condition and donor.

2.2. Ex Vivo Human Skin Explants Ozone (O_3) Exposure

A full 24 h after skin biopsy collection, ex vivo explants were allocated into a plexiglass sealed chamber, connected to the ozone generator machine (ECO3 model CUV-01, Model 306 Ozone Calibration Source, 2B Technologies, Ozone solution, ITA), and exposed to 0.2 ppm for 4 h. Sample biopsies were then collected following ozone exposure (T0) or after 24 h (T24).

2.3. Ex Vivo Human Skin Explants Diesel Engine Exhaust (Diesel) Exposure

Another set of skin biopsies was exposed to diesel engine exhaust by letting the engine run for 10 s and allowing the exhaust to reach the sealed exposure chamber where the skin biopsies remained for 30 min. Specifically, the skin explants were placed into a sealed plexiglass box connected to a Kubota RTV-X900 diesel engine (3-cylinder, 4-cycle diesel with overhead valves, 1123 cc with 24.8 HP at 3000 rpm). After the 30 min of Diesel exposure, the exposure medium was changed with a fresh one, and the biopsies were either collected (T0) or moved back into the incubator at 37 °C in 5% CO_2 for 24 h (T24).

2.4. Ex Vivo Human Skin Explants Ultraviolet Light (UV) Exposure

The other human skin biopsies were exposed to 200 milli Joule (mJ) UVA/UVB light, which equates to circa 2 h at solar apex and corresponding to 10 minimal erythemal doses (MED, 1 MED = 20 mJ/cm^2) [22]. UVA/UVB light (exposure of circa 20 s) was generated by a Sol1A Class ABB Solar Simulator, equipped with a xenon lamp (Newport Oriel Sol1A, CA, USA). Samples were collected after UV exposure (T0), or after 24 h (T24).

To match the real solar spectrum at the condition of the sun at the Zenith angle of 0, we performed UV exposure with a UVA/UVB ratio of 21:1 measured with a radiometer ILT2400 Hang-Held Light Meter/Optometer (International Light Technologies, Inc., Peabody, MA, USA).

2.5. Total RNA Extraction and Lyophilization

Total RNA extraction was performed using a miRNeasy Mini kit QIAGEN (Hilgen, DE, cat. 1038703) and Qiazol Lysis Reagent 50 QIAGEN (Hilgen, DE, cat. 1023537), according to the manufacturer's protocol. Briefly, skin biopsies were homogenized in 700 µL of Qiazol Lysis Reagent, with a tissue homogenizer (Precellys 24 homogenizer, 5 cycles 6500 rpm 3 × 30 s, at 4 °C). Samples were then centrifuged (12,700 rpm, 5 min at 4 °C), the supernatant was collected and transferred to a new tube containing 140 µL of Chloroform, and then centrifuged again (12,000 g, 15 min at 4 °C). The upper aqueous phase was transferred to a new tube containing 1.5 volumes of ethanol 100% and mixed thoroughly. Then, half of the volume was moved into the RNeasy Mini spin column and centrifuged (8000× g, 30 s, RT). This last step was repeated for the other half of the volume.

Next, 700 µL of diluter Buffer RWT was added to the column, centrifuged (8000× g, 30 s, RT), and then the liquid was discarded. Next, the addition of 500 µL of diluted Buffer RPE to the column, centrifugation (8000× g, 30 s, RT), and discarding of the liquid was repeated twice. Finally, the columns were moved into new Rnase free tubes, centrifuged at maximum speed for 1 min, and 30 µL of RNase free water was added to the spin column membrane. Elution of RNA was performed by centrifugation at 8000 g, 1 min, RT.

Then, the eluted RNA was concentrated via a lyophilization process (1.5 h, Low Setting, RT) using a Savant DNA SpeedVac Concentrator (Savant DNA120, DNA 120 OP, Thermo Electron Corporation, Waltham, MA, USA).

2.6. miRNA-Microarray and Bioinformatic Analyses

miRNA expression profiling was carried out by an Agilent platform, following the miRNA Microarray protocol v.3.1.1 (Agilent Technologies, Santa Clara, CA, USA). Briefly, 50 ng of total RNA containing miRNAs and Spike-in controls underwent dephosphorylation and a labeling step with Cyanine 3-pCp. The Cy3-labeled RNA was then purified using Micro Bio-Spin P-6 Gel Column (Bio-Rad Laboratories, Inc., Hercules, CA, USA) and hybridized on a Human miRNA microarray slide 8 × 60K (Agilent Technologies; including 2549 miRNAs, miRBase 21.0) at 55 °C for 20 h. After washing, the slides were scanned by a G2565CA scanner (Agilent Technologies), and the images were extracted by Feature Extraction software v.10 (Agilent Technologies). Microarray raw data were deposited in the Gene Expression Omnibus (http://www.ncbi.nlm.nih.gov/geo); GEO number accession requested, 15 March 2022).

Bioinformatic analyses were performed using the GeneSpring software (GeneSpring Multi-Omic Analysis v 14.9 by Agilent Technologies). For each sample, the intensities of replicated spots on each array were log transformed and averaged. Data processing was performed by 3D principal component analysis (PCA) scores and Hierarchical Clustering.

Comparisons between sets of data were performed by evaluating the fold changes. A volcano Plot T-Test analysis for all miRNA entities was run, using Fold Change ≥ 2 and p-value ≤ 0.05. Because log transformed data were used, negative and zero signals were transformed into 0.01 values. This approach could result in artificially high-fold variations. To correct this artifact, we now report in Tables that fold variation values upregulated more than 10 times into '>10-fold' and fold variation values downregulated more than 10 times into <0.1-fold.

miRNAs related to three different environmental exposures (Environmental Exposure miRNA Signature) were determined by analyzing miRNAs comparatively in exposed vs. non-exposed subjects. Environmental exposures were determined for each sample according to (a) Diesel, (b) Ozone, and (c) UV.

To understand the relationship between environmental exposure signatures and their biological significance in human tissues, a target detection for each environmental exposure signature was performed using the TargetScan prediction database.

3. Results

Comparison of miRNA Expression Profile between Pollutants

The overall trend of miRNA expression in human skin either untreated or exposed to diesel, ozone, and UV was evaluated at 0 and 24 h by Line plot analysis. (Figure 1).

The expression line plot was similar at 0 and 24 h in unexposed skin. Diesel induced dramatic alteration of miRNA profile compared to air but mainly after 24 h. Conversely, miRNA alteration induced by ozone was remarkable at time 0 while being much more attenuated compared to untreated skin at 24 h. miRNA profiles were slightly increased by UV exposure, mostly at 24 h compared to unexposed skin.

Scatter plot analyses were performed to assess the number of miRNAs with more than two-fold profile alteration compared to untreated (air-exposed), Figure 2.

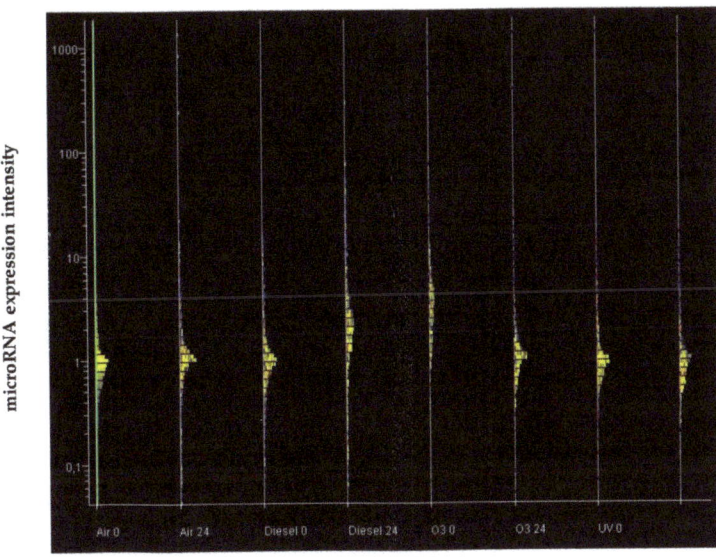

Figure 1. Line plot analysis of the overall expression of the 2549 human miRNAs analyzed under each experimental condition tested. The expression of 2549 human miRNAs was evaluated at 0 and 24 h in skin either unexposed (Air) or exposed to diesel, ozone, and UV. miRNAs are distributed in horizontal lines according to their level of expression, the majority being located at intermediate levels of expression (central part of the distribution), and the minority being located at high and low levels of expression (lower and upper part of the distribution). The distribution profile is progressively modified according to the treatment used.

Each miRNA is represented by colored dots, whose expression intensity can be inferred from the position on the horizontal and vertical axes. The horizontal axis indicates the miRNA expression level in untreated samples and the vertical axis in treated (diesel, ozone, and UV) samples. The central diagonal lines indicate the equivalence (<two-fold variation) in the intensity of miRNA expression in treated as compared to untreated samples. miRNA dots falling outside the green diagonal lines indicate higher than two-fold differences in miRNA expression between the tested experimental conditions. Scatter plot analyses compared untreated (air) and treated (diesel, ozone, and UV) samples both at 0 and 24 h. miRNA colors reflect the signal intensity in the treated samples (red is high, yellow is intermediate, and blue is low). Upregulated miRNAs are located in the upper-right area, and downregulated miRNAs are in the lower-right area of the scatter plots.

For diesel and to a lesser extent for UV, a cloud of downregulated miRNAs was detected already at 0 h, while the additional cloud of upregulated miRNAs was detected only at 24 h.

Conversely, for ozone, two clouds of both upregulated and downregulated miRNAs were already detected at time 0.

At time 0, out of the 2549 miRNAs tested, 100 (2.5%) were downregulated (blue dots) while 122 (4.8%) were upregulated (red dots) after exposure to diesel. Immediately after ozone exposure, we evidenced 262 (10.3%) downregulated miRNAs and 297 (11.6%) upregulated; however, upon UV exposure, we detected that 238 (9.3%) were downregulated and 294 (11.5%) upregulated.

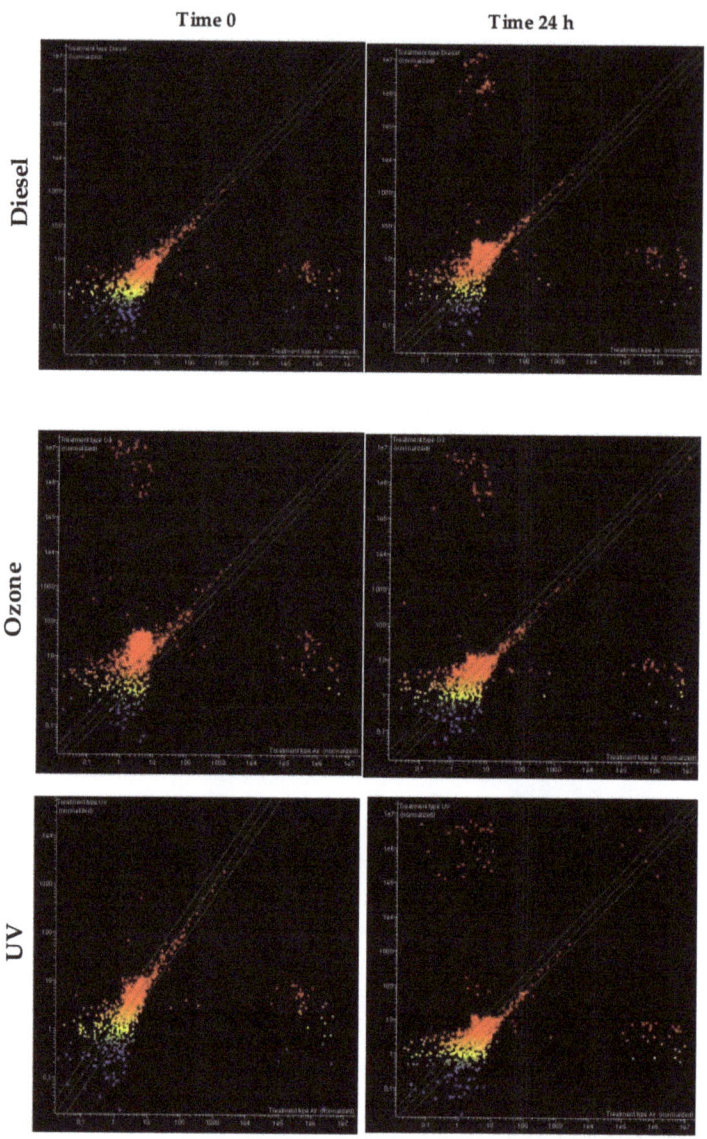

Figure 2. Scatter plot analysis of changes in miRNA-expression in human skin upon exposure to diesel, ozone, and UV at different times (0 and 24 h).

At 24 h, out of the 2549 miRNAs tested, 219 (8.6%) were downregulated (blue dots), and 251 (9.8%) were upregulated (red dots) after exposure to diesel; 229 (8.9%) were downregulated, and 238 (9.3%) upregulated after ozone exposure; and 174 (6.8%) were downregulated and 241 (9.4%) upregulated after UV exposure.

The effects of the tested pollutants on the whole miRNA expression profile were compared by unsupervised principal component analysis of variance (PCA) and supervised hierarchical cluster (HCA) analyses.

The PCA at 0 h (Figure 3) showed that the miRNA profiles of ozone and UV treated samples were remarkably altered, being located far away and in another quadrant, as compared to the untreated (air) samples. Conversely, the miRNA profile in diesel-treated samples was only slightly distant from the untreated samples, being located in the same quadrant.

Time 0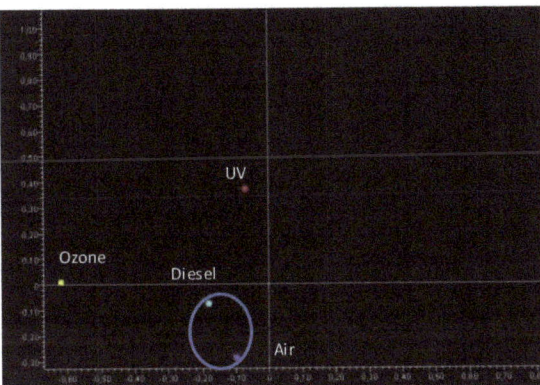

Time 24h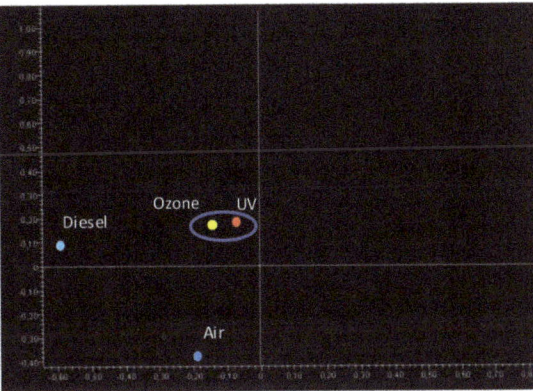

Figure 3. Bidimensional principal component analysis (PCA) of miRNA profiles of skin samples either untreated (air) or treated with diesel, ozone, and UV at 0 (**left panel**) and 24 h (**right panel**). PCA1 (X axis), PCA2 (Y axis).

The PCA at 24 h (Figure 3) reported that the miRNA profiles of all pollutant-treated samples (including diesel) were located far away and in another quadrant compared to the untreated sample. The samples treated with diesel and ozone were close to each other but far away from the UV-treated sample. This finding indicates that the pattern of miRNAs altered by UV is quite different from those induced by ozone and diesel exposure. This situation is likely due to the different pathogenic mechanisms induced by exciting radiation (UV) as compared to gaseous (ozone) and mixed gaseous-particulate pollutants (diesel).

The HCA at 0 h (Figure 4) showed that the most remarkable alterations in miRNA profiles were induced by ozone, whose expression profile was located at the right of the hierarchical tree far away from the untreated (air) sample. An intermediate situation occurred for UV, whose alteration profile was in the central part of the hierarchical tree. miRNA alterations induced by diesel were less remarkable; indeed, the profile was linked to the untreated (air) sample in the hierarchical tree.

The HCA at 24 h (Figure 4) indicated that the most remarkable alterations in miRNA profiles were induced by diesel, whose expression profile was located at the right of the hierarchical tree far away from the untreated (air) sample. An intermediate response was visible for UV, whose alteration profile was located in the central part of the hierarchical tree. On the other hand, the changes in miRNA profiles induced by ozone exposure were less remarkable; in fact, this profile was linked to the untreated (air) sample in the hierarchical tree.

A Venn diagram data representation was used to identify microRNAs presented in both lists, i.e., altered by each pollutant both at 0 and 24 h.

These miRNAs represent the specific miRNA signature induced by each pollutant. Their identity is reported in Table 1 (diesel), Table 2 (ozone), and Table 3 (UV). These Tables enlist miRNAs modulating their expression more than two-fold and above the statistical significance threshold of $p < 0.05$ considering the four replicates spotted in each microarray. A comparison of fold variation was made by dividing the signal intensity detected in treated skin by those detected in untreated skin. Fold variation values >2.0 indicate upregulation after treatment and <0.5 downregulation after treatment. Available information for the main biological pathways regulated by modulated microRNAs is also reported (column Function), as well as the reference from where this information was collected.

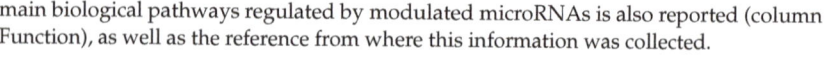

Figure 4. Hierarchical Cluster Analysis (HCA) reporting the expression of the 2549 miRNAs (colored horizontal bars) tested at time 0 (**left panel**) and 24 h (**right panel**) in samples either untreated (air) or treated with pollutants (ozone, diesel, and UV). Columns report miRNA expression profiles for each experimental condition. Similar expression profiles are linked in the upper hierarchical tree (green), thus being located nearby, while different expression profiles are located far away in the hierarchical tree.

Table 1. Diesel.

MicroRNA	Fold Change	Function	Reference
hsa-miR-495-5p	>10	Promotes Th2 differentiation in allergic rhinitis, as a tumor suppressor	[23]
hsa-miR-628-5p	>10	Inhibits osteoblast differentiation via RUNX2	[24]
hsa-miR-361-3p	>10	Suppresses proliferation, invasion inhibited cells invasive and proliferative abilities, and cell lines invasion and proliferation	[25,26]
hsa-miR-875-5p	>10	Promotes cellular apoptosis and proliferation	[27]
hsa-miR-509-3p	>10	Tumor suppressor	[28,29]
hsa-miR-518b	>10	Suppresses cell proliferation, invasiveness, and migration in colorectal cancer	[30,31]
hsa-miR-516b-5p	>10	Cell proliferation, inducing G1 cell cycle arrest and apoptosis	[32]
hsa-miR-381-5p	>10	Induces apoptosis	[33]
hsa-miR-661	>10	Promotes proliferation, migration, and metastasis of NSCLC	[34]
hsa-miR-216a-3p	>10	Antitumor functions	[35]
hsa-miR-548c-3p	>10	Inflammatory responses and potential estrogen receptor sensitivity	[36]
hsa-miR-106a-3p	>10	Cell proliferation and autophagy	[37]
hsa-miR-616-5p	>10	Promotes angiogenesis and modulates cell proliferation	[38]

Table 1. Cont.

MicroRNA	Fold Change	Function	Reference
hsa-miR-671-3p	>10	Suppresses proliferation and invasion of breast cancer cells and regulates metabolic processes	[39,40]
hsa-miR-544a	>10	Regulates migration and invasion in colorectal cancer cells	[41]
hsa-miR-614	>10	Inflammatory process	[42]
hsa-miR-525-3p	<10	Modifies the expression of proinflammatory cytokines; apoptosis	[43]
hsa-miR-378c	<10	Regulates the angiogenic capacity of CD34(+) progenitor cells	[44]
hsa-miR-924	<10	Suppresses the proliferation, migration, and invasion of NSCLC cells	[45]
hsa-miR-522-3p	<10	Cell proliferation of human glioblastoma cells; modulates the expression of proinflammatory cytokines	[46]
hsa-miR-431-5p	<10	Promotes differentiation and regeneration of cells	[47,48]
hsa-miR-770-5p	<10	Suppresses cell apoptosis and the release of proinflammatory factors	[49]
hsa-miR-183-5p	<10	Tumor suppressor inflammation and alters miRNA expression in the airway epithelium	[50]
hsa-miR-598-5p	<10	Promotes cell proliferation and cell cycle progression in human colorectal carcinoma; elevates apoptosis	[51]
hsa-miR-486-5p	<10	Regulation of heart contraction, muscle contraction, and ion channel activity	[52]
hsa-miR-125a-5p	<10	Regulates stress response, apoptosis, proliferation, angiogenesis, and expression of genes, associated with human lung cancer	[53]
hsa-miR-34b-5p	<10	Regulates stress response, apoptosis, proliferation, angiogenesis, and expression of genes, and is upregulated during cardiac hypertrophy	[54]
hsa-miR-301a-3p	<10	Promotes autophagy and inhibits apoptosis	[55,56]
hsa-miR-23c	<10	Inhibits cell proliferation and induces apoptosis of hepatocellular carcinoma cells; cell growth arrest and apoptosis.	[57]
hsa-miR-383-5p	<10	Oxidative stress and inflammation-related factors	[58]
hsa-miR-574-5p	<10	Promotes the differentiation of human cardiac fibroblasts	[59]
hsa-miR-151a-5p	<10	Regulation of cellular respiration and ATP production through targeting Cytb	[60]
hsa-miR-514a-3p	<10	Attenuates proliferation and increases chemoresistance	[61]
hsa-miR-136-3p	<10	Promotes apoptosis in gastric cancer cells	[62]
hsa-miR-1-3p	<10	Inflammation; regulator of heart adaption after ischemia or ischemic stress	[63]
hsa-miR-18a-3p	<10	Downregulated in aging cells; induces the apoptosis of colon cancer cells	[64]
hsa-miR-502-5p	<10	Enhances early apoptosis and inhibits proliferation of breast cancer cells	[65]
hsa-miR-451a	<10	Apoptosis; inhibits autophagy	[66]
hsa-miR-19b-1-5p	<10	Linked to oxidative stress, inflammation, and atherosclerosis	[67]
hsa-miR-873-5p	<0.1	Tumor suppressor in thyroid cancer by inhibiting the proliferation, migration, and invasion of the cancer cells	[68]
hsa-miR-212-5p	<0.1	Promotes cancer cell apoptosis and suppresses cancer cell proliferation and invasion	[69]
hsa-miR-552-5p	<0.1	Tumorigenesis; progression	[70]
hsa-let-7a-3p	<0.1	Linked to oxidative stress, inflammation, and atherosclerosis	[71]
hsa-miR-495-3p	<0.1	Regulates proliferation, apoptosis, migration, and invasion in metastatic prostate cancer cells.	[68]

Table 1. Cont.

MicroRNA	Fold Change	Function	Reference
hsa-miR-767-3p	<0.1	Promoted cell proliferation in human melanoma cell lines	[72]
hsa-miR-27b-5p	<0.1	Involved in beige and brown adipogenesis after cold exposure	[73]
hsa-miR-26a-2-3p	<0.1	Regulated stress response, apoptosis, proliferation, angiogenesis, and expression of genes	[74]
hsa-miR-629-5p	<0.1	Action on tumor growth and metastasis in hepatocellular carcinoma	[75]
hsa-miR-543	<0.1	Cell oxidative phosphorylation	[76]
hsa-miR-515-5p	<0.1	Upregulated in placentas from women with preeclampsia	[77]
hsa-miR-708-5p	<0.1	Induces apoptosis and suppresses tumorigenicity in renal cancer cells	[78]
hsa-miR-378j	<0.1	Tumor suppressor	[79]
hsa-miR-548az-3p	<0.1	Alters inflammation	[80]
hsa-miR-876-5p	<0.1	Regulates regulation proliferation, migration, invasion, and glutaminolysis in gastric cancer cells	[37]
hsa-miR-656-3p	<0.1	Suppresses glioma cell proliferation, neurosphere formation, migration, and invasion	[81]
hsa-miR-944	<0.1	Increases p53 expression in cancer cells	[82]
hsa-miR-518e-3p	<0.1	Tumor suppressor	[83]
hsa-miR-373-3p	<0.1	Promotes the invasion and migration of breast cancer; regulates inflammatory cytokine-mediated chondrocyte proliferation	[32]

Table 2. Ozone exposure.

MicroRNA	Fold Change	Function	Reference
hsa-miR-628-5p	>10	Inhibits osteoblast differentiation	[84]
hsa-miR-15a-3p	>10	Proliferation; inflammation; apoptosis	[25,26]
hsa-miR-548am-3p	>10	Induces proliferation and migration	[85]
hsa-miR-550b-2-5p	>10	Cancer promotion	[86]
hsa-miR-495-5p	>10	Tumor suppressor; proliferation and differentiation of osteoblasts in mice; inhibits the growth of fibroblasts in hypertrophic scar	[87]
hsa-miR-345-3p	>10	Apoptosis and inflammation	[24,88]
hsa-miR-548q	>10	Induces proliferation and migration	[89]
hsa-miR-887-3p	>10	Pathways in cancer	[86]
hsa-miR-877-5p	>10	Pathways in cancer	[90]
hsa-miR-513c-5p	>10	Pathways in cancer	[91]
hsa-miR-422a	>10	Pathways in cancer	[92]
hsa-miR-194-5p	>10	Pathways in cancer	[93]
hsa-miR-378b	>10	Inflammation and cell cycle	[94]
hsa-miR-610	>10	Pathways in cancer	[95]
hsa-miR-519e-5p	>10	Atherosclerosis and pathways in cancer	[96]
hsa-miR-627-5p	>10	Cell proliferation and cancer promotion	[97,98]
hsa-miR-548au-5p	>10	Pathways in cancer	[99]

Table 2. Cont.

MicroRNA	Fold Change	Function	Reference
hsa-miR-770-5p	>10	Apoptosis and inflammation	[100]
hsa-miR-196b-3p	>10	Cell proliferation	[101]
hsa-miR-330-3p	>10	Apoptosis and cell proliferation	[102]
hsa-miR-617	>10	Pathways in cancer	[103]
hsa-miR-375	>10	Cell proliferation and pathways in cancer	[104]
hsa-miR-936	>10	Cell proliferation, pathways in cancer, and apoptosis	[105]
hsa-miR-657	>10	Inflammation	[106]
hsa-miR-542-5p	>10	Mitochondrial dysfunction and inflammation	[107]
hsa-miR-136-3p	>10	Vascularization and pathways in cancer	[108]
hsa-miR-409-5p	>10	Cardiovascular process, proliferation, migration, and cell cycle.	[109,110]
hsa-miR-154-3p	>10	Pathways in cancer	[111,112]
hsa-miR-378c	>10	Proliferation and inhibited apoptosis	[113]
hsa-miR-93-3p	>10	Inflammation and apoptosis	[114]
hsa-miR-556-3p	>10	Cell proliferation and apoptosis	[115]
hsa-miR-518c-5p	>10	Tumor suppressor	[116]
hsa-miR-23b-5p	>10	Cell proliferation and cancer	[32]
hsa-miR-504-5p	>10	Cell proliferation and differentiation	[117]
hsa-miR-509-3p	>10	Cardiovascular process	[118]
hsa-miR-514a-3p	>10	Tumor suppressor	[119]
hsa-miR-431-5p	>10	Cell proliferation and apoptosis	[120]
hsa-miR-506-3p	>10	Cell proliferation and cancer	[121]
hsa-miR-645	>10	Cell proliferation and cancer	[122]
hsa-miR-129-5p	>10	Inhibits the proliferation and metastasis of gastric cancer cells	[123]
hsa-miR-516b-5p	>10	Migration, cell proliferation, and cancer process	[124]
hsa-miR-512-3p	>10	Apoptosis and cell cycle	[125]
hsa-miR-101-5p	>10	Apoptosis and promotes cell proliferation	[126]
hsa-miR-561-5p	>10	Cell proliferation, G(1)/S transition, and suppresses apoptosis	[127]
hsa-miR-194-5p	>10	Cell proliferation and cancer	[128]
hsa-miR-329-3p	>10	Proliferation, invasion, and suppresses cell apoptosis	[129]
hsa-let-7i-3p	>10	Coronary disease and cancer	[130]
hsa-miR-129-2-3p	>10	Proliferation, invasion, and apoptosis	[131]
hsa-miR-548a-5p	>10	Proliferation and inhibits apoptosis	[132]
hsa-miR-887-5p	>10	Pathways in cancer	[133]
hsa-miR-99a-3p	>10	Cell proliferation and pathways in cancer	[134]
hsa-miR-487a-3p	>10	Cell proliferation and cancer	[135]
hsa-miR-378g	>10	Cancer promotion	[136]
hsa-miR-548at-5p	>10	Neurodegenerative disease	[137]
hsa-miR-374c-5p	>10	Proliferation, apoptosis, and autophagy	[138]
hsa-miR-106a-3p	>10	Proliferation and apoptosis	[139]
hsa-miR-92a-2-5p	>10	Apoptosis and cell proliferation	[140]

Table 2. Cont.

MicroRNA	Fold Change	Function	Reference
hsa-miR-616-5p	>10	Invasion, cell migration, and cancer	[141]
hsa-miR-509-5p	>10	Tumor suppressor	[142]
hsa-miR-598-3p	>10	Cancer process	[21]
hsa-miR-873-5p	>10	Cell migration and cancer	[143]
hsa-miR-525-3p	<10	Cancer cell migration	[21]
hsa-miR-500a-5p	<10	Cell apoptosis and proliferation	[144]
hsa-miR-659-3p	<10	Cell proliferation and cancer; apoptosis	[145]
hsa-miR-526b-5p	<10	Cell proliferation and cancer	[146]
hsa-miR-764	<10	Cardiac diseases and cancer	[147]
hsa-miR-934	<10	Cancer progression and inflammation	[148]
hsa-miR-516a-5p	<10	Cell proliferation and cancer	[149]
hsa-miR-520f-3p	<10	DNA repair	[150]
hsa-miR-369-5p	<10	Aerobic glycolysis and pathways in cancer	[151]
hsa-miR-613	<10	Invasion and cell proliferation	[152]
hsa-miR-411-3p	<10	Proliferation and cancer	[153]
hsa-miR-432-3p	<10	Inflammation	[154]
hsa-let-7c-3p	<10	Apoptosis	[155]
hsa-miR-671-5p	<10	Proliferation and cell cycle	[156]
hsa-miR-181d-5p	<10	Proliferation and angiogenesis	[157]
hsa-miR-192-5p	<10	Hypertension and cancer	[158]
hsa-let-7g-3p	<10	Linked to oxidative stress, inflammation, and atherosclerosis	[159]
hsa-miR-1-3p	<10	Decreases tumor volume in a xenograft model	[68]
hsa-miR-515-3p	<10	Cell proliferation, migration, invasion, and induced apoptosis	[160]
hsa-miR-320d	<10	Apoptosis and cancer	[161]
hsa-miR-548aa	<10	Can alter the inflammatory responses	[162]
hsa-miR-502-5p	<10	Cell proliferation and invasion	[37]
hsa-miR-758	<10	Proliferation and invasion	[163]
hsa-miR-7-1-3p	<10	Autophagy and cancer process	[164]
hsa-miR-324-3p	<10	Cell proliferation and cancer	[165]
hsa-miR-520g-3p	<10	DNA repair	[166]
hsa-miR-576-5p	<10	Cell invasion and cancer	[151]
hsa-miR-520a-3p	<10	Inhibits tumor progression, indicating its potential role as a tumor suppressor.	[167]
hsa-miR-449b-3p	<10	Proliferation	[168]
hsa-miR-211-5p	<10	Pathways in cancer	[169]
hsa-miR-376a-3p	<10	Coronary artery disease	[170]
hsa-miR-939-3p	<10	Pathways in cancer	[171]
hsa-miR-214-3p	<10	Inhibition of migration and proliferation	[172]
hsa-miR-609	<10	Cardiovascular process	[173]
hsa-miR-29a-5p	<10	Cardiac myocytes and overall cardiac dysfunction	[174]

Table 2. Cont.

MicroRNA	Fold Change	Function	Reference
hsa-miR-449c-3p	<10	Inhibits NSCLC cell progression	[175]
hsa-miR-185-3p	<10	Proliferation and invasion of cell	[176]
hsa-miR-766-3p	<10	Suppresses apoptosis and facilitates autophagy	[177]
hsa-miR-486-5p	<10	Regulation of heart contraction, muscle contraction, and ion channel activity	[53]
hsa-miR-144	<10	Tumor inhibitors or tumor suppressors, proliferation, and apoptosis	[53]
hsa-miR-664a-5p	<10	Induces cell differentiation	[178]
hsa-miR-32-3p	<10	Atherosclerosis	[179]
hsa-miR-224-3p	<10	Cell proliferation and promotes apoptosis	[180]
hsa-miR-130a-5p	<10	Myocardial infarction	[181]
hsa-miR-378i	<10	Metabolic pathways, mitochondrial energy homeostasis, and related biological processes	[182]
hsa-miR-642b-5p	<10	Inflammation	[183]
hsa-miR-668-3p	<10	Progression of different types of cancer	[184]
hsa-miR-18b-5p	<10	Progression of different types of cancer; cardiac function	[185]
hsa-miR-483-3p	<10	Apoptosis	[186]
hsa-miR-485-3p	<10	Cell proliferation; pathways in cancer	[187]
hsa-miR-200c-5p	<10	Oxidative stress and cell apoptosis	[188]
hsa-miR-126-5p	<10	Linked to oxidative stress, inflammation, and atherosclerosis	[189]
hsa-miR-26b-3p	<10	Cell proliferation and invasion	[190]
hsa-miR-378d	<10	Proliferation and migration of cancer	[191]
hsa-miR-526b-3p	<10	Regulates the proliferation, invasion, and migration of cancer cells	[192]
hsa-miR-575	<10	Oncogene	[193]
hsa-miR-564	<10	Cell proliferation and invasion	[194]
hsa-miR-513a-5p	<10	Induced apoptosis	[195]
hsa-miR-548i	<10	Downregulates the inflammatory cytokines	[196]
hsa-miR-188-5p	<10	Cell proliferation and cancer promotion	[197]
hsa-miR-563	<10	Cell proliferation and cancer promotion	[198]
hsa-miR-139-3p	<10	Proliferation and invasion	[199]
hsa-miR-34a-5p	<0.1	Inflammation	[200]
hsa-miR-34b-5p	<0.1	P53 effector, cell proliferation, and apoptosis	[201]
hsa-miR-371b-5p	<0.1	Cell proliferation and apoptosis	[202]
hsa-let-7f-2-3p	<0.1	Cell proliferation and apoptosis	[203,204]
hsa-miR-557	<0.1	Tumor suppressor	[205]
hsa-miR-574-5p	<0.1	Cell cycle and cancer process	[206]
hsa-miR-216a-3p	<0.1	Cell proliferation and apoptosis	[207]
hsa-miR-466	<0.1	Tumor suppressor	[208]
hsa-miR-222-3p	<0.1	Cell viability, migration, and invasion	[209]
hsa-miR-586	<0.1	Cell proliferation, invasion, metastasis, and apoptosis	[210]
hsa-miR-939-5p	<0.1	Inflammation	[211]

Table 2. *Cont.*

MicroRNA	Fold Change	Function	Reference
hsa-miR-548b-3p	<0.1	Proliferation, apoptosis, and mitochondrial function	[212]
hsa-miR-517c-3p	<0.1	Responses to stress; alterations in circulating glucose levels	[213]
hsa-miR-630	<0.1	Oxidative damage and cell migration	[214]
hsa-miR-544a	<0.1	Pathways in cancer	[215]
hsa-miR-603	<0.1	Proliferation, migration, invasion, and metastasis	[216]
hsa-miR-552-5p	<0.1	Cell proliferation	[217]
hsa-miR-562	<0.1	Tumor suppressor	[218]
hsa-miR-548	<0.1	Cancer cell proliferation, migration, and invasion	[219]
hsa-miR-518a-	<0.1	Tumor suppressor	[220]
hsa-miR-433-5p	<0.1	Cardiovascular process	[32]
hsa-miR-138-5p	<0.1	Cardiac function and pathological damage	[221]
hsa-miR-548ad-5p	<0.1	Cancer cell proliferation, migration, and invasion	[222]
hsa-miR-450a-2-3p	<0.1	Cell proliferation and cancer	[220]
hsa-miR-548av-3p	<0.1	Cancer cell proliferation, migration, and invasion	[223]
hsa-miR-624-5p	<0.1	Cell proliferation and cancer	[220]
hsa-miR-553	<0.1	Cell proliferation and cancer	[224]
hsa-miR-876-5p	<0.1	Cell proliferation and cancer	[225]
hsa-miR-190b	<0.1	Autophagy and cell cycle	[226]
hsa-miR-26a-2-3p	<0.1	Cell cycle and cancer process	[227]
hsa-miR-515-5p	<0.1	Cardiac function and proliferation cells	[75]
hsa-miR-195-3p	<0.1	Cardiac function and proliferation cells	[228]
hsa-miR-365b-5p	<0.1	Inflammation and cell proliferation	[229]
Hsa-miR-885-3p	<0.1	Inflammation	[230]

Table 3. UV exposure.

MicroRNA	Fold Variation	Functions	Reference
hsa-miR-329-3p	>10	Inhibits cell proliferation in glioma cells	[231]
hsa-miR-520g-5p	>10	DNA repair	[232]
hsa-miR-216a-	>10	Regulates the proliferation, apoptosis, migration, and invasion of lung cancer cells	[151]
hsa-miR-548c-3p	>10	Cancer cell proliferation, migration, and invasion	[233]
hsa-miR-129-2-3p	>10	Inhibits the proliferation and metastasis of gastric cancer cells	[220]
hsa-miR-887-5p	<10	Pathways in cancer	[124]
hsa-miR-106a-3p	>10	Involved in tumorigenesis and highly expressed in gastric cancer	[234]
hsa-miR-616-5p	>10	Progression of bladder cancer by regulating cell proliferation, migration, and apoptosis	[235]
hsa-miR-509-5p	>10	Tumor suppressive effects	[236]
hsa-miR-648	>10	Post-transcriptional regulators of glioblastoma	[237]

Table 3. *Cont.*

MicroRNA	Fold Variation	Functions	Reference
hsa-miR-378h	>10	Metabolic pathways, mitochondrial energy homeostasis, and angiogenic network in tumors	[238]
hsa-miR-200c-5p	>10	Upregulated by oxidative stress and induces endothelial cell apoptosis	[183]
hsa-miR-525-3p	<10	Pathways in cancer	[239]
hsa-miR-488-3p	<10	Pathways in cancer	[44]
hsa-miR-101-5p	<10	Regulates cell proliferation	[240]
hsa-let-7g-3p	<10	Modulates inflammatory responses; pathways in cancer	[241]
hsa-miR-376a-2-5p	<10	Pathways in cancer	[242]
hsa-miR-640	<10	Pathways in cancer	[243]
hsa-miR-300	<10	Controls stem cell function and inhibits differentiation	[244]
hsa-miR-509-3p	<10	Pathways in cancer	[245]
hsa-miR-548au-5p	<10	Pathways in cancer	[246]
hsa-miR-337-3p	<10	Pathways in cancer	[100]
hsa-miR-411-3p	<10	Pathways in cancer	[247]
hsa-miR-494-3p	<10	Mitochondrial biogenesis and pathways in cancer	[248]
hsa-let-7e-3p	<10	Pathways in cancer	[249]
hsa-miR-144-3p	<10	Regulates adipogenesis and pathways in cancer	[250]
hsa-miR-196b-3p	<10	Cell proliferation	[251]
hsa-miR-10b-5p	<10	Pathways in cancer	[102]
hsa-miR-33a-5p	<10	Associated with carcinogenesis	[252]
hsa-miR-136-3p	<10	Cardiac function and pathological damage in myocardial tissue, cardiomyocyte apoptosis, oxidative stress, and inflammatory response	[253]
hsa-miR-143-3p	<10	Pathways in cancer	[254]
hsa-miR-762	<10	Modulates thyroxine-induced cardiomyocyte and pathways in cancer	[255]
hsa-miR-582-5p	<10	Cell proliferation	[256]
hsa-miR-645	<10	Cell proliferation and apoptosis	[21]
hsa-miR-411-5p	<10	Cell proliferation and pathways in cancer	[257]
hsa-miR-7-1-3p	<10	Inhibits autophagy and induces apoptosis in glioblastoma	[258]
hsa-miR-18a-3p	<10	Progression of different types of cancer; cardiac function.	[259]
hsa-miR-99a-3p	<10	Cell proliferation and pathways in cancer	[186]
hsa-miR-491-5p	<10	Cell proliferation and pathways in cancer	[135]
hsa-miR-19b-1-5p	<10	Pathways in cancer	[260,261]
hsa-miR-614	<10	Cell proliferation and pathways in cancer	[262]
hsa-miR-493-5p	<0.1	Cell proliferation	[263]
hsa-miR-15b-3p	<0.1	Proliferation, inflammation, and apoptosis	[264]
hsa-miR-510-5p	<0.1	Cell proliferation	[265]
hsa-miR-485-5p	<0.1	Cell proliferation and pathways in cancer	[266]
hsa-miR-581	<0.1	Induces proliferation and migration	[188]
hsa-miR-340-3p	<0.1	Cell proliferation and pathways in cancer	[267]
hsa-miR-708-5p	<0.1	Cell proliferation and pathways in cancer	[268]

Table 3. Cont.

MicroRNA	Fold Variation	Functions	Reference
hsa-miR-548j-3p	<0.1	Induces proliferation and migration	[269]
hsa-miR-618	<0.1	Cell proliferation and pathways in cancer	[270]
hsa-miR-885-3p	<0.1	Inflammatory response and pathways in cancer	[271]
hsa-miR-297	<0.1	Oncogene, inflammatory response, and apoptosis	[231]
hsa-miR-518a-5p	<0.1	Tumor suppressor	[272,273]
hsa-let-7f-2-3p	<0.1	Proliferation and apoptosis	[32]
hsa-miR-519b-3p	<0.1	Radiosensitivity of radio-resistant cells and pathways in cancer	[205]
hsa-miR-27b-5p	<0.1	Prevents atherosclerosis by inhibiting inflammatory responses	[274]
hsa-miR-625-5p	<0.1	Inflammation and inhibits cardiac hypertrophy	[275]
hsa-miR-548ah-5p	<0.1	Induces proliferation and migration	[276]
hsa-miR-892c-3p	<0.1	Pathways in cancer	[86]
hsa-miR-373-3p	<0.1	Inhibits autophagy	[277]
hsa-miR-656-3p	<0.1	Induces proliferation and migration	[278]
hsa-miR-20a-3p	<0.1	Proliferation and autophagy	[279]
hsa-miR-518a-3p	<0.1	Tumor suppressor	[280]
hsa-miR-649	<0.1	Pathways in cancer	[32]
hsa-miR-483-3p	<0.1	Pathways in cancer and cardiac response	[281]
hsa-miR-501-3p	<0.1	Cell proliferation, clonogenicity, migration, and invasion	[282]
hsa-miR-335-5p	<0.1	Cell proliferation, migration, and invasion.	[283]
hsa-miR-129-5p	<0.1	Proliferation, invasion, and apoptosis	[284]
hsa-miR-34c-5p	<0.1	Proliferation and apoptosis	[132]
hsa-miR-548ao-5p	<0.1	Promotes proliferation and inhibits apoptosis	[202]
hsa-miR-624-5p	<0.1	Cell proliferation and pathways in cancer	[133]

MicroRNAs reported in Tables 1–3 were selected by both volcano plot analysis and Venn diagram data representation. These miRNAs represent the specific signature of each pollutant, being modulated both after short-term exposure (UV 20 s, diesel 30 min, and ozone 4 h) and long-term exposure (24 h for all pollutants).

Fold variations reported in Tables 1–3 are the rate of signal intensity changes between treated and untreated samples at 24 h.

The main biological pathways regulated by these miRNAs, as inferred from available literature, are also reported.

The main pathways targeted by tested pollutants were: apoptosis, cell cycle, and inflammation (Table 4).

Table 4. Number of the miRNAs involved in the pathways deregulated by each pollutant tested. Only miRNAs demonstrated to be involved in the pathways are included.

	Diesel	Ozone	UV
Apoptosis	16	36	12
Cell cycle	7	24	11
Inflammation	11	21	7
DNA repair	1	4	2
Pathways in cancer	23	72	39

4. Discussion and Conclusions

The constant exposure to oxidants, including ultraviolet (UV) radiation and other environmental pollutants, such as diesel fuel exhaust and ozone, makes the skin our first defense against the outdoor environment, and it is also the tissue more affected by outdoor stressors. The contribution of the now defined "exposome" to extrinsic skin aging and skin conditions is well accepted. Pollution is one of the main players included in the skin exposome [224]. It has been recently shown [285] that exposure to more pollutants can have an additive effect. This could be a consequence of the different mechanisms of action of each stressor based on its chemical/physical properties.

It is generally understood that the toxic effects of O_3, although it is not a radical species, per se, are mediated through free radical reactions either directly by the oxidation of biomolecules to give classical radical species (hydroxyl radical) or by driving the radical-dependent production of cytotoxic nonradical species (aldehydes) [286].

O_3 cannot penetrate the SC, so it first interacts with the lipids present in the outermost layer of the skin, leading to the generation of a number of bioreactive species [287]. It can be suggested that reaction with the well-organized interstitial lipids and protein constituents of the outermost stratum corneum barrier, and the diffusion of bioreactive products from this tissue into the viable layers of the epidermis, may represent a contribution to the development/exacerbation of skin disorders associated with O_3 exposure. Indeed, once these "mediators" can reach live cells (keratinocytes, fibroblasts, etc.), they can induce a cellular defensive and inflammatory response that leads to an inflammatory/oxidative vicious cycle, called OxInflammation [288]. Unless quenched by endogenous or exogenous mechanisms, this will damage the skin and compromise its barrier functions, contributing to extrinsic skin aging.

Different hypotheses have been proposed concerning the initiation of the PM's detrimental effects on cutaneous tissues. This could be due to an indirect effect by an outside-inside signaling cascade. PM, especially smaller particles, may carry metal ions and/or organic compounds such as polycyclic aromatic hydrocarbons (PAHs), which are highly lipophilic and can penetrate the skin surface [287]. This is in agreement with our observations. Moreover, PAHs are potent ligands for the AhR receptor, expressed by both keratinocytes and melanocytes, which upregulates proinflammatory mediators and increases ROS production [289].

In a previous study, we provided evidence that PM develops cutaneous damage not only directly once particles reach deeper layers in the epidermis but also indirectly by triggering a signaling pathway [290]. Oxidative stress and an inflammatory response seem to be important steps in the PM toxic mechanisms.

The solar spectrum reaching the surface of the earth is divided into three main segments based on wavelength: UVC (100–290 nm), UVB (290–320 nm), and UVA (320–400 nm). Both UVA and UVB have acute and chronic effects on human skin [287]. It has been established that approximately 50% of UV-induced direct cellular injury accounts for the remainder of the damage [291–293].

Therefore, although UV, PM, and ozone have different mechanisms of action, they all have the common denominator of damage that can be summarized as oxidative stress.

This effect is not limited to a biochemical effect, but it has been shown that air pollutants modulate epigenetic states, ranging from DNA methylation to miRNAs expression [294].

The aim of this study was to evaluate the different miRNA cutaneous responses to the main pollutants to which our skin is exposed daily.

It was not surprising that there was a clear difference among the pollutants in terms of the modulated miRNAs and the pathways associated with the epigenetic variation.

We found that the main pathways affected by the analyzed pollutants were: apoptosis, cell cycle, inflammation, DNA repair, and cancer. Of note, apoptosis was not associated with O_3 exposure, and this could be a consequence of the O_3 mechanism of action, which leads to the generation of proinflammatory mediators (H_2O_2 and aldehydes) less aggressively compared to UV and PM [89,100]

The ability of UV to induce DNA damage and subsequent apoptosis has been well demonstrated in the past, and our data confirm these results under the epigenetic mechanism as well. In addition, our data confirmed the involvement of O_3 exposure in cutaneous inflammation, as previously demonstrated by Xu et al., where ER visit for skin inflammatory conditions perfectly correlated with increased ozone levels in urban cities [17,20].

To confirm that the O_3 epigenetic effect is tissue-specific (due to the different mediators generated by the interaction with different tissues), the work by [295] showed that the expression analysis of sputum samples revealed that O_3 exposure significantly increased the expression levels of several miRNAs, namely miR-132, miR-143, miR-145, miR-199b-5p, miR-222, miR-223, miR-25, miR-424, and miR-582-5p that while not detected in our analysis were still involved in inflammation. A quite recent work suggests that the main effect of PM on the skin is due to the absorption of PAHs, which can lead to skin barrier perturbation and damage [296]. PAH exposure has been already associated with epigenetic variation related mainly to DNA methylation.

In the present study, we have shown for the first time that PAH (present in diesel particles) can affect cutaneous epigenetics related to miRNA expression, highlighting the possible detrimental effect that those compounds can have on the skin [61]. The time-related kinetic differences in miRNA expression at 0 and 24 h reflect the different nature of the tested pollutants.

Ozone is a volatile gas; accordingly, its interaction with the skin induces effects on a short–term basis because this gas is neither metabolized nor entrapped into skin layers. UV radiation induces short-term alteration triggering reactive mechanisms (DNA repair, etc.), requiring at least 8 h to be activated by the modulation of the microRNA machinery. MicroRNAs are highly sensitive to environmental stressors, as is well demonstrated in the lung for cigarette smoke [297] and airborne pollutants [298]. However, this issue has not yet been explored in the skin. The presented results herein provide experimental evidence that human skin undergoes dramatic changes in its physiological microRNA profile when exposed to environmental pollutants, either physical or chemical.

Diesel fumes are well known to induce genotoxic damage and DNA adduct formation [299], as well as microRNA alteration in the lung [300]. Diesel extracts can induce cancer in mouse skin [301]. The carcinogenic effect of diesel fumes is mainly due to the presence in this mixture of potent chemical genotoxic carcinogens such as nitropyrenes [302]. Indeed, epigenome regulation performed by the microRNA machinery can silence the expression of mutated oncogenes, thus defending our organism from the progression of the carcinogenic process. Only when genomic damage accumulates in the presence of irreversible alteration of the microRNA machinery does cancer occur [303].

Accordingly, the demonstration that microRNA are dramatically altered in human skin shows that diesel fumes are a complete skin carcinogen inducing both genomic and epigenomic alterations. The carcinogenicity of diesel fumes is exerted by the phase I and II metabolic reaction of its chemical components with particular reference to polycyclic aromatic hydrocarbons. This situation, together with the limited metabolic potential of the skin as compared to other tissues, explains why microRNA alterations reach the maximum level only after 40 h of exposure. The carcinogenicity of diesel fumes is confirmed by the finding that the majority (40%) of altered microRNA is involved in carcinogenesis processes, while only a minority is involved in defensive processes such as apoptosis (22%) and DNA repair (4%) [73,76].

Ozone displays an immediate effect on skin microRNA that does not increase after 24 h from the exposure. This finding indicates that adaptive mechanisms are triggered by ozone. Skin is well equipped with antioxidant defenses requiring some time to be activated. This situation is confirmed by the finding that the majority (31%) of altered microRNA is involved in defensive mechanisms allowing removal of damaged cells (apoptosis) and DNA repair (8%, i.e., two-fold more than diesel fumes), while only a minority in carcinogenesis (20%, i.e., two-fold less than diesel fumes).

UV radiation is carcinogenic, as demonstrated by the finding that this exposure induces the most dramatic alterations of microRNA involved in carcinogenesis (45%) compared to diesel fume and ozone.

Furthermore, UV displays a variety of other adverse biological effects, including cell loss by apoptosis, cell proliferation to replace lost cells, and inflammation. In this regard, microRNA alteration overlaps the main function of genes whose expression undergoes upregulation, as demonstrated in mouse skin [299].

Conversely, only a minority (7%) of microRNA involved in DNA repair are activated in human skin after 24 and 48 h. This situation is different from those reported in vivo in mouse skin after long-term exposure that activated a variety of genes involved in base excision (XP) and nucleotide excision (OGG1) DNA repair [304]. This finding indicates that only long-term exposure to UV is effective in activating defensive DNA repair, while exposures to high doses for a short time results in a lack of DNA repair activation. Because of this situation, sunburns, indicating the occurrence of UV exposure in the absence of effective activation of DNA and protein repair, represent a major risk factor for cancer development.

A limitation of the presented study is that skin biopsies were collected from three subjects only. Future studies using a wider number of subjects are necessary to explore the interindividual variation occurring in the miRNA of human skin when exposed to environmental pollutants.

5. Conclusions

In conclusion, our results provide experimental evidence in human skin that microRNA machinery is altered by exposure to environmental pollutants. This situation occurs regarding either chemical pollutants, such as diesel fumes and ozone, or exciting radiation, such as UV. MicroRNA alteration, on a short-term basis, represents an adaptive event triggering defensive mechanisms such as DNA repair and apoptosis, attenuating the consequences of molecular damage induced in the skin by environmental stressors. Whenever microRNA alterations persist for a long time because of continuous exposure to environmental stressors, microRNA defensive function is neutralized, thus leaving the pathology or even carcinogenesis process to develop. Our findings demonstrate that skin has potent microRNA machinery used to face exposure to environmental pollutants. The alteration induced in skin microRNA undergoes a signature specific to the environmental pollutant involved.

Author Contributions: Conceptualization, G.V. and A.I.; methodology A.P., S.C. and E.P. validation A.P. and A.I.; investigation G.V., resources, and data curation, and; writing—original draft preparation A.P., G.V. and A.I. and writing—review and editing all authors; visualization all authors, supervision A.I.; project administration, A.I. and G.V. and funding acquisition A.I. All authors have read and agreed to the published version of the manuscript.

Funding: This research was partially supported by the Italian Association for Cancer Research (AIRC, IG2017-20699 to A.I.).

Institutional Review Board Statement: Ethical review was waived for this study, due to the fact that human skin was obtained from cosmetic/elective surgery and was collected from consented donors under IRB approved protocols at facilities located in the continental United States.

Informed Consent Statement: As reported already in our recent Pambianchi E. et al., Antioxidants (Basel). 2021 Nov 30;10(12):1928, doi:10.3390/antiox10121928.

Data Availability Statement: The datasets used and/or analyzed during the current study are available in Gene Expression Omnibus (http://www.ncbi.nlm.nih.gov/geo); GEO number accession requested, 15 March 2022).

Conflicts of Interest: The authors declare no conflict of interest.

References

1. Lelieveld, J.; Pozzer, A.; Pöschl, U.; Fnais, M.; Haines, A.; Münzel, T. Loss of life expectancy from air pollution compared to other risk factors: A worldwide perspective. *Cardiovasc. Res.* **2020**, *116*, 1910–1917. [CrossRef] [PubMed]
2. World Health Organization (WHO). *WHO's Urban Ambient Air Pollution Database—Update 2016*; WHO: Geneva, Switzerland, 2016.
3. Fuchs, E. Epithelial Skin Biology. Three Decades of Developmental Biology, a Hundred Questions Answered and a Thousand New Ones to Address. *Curr. Top. Dev. Biol.* **2016**, *116*, 357–374. [CrossRef] [PubMed]
4. Feingold, K.R.; Schmuth, M.; Elias, P.M. The regulation of permeability barrier homeostasis. *J. Investig. Dermatol.* **2007**, *127*, 1574–1576. [CrossRef]
5. Valacchi, G.; Magnani, N.; Woodby, B.; Ferreira, S.M.; Evelson, P. Particulate Matter Induces Tissue OxInflammation: From Mechanism to Damage. *Antioxid. Redox Signal.* **2020**, *33*, 308–326. [CrossRef] [PubMed]
6. Criteria Air Pollutants. Available online: https://www.epa.gov/criteria-air-pollutants (accessed on 30 September 2021).
7. Fuks, K.B.; Hüls, A.; Sugiri, D.; Altug, H.; Vierkötter, A.; Abramson, M.J.; Goebel, J.; Wagner, G.G.; Demuth, I.; Krutmann, J.; et al. Tropospheric ozone and skin aging: Results from two German cohort studies. *Environ. Int.* **2019**, *124*, 139–144. [CrossRef]
8. Xu, F.; Yan, S.; Wu, M.; Li, F.; Xu, X.; Song, W.; Zhao, J.; Xu, J.; Kan, H. Ambient ozone pollution as a risk factor for skin disorders. *Br. J. Dermatol.* **2011**, *165*, 224–225. [CrossRef]
9. Kousha, T.; Valacchi, G. The air quality health index and emergency department visits for urticaria in Windsor, Canada. *J. Toxicol. Environ. Health Part A Curr. Issues* **2015**, *78*, 524–533. [CrossRef]
10. Valacchi, G.; Porada, E.; Rowe, B.H. Ambient ozone and bacterium streptococcus: A link between cellulitis and pharyngitis. *Int. J. Occup. Med. Environ. Health* **2015**, *28*, 771–774. [CrossRef]
11. Lademann, J.; Otberg, N.; Jacobi, U.; Hoffman, R.M.; Blume-Peytavi, U. Follicular penetration and targeting. *J. Investig. Dermatol. Symp. Proc.* **2005**, *10*, 301–303. [CrossRef]
12. Dijkhoff, I.M.; Drasler, B.; Karakocak, B.B.; Petri-Fink, A.; Valacchi, G.; Eeman, M.; Rothen-Rutishauser, B. Impact of airborne particulate matter on skin: A systematic review from epidemiology to in vitro studies. *Part. Fibre Toxicol.* **2020**, *17*, 35. [CrossRef]
13. Ferrara, F.; Woodby, B.; Pecorelli, A.; Schiavone, M.L.; Pambianchi, E.; Messano, N.; Therrien, J.P.; Choudhary, H.; Valacchi, G. Additive effect of combined pollutants to UV induced skin OxInflammation damage. Evaluating the protective topical application of a cosmeceutical mixture formulation. *Redox Biol.* **2020**, *34*, 1014481. [CrossRef] [PubMed]
14. Plusquin, M.; Guida, F.; Polidoro, S.; Vermeulen, R.; Raaschou-Nielsen, O.; Campanella, G.; Hoek, G.; Kyrtopoulos, S.A.; Georgiadis, P.; Naccarati, A.; et al. DNA methylation and exposure to ambient air pollution in two prospective cohorts. *Environ. Int.* **2017**, *108*, 127–136. [CrossRef] [PubMed]
15. Ding, R.; Jin, Y.; Liu, X.; Zhu, Z.; Zhang, Y.; Wang, T.; Xu, Y. Characteristics of DNA methylation changes induced by traffic-related air pollution. *Mutat. Res. Genet. Toxicol. Environ. Mutagen.* **2016**, *15*, 46–53. [CrossRef] [PubMed]
16. Xu, C.J.; Söderhäll, C.; Bustamante, M.; Baïz, N.; Gruzieva, O.; Gehring, U.; Mason, D.; Chatzi, L.; Basterrechea, M.; Llop, S.; et al. DNA methylation in childhood asthma: An epigenome-wide meta-analysis. *Lancet Respir. Med.* **2018**, *6*, 379–388. [CrossRef]
17. Alfano, R.; Herceg, Z.; Nawrot, T.S.; Chadeau-Hyam, M.; Ghantous, A.; Plusquin, M. The Impact of Air Pollution on Our Epigenome: How Far Is the Evidence? (A Systematic Review). *Curr. Environ. Health Rep.* **2018**, *5*, 544–578. [CrossRef]
18. Weinhold, B. Epigenetics: The science of change. *Environ. Health Perspect.* **2006**, *114*, 160–167. [CrossRef]
19. Jin, B.; Li, Y.; Robertson, K.D. DNA methylation: Superior or subordinate in the epigenetic hierarchy? *Genes Cancer* **2011**, *2*, 607–617. [CrossRef]
20. Breton, C.V.; Marutani, A.N. Air Pollution and Epigenetics: Recent Findings. *Curr. Environ. Health Rep.* **2014**, *1*, 35–45. [CrossRef]
21. Chuang, J.C.; Jones, P.A. Epigenetics and microRNAs. *Pediatr. Res.* **2007**, *61*, 24–29. [CrossRef]
22. Cancer, I.A. *IARC Monographs on the Evaluation of Carcinogenic Risks to Humans, No. 100D.*; World Health Organization: Geneva, Switzerland, 2012; Volume 100D, p. 341. ISBN 978-9283213215.
23. Rooks, M.G.; Veiga, P.; Wardwell-Scott, L.H.; Tickle, T.; Segata, N.; Michaud, M.; Gallini, C.A.; Beal, C.; Van Hylckama-Vlieg, J.E.T.; Ballal, S.A.; et al. Gut microbiome composition and function in experimental colitis during active disease and treatment-induced remission. *ISME J.* **2014**, *8*, 1403–1417. [CrossRef]
24. Guo, B.; Hui, Q.; Xu, Z.; Chang, P.; Tao, K. miR-495 inhibits the growth of fibroblasts in hypertrophic scars. *Aging* **2019**, *11*, 2898–2910. [CrossRef]
25. Jun, H.; Ying, H.; Daiwen, C.; Bing, Y.; Xiangbing, M.; Ping, Z.; Jie, Y.; Zhiqing, H.; Junqiu, L. MIR-628, a microRNA that is induced by Toll-like receptor stimulation, regulates porcine innate immune responses. *Sci. Rep.* **2015**, *5*, 1–10. [CrossRef]
26. Chen, H.; Ji, X.; She, F.; Gao, Y.; Tang, P. MIR-628-3p regulates osteoblast differentiation by targeting RUNX2: Possible role in atrophic non-union. *Int. J. Mol. Med.* **2017**, *39*, 279–286. [CrossRef] [PubMed]
27. Dong, P.; Xiong, Y.; Yue, J.; Xu, D.; Ihira, K.; Konno, Y.; Kobayashi, N.; Todo, Y.; Watari, H. Long noncoding RNA NEAT1 drives aggressive endometrial cancer progression via miR-361-regulated networks involving STAT3 and tumor microenvironment-related genes. *J. Exp. Clin. Cancer Res.* **2019**, *8*, 38–295. [CrossRef] [PubMed]
28. Zhang, T.; Cai, X.; Li, Q.; Xue, P.; Chen, Z.; Dong, X.; Xue, Y. Hsa-miR-875-5p exerts tumor suppressor function through down-regulation of EGFR in colorectal carcinoma (CRC). *Oncotarget* **2016**, *7*, 42225–42240. [CrossRef]
29. Kang, N.; Ou, Y.; Wang, G.; Chen, J.; Li, D.; Zhan, Q. miR-875-5p exerts tumor-promoting function via down-regulation of CAPZA1 in esophageal squamous cell carcinoma. *PeerJ* **2021**, *9*, e10020. [CrossRef]

30. Liang, J.-J.; Wang, J.-Y.; Zhang, T.-J.; An, G.-S.; Ni, J.-H.; Li, S.-Y.; Jia, H.-T. MiR-509-3-5p-NONHSAT112228.2 Axis Regulates p21 and Suppresses Proliferation and Migration of Lung Cancer Cells. *Curr. Top. Med. Chem.* **2020**, *20*, 835–846. [CrossRef]
31. Ram Kumar, R.M.; Boro, A.; Fuchs, B. Involvement and Clinical Aspects of MicroRNA in Osteosarcoma. *Int. J. Mol. Sci.* **2016**, *17*, 877. [CrossRef]
32. Yang, H.; Ren, J.; Bai, Y.; Jiang, J.; Xiao, S. Microrna-518-3p suppresses cell proliferation, invasiveness, and migration in colorectal cancer via targeting trip4. *Biochem. Cell Biol.* **2020**, *98*, 575–582. [CrossRef]
33. Zhao, Y.; Lukiw, W.J. Bacteroidetes Neurotoxins and Inflammatory Neurodegeneration. *Mol. Neurobiol.* **2018**, *55*, 9100–9107. [CrossRef]
34. Lu, L.; Zhang, H.; Dong, W.; Peng, W.; Yang, J. MiR-381 negatively regulates cardiomyocyte survival by suppressing Notch signaling. *Vitr. Cell. Dev. Biol. Anim.* **2018**, *54*, 610–619. [CrossRef]
35. Reddy, S.D.N.; Pakala, S.B.; Ohshiro, K.; Rayala, S.K.; Kumar, R. MicroRNA-661, a c/EBPα target, inhibits metastatic tumor antigen 1 and regulates its functions. *Cancer Res.* **2009**, *69*, 5639–5642. [CrossRef] [PubMed]
36. Yonemori, K.; Seki, N.; Idichi, T.; Kurahara, H.; Osako, Y.; Koshizuka, K.; Arai, T.; Okato, A.; Kita, Y.; Arigami, T.; et al. The microRNA expression signature of pancreatic ductal adenocarcinoma by RNA sequencing: Anti-tumour functions of the microRNA-216 cluster. *Oncotarget* **2017**, *8*, 70097–70115. [CrossRef] [PubMed]
37. Son, G.H.; Kim, Y.; Lee, J.J.; Lee, K.Y.; Ham, H.; Song, J.E.; Park, S.T.; Kim, Y.H. MicroRNA-548 regulates high mobility group box 1 expression in patients with preterm birth and chorioamnionitis. *Sci. Rep.* **2019**, *9*, 19746. [CrossRef] [PubMed]
38. Treiber, T.; Treiber, N.; Meister, G. Regulation of microRNA biogenesis and its crosstalk with other cellular pathways. *Nat. Rev. Mol. Cell Biol.* **2019**, *20*, 5–20. [CrossRef] [PubMed]
39. Wu, Z.H.; Huang, K.H.; Liu, K.; Wang, G.T.; Sun, Q. DGCR5 induces osteogenic differentiation by up-regulating Runx2 through miR-30d-5p. *Biochem. Biophys. Res. Commun.* **2018**, *505*, 426–431. [CrossRef] [PubMed]
40. Xu, Y.; Wu, D.; Jiang, Z.; Zhang, Y.; Wang, S.; Ma, Z.; Hui, B.; Wang, J.; Qian, W.; Ge, Z.; et al. MiR-616-3p modulates cell proliferation and migration through targeting tissue factor pathway inhibitor 2 in preeclampsia. *Cell Prolif.* **2018**, *51*, e12490. [CrossRef]
41. Ntoumou, E.; Tzetis, M.; Braoudaki, M.; Lambrou, G.; Poulou, M.; Malizos, K.; Stefanou, N.; Anastasopoulou, L.; Tsezou, A. Serum microRNA array analysis identifies miR-140-3p, miR-33b-3p and miR-671-3p as potential osteoarthritis biomarkers involved in metabolic processes. *Clin. Epigenetics* **2017**, *12*, 9–127. [CrossRef]
42. Sun, S.; Su, C.; Zhu, Y.; Li, H.; Liu, N.; Xu, T.; Sun, C.; Lv, Y. MicroRNA-544a Regulates Migration and Invasion in Colorectal Cancer Cells via Regulation of Homeobox A10. *Dig. Dis. Sci.* **2016**, *61*, 2535–2544. [CrossRef]
43. Shin, C.-H.; Byun, J.; Lee, K.; Kim, B.; Noh, Y.K.; Tran, N.L.; Park, K.; Kim, S.-H.; Kim, T.H.; Oh, S.J. Exosomal miRNA-19a and miRNA-614 Induced by Air Pollutants Promote Proinflammatory M1 Macrophage Polarization via Regulation of RORα Expression in Human Respiratory Mucosal Microenvironment. *J. Immunol.* **2020**, *205*, 3179–3190. [CrossRef]
44. Xiong, G.; Zhang, J.; Zhang, Y.; Pang, X.; Wang, B.; Zhang, Y. Circular RNA_0074027 participates in cell proliferation, apoptosis and metastasis of colorectal cancer cells through regulation of miR-525-3p. *Mol. Med. Rep.* **2021**, *23*, 324. [CrossRef] [PubMed]
45. Templin, C.; Volkmann, J.; Emmert, M.Y.; Mocharla, P.; Müller, M.; Kraenkel, N.; Ghadri, J.R.; Meyer, M.; Styp-Rekowska, B.; Briand, S.; et al. Increased proangiogenic activity of mobilized CD34 + progenitor cells of patients with acute ST-segment-elevation myocardial infarction: Role of differential MicroRNA-378 expression. *Arterioscler. Thromb. Vasc. Biol.* **2017**, *37*, 341–349. [CrossRef]
46. Wang, H.; Chen, X.; Yang, B.; Xia, Z.; Chen, Q. MiR-924 as a tumor suppressor inhibits non-small cell lung cancer by inhibiting RHBDD1/Wnt/β-catenin signaling pathway. *Cancer Cell Int.* **2020**, *8*, 20–49. [CrossRef] [PubMed]
47. Wang, X.; Tan, Y.; Xu, B.; Lu, L.; Zhao, M.; Ma, J.; Liang, H.; Liu, J.; Yu, S. GPR30 Attenuates Myocardial Fibrosis in Diabetic Ovariectomized Female Rats: Role of iNOS Signaling. *DNA Cell Biol.* **2018**, *37*, 821–830. [CrossRef] [PubMed]
48. Shuai, F.; Wang, B.; Dong, S. MiR-522-3p promotes tumorigenesis in human colorectal cancer via targeting bloom syndrome protein. *Oncol. Res.* **2018**, *26*, 1113–1121. [CrossRef]
49. Vettori, A.; Pompucci, G.; Paolini, B.; Del Ciondolo, I.; Bressan, S.; Dundar, M.; Kenanoğlu, S.; Unfer, V.; Bertelli, M. Genetic background, nutrition and obesity: A review. *Eur. Rev. Med. Pharmacol. Sci.* **2019**, *23*, 1751–1761. [CrossRef]
50. Wang, L.; Sun, M.; Cao, Y.; Ma, L.; Shen, Y.; Velikanova, A.A.; Li, X.; Sun, C.; Zhao, Y. miR-34a regulates lipid metabolism by targeting SIRT1 in non-alcoholic fatty liver disease with iron overload. *Arch. Biochem. Biophys.* **2020**, *695*, 108642. [CrossRef]
51. Xiao, K.; Luo, X.; Wang, X.; Gao, Z. MicroRNA-185 regulates transforming growth factor-β1 and collagen-1 in hypertrophic scar fibroblasts. *Mol. Med. Rep.* **2017**, *15*, 1489–1496. [CrossRef]
52. Li, K.P.; Fang, Y.P.; Liao, J.Q.; Duan, J.D.; Feng, L.G.; Luo, X.Z.; Liang, Z.J. Upregulation of miR-598 promotes cell proliferation and cell cycle progression in human colorectal carcinoma by suppressing INPP5E expression. *Mol. Med. Rep.* **2018**, *17*, 2991–2997. [CrossRef]
53. Xiao, Y. MiR-486-5p inhibits the hyperproliferation and production of collagen in hypertrophic scar fibroblasts via IGF1/PI3K/AKT pathway. *J. Dermatolog. Treat.* **2020**, *32*, 973–982. [CrossRef]
54. Pedersen, I.M.; Cheng, G.; Wieland, S.; Volinia, S.; Croce, C.M.; Chisari, F.V.; David, M. Interferon modulation of cellular microRNAs as an antiviral mechanism. *Nature* **2007**, *449*, 919–922. [CrossRef] [PubMed]
55. Feng, H.J.; Ouyang, W.; Liu, J.H.; Sun, Y.G.; Hu, R.; Huang, L.H.; Xian, J.L.; Jing, C.F.; Zhou, M.J. Global microRNA profiles and signaling pathways in the development of cardiac hypertrophy. *Braz. J. Med. Biol. Res.* **2014**, *47*, 361–368. [CrossRef] [PubMed]

56. Chaudhari, U.; Nemade, H.; Gaspar, J.A.; Hescheler, J.; Hengstler, J.G.; Sachinidis, A. MicroRNAs as early toxicity signatures of doxorubicin in human-induced pluripotent stem cell-derived cardiomyocytes. *Arch. Toxicol.* **2016**, *90*, 3087–3098. [CrossRef]
57. Xia, X.; Wang, S.; Ni, B.; Xing, S.; Cao, H.; Zhang, Z.; Yu, F.; Zhao, E.; Zhao, G. Hypoxic gastric cancer-derived exosomes promote progression and metastasis via MiR-301a-3p/PHD3/HIF-1α positive feedback loop. *Oncogene* **2020**, *39*, 6231–6244. [CrossRef]
58. Zhang, L.; Li, J.; Cui, L.; Shang, J.; Tian, F.; Wang, R.; Xing, G. Retraction notice to MicroRNA-30b promotes lipopolysaccharide-induced in fl ammatory injury and alleviates autophagy through JNK and NF- κ B. *Biomed. Pharmacother.* **2020**, *128*, 266021.
59. Guan, C.; Wang, Y. LncRNA CASC9 attenuates lactate dehydrogenase-mediated oxidative stress and inflammation in spinal cord injury via sponging miR-383-5p. *Inflammation* **2021**, *44*, 923–933. [CrossRef]
60. Sun, R.; Ge, L.; Cao, Y.; Wu, W.; Wu, Y.; Zhu, H.; Li, J.; Yu, D. Corrigendum to "MiR-429 regulates blood-spinal cord barrier permeability by targeting Krüppel-like factor 6". *Biochem. Biophys. Res. Commun.* **2020**, *525*, 740–746. [CrossRef]
61. Chen, X.F.; Zhang, L.J.; Zhang, J.; Dou, X.; Shao, Y.; Jia, X.J.; Zhang, W.; Yu, B. MiR-151a is involved in the pathogenesis of atopic dermatitis by regulating interleukin-12 receptor β2. *Exp. Dermatol.* **2018**, *27*, 427–432. [CrossRef]
62. Xiao, S.; Zhang, M.; Liu, C.; Wang, D. MiR-514 attenuates proliferation and increases chemoresistance by targeting ATP binding cassette subfamily in ovarian cancer. *Mol. Genet. Genom.* **2018**, *293*, 1159–1167. [CrossRef]
63. Chu, H.T.; Li, L.; Jia, M.; Diao, L.L.; Li, Z.B. Correlation between serum microRNA-136 levels and RAAS biochemical markers in patients with essential hypertension. *Eur. Rev. Med. Pharmacol. Sci.* **2020**, *24*, 11761–11767. [CrossRef]
64. Mishima, Y.; Stahlhut, C.; Giraldez, A.J. miR-1-2 Gets to the Heart of the Matter. *Cell* **2007**, *20*, 247–249. [CrossRef] [PubMed]
65. Qi, B.; Dong, Y.; Qiao, X.L. Effects of miR-18a on proliferation and apoptosis of gastric cancer cells by regulating RUNX1. *Eur. Rev. Med. Pharmacol. Sci.* **2020**, *24*, 9957–9964. [CrossRef] [PubMed]
66. Jin, H.; Yu, M.; Lin, Y.; Hou, B.; Wu, Z.; Li, Z.; Sun, J. MiR-502-3P suppresses cell proliferation, migration, and invasion in hepatocellular carcinoma by targeting SET. *Onco. Targets. Ther.* **2016**, *9*, 3281–3289. [CrossRef] [PubMed]
67. Zhang, Y.; Chu, X.; Wei, Q. Mir-451 promotes cell apoptosis and inhibits autophagy in pediatric acute myeloid leukemia by targeting hmgb1. *J. Environ. Pathol. Toxicol. Oncol.* **2021**, *40*, 45–53. [CrossRef]
68. Rodosthenous, R.S.; Coull, B.A.; Lu, Q.; Vokonas, P.S.; Schwartz, J.D.; Baccarelli, A.A. Ambient particulate matter and microRNAs in extracellular vesicles: A pilot study of older individuals. *Part. Fibre Toxicol.* **2016**, *13*, 13. [CrossRef]
69. Wang, Z.; Liu, W.; Wang, C.; Ai, Z. Mir-873-5p inhibits cell migration and invasion of papillary thyroid cancer via regulation of CXCL16. *Onco. Targets. Ther.* **2020**, *13*, 1037–1046. [CrossRef]
70. Tu, H.; Wei, G.; Cai, Q.; Chen, X.X.; Sun, Z.; Cheng, C.; Zhang, L.; Feng, Y.; Zhou, H.; Zhou, B.; et al. MicroRNA-212 inhibits hepatocellular carcinoma cell proliferation and induces apoptosis by targeting FOXA1. *Onco. Targets. Ther.* **2015**, *24*, 2227–2235. [CrossRef]
71. Zhang, X.; Zhang, Y.; Dou, L. MiR-552 promotes the proliferation and metastasis of cervical cancer cells through targeting MUC15 pathway. *J. Cancer* **2021**, *12*, 6094–6104. [CrossRef]
72. Fang, L.; Xu, X.; Lu, Y.; Wu, Y.Y.; Li, J.J. MicroRNA-495 attenuates proliferation and inflammatory response in rheumatoid arthritis fibroblast-like synoviocytes through attenuating β-catenin pathway. *J. Biol. Regul. Homeost. Agents* **2020**, *34*, 837–844. [CrossRef]
73. Zhang, K.; Guo, L. MiR-767 promoted cell proliferation in human melanoma by suppressing CYLD expression. *Gene* **2018**, *641*, 272–278. [CrossRef]
74. Sun, L.; Trajkovski, M. MiR-27 orchestrates the transcriptional regulation of brown adipogenesis. *Metabolism* **2014**, *63*, 272–282. [CrossRef] [PubMed]
75. Si, Z.; Yu, L.; Jing, H.; Wu, L.; Wang, X. Oncogenic lncRNA ZNF561-AS1 is essential for colorectal cancer proliferation and survival through regulation of miR-26a-3p/miR-128-5p-SRSF6 axis. *J. Exp. Clin. Cancer Res.* **2021**, *40*, 78. [CrossRef] [PubMed]
76. Tao, X.; Yang, X.; Wu, K.; Yang, L.; Huang, Y.; Jin, Q.; Chen, S. miR-629-5p promotes growth and metastasis of hepatocellular carcinoma by activating β-catenin. *Exp. Cell Res.* **2019**, *15*, 124–130. [CrossRef] [PubMed]
77. Liu, X.; Gan, L.; Zhang, J. miR-543 inhibits cervical cancer growth and metastasis by targeting TRPM7. *Chem. Biol. Interact.* **2019**, *302*, 83–92. [CrossRef]
78. Zhang, M.; Muralimanoharan, S.; Wortman, A.C.; Mendelson, C.R. Primate-specific miR-515 family members inhibit key genes in human trophoblast differentiation and are upregulated in preeclampsia. *Proc. Natl. Acad. Sci. USA* **2016**, *113*, 7069–7076. [CrossRef]
79. Witwer, K.W.; Sarbanes, S.L.; Liu, J.; Clements, J.E. A plasma microRNA signature of acute lentiviral infection: Biomarkers of central nervous system disease. *AIDS* **2011**, *25*, 2057–2067. [CrossRef]
80. Li, B.; Wang, Y.; Li, S.; He, H.; Sun, F.; Wang, C.; Lu, Y.; Wang, X.; Tao, B. Decreased expression of miR-378 correlates with tumor invasiveness and poor prognosis of patients with glioma. *Int. J. Clin. Exp. Pathol.* **2015**, *8*, 7016–7021.
81. Li, Q.; Tian, Y.; Liang, Y.; Li, C. CircHIPK3/miR-876-5p/PIK3R1 axis regulates regulation proliferation, migration, invasion, and glutaminolysis in gastric cancer cells. *Cancer Cell Int.* **2020**, *13*, 391. [CrossRef]
82. Guo, M.; Jiang, Z.; Zhang, X.; Lu, D.; Ha, A.D.; Sun, J.; Du, W.; Wu, Z.; Hu, L.; Khadarian, K.; et al. miR-656 inhibits glioma tumorigenesis through repression of BMPR1A. *Carcinogenesis* **2014**, *35*, 1698–1706. [CrossRef]
83. Lv, L.; Wang, X.; Ma, T. MicroRNA-944 inhibits the malignancy of hepatocellular carcinoma by directly targeting IGF-1R and deactivating the PI3K/Akt signaling pathway. *Cancer Manag. Res.* **2019**, *11*, 2531–2543. [CrossRef]
84. Zhang, W.; Zhong, B.; Zhang, C.; Luo, C.; Zhan, Y. miR-373 regulates inflammatory cytokine-mediated chondrocyte proliferation in osteoarthritis by targeting the P2X7 receptor. *FEBS Open Bio* **2018**, *8*, 325–331. [CrossRef] [PubMed]

85. Aqeilan, R.I.; Calin, G.A.; Croce, C.M. MiR-15a and miR-16-1 in cancer: Discovery, function and future perspectives. *Cell Death Differ.* **2010**, *17*, 215–220. [CrossRef] [PubMed]
86. Yang, Z.; Wei, Z.; Wu, X.; Yang, H. Screening of exosomal miRNAs derived from subcutaneous and visceral adipose tissues: Determination of targets for the treatment of obesity and associated metabolic disorders. *Mol. Med. Rep.* **2018**, *18*, 3314–3324. [CrossRef] [PubMed]
87. Xu, Y.; Wang, L.; Jiang, L.; Zhang, X. Novel MicroRNA Biomarkers, miR-142-5p, miR-550a, miR-1826, and miR-1201, Were Identified for Primary Melanoma. *J. Comput. Biol.* **2020**, *27*, 815–824. [CrossRef]
88. Jiang, X.; Huang, H.; Li, Z.; He, C.; Li, Y.; Chen, P.; Gurbuxani, S.; Arnovitz, S.; Hong, G.M.; Price, C.; et al. miR-495 is a tumor-suppressor microRNA down-regulated in MLL-rearranged leukemia. *Proc. Natl. Acad. Sci. USA* **2012**, *109*, 19397–19402. [CrossRef]
89. Wei, Q.; Tu, Y.; Zuo, L.; Zhao, J.; Chang, Z.; Zou, Y.; Qiu, J. MiR-345-3p attenuates apoptosis and inflammation caused by oxidized low-density lipoprotein by targeting TRAF6 via TAK1/p38/NF-kB signaling in endothelial cells. *Life Sci.* **2020**, *241*, 117142. [CrossRef]
90. Xu, X.; Zheng, S. MiR-887-3p negatively regulates StARD13 and promotes pancreatic cancer progression. *Cancer Manag. Res.* **2020**, *12*, 6137–6147. [CrossRef]
91. Wu, K.; Yu, Z.; Tang, Z.; Wei, W.; Xie, D.; Xie, Y.; Xiao, Q. MiR-877-5p suppresses gastric cancer cell proliferation through targeting FOXM1. *Onco. Targets. Ther.* **2020**, *13*, 4731–4742. [CrossRef]
92. Muti, P.; Donzelli, S.; Sacconi, A.; Hossain, A.; Ganci, F.; Frixa, T.; Sieri, S.; Krogh, V.; Berrino, F.; Biagioni, F.; et al. MiRNA-513a-5p inhibits progesterone receptor expression and constitutes a risk factor for breast cancer: The hOrmone and Diet in the ETiology of breast cancer prospective study. *Carcinogenesis* **2018**, *39*, 98–108. [CrossRef]
93. Zhu, F.; Li, H.; Ding, F.; Guo, H.; Mou, H.; Ma, J. MiR-422a in gastric cancer cells directly targets CDC40 and modulates cell proliferation. *Am. J. Transl. Res.* **2020**, *12*, 4693.
94. Wang, Y.; Yang, L.; Chen, T.; Liu, X.; Guo, Y.; Zhu, Q.; Tong, X.; Yang, W.; Xu, Q.; Huang, D.; et al. A novel lncRNA MCM3AP-AS1 promotes the growth of hepatocellular carcinoma by targeting miR-194-5p/FOXA1 axis. *Mol. Cancer* **2019**, *18*, 28. [CrossRef] [PubMed]
95. Zhang, T.; Hu, J.; Wang, X.; Zhao, X.; Li, Z.; Niu, J.; Steer, C.J.; Zheng, G.; Song, G. MicroRNA-378 promotes hepatic inflammation and fibrosis via modulation of the NF-κB-TNFα pathway. *J. Hepatol.* **2019**, *70*, 87–96. [CrossRef] [PubMed]
96. Zhao, J.P.; Chen, L.L. Circular rna mat2b induces colorectal cancer proliferation via sponging mir-610, resulting in an increased e2f1 expression. *Cancer Manag. Res.* **2020**, *12*, 7107. [CrossRef] [PubMed]
97. Wang, F.; Long, G.; Zhao, C.; Li, H.; Chaugai, S.; Wang, Y.; Chen, C.; Wang, D.W. Atherosclerosis-related circulating miRNAs as novel and sensitive predictors for acute myocardial infarction. *PLoS ONE* **2014**, *9*, e105734. [CrossRef]
98. Chen, Z.; Li, Y.; Tan, B.; Li, F.; Zhao, Q.; Fan, L.; Zhang, Z.; Zhao, X.; Liu, Y.; Wang, D. Long Non-coding RNA ASNR Targeting miR-519e-5p Promotes Gastric Cancer Development by Regulating FGFR2. *Front. Cell Dev. Biol.* **2021**, *9*, 679176. [CrossRef]
99. Chen, F.; Liu, M.; Yu, Y.; Sun, Y.; Li, J.; Hu, W.; Wang, X.; Tong, D. LINC00958 regulated miR-627-5p/YBX2 axis to facilitate cell proliferation and migration in oral squamous cell carcinoma. *Cancer Biol. Ther.* **2019**, *20*, 1270–1280. [CrossRef]
100. Liang, T.; Guo, L.; Liu, C. Genome-wide analysis of mir-548 gene family reveals evolutionary and functional implications. *J. Biomed. Biotechnol.* **2012**, *2012*, 679563. [CrossRef]
101. Wang, L.; Li, H. MiR-770-5p facilitates podocyte apoptosis and inflammation in diabetic nephropathy by targeting TIMP3. *Biosci. Rep.* **2020**, *40*, BSR20193653. [CrossRef]
102. Li, J.; Wang, L.; He, F.; Li, B.; Han, R. Long noncoding RNA LINC00629 restrains the progression of gastric cancer by upregulating AQP4 through competitively binding to miR-196b-5p. *J. Cell. Physiol.* **2020**, *235*, 2973–2985. [CrossRef]
103. Zhu, H.; Hu, Y.; Wang, C.; Zhang, X.; He, D. CircGCN1L1 promotes synoviocyte proliferation and chondrocyte apoptosis by targeting miR-330-3p and TNF-α in TMJ osteoarthritis. *Cell Death Dis.* **2020**, *11*, 284. [CrossRef]
104. Liu, T.; Feng, X.; Liao, Y. miR-617 Promotes the Growth of IL-22-Stimulated Keratinocytes Through Regulating FOXO4 Expression. *Biochem. Genet.* **2021**, *59*, 547–559. [CrossRef] [PubMed]
105. Chen, S.; Tang, Y.; Liu, Y.; Zhang, P.; Lv, L.; Zhang, X.; Jia, L.; Zhou, Y. Exosomes derived from miR-375-overexpressing human adipose mesenchymal stem cells promote bone regeneration. *Cell Prolif.* **2019**, *52*, e12669. [CrossRef] [PubMed]
106. Liu, S.; Gong, Y.; Xu, X.D.; Shen, H.; Gao, S.; Bao, H.D.; Guo, S.B.; Yu, X.F.; Gong, J. MicroRNA-936/ERBB4/Akt axis exhibits anticancer properties of gastric cancer through inhibition of cell proliferation, migration, and invasion. *Kaohsiung J. Med. Sci.* **2021**, *37*, 111–120. [CrossRef]
107. Wang, P.; Wang, Z.; Liu, G.; Jin, C.; Zhang, Q.; Man, S.; Wang, Z. MiR-657 promotes macrophage polarization toward M1 by targeting FAM46C in gestational diabetes mellitus. *Mediat. Inflamm.* **2019**, *2019*, 4851214. [CrossRef] [PubMed]
108. Garros, R.F.; Paul, R.; Connolly, M.; Lewis, A.; Garfield, B.E.; Natanek, S.A.; Bloch, S.; Mouly, V.; Griffiths, M.J.; Polkey, M.I.; et al. MicroRNA-542 promotes mitochondrial dysfunction and SMAD activity and is elevated in intensive care unit–acquired weakness. *Am. J. Respir. Crit. Care Med.* **2017**, *196*, 1422–1433. [CrossRef]
109. Chen, Y.; Yu, H.; Zhu, D.; Liu, P.; Yin, J.; Liu, D.; Zheng, M.; Gao, J.; Zhang, C.; Gao, Y. miR-136-3p targets PTEN to regulate vascularization and bone formation and ameliorates alcohol-induced osteopenia. *FASEB J.* **2020**, *34*, 5348–5362. [CrossRef] [PubMed]

110. Xu, Y. MicroRNA-136-3p inhibits glioma tumorigenesis in vitro and in vivo by targeting KLF7. *World J. Surg. Oncol.* **2020**, *18*, 1–10. [CrossRef]
111. Xue, Q.; Yang, D.; Zhang, J.; Gan, P.; Lin, C.; Lu, Y.; Zhang, W.; Zhang, L.; Guang, X. USP7, negatively regulated by miR-409-5p, aggravates hypoxia-induced cardiomyocyte injury. *APMIS* **2021**, *129*, 152–162. [CrossRef]
112. Wang, Y.; Lin, W.; Ju, J. MicroRNA-409-5p promotes retinal neovascularization in diabetic retinopathy. *Cell Cycle* **2020**, *19*, 1314–1325. [CrossRef]
113. Fan, X.D.; Luo, Y.; Wang, J.; An, N. MiR-154-3p and miR-487-3p synergistically modulate RHOA signaling in the carcinogenesis of thyroid cancer. *Biosci. Rep.* **2020**, *40*, BSR20193158. [CrossRef]
114. Ma, J.; Wu, D.; Yi, J.; Yi, Y.; Zhu, X.; Qiu, H.; Kong, R.; Lin, J.; Qian, J.; Deng, Z. MiR-378 promoted cell proliferation and inhibited apoptosis by enhanced stem cell properties in chronic myeloid leukemia K562 cells. *Biomed. Pharmacother.* **2019**, *112*, 108623. [CrossRef] [PubMed]
115. Tang, B.; Xuan, L.; Tang, M.; Wang, H.; Zhou, J.; Liu, J.; Wu, S.; Li, M.; Wang, X.; Zhang, H. miR-93-3p alleviates lipopolysaccharide-induced inflammation and apoptosis in H9c2 cardiomyocytes by inhibiting toll-like receptor 4. *Pathol. Res. Pract.* **2018**, *214*, 1686–1693. [CrossRef] [PubMed]
116. Jin, W.; Chen, L.; Gao, F.; Yang, M.; Liu, Y.; Wang, B. Down-regulation of miR-556-3p inhibits hemangioma cell proliferation and promotes apoptosis by targeting VEGFC. *Cell. Mol. Biol.* **2020**, *66*, 204–207. [CrossRef] [PubMed]
117. Yang, X.; Yang, S.; Song, J.; Yang, W.; Ji, Y.; Zhang, F.; Rao, J. Dysregulation of miR-23b-5p promotes cell proliferation via targeting FOXM1 in hepatocellular carcinoma. *Cell Death Discov.* **2021**, *7*, 1–12. [CrossRef] [PubMed]
118. Zhou, R.; Mao, Y.; Xiong, L.; Li, L. Integrated Transcriptome Analysis of microRNA and mRNA in Mouse Skin Derived Precursors (SKPs) and SKP Derived Fibroblast (SFBs) by RNA-Seq. *Curr. Genomics* **2018**, *20*, 49–60. [CrossRef] [PubMed]
119. Tang, P. Clinical diagnostic value of circulating serum miR-509-3p in pulmonary arterial hypertension with congenital heart disease. *Hell. J. Cardiol.* **2020**, *61*, 26–30. [CrossRef]
120. Stark, M.S.; Bonazzi, V.F.; Boyle, G.M.; Palmer, J.M.; Symmons, J.; Lanagan, C.M.; Schmidt, C.W.; Herington, A.C.; Ballotti, R.; Pollock, P.M.; et al. miR-514a regulates the tumour suppressor NF1 and modulates BRAFi sensitivity in melanoma. *Oncotarget* **2015**, *6*, 17753. [CrossRef]
121. Wang, Y.; Zhang, K.; Yuan, X.; Xu, N.; Zhao, S.; Hou, L.; Yang, L.; Zhang, N. MiR-431-5p regulates cell proliferation and apoptosis in fibroblast-like synoviocytes in rheumatoid arthritis by targeting XIAP. *Arthritis Res. Ther.* **2020**, *22*, 231. [CrossRef]
122. Wang, Y.; Lei, X.; Gao, C.; Xue, Y.; Li, X.; Wang, H.; Feng, Y. MiR-506-3p suppresses the proliferation of ovarian cancer cells by negatively regulating the expression of MTMR6. *J. Biosci.* **2019**, *44*, 126. [CrossRef]
123. Zhu, B.; Tian, T.; Zhao, M. MiR-645 promotes proliferation and migration of non-small cell lung cancer cells by targeting TP53I11. *Eur. Rev. Med. Pharmacol. Sci.* **2020**, *24*, 6150–6156. [CrossRef]
124. Zhang, Y.; Wang, Y.; Wei, Y.; Li, M.; Yu, S.; Ye, M.; Zhang, H.; Chen, S.; Liu, W.; Zhang, J. MiR-129-3p promotes docetaxel resistance of breast cancer cells via CP110 inhibition. *Sci. Rep.* **2015**, *5*, 15424. [CrossRef] [PubMed]
125. Huang, Y.; Jiang, L.; Wei, G. Circ_0006168 promotes the migration, invasion and proliferation of esophageal squamous cell carcinoma cells via mir-516b-5p-dependent regulation of xbp1. *Onco. Targets. Ther.* **2021**, *14*, 475–2488. [CrossRef] [PubMed]
126. Kong, M.; Han, Y.; Zhao, Y.; Zhang, H. miR-512-3p Overcomes Resistance to Cisplatin in Retinoblastoma by Promoting Apoptosis Induced by Endoplasmic Reticulum Stress. *Med. Sci. Monit.* **2020**, *26*, 923817. [CrossRef] [PubMed]
127. Wang, H.; Guo, Y.; Mi, N.; Zhou, L. miR-101-3p and miR-199b-5p promote cell apoptosis in oral cancer by targeting BICC1. *Mol. Cell. Probes* **2020**, *52*, 101567. [CrossRef]
128. Liao, Z.J.; Zheng, Q.; Wei, T.; Zhang, Y.B.; Ma, J.Q.; Zhao, Z.; Sun, H.F.; Nan, K.J. MicroRNA-561 Affects Proliferation and Cell Cycle Transition through PTEN/AKT Signaling Pathway by Targeting P-REX2a in NSCLC. *Oncol. Res.* **2020**, *28*, 147–159. [CrossRef]
129. He, Q.; Liu, N.; Hu, F.; Shi, Q.; Pi, X.; Chen, H.; Li, J.; Zhang, B. Circ_0061012 contributes to IL-22-induced proliferation, migration and invasion in keratinocytes through miR-194-5p/GAB1 axis in psoriasis. *Biosci. Rep.* **2021**, *4*, BSR20203130. [CrossRef]
130. Wang, Y.P.; Li, H.Q.; Chen, J.X.; Kong, F.G.; Mo, Z.H.; Wang, J.Z.; Huang, K.M.; Li, X.N.; Yan, Y. Overexpression of XIST facilitates cell proliferation, invasion and suppresses cell apoptosis by reducing radio-sensitivity of glioma cells via miR-329-3p/CREB1 axis. *Eur. Rev. Med. Pharmacol. Sci.* **2020**, *24*, 3190–3203. [CrossRef]
131. Wang, Y.F.; Lian, X.L.; Zhong, J.Y.; Su, S.X.; Xu, Y.F.; Xie, X.F.; Wang, Z.P.; Li, W.; Zhang, L.; Che, D.; et al. Serum exosomal microRNA let-7i-3p as candidate diagnostic biomarker for Kawasaki disease patients with coronary artery aneurysm. *IUBMB Life* **2019**, *71*, 891–900. [CrossRef]
132. Liu, Z.; Dou, C.; Yao, B.; Xu, M.; Ding, L.; Wang, Y.; Jia, Y.; Li, Q.; Zhang, H.; Tu, K.; et al. Methylation-mediated repression of microRNA-129-2 suppresses cell aggressiveness by inhibiting high mobility group box 1 in human hepatocellular carcinoma. *Oncotarget* **2016**, *7*, 36909–36923. [CrossRef]
133. Zhao, G.; Wang, T.; Huang, Q.K.; Pu, M.; Sun, W.; Zhang, Z.C.; Ling, R.; Tao, K.S. MicroRNA-548a-5p promotes proliferation and inhibits apoptosis in hepatocellular carcinoma cells by targeting Tg737. *World J. Gastroenterol.* **2016**, *22*, 5364–5373. [CrossRef]
134. Jiang, Y.; Wang, N.; Yin, D.; Li, Y.K.; Guo, L.; Shi, L.P.; Huang, X. Changes in the Expression of Serum MiR-887-5p in Patients with Endometrial Cancer. *Int. J. Gynecol. Cancer* **2016**, *26*, 1143–1147. [CrossRef] [PubMed]
135. Moura, S.R.; Bras, J.P.; Freitas, J.; Osório, H.; Barbosa, M.A.; Santos, S.G.; Almeida, M.I. miR-99a in bone homeostasis: Regulating osteogenic lineage commitment and osteoclast differentiation. *Bone* **2020**, *134*, 115303. [CrossRef] [PubMed]

136. Fan, Y.; Hao, J.; Cen, X.; Song, K.; Yang, C.; Xiao, S.; Cheng, S. Downregulation of miR-487a-3p suppresses the progression of non-small cell lung cancer via targeting Smad7. *Drug Dev. Res.* **2021**. [CrossRef]
137. Liu, W.; Yang, Y.J.; An, Q. LINC00963 promotes ovarian cancer proliferation, migration and EMT via the miR-378g/CHI3L1 axis. *Cancer Manag. Res.* **2020**, *12*, 463–473. [CrossRef] [PubMed]
138. Li, F.; Liu, H.; Cheng, Y.; Yang, J.; Liu, Y.; Wang, Y.; Yang, Z.; Shi, C.; Xu, Y. Association of variants in microRNA with Parkinson's disease in Chinese Han population. *Neurol. Sci.* **2018**, *39*, 353–357. [CrossRef]
139. Dong, L.; Zheng, Y.; Gao, L.; Luo, X. lncRNA NEAT1 prompts autophagy and apoptosis in MPTP-induced Parkinson's disease by impairing miR-374c-5p. *Acta Biochim. Biophys. Sin.* **2021**, *53*, 870–882. [CrossRef]
140. Zhu, M.; Zhang, N.; He, S.; Yan, R.; Zhang, J. MicroRNA-106a functions as an oncogene in human gastric cancer and contributes to proliferation and metastasis in vitro and in vivo. *Clin. Exp. Metastasis* **2016**, *3*, 509–519. [CrossRef]
141. Long, C.Y.; Xiao, Y.X.; Li, S.Y.; Tang, X.B.; Yuan, Z.W.; Bai, Y.Z. Upregulation of miR-92a-2-5p potentially contribute to anorectal malformations by inhibiting proliferation and enhancing apoptosis via PRKCA/β-catenin. *Biomed. Pharmacother.* **2020**, *127*, 110117. [CrossRef]
142. Zhu, L.M.; Li, N. Downregulation of long noncoding RNA TUSC7 promoted cell growth, invasion and migration through sponging with miR-616-5p/GSK3β pathway in ovarian cancer. *Eur. Rev. Med. Pharmacol. Sci.* **2020**, *24*, 7253–7265. [CrossRef]
143. Fu, L.; Li, Z.; Zhu, J.; Wang, P.; Fan, G.; Dai, Y.; Zheng, Z.; Liu, Y. Serum expression levels of microRNA-382-3p, -598-3p, -1246 and -184 in breast cancer patients. *Oncol. Lett.* **2016**, *12*, 269–274. [CrossRef]
144. Li, G.; Xu, Y.; Wang, S.; Yan, W.; Zhao, Q.; Guo, J. MiR-873-5p inhibits cell migration, invasion and epithelial-mesenchymal transition in colorectal cancer via targeting ZEB1. *Pathol. Res. Pract.* **2019**, *215*, 34–39. [CrossRef] [PubMed]
145. Liu, Z.; Su, D.; Qi, X.; Ma, J. MiR-500a-5p promotes glioblastoma cell proliferation, migration and invasion by targeting chromodomain helicase DNA binding protein 5. *Mol. Med. Rep.* **2018**, *18*, 2689–2696. [CrossRef] [PubMed]
146. Liu, Z.; He, C.; Qu, Y.; Chen, X.; Zhu, H.; Xiang, B. MiR-659-3p regulates the progression of chronic myeloid leukemia by targeting SPHK1. *Int. J. Clin. Exp. Pathol.* **2018**, *11*, 2470.
147. Lin, Q.; Jia, Y.; Zhang, D.; Jin, H. NCK1-AS1 promotes the progression of melanoma by accelerating cell proliferation and migration via targeting miR-526b-5p/ADAM15 axis. *Cancer Cell Int.* **2021**, *21*, 1–10. [CrossRef]
148. Zhu, F.; Li, Q.; Li, J.; Li, B.; Li, D. Long noncoding Mirt2 reduces apoptosis to alleviate myocardial infarction through regulation of the miR-764/PDK1 axis. *Lab. Investig.* **2021**, *101*, 165–176. [CrossRef] [PubMed]
149. Zhao, S.; Mi, Y.; Guan, B.; Zheng, B.; Wei, P.; Gu, Y.; Zhang, Z.; Cai, S.; Xu, Y.; Li, X.; et al. Tumor-derived exosomal miR-934 induces macrophage M2 polarization to promote liver metastasis of colorectal cancer. *J. Hematol. Oncol.* **2020**, *13*, 156. [CrossRef]
150. Ye, X.Y.; Xu, L.; Lu, S.; Chen, Z.W. Mir-516a-5p inhibits the proliferation of non-small cell lung cancer by targeting hist3h2a. *Int. J. Immunopathol. Pharmacol.* **2019**, *33*, 2058738419841481. [CrossRef] [PubMed]
151. Yuan, X.; Ma, R.; Yang, S.; Jiang, L.; Wang, Z.; Zhu, Z.; Li, H. miR-520g and miR-520h overcome bortezomib resistance in multiple myeloma via suppressing APE1. *Cell Cycle* **2019**, *18*, 1660–1669. [CrossRef]
152. Wang, J.; Wang, H.; Liu, A.; Fang, C.; Hao, J.; Wang, Z. Lactate dehydrogenase A negatively regulated by miRNAs promotes aerobic glycolysis and is increased in colorectal cancer. *Oncotarget* **2015**, *6*, 19465. [CrossRef]
153. Su, X.; Gao, C.; Feng, X.; Jiang, M. miR-613 suppresses migration and invasion in esophageal squamous cell carcinoma via the targeting of G6PD. *Exp. Ther. Med.* **2020**, *19*, 3081–3089. [CrossRef]
154. Wang, M.; Zhao, H.Y.; Zhang, J.L.; Wan, D.M.; Li, Y.M.; Jiang, Z.X. Dysregulation of LncRNA ANRIL mediated by miR-411-3p inhibits the malignant proliferation and tumor stem cell like property of multiple myeloma via hypoxia-inducible factor 1α. *Exp. Cell Res.* **2020**, *396*, 112280. [CrossRef] [PubMed]
155. Hou, J.; Li, A.L.; Xiong, W.Q.; Chen, R. Hsa Circ 001839 Promoted Inflammation in Renal Ischemia-Reperfusion Injury through NLRP3 by miR-432-3p. *Nephron* **2021**, *145*, 540–552. [CrossRef] [PubMed]
156. Fan, R.F.; Cao, C.Y.; Chen, M.H.; Shi, Q.X.; Xu, S.W. Gga-let 7f 3p promotes apoptosis in selenium deficiency induced skeletal muscle by targeting selenoprotein K. *Metallomics* **2018**, *10*, 941–952. [CrossRef] [PubMed]
157. Zhang, B. Guizhi Fuling pills inhibit the proliferation, migration and invasion of human cutaneous malignant melanoma cells by regulating the molecular axis of LncRNA TPT1-AS1/miR-671-5p. *Cell. Mol. Biol.* **2020**, *66*, 148–154. [CrossRef]
158. Li, Y.; Kuscu, C.; Banach, A.; Zhang, Q.; Pulkoski-Gross, A.; Kim, D.; Liu, J.; Roth, E.; Li, E.; Shroyer, K.R.; et al. miR-181a-5p inhibits cancer cell migration and angiogenesis via downregulation of matrix metalloproteinase-14. *Cancer Res.* **2015**, *75*, 2674–2685. [CrossRef] [PubMed]
159. Baker, M.A.; Wang, F.; Liu, Y.; Kriegel, A.J.; Geurts, A.M.; Usa, K.; Xue, H.; Wang, D.; Kong, Y.; Liang, M. MiR-192-5p in the Kidney Protects Against the Development of Hypertension. *Hypertension* **2019**, *73*, 399–406. [CrossRef]
160. Zhang, H.; Zhang, Z.; Gao, L.; Qiao, Z.; Yu, M.; Yu, B.; Yang, T. miR-1-3p suppresses proliferation of hepatocellular carcinoma through targeting SOX9. *Onco. Targets. Ther.* **2019**, *12*, 2149–2157. [CrossRef]
161. Wang, Y.; Zhang, Q. Long Noncoding RNA MALAT1 Knockdown Inhibits Proliferation, Migration, and Invasion and Promotes Apoptosis in Non-Small-Cell Lung Cancer Cells Through Regulating miR-515-3p/TRIM65 Axis. *Cancer Biother. Radiopharm.* **2020**. [CrossRef]
162. Liu, L.; Zhang, H.; Mao, H.; Li, X.; Hu, Y. Exosomal miR-320d derived from adipose tissue-derived MSCs inhibits apoptosis in cardiomyocytes with atrial fibrillation (AF). *Artif. Cells Nanomed. Biotechnol.* **2019**, *47*, 3976–3984. [CrossRef]

163. Peng, X.; Wu, M.; Liu, W.; Guo, C.; Zhan, L.; Zhan, X. MiR-502-5p inhibits the proliferation, migration and invasion of gastric cancer cells by targeting SP1. *Oncol. Lett.* **2020**, *20*, 2757–2762. [CrossRef]
164. Wu, X.; Chen, B.; Shi, H.; Zhou, J.; Zhou, F.; Cao, J.; Sun, X. miR-758-3p suppresses human bladder cancer cell proliferation, migration and invasion by targeting NOTCH2. *Exp. Ther. Med.* **2019**, *17*, 4273–4278. [CrossRef]
165. Pourhanifeh, M.H.; Mahjoubin-Tehran, M.; Karimzadeh, M.R.; Mirzaei, H.R.; Razavi, Z.S.; Sahebkar, A.; Hosseini, N.; Mirzaei, H.; Hamblin, M.R. Autophagy in cancers including brain tumors: Role of MicroRNAs. *Cell Commun. Signal.* **2020**, *18*, 88. [CrossRef] [PubMed]
166. Xu, J.; Lei, S.; Sun, S.; Zhang, W.; Zhu, F.; Yang, H.; Xu, Q.; Zhang, B.; Li, H.; Zhu, M.; et al. Mir-324-3p regulates fibroblast proliferation via targeting tgf-β1 in atrial fibrillation. *Int. Heart J.* **2020**, *61*, 20–423. [CrossRef] [PubMed]
167. Kordaß, T.; Weber, C.E.M.; Eisel, D.; Pane, A.A.; Osen, W.; Eichmüller, S.B. miR-193b and miR-30c-1* inhibit, whereas miR-576-5p enhances melanoma cell invasion in vitro. *Oncotarget* **2018**, *9*, 32507–32522. [CrossRef] [PubMed]
168. Li, J.; Shao, W.; Zhao, J. MiR-520a-3p inhibits malignant progression of epithelial ovarian cancer by targeting SUV39H1 expression. *Hum. Cell* **2021**, *34*, 570–578. [CrossRef]
169. Fang, Y.; Gu, X.; Li, Z.; Xiang, J.; Chen, Z. miR-449b inhibits the proliferation of SW1116 colon cancer stem cells through downregulation of CCND1 and E2F3 expression. *Oncol. Rep.* **2013**, *30*, 399–506. [CrossRef] [PubMed]
170. Díaz-Martínez, M.; Benito-Jardon, L.; Alonso, L.; Koetz-Ploch, L.; Hernando, E.; Teixido, J. miR-204-5p and miR-211-5p contribute to BRAF inhibitor resistance in melanoma. *Cancer Res.* **2018**, *78*, 1017–1030. [CrossRef] [PubMed]
171. Du, L.; Xu, Z.; Wang, X.; Liu, F. Integrated bioinformatics analysis identifies microRNA-376a-3p as a new microRNA biomarker in patient with coronary artery disease. *Am. J. Transl. Res.* **2020**, *12*, 633–648.
172. Han, X.; Du, C.; Chen, Y.; Zhong, X.; Wang, F.; Wang, J.; Liu, C.; Li, M.; Chen, S.; Li, B. Overexpression of miR-939-3p predicts poor prognosis and promotes progression in lung cancer. *Cancer Biomark.* **2019**, *25*, 335–342. [CrossRef]
173. Xu, M.; Sun, J.; Yu, Y.; Pang, Q.; Lin, X.; Barakat, M.; Lei, R.; Xu, J. TM4SF1 involves in miR-1-3p/miR-214-5p-mediated inhibition of the migration and proliferation in keloid by regulating AKT/ERK signaling. *Life Sci.* **2020**, *254*, 117746. [CrossRef]
174. Van Solingen, C.; Oldebeken, S.R.; Salerno, A.G.; Wanschel, A.C.B.A.; Moore, K.J. High-Throughput Screening Identifies MicroRNAs Regulating Human PCSK9 and Hepatic Low-Density Lipoprotein Receptor Expression. *Front. Cardiovasc. Med.* **2021**, *8*, 701. [CrossRef] [PubMed]
175. Sassi, Y.; Avramopoulos, P.; Ramanujam, D.; Grüter, L.; Werfel, S.; Giosele, S.; Brunner, A.D.; Esfandyari, D.; Papadopoulou, A.S.; De Strooper, B.; et al. Cardiac myocyte miR-29 promotes pathological remodeling of the heart by activating Wnt signaling. *Nat. Commun.* **2017**, *8*, 1614. [CrossRef] [PubMed]
176. Miao, L.J.; Huang, S.F.; Sun, Z.T.; Gao, Z.Y.; Zhang, R.X.; Liu, Y.; Wang, J. MiR-449c targets c-Myc and inhibits NSCLC cell progression. *FEBS Lett.* **2013**, *587*, 1359–1365. [CrossRef] [PubMed]
177. Deng, Z.H.; Yu, G.S.; Deng, K.L.; Feng, Z.H.; Huang, Q.; Pan, B.; Deng, J.Z. Hsa_circ_0088233 Alleviates Proliferation, Migration, and Invasion of Prostate Cancer by Targeting hsa-miR-185-3p. *Front. Cell Dev. Biol.* **2020**, *8*, 528155. [CrossRef]
178. Ye, W.; Ma, J.; Wang, F.; Wu, T.; He, M.; Li, J.; Pei, R.; Zhang, L.; Wang, Y.; Zhou, J. LncRNA MALAT 1 Regulates miR-144-3p to Facilitate Epithelial-Mesenchymal Transition of Lens Epithelial Cells via the ROS/NRF2/Notch1/Snail Pathway. *Oxid. Med. Cell. Longev.* **2020**, *2020*, 8184314. [CrossRef]
179. Watanabe, K.; Yamaji, R.; Ohtsuki, T. MicroRNA-664a-5p promotes neuronal differentiation of SH-SY5Y cells. *Genes Cells* **2018**, *23*, 225–233. [CrossRef]
180. Huang, D.; Liu, Y.; Gao, L.; Wei, X.; Xu, Y.; Cai, R.; Su, Q. MiR-32-3p Regulates Myocardial Injury Induced by Microembolism and Microvascular Obstruction by Targeting RNF13 to Regulate the Stability of Atherosclerotic Plaques. *J. Cardiovasc. Transl. Res.* **2021**, 1–24. [CrossRef]
181. Wang, G.; Liu, L.; Zhang, J.; Huang, C.; Chen, Y.; Bai, W.; Wang, Y.; Zhao, K.; Li, S. Lncrna hcg11 suppresses cell proliferation and promotes apoptosis via sponging mir-224-3p in non-small-cell lung cancer cells. *Onco. Targets. Ther.* **2020**, *3*, 6553–6563. [CrossRef]
182. Pan, X.; He, Y.; Chen, Z.; Yan, G.; Ma, G. Circulating miR-130 is a potential bio signature for early prognosis of acute myocardial infarction. *J. Thorac. Dis.* **2020**, *12*, 7320–7325. [CrossRef]
183. Krist, B.; Florczyk, U.; Pietraszek-Gremplewicz, K.; Józkowicz, A.; Dulak, J. The role of miR-378a in metabolism, angiogenesis, and muscle biology. *Int. J. Endocrinol.* **2015**, *2015*, 281756. [CrossRef]
184. Kurowska, W.; Kuca-Warnawin, E.; Radzikowska, A.; Jakubaszek, M.; Maślińska, M.; Kwiatkowska, B.; Maśliński, W. Monocyte-related biomarkers of rheumatoid arthritis development in undifferentiated arthritis patients—A pilot study. *Reumatologia* **2018**, *56*, 10–16. [CrossRef] [PubMed]
185. Ma, H.; Huang, C.; Huang, Q.; Li, G.; Li, J.; Huang, B.; Zhong, Q.; Cao, C. Circular RNA circ_0014717 Suppresses Hepatocellular Carcinoma Tumorigenesis Through Regulating miR-668-3p/BTG2 Axis. *Front. Oncol.* **2021**, *10*, 3013. [CrossRef] [PubMed]
186. Jiang, M.; Yin, Y.; Xie, L.; He, H. Plasma miR-18 screens acute myocardial infarction from healthy controls by targeting hypoxia inducible factor 1α. *Clin. Lab.* **2018**, *64*, 1207–1212. [CrossRef]
187. Lupini, L.; Pepe, F.; Ferracin, M.; Braconi, C.; Callegari, E.; Pagotto, S.; Spizzo, R.; Zagatti, B.; Lanuti, P.; Fornari, F.; et al. Over-expression of the miR-483-3p overcomes the miR-145/TP53 pro-apoptotic loop in hepatocellular carcinoma. *Oncotarget* **2016**, *7*, 31361. [CrossRef] [PubMed]
188. Pan, Y.; Qin, J.; Sun, H.; Xu, T.; Wang, S.; He, B. MiR-485-5p as a potential biomarker and tumor suppressor in human colorectal cancer. *Biomark. Med.* **2020**, *14*, 239–248. [CrossRef]

189. Carlomosti, F.; D'Agostino, M.; Beji, S.; Torcinaro, A.; Rizzi, R.; Zaccagnini, G.; Maimone, B.; Di Stefano, V.; De Santa, F.; Cordisco, S.; et al. Oxidative Stress-Induced miR-200c Disrupts the Regulatory Loop among SIRT1, FOXO1, and eNOS. *Antioxid. Redox Signal.* **2017**, *27*, 328–344. [CrossRef]
190. Li, S.N.; Li, P.; Liu, W.H.; Shang, J.J.; Qiu, S.L.; Zhou, M.X.; Liu, H.X. Danhong injection enhances angiogenesis after myocardial infarction by activating MiR-126/ERK/VEGF pathway. *Biomed. Pharmacother.* **2019**, *120*, 109538. [CrossRef]
191. Tsai, M.M.; Huang, H.W.; Wang, C.S.; Lee, K.F.; Tsai, C.Y.; Lu, P.H.; Chi, H.C.; Lin, Y.H.; Kuo, L.M.; Lin, K.H. MicroRNA-26b inhibits tumor metastasis by targeting the KPNA2/c-jun pathway in human gastric cancer. *Oncotarget* **2016**, *7*, 39511–39526. [CrossRef]
192. Skrzypek, K.; Tertil, M.; Golda, S.; Ciesla, M.; Weglarczyk, K.; Collet, G.; Guichard, A.; Kozakowska, M.; Boczkowski, J.; Was, H.; et al. Interplay between heme oxygenase-1 and miR-378 affects non-small cell lung carcinoma growth, vascularization, and metastasis. *Antioxid. Redox Signal.* **2013**, *19*, 644–660. [CrossRef]
193. Wu, M.; Li, X.; Liu, Q.; Xie, Y.; Yuan, J.; Wanggou, S. miR-526b-3p serves as a prognostic factor and regulates the proliferation, invasion, and migration of glioma through targeting WEEI. *Cancer Manag. Res.* **2019**, *11*, 3099–3110. [CrossRef]
194. Wang, Y.N.; Xu, F.; Zhang, P.; Wang, P.; Wei, Y.N.; Wu, C.; Cheng, S.J. MicroRNA-575 regulates development of gastric cancer by targeting PTEN. *Biomed. Pharmacother.* **2019**, *113*, 108716. [CrossRef] [PubMed]
195. Liang, C.; Xu, Y.; Ge, H.; Xing, B.; Li, G.; Li, G.; Wu, J. MiR-564 inhibits hepatocellular carcinoma cell proliferation and invasion by targeting the GRB2-ERK1/2-AKT axis. *Oncotarget* **2017**, *8*, 107543–107557. [CrossRef] [PubMed]
196. Li, S.; Xu, Y.N.; Niu, X.; Li, Z.; Wang, J.F. miR-513a-5p targets Bcl-2 to promote dichlorvos induced apoptosis in HK-2 cells. *Biomed. Pharmacother.* **2018**, *108*, 876–882. [CrossRef] [PubMed]
197. Shu, W.; Zhang, Y.; Zhang, C.; You, Q.; Zhou, H.; Wen, S. Triclosan inhibits the activation of human periodontal ligament fibroblasts induced by lipopolysaccharide from Porphyromonas gingivalis. *J. Biomed. Res.* **2021**, *35*, 206. [CrossRef]
198. Wang, M.; Qiu, R.; Gong, Z.; Zhao, X.; Wang, T.; Zhou, L.; Lu, W.; Shen, B.; Zhu, W.; Xu, W. miR-188-5p emerges as an oncomiRNA to promote gastric cancer cell proliferation and migration via upregulation of SALL4. *J. Cell. Biochem.* **2019**, *120*, 15027–15037. [CrossRef] [PubMed]
199. Zhang, X.; Li, M.; Sun, G.; Bai, Y.; Lv, D.; Liu, C. MiR-563 restrains cell proliferation via targeting LIN28B in human lung cancer. *Thorac. Cancer* **2020**, *11*, 55–61. [CrossRef]
200. Zhang, W.; Xu, J.; Wang, K.; Tang, X.; He, J. MIR-139-3p suppresses the invasion and migration properties of breast cancer cells by targeting RAB1A. *Oncol. Rep.* **2019**, *42*, 1699–1708. [CrossRef] [PubMed]
201. Pan, Y.; Hui, X.; Chong Hoo, R.L.; Ye, D.; Cheung Chan, C.Y.; Feng, T.; Wang, Y.; Ling Lam, K.S.; Xu, A. Adipocyte-secreted exosomal microRNA-34a inhibits M2 macrophage polarization to promote obesity-induced adipose inflammation. *J. Clin. Investig.* **2019**, *129*, 834–849. [CrossRef]
202. Liu, X.; Feng, J.; Tang, L.; Liao, L.; Xu, Q.; Zhu, S. The regulation and function of mir-21-foxo3a-mir-34b/c signaling in breast cancer. *Int. J. Mol. Sci.* **2015**, *16*, 3148–3162. [CrossRef]
203. Luo, X.; Zhang, X.; Peng, J.; Chen, Y.; Zhao, W.; Jiang, X.; Su, L.; Xie, M.; Lin, B. miR-371b-5p promotes cell proliferation, migration and invasion in non-small cell lung cancer via SCAI. *Biosci. Rep.* **2020**, *40*, BSR290200163. [CrossRef]
204. Zhu, G.; Zhang, W.; Liu, Y.; Wang, S. MiR-371b-5p inhibits endothelial cell apoptosis in monocrotaline-induced pulmonary arterial hypertension via PTEN/PI3K/Akt signaling pathways. *Mol. Med. Rep.* **2018**, *8*, 5489–5501. [CrossRef] [PubMed]
205. Li, D.; Chen, L.; Zhao, W.; Hao, J.; An, R. MicroRNA-let-7f-1 is induced by lycopene and inhibits cell proliferation and triggers apoptosis in prostate cancer. *Mol. Med. Rep.* **2016**, *13*, 2708–2714. [CrossRef] [PubMed]
206. Qiu, J.; Hao, Y.; Huang, S.; Ma, Y.; Li, X.; Li, D.; Mao, Y. MIR-557 works as a tumor suppressor in human lung cancers by negatively regulating LEF1 expression. *Tumor Biol.* **2017**, *39*, 1010428317709467. [CrossRef] [PubMed]
207. Cui, J.; Qi, S.; Liao, R.; Su, D.; Wang, Y.; Xue, S. MiR-574–5p promotes the differentiation of human cardiac fibroblasts via regulating ARID3A. *Biochem. Biophys. Res. Commun.* **2020**, *521*, 427–433. [CrossRef]
208. Wang, X.; Shi, J.; Niu, Z.; Wang, J.; Zhang, W. MiR-216a-3p regulates the proliferation, apoptosis, migration, and invasion of lung cancer cells via targeting COPB2. *Biosci. Biotechnol. Biochem.* **2020**, *84*, 2014–2027. [CrossRef]
209. Tong, F.; Ying, Y.; Pan, H.; Zhao, W.; Li, H.; Zhan, X. Microrna-466 (Mir-466) functions as a tumor suppressor and prognostic factor in colorectal cancer (CRC). *Bosn. J. Basic Med. Sci.* **2018**, *18*, 252–259. [CrossRef]
210. He, N.; Liu, L.; Ding, J.; Sun, Y.; Xing, H.; Wang, S. MiR-222-3p ameliorates glucocorticoid-induced inhibition of airway epithelial cell repair through down-regulating GILZ expression. *J. Recept. Signal Transduct.* **2020**, *40*, 301–312. [CrossRef]
211. Yang, L.; Liu, Z.M.; Rao, Y.W.; Cui, S.Q.; Wang, H.; Jia, X.J. Downregulation of microRNA-586 Inhibits Proliferation, Invasion and Metastasis and Promotes Apoptosis in Human Osteosarcoma U2-OS Cell Line. *Cytogenet. Genome Res.* **2015**, *146*, 268–278. [CrossRef]
212. Ramanathan, S.; Shenoda, B.B.; Lin, Z.; Alexander, G.M.; Huppert, A.; Sacan, A.; Ajit, S.K. Inflammation potentiates miR-939 expression and packaging into small extracellular vesicles. *J. Extracell. Vesicles* **2019**, *8*, 1650595. [CrossRef]
213. Lin, L.; Wang, Y. MiR-548b-3p regulates proliferation, apoptosis, and mitochondrial function by targeting CIP2A in hepatocellular carcinoma. *Biomed Res. Int.* **2018**, *2018*, 7385426. [CrossRef]

214. Herrera-Van Oostdam, A.S.; Toro-Ortíz, J.C.; López, J.A.; Noyola, D.E.; García-López, D.A.; Durán-Figueroa, N.V.; Martínez-Martínez, E.; Portales-Pérez, D.P.; Salgado-Bustamante, M.; López-Hernández, Y. Placental exosomes isolated from urine of patients with gestational diabetes exhibit a differential profile expression of microRNAs across gestation. *Int. J. Mol. Med.* **2020**, *46*, 546–560. [CrossRef] [PubMed]
215. Mei, L.; Yan, H.; Wang, S.; Guo, C.; Zheng, X.; Yan, B.; Zhao, J.; Yang, A. Upregulation of miR-630 Induced by Oxidative Damage Resists Cell Migration Through Targeting ALCAM in Human Lens Epithelium Cells. *Curr. Eye Res.* **2020**, *45*, 153–161. [CrossRef] [PubMed]
216. Yanaka, Y.; Muramatsu, T.; Uetake, H.; Kozaki, K.I.; Inazawa, J. miR-544a induces epithelial-mesenchymal transition through the activation of WNT signaling pathway in gastric cancer. *Carcinogenesis* **2015**, *36*, 1363–1371. [CrossRef] [PubMed]
217. Lin, Y.X.; Wu, X.B.; Zheng, C.W.; Zhang, Q.L.; Zhang, G.Q.; Chen, K.; Zhan, Q.; An, F.M. Mechanistic Investigation on the Regulation of FABP1 by the IL-6/miR-603 Signaling in the Pathogenesis of Hepatocellular Carcinoma. *Biomed Res. Int.* **2021**, *2021*, 8579658. [CrossRef]
218. Cai, W.; Xu, Y.; Yin, J.; Zuo, W.; Su, Z. miR-552-5p facilitates osteosarcoma cell proliferation and metastasis by targeting WIF1. *Exp. Ther. Med.* **2019**, *17*, 3781–3788. [CrossRef]
219. Chen, Y.; Lei, Y.; Lin, J.; Huang, Y.; Zhang, J.; Chen, K.; Sun, S.; Lin, X. The Linc01260 functions as a tumor suppressor via the miR-562/CYLD/NF-κB pathway in non-small cell lung cancer. *Onco. Targets. Ther.* **2020**, *13*, 10707–10719. [CrossRef] [PubMed]
220. Christofides, A.; Papagregoriou, G.; Dweep, H.; Makrides, N.; Gretz, N.; Felekkis, K.; Deltas, C. Evidence for miR-548c-5p regulation of FOXC2 transcription through a distal genomic target site in human podocytes. *Cell. Mol. Life Sci.* **2020**, *77*, 2441–2459. [CrossRef]
221. Kijpaisalratana, N.; Nimsamer, P.; Khamwut, A.; Payungporn, S.; Pisitkun, T.; Chutinet, A.; Utoomprurkporn, N.; Kerr, S.J.; Vongvasinkul, P.; Suwanwela, N.C. Serum miRNA125a-5p, miR-125b-5p, and miR-433-5p as biomarkers to differentiate between posterior circulation stroke and peripheral vertigo. *BMC Neurol.* **2020**, *20*, 372. [CrossRef]
222. Mao, Q.; Liang, X.L.; Zhang, C.L.; Pang, Y.H.; Lu, Y.X. LncRNA KLF3-AS1 in human mesenchymal stem cell-derived exosomes ameliorates pyroptosis of cardiomyocytes and myocardial infarction through miR-138-5p/Sirt1 axis. *Stem Cell Res. Ther.* **2019**, *10*, 393. [CrossRef]
223. Liu, F.; Yu, X.; Huang, H.; Chen, X.; Wang, J.; Zhang, X.; Lin, Q. Upregulation of microRNA-450 inhibits the progression of lung cancer in vitro and in vivo by targeting interferon regulatory factor 2. *Int. J. Mol. Med.* **2016**, *38*, 283–290. [CrossRef]
224. Luo, Y.; Liu, W.; Tang, P.; Jiang, D.; Gu, C.; Huang, Y.; Gong, F.; Rong, Y.; Qian, D.; Chen, J.; et al. MiR-624-5p promoted tumorigenesis and metastasis by suppressing hippo signaling through targeting PTPRB in osteosarcoma cells. *J. Exp. Clin. Cancer Res.* **2019**, *38*, 488. [CrossRef] [PubMed]
225. Liang, Y.; Song, X.; Li, Y.; Ma, T.; Su, P.; Guo, R.; Chen, B.; Zhang, H.; Sang, Y.; Liu, Y.; et al. Targeting the circBMPR2/miR-553/USP4 Axis as a Potent Therapeutic Approach for Breast Cancer. *Mol. Ther. Nucleic Acids* **2019**, *17*, 347–361. [CrossRef] [PubMed]
226. Rongna, A.; Yu, P.; Hao, S.; Li, Y. MiR-876-5p suppresses cell proliferation by targeting Angiopoietin-1 in the psoriasis. *Biomed. Pharmacother.* **2018**, *103*, 1163–1169. [CrossRef]
227. Pei, X.; Li, Y.; Zhu, L.; Zhou, Z. Astrocyte-derived exosomes transfer miR-190b to inhibit oxygen and glucose deprivation-induced autophagy and neuronal apoptosis. *Cell Cycle* **2020**, *19*, 906–917. [CrossRef] [PubMed]
228. Xie, Q.; Li, F.; Shen, K.; Luo, C.; Song, G. LOXL1-AS1/miR-515-5p/STAT3 Positive Feedback Loop Facilitates Cell Proliferation and Migration in Atherosclerosis. *J. Cardiovasc. Pharmacol.* **2020**, *76*, 151–158. [CrossRef] [PubMed]
229. He, X.; Ji, J.; Wang, T.; Wang, M.B.; Chen, X.L. Upregulation of Circulating miR-195-3p in Heart Failure. *Cardiology* **2017**, *138*, 107–114. [CrossRef] [PubMed]
230. Li, C.; Han, H.; Li, X.; Wu, J.; Li, X.; Niu, H.; Li, W. Analysis of lncRNA, miRNA, and mRNA Expression Profiling in Type i IFN and Type II IFN Overexpressed in Porcine Alveolar Macrophages. *Int. J. Genomics* **2021**, *2021*, 6666160. [CrossRef] [PubMed]
231. Zhang, X.; Gu, H.; Wang, L.; Huang, F.; Cai, J. MiR-885-3p is down-regulated in peripheral blood mononuclear cells from T1D patients and regulates the inflammatory response via targeting TLR4/NF-κB signaling. *J. Gene Med.* **2020**, *22*, 3145. [CrossRef]
232. Liao, C.H.; Liu, Y.; Wu, Y.F.; Zhu, S.W.; Cai, R.Y.; Zhou, L.; Yin, X.M. microRNA-329 suppresses epithelial-to-mesenchymal transition and lymph node metastasis in bile duct cancer by inhibiting laminin subunit beta 3. *J. Cell. Physiol.* **2019**, *234*, 17786–17799. [CrossRef]
233. Wang, W.; Zhao, E.; Yu, Y.; Geng, B.; Zhang, W.; Li, X. MiR-216a exerts tumor-suppressing functions in renal cell carcinoma by targeting TLR4. *Am. J. Cancer Res.* **2018**, *8*, 476–488.
234. Goodwin, A.J.; Li, P.; Halushka, P.V.; Cook, J.A.; Sumal, A.S.; Fan, H. Circulating miRNA 887 is differentially expressed in ARDS and modulates endothelial function. *Am. J. Physiol. Lung Cell. Mol. Physiol.* **2020**, *318*, L1261–L1269. [CrossRef] [PubMed]
235. Guo, W.; Li, W.; Yuan, L.; Mei, X.; Hu, W. MicroRNA-106a-3p induces apatinib resistance and activates Janus-Activated Kinase 2 (JAK2)/Signal Transducer and Activator of Transcription 3 (STAT3) by targeting the SOCS system in gastric cancer. *Med. Sci. Monit.* **2019**, *25*, 10122–10128. [CrossRef] [PubMed]
236. Zhao, X.; Li, D.; Zhao, S.T.; Zhang, Y.; Xu, A.; Hu, Y.Y.; Fang, Z. MiRNA-616 aggravates the progression of bladder cancer by regulating cell proliferation, migration and apoptosis through downregulating SOX7. *Eur. Rev. Med. Pharmacol. Sci.* **2019**, *23*, 9304–9312. [CrossRef] [PubMed]

237. Song, Y.H.; Wang, J.; Nie, G.; Chen, Y.J.; Li, X.; Jiang, X.; Cao, W.H. MicroRNA-509-5p functions as an anti-oncogene in breast cancer via targeting SOD2. *Eur. Rev. Med. Pharmacol. Sci.* **2017**, *21*, 3617–3625. [CrossRef]
238. Siege, S.R.; MacKenzie, J.; Chaplin, G.; Jablonski, N.G.; Griffiths, L. Circulating microRNAs involved in multiple sclerosis. *Mol. Biol. Rep.* **2012**, *39*, 6219–6225. [CrossRef]
239. Magenta, A.; Cencioni, C.; Fasanaro, P.; Zaccagnini, G.; Greco, S.; Sarra-Ferraris, G.; Antonini, A.; Martelli, F.; Capogrossi, M.C. MiR-200c is upregulated by oxidative stress and induces endothelial cell apoptosis and senescence via ZEB1 inhibition. *Cell Death Differ.* **2011**, *18*, 1628–1639. [CrossRef]
240. Chen, Y.; Li, Y.; Gao, H. Long noncoding RNA CASC9 promotes the proliferation and metastasis of papillary thyroid cancer via sponging miR-488-3p. *Cancer Med.* **2020**, *9*, 1830–1841. [CrossRef]
241. Shibayama, Y.; Kubo, Y.; Nakagawa, T.; Iseki, K. MicroRNA-101-5p suppresses the expression of the ras-related protein RAP1A. *Biol. Pharm. Bull.* **2019**, *42*, 1332–1336. [CrossRef]
242. Chhabra, R. Let-7i-5p, miR-181a-2-3p and EGF/PI3K/SOX2 axis coordinate to maintain cancer stem cell population in cervical cancer. *Sci. Rep.* **2018**, *18*, 7840. [CrossRef]
243. Li, Y.; Wu, Y.; Sun, Z.; Wang, R.; Ma, D. MicroRNA-376a inhibits cell proliferation and invasion in glioblastoma multiforme by directly targeting specificity protein 1. *Mol. Med. Rep.* **2018**, *17*, 1583–1590. [CrossRef]
244. Tang, C.; Wang, X.; Ji, C.; Wang, X.; Yu, Y.; Deng, X.; Zhou, X.; Fang, L. The Role of miR-640: A Potential Suppressor in Breast Cancer via Wnt7b/β-catenin Signaling Pathway. *Front. Oncol.* **2021**, *11*, 1142. [CrossRef] [PubMed]
245. Liang, D.; Wu, X.; Bai, J.; Zhang, L.; Yin, C.; Zhong, W. MiR-300 inhibits invasion and metastasis of osteosarcoma cell MG63 by negatively regulating PTTG1. *Nan Fang Yi Ke Da Xue Xue Bao* **2021**, *41*, 285–291. [CrossRef] [PubMed]
246. Pan, Y.; Robertson, G.; Pedersen, L.; Lim, E.; Hernandez-Herrera, A.; Rowat, A.C.; Patil, S.L.; Chan, C.K.; Wen, Y.; Zhang, X.; et al. miR-509-3p is clinically significant and strongly attenuates cellular migration and multi-cellular spheroids in ovarian cancer. *Oncotarget* **2016**, *7*, 25930. [CrossRef] [PubMed]
247. Xiao, W.; Yao, E.; Zheng, W.; Tian, F.; Tian, L. miR-337 can be a key negative regulator in melanoma. *Cancer Biol. Ther.* **2017**, *18*, 392–399. [CrossRef]
248. Gao, X.; Xu, D.; Li, S.; Wei, Z.; Li, S.; Cai, W.; Mao, N.; Jin, F.; Li, Y.; Yi, X.; et al. Pulmonary Silicosis Alters MicroRNA Expression in Rat Lung and miR-411-3p Exerts Anti-fibrotic Effects by Inhibiting MRTF-A/SRF Signaling. *Mol. Ther. Nucleic Acids* **2020**, *20*, 851–865. [CrossRef]
249. Lemecha, M.; Morino, K.; Imamura, T.; Iwasaki, H.; Ohashi, N.; Ida, S.; Sato, D.; Sekine, O.; Ugi, S.; Maegawa, H. MiR-494-3p regulates mitochondrial biogenesis and thermogenesis through PGC1-α signalling in beige adipocytes. *Sci. Rep.* **2018**, *8*, 15096. [CrossRef]
250. Yu, D.; Liu, X.; Han, G.; Liu, Y.; Zhao, X.; Wang, D.; Bian, X.; Gu, T.; Wen, L. The let-7 family of microRNAs suppresses immune evasion in head and neck squamous cell carcinoma by promoting PD-L1 degradation. *Cell Commun. Signal.* **2019**, *17*, 173. [CrossRef]
251. Lin, W.; Tang, Y.; Zhao, Y.; Zhao, J.; Zhang, L.; Wei, W.; Chen, J. MiR-144-3p Targets FoxO1 to Reduce Its Regulation of Adiponectin and Promote Adipogenesis. *Front. Genet.* **2020**, *11*, 603144. [CrossRef]
252. Sheedy, P.; Medarova, Z. The fundamental role of miR-10b in metastatic cancer. *Am. J. Cancer Res.* **2018**, *8*, 1674–1688.
253. Gao, C.; Wei, J.; Tang, T.; Huang, Z. Role of microRNA-33a in malignant cells (review). *Oncol. Lett.* **2020**, *20*, 2537–2556. [CrossRef]
254. Lin, Y.; Dan, H.; Lu, J. Overexpression of microRNA-136-3p Alleviates Myocardial Injury in Coronary Artery Disease via the Rho A/ROCK Signaling Pathway. *Kidney Blood Press. Res.* **2020**, *45*, 477–496. [CrossRef] [PubMed]
255. Wang, H.; Deng, Q.; Lv, Z.; Ling, Y.; Hou, X.; Chen, Z.; Dinglin, X.; Ma, S.; Li, D.; Wu, Y.; et al. N6-methyladenosine induced miR-143-3p promotes the brain metastasis of lung cancer via regulation of VASH1. *Mol. Cancer* **2019**, *18*, 181. [CrossRef] [PubMed]
256. Qiang, Z.; Jin, B.; Peng, Y.; Zhang, Y.; Wang, J.; Chen, C.; Wang, X.; Liu, F. miR-762 modulates thyroxine-induced cardiomyocyte hypertrophy by inhibiting Declin-1. *Endocrine* **2019**, *66*, 585–595. [CrossRef] [PubMed]
257. Li, S.; Hou, X.; Wu, C.; Han, L.; Li, Q.; Wang, J.; Luo, S. MiR-645 promotes invasiveness, metastasis and tumor growth in colorectal cancer by targeting EFNA5. *Biomed. Pharmacother.* **2020**, *125*, 109889. [CrossRef]
258. Xia, L.H.; Yan, Q.H.; Sun, Q.D.; Gao, Y.P. MiR-411-5p acts as a tumor suppressor in non-small cell lung cancer through targeting PUM1. *Eur. Rev. Med. Pharmacol. Sci.* **2018**, *22*, 5546–5553. [CrossRef]
259. Chakrabarti, M.; Ray, S.K. Anti-tumor activities of luteolin and silibinin in glioblastoma cells: Overexpression of miR-7-1-3p augmented luteolin and silibinin to inhibit autophagy and induce apoptosis in glioblastoma in vivo. *Apoptosis* **2016**, *21*, 312–328. [CrossRef]
260. Liu, F.; Zhang, H.; Xie, F.; Tao, D.; Xiao, X.; Huang, C.; Wang, M.; Gu, C.; Zhang, X.; Jiang, G. Hsa_circ_0001361 promotes bladder cancer invasion and metastasis through miR-491-5p/MMP9 axis. *Oncogene* **2020**, *39*, 1696–1709. [CrossRef]
261. Yu, T.; Wang, L.N.; Li, W.; Zuo, Q.F.; Li, M.M.; Zou, Q.M.; Xiao, B. Downregulation of miR-491-5p promotes gastric cancer metastasis by regulating SNAIL and FGFR4. *Cancer Sci.* **2018**, *109*, 1393–1403. [CrossRef]
262. Li, J.; Lin, T.Y.; Chen, L.; Liu, Y.; Dian, M.J.; Hao, W.C.; Lin, X.L.; Li, X.Y.; Li, Y.L.; Lian, M.; et al. Mir-19 regulates the expression of interferon-induced genes and mhc class i genes in human cancer cells. *Int. J. Med. Sci.* **2020**, *17*, 953. [CrossRef]
263. Zhang, J.; Gao, D.; Zhang, H. Upregulation of miR-614 promotes proliferation and inhibits apoptosis in ovarian cancer by suppressing PPP2R2A expression. *Mol. Med. Rep.* **2018**, *17*, 6285–6292. [CrossRef]

264. Gu, Y.; Cheng, Y.; Song, Y.; Zhang, Z.; Deng, M.; Wang, C.; Zheng, G.; He, Z. MicroRNA-493 suppresses tumor growth, invasion and metastasis of lung cancer by regulating E2F1. *PLoS ONE* **2014**, *9*, 102602. [CrossRef] [PubMed]
265. Cimmino, A.; Calin, G.A.; Fabbri, M.; Iorio, M.V.; Ferracin, M.; Shimizu, M.; Wojcik, S.E.; Aqeilan, R.I.; Zupo, S.; Dono, M.; et al. miR-15 and miR-16 induce apoptosis by targeting BCL2. *Proc. Natl. Acad. Sci. USA* **2005**, *102*, 13944–13949. [CrossRef] [PubMed]
266. Liu, Y.; Li, J.; Li, M.; Li, F.; Shao, Y.; Wu, L. microRNA-510-5p promotes thyroid cancer cell proliferation, migration, and invasion through suppressing SNHG15. *J. Cell. Biochem.* **2019**, *120*, 11738–11744. [CrossRef] [PubMed]
267. Zhao, X.; Liu, S.; Yan, B.; Yang, J.; Chen, E. Mir-581/smad7 axis contributes to colorectal cancer metastasis: A bioinformatic and experimental validation-based study. *Int. J. Mol. Sci.* **2020**, *21*, 6499. [CrossRef]
268. Ren, K.; Yu, Y.; Wang, X.; Liu, H.; Zhao, J. MiR-340-3p-HUS1 axis suppresses proliferation and migration in lung adenocarcinoma cells. *Life Sci.* **2021**, *274*, 119330. [CrossRef]
269. Monteleone, N.J.; Lutz, C.S. miR-708-5p: A microRNA with emerging roles in cancer. *Oncotarget* **2017**, *8*, 71292–71316. [CrossRef]
270. Ramírez-Salazar, E.G.; Almeraya, E.V.; López-Perez, T.V.; Patiño, N.; Salmeron, J.; Velázquez-Cruz, R. MicroRNA-548-3p overexpression inhibits proliferation, migration and invasion in osteoblast-like cells by targeting STAT1 and MAFB. *J. Biochem.* **2020**, *168*, 203–211. [CrossRef]
271. Shi, J.; Gong, L.; Chen, L.; Luo, J.; Song, G.; Xu, J.; Lv, Z.; Tao, H.; Xia, Y.; Ye, Z. miR-618 Suppresses Metastasis in Gastric Cancer by Downregulating the Expression of TGF-β2. *Anat. Rec.* **2019**, *302*, 931–940. [CrossRef]
272. Sun, Y.; Zhao, J.; Yin, X.; Yuan, X.; Guo, J.; Bi, J. miR-297 acts as an oncogene by targeting GPC5 in lung adenocarcinoma. *Cell Prolif.* **2016**, *49*, 636–643. [CrossRef]
273. Yao, Y.; Jia, H.; Wang, G.; Ma, Y.; Sun, W.; Li, P. MiR-297 protects human umbilical vein endothelial cells against LPS-induced inflammatory response and apoptosis. *Cell. Physiol. Biochem.* **2019**, *52*, 696–707. [CrossRef]
274. Liu, Z.; Lu, X.; Wen, L.; You, C.; Jin, X.; Liu, J. Hsa_circ_0014879 regulates the radiosensitivity of esophageal squamous cell carcinoma through miR-519-3p/CDC25A axis. *Anticancer. Drugs* **2021**, *33*, e349–e361. [CrossRef] [PubMed]
275. Zhang, X.L.; An, B.F.; Zhang, G.C. MiR-27 alleviates myocardial cell damage induced by hypoxia/reoxygenation via targeting TGFBR1 and inhibiting NF-κB pathway. *Kaohsiung J. Med. Sci.* **2019**, *35*, 607–614. [CrossRef] [PubMed]
276. Qian, F.H.; Deng, X.; Zhuang, Q.X.; Wei, B.; Zheng, D.D. MiR-625-5p suppresses inflammatory responses by targeting AKT2 in human bronchial epithelial cells. *Mol. Med. Rep.* **2019**, *19*, 1951–1957. [CrossRef] [PubMed]
277. Yoshida, K.; Yokoi, A.; Yamamoto, Y.; Kajiyama, H. ChrXq27.3 miRNA cluster functions in cancer development. *J. Exp. Clin. Cancer Res.* **2021**, *40*, 1–11. [CrossRef] [PubMed]
278. Lv, P.; Luo, Y.F.; Zhou, W.Y.; Liu, B.; Zhou, Z.; Shi, Y.Z.; Huang, R.; Peng, C.; He, Z.L.; Wang, J.; et al. miR-373 inhibits autophagy and further promotes apoptosis of cholangiocarcinoma cells by targeting ULK1. *Kaohsiung J. Med. Sci.* **2020**, *36*, 429–440. [CrossRef] [PubMed]
279. Chen, T.; Qin, S.; Gu, Y.; Pan, H.; Bian, D. Long non-coding RNA NORAD promotes the occurrence and development of non-small cell lung cancer by adsorbing MiR-656-3p. *Mol. Genet. Genomic Med.* **2019**, *7*, e757. [CrossRef] [PubMed]
280. He, W.; Cheng, Y. Inhibition of miR-20 promotes proliferation and autophagy in articular chondrocytes by PI3K/AKT/mTOR signaling pathway. *Biomed. Pharmacother.* **2018**, *97*, 607–615. [CrossRef]
281. Zhang, Y.; Dai, J.; Tang, J.; Zhou, L.; Zhou, M. MicroRNA-649 promotes HSV-1 replication by directly targeting MALT1. *J. Med. Virol.* **2017**, *89*, 1069–1079. [CrossRef]
282. Pepe, F.; Visone, R.; Veronese, A. The glucose-regulated MiR-483-3p influences key signaling pathways in cancer. *Cancers* **2018**, *10*, 181. [CrossRef]
283. Lu, J.; Zhou, L.; Wu, B.; Duan, Y.; Sun, Y.; Gu, L.; Xu, D.; Du, C. MiR-501-3p functions as a tumor suppressor in non-small cell lung cancer by downregulating RAP1A. *Exp. Cell Res.* **2020**, *387*, 111752. [CrossRef]
284. Zhang, D.; Yang, N. MiR-335-5p inhibits cell proliferation, migration and invasion in colorectal cancer through downregulating LDHB. *J. Buon* **2019**, *24*, 1128–1136. [PubMed]
285. Gracia-Cazaña, T.; González, S.; Parrado, C.; Juarranz, Á.; Gilaberte, Y. Influence of the Exposome on Skin Cancer. *Actas Dermosifiliogr.* **2020**, *111*, 460–470. [CrossRef] [PubMed]
286. Pecorelli, A.; Cordone, V.; Messano, N.; Zhang, C.; Falone, S.; Amicarelli, F.; Hayek, J.; Valacchi, G. Altered inflammasome machinery as a key player in the perpetuation of Rett syndrome oxinflammation. *Redox Biol.* **2020**, *28*, 101334. [CrossRef] [PubMed]
287. Valacchi, G.; Sticozzi, C.; Pecorelli, A.; Cervellati, F.; Cervellati, C.; Maioli, E. Cutaneous responses to environmental stressors. *Ann. N. Y. Acad. Sci.* **2012**, *1271*, 75–81. [CrossRef] [PubMed]
288. Valacchi, G.; Virgili, F.; Cervellati, C.; Pecorelli, A. OxInflammation: From subclinical condition to pathological biomarker. *Front. Physiol.* **2018**, *9*, 858. [CrossRef] [PubMed]
289. Vierkötter, A.; Schikowski, T.; Ranft, U.; Sugiri, D.; Matsui, M.; Krämer, U.; Krutmann, J. Airborne particle exposure and extrinsic skin aging. *J. Investig. Dermatol.* **2010**, *130*, 2719–2726. [CrossRef]
290. Magnani, N.D.; Muresan, X.M.; Belmonte, G.; Cervellati, F.; Sticozzi, C.; Pecorelli, A.; Miracco, C.; Marchini, T.; Evelson, P.; Valacchi, G. Skin damage mechanisms related to airborne particulate matter exposure. *Toxicol. Sci.* **2016**, *149*, 227–236. [CrossRef] [PubMed]

291. Furukawa, J.Y.; Martinez, R.M.; Morocho-Jácome, A.L.; Castillo-Gómez, T.S.; Pereda-Contreras, V.J.; Rosado, C.; Velasco, M.V.R.; Baby, A.R. Skin impacts from exposure to ultraviolet, visible, infrared, and artificial lights—A review. *J. Cosmet. Laser Ther.* **2021**, *23*, 1–7. [CrossRef]
292. Pattison, D.I.; Davies, M.J. Actions of ultraviolet light on cellular structures. *EXS* **2006**, *96*, 131–157. [CrossRef]
293. Svobodova, A.; Walterova, D.; Vostalova, J. Ultraviolet light induced alteration to the skin. *Biomed. Pap. Med. Fac. Univ. Palacky. Olomouc. Czech. Repub.* **2006**, *150*, 25–38. [CrossRef]
294. Fritsche, K. Important differences exist in the dose-response relationship between diet and immune cell fatty acids in humans and rodents. *Lipids* **2007**, *42*, 961–979. [CrossRef] [PubMed]
295. Xu, J.; Li, C.X.; Li, Y.S.; Lv, J.Y.; Ma, Y.; Shao, T.T.; Xu, L.D.; Wang, Y.Y.; Du, L.; Zhang, Y.P.; et al. MiRNA-miRNA synergistic network: Construction via co-regulating functional modules and disease miRNA topological features. *Nucleic Acids Res.* **2011**, *39*, 825–836. [CrossRef] [PubMed]
296. Fry, R.C.; Rager, J.E.; Bauer, R.; Sebastian, E.; Peden, D.B.; Jaspers, I.; Alexis, N.E. Air toxics and epigenetic effects: Ozone altered microRNAs in the sputum of human subjects. *Am. J. Physiol. Lung Cell. Mol. Physiol.* **2014**, *306*, L1129–L1137. [CrossRef] [PubMed]
297. Abdel-Shafy, H.I.; El-Khateeb, M.A.; Mansour, M.S.M. Treatment of leather industrial wastewater via combined advanced oxidation and membrane filtration. *Water Sci. Technol.* **2016**, *74*, 586–594. [CrossRef] [PubMed]
298. Izzotti, A.; Calin, G.A.; Arrigo, P.; Steele, V.E.; Croce, C.M.; De Flora, S. Downregulation of microRNA expression in the lungs of rats exposed to cigarette smoke. *FASEB J.* **2009**, *23*, 806–812. [CrossRef] [PubMed]
299. Izzotti, A.; Pulliero, A. The effects of environmental chemical carcinogens on the microRNA machinery. *Int. J. Hyg. Environ. Health* **2014**, *217*, 601–627. [CrossRef] [PubMed]
300. Huang, Y.; Unger, N.; Harper, K.; Heyes, C. Global Climate and Human Health Effects of the Gasoline and Diesel Vehicle Fleets. *GeoHealth* **2020**, *4*, e2019GH000240. [CrossRef]
301. Izzotti, A.; Pulliero, A. Molecular damage and lung tumors in cigarette smoke-exposed mice. *Ann. N. Y. Acad. Sci.* **2015**, *1340*, 75–83. [CrossRef]
302. Meek, M.D. Ah receptor and estrogen receptor-dependent modulation of gene expression by extracts of diesel exhaust particles. *Environ. Res.* **1998**, *79*, 114–121. [CrossRef]
303. Hoskin, R.; Pambianchi, E.; Pecorelli, A.; Grace, M.; Therrien, J.P.; Valacchi, G.; Lila, M.A. Novel spray dried algae-rosemary particles attenuate pollution-induced skin damage. *Molecules* **2021**, *26*, 3781. [CrossRef]
304. Izzotti, A.; Calin, G.A.; Steele, V.E.; Croce, C.M.; De Flora, S. Relationships of microRNA expression in mouse lung with age and exposure to cigarette smoke and light. *FASEB J.* **2009**, *23*, 3243–3250. [CrossRef] [PubMed]

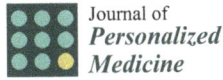

Journal of
Personalized
Medicine

Review

The Interaction among Microbiota, Epigenetic Regulation, and Air Pollutants in Disease Prevention

Alessandra Pulliero [1,*], Deborah Traversi [2], Elena Franchitti [2], Martina Barchitta [3], Alberto Izzotti [4,5] and Antonella Agodi [3]

1. Department of Health Sciences, School of Medicine, University of Genoa, 16132 Genoa, Italy
2. Department of Public Health and Pediatrics, School of Medicine, University of Torino, 10126 Torino, Italy; deborah.traversi@unito.it (D.T.); elena.franchitti@edu.unito.it (E.F.)
3. Department of Medical and Surgical Sciences and Advanced Technologies "GF Ingrassia", University of Catania, 95123 Catania, Italy; mbarchitta@unict.it (M.B.); agodi@unict.it (A.A.)
4. Department of Experimental Medicine, School of Medicine, University of Genoa, 16132 Genoa, Italy; izzotti@unige.it
5. UOC Mutagenesis and Cancer Prevention, IRCCS Ospedale Policlinico San Martino, 16132 Genoa, Italy
* Correspondence: alessandra.pulliero@unige.it; Tel.: +39-010-3538509

Abstract: Environmental pollutants can influence microbiota variety, with important implications for the general wellbeing of organisms. In subjects at high-risk of cancer, gut, and lung microbiota are distinct from those of low-risk subjects, and disease progression is associated with microbiota alterations. As with many inflammatory diseases, it is the combination of specific host and environmental factors in certain individuals that provokes disease outcomes. The microbiota metabolites influence activity of epigenetic enzymes. The knowledge of the mechanisms of action of environmental pollution now includes not only the alteration of the gut microbiota but also the interaction between different human microbiota niches such as the lung–gut axis. The epigenetic regulations can reprogram differentiated cells in response to environmental changes. The microbiota can play a major role in the progression and suppression of several epigenetic diseases. Accordingly, the maintenance of a balanced microbiota by monitoring the environmental stimuli provides a novel preventive approach for disease prevention. Metagenomics technologies can be utilized to establish new mitigation approaches for diseases induced by polluted environments. The purpose of this review is to examine the effects of particulate matter exposure on the progression of disease outcomes as related to the alterations of gut and lung microbial communities and consequent epigenetic modifications.

Keywords: cancer prevention; microbiota; epigenetics; environmental pollutants

Citation: Pulliero, A.; Traversi, D.; Franchitti, E.; Barchitta, M.; Izzotti, A.; Agodi, A. The Interaction among Microbiota, Epigenetic Regulation, and Air Pollutants in Disease Prevention. *J. Pers. Med.* **2022**, *12*, 14. https://doi.org/10.3390/jpm12010014

Academic Editor: Susan M. Bailey

Received: 4 October 2021
Accepted: 22 December 2021
Published: 29 December 2021

Publisher's Note: MDPI stays neutral with regard to jurisdictional claims in published maps and institutional affiliations.

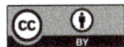

Copyright: © 2021 by the authors. Licensee MDPI, Basel, Switzerland. This article is an open access article distributed under the terms and conditions of the Creative Commons Attribution (CC BY) license (https://creativecommons.org/licenses/by/4.0/).

1. Introduction

The microbiota, present in various regions of the human body (intestine, lung, skin, etc.), is exposed to the action of environmental pollutants and contaminants present in food (preservatives, residues of antibiotics or pesticides, etc.). These environmental factors can influence microbiota variety, viability, and functionality in the long term. Some effects of the environment on the microbiota have important implications for the general wellbeing of organisms. The "microbiome", meaning the genome of the microbiota combined with its environmental interactions, includes more than 3 million genes and is 150 times the size of the human genome [1].

Alterations of the pulmonary microbiota induced by inhalation of pollutants are related to the appearance of chronic obstructive respiratory diseases (COPDs) [2].

The lung microbiota can also be the target (or at least one of the targets) of the injury induced by airborne particles of assorted sizes, as well as by toxins derived from atmospheric pollution (NO, NO_2, SO_2, etc.) [3].

Exposure to elevated levels of airborne pollution increases the abundance in the lung microbiota of potential pathogens such as *Streptococcus pneumoniae* and *Neisseria* sp. [4]. It is now well known that environmental pollution represents an important risk factor for cardiovascular diseases, but the mechanisms of this effect are poorly known. Atmospheric pollution can activate local inflammatory responses as a direct effect of inhaled particles and toxic gas [5]. Local lung inflammation can become systemic due to the release of immunological and biological mediators, thus increasing the cardiovascular risk. Airborne oxidizing gaseous pollutants damage the membrane of lung macrophages in the alveoli determining the release of thromboxane from the intracellular vacuoles into the bloodstream [6]. This situation increases plasma viscosity and thrombo-philicity, facilitating platelet aggregation and clot formation, thus increasing the risk of infarction. In this scenario, similar adverse effects can be mediated by the alteration of lung microbiota, including eubiosis and dysbiosis [7]. The exact differentiation between eubiosis and dysbiosis is not yet established; however, some microbiota characteristics, such as biodiversity and ratio between microorganism groups, have been proposed [8]. Exposure to environmental pollutants, especially in early life, can lead to variations in the microbiota not only in the lung but also in the entire body, establishing a generalized dysbiosis that correlates with the incidence of a series of pathological issues at later ages such as those of an immune (such as atopic), metabolic, epigenomic, or neurological nature [9]. The maintenance of the state of wellbeing of microbiota (intestinal or otherwise) is a more complex issue than the assumption of a healthy diet rich in dietary fiber. Components of a healthy diet (such as five courses of fruit or vegetables per day) represent the preferred metabolic substrate of fermentative saprophyte intestinal bacteria allowing xenobiotic (carcinogen and pollutant) metabolization and detoxification [9,10]. Conversely, components of an unhealthy diet (such as those abundant in nitrosable substrates or amino acid pyrolysates) represent the preferred metabolic substrate of bacteria producing endogenous putrescins, mutagens, and carcinogens [11]. The knowledge of the mechanisms of action of environmental pollution should now include the alteration of the gut microbiota as well as the interaction between different human microbiota niches such as the lung–gut axis [2]. In this regard, particular emphasis should be given to new trace pollutants such as drugs, antibiotics, and disinfectants that are detected in soil, water, and air in continuously increasing amounts.

This work aims to review the existing evidence dealing with microbiota modulation and epigenetic regulation as intermediate actors between air pollution and lung cancer. The interactions between microbiota and epigenetic modulations resulting from air pollution exposure are discussed with focus on the lung–gut microbiota axis and its influence on the immune system especially during early human development.

2. Early Exposure to Environmental Pollutants, and Dysbiosis as Risk Factor for Late Onset Diseases

Environmental exposure, particularly in early life, can result in the development of dysbiosis and consequent diseases [12]. Chemicals, including xenoestrogens, pesticides, and heavy metals, as well as tobacco smoking, alcohol consumption, and medical drug abuse, are major factors that unfavorably influence prenatal development and increase the susceptibility of offspring to later disease development [13]. Exposure to unhealthy lifestyle factors and environmental human-made chemical pollutants often results in the generation of reactive oxygen species (ROS) and cellular oxidative damage [14]. Oxidative stress is involved in pregnancy disorders such as abortion, intrauterine growth retardation, and prenatal mortality [15]. Upper airway microbiota assemblage begins at birth and is thus affected by the environmental exposure occurring during birth (i.e., maternal vaginal (normal birth) or skin microbiota (cesarean)). If an infant is born via cesarean, their nasopharyngeal microbiota represents their mother's skin microbiota, whereas if born via the vaginal route, their microbiota will resemble the maternal urogenital microbiota [16]. Positive and negative changes to the microbiota may be attributed to intramicrobial interaction and the immune response to a pathogen [17]. Influenza A infections modify the lung microbiota by increasing the presence of pathogenic bacteria. Probiotics are a promising therapeutic for dysbiosis and are used in many diseases, such as asthma. Distinct nasopharyngeal microbiota predicts the risk and severity of asthma-related inflammation [18]. During the first year of life, increased nasopharyngeal colonization of *Streptococcus sp.* occurs. Individuals suffering from obstructive sleep apnea have a distinct nasal microbiota, the microbial diversity and composition distinctions in patients correlating with inflammatory biomarkers. A recent study in children presenting SARS-CoV-2 infection demonstrated that both the upper respiratory tract and the gut microbiota were altered. The alteration of the microbiota in these children was dominated by the genus *Pseudomonas* and remained altered up to 25–58 days in different individuals [19]. As children do not experience the same complications associated with COVID-19 as adults do, these microbiota profiles give important insight into the role of the microbiota in disease susceptibility. The pollution and prolonged stress change the balance of the systems, in particular the immune system, which obviously dialogues with all other systems. In fact, the basic condition common to many diseases, including cancer, is mild and silent but chronic systemic inflammation.

Insults provided by pollutants—from motor vehicles, incinerators, particulate matter, heavy metals, pesticides, or electromagnetic fields—are more harmful if the exposure occurs during gestation or in the very first years of life. At this point the epigenetic programming takes place that even 10 or 20 years later or in subsequent generations could lead to serious pathologies [20]. The entire genome is a unitary, dynamic, fluid, and systemic molecular network in a continuous relationship with the environment. The flow of information from the outside meets the information that has been encoded for millions of years in DNA, organizing the main molecular processes that determine the structure and functions of cells and tissues. Thus, the human microbiota is constantly changing because of the information it receives from the outside resulting in a physiological (or pathological) adaptive reactivity.

The Microbiota and Epigenetic Regulation

Since the beginning of their evolution, humans have lived in constant association with bacteria. The number of bacteria in the human body exceeds the number of human cells. The bacteria genome (metagenome) is about 100 times the size of the human genome. The total weight of the bacteria contained in our body is about 1.5 kg. This massive bacteria presence has been neglected by research for many years and its importance underestimated in the therapeutic protocols [21].

The microbiota is present in five macro-areas of the human body, all in continuity with the outer environment, oral nasal cavity, skin, and gastrointestinal and urogenital tracts. Ongoing research programs aim at sequencing the metagenome, examining the relationship between bacterial species and human health by computational analyses. About 70% of the bacteria composing the human microbiota is in the gastrointestinal tract, with a concentration increasing in an exponential way in the oral–fecal sense. Bacteria colonization happens at the moment of birth, and the initial pattern of bacteria depends on the type of birth [22], even if such diversity disappeared early. Indeed, a natural birth allows high number of maternal bacteria to be transmitted to the newborn, while this situation does not occur in the cesarean delivery [23].

From the first 4 weeks of life onwards, especially after weaning, the composition of the bacterial microbiota tends to be pretty stable but may remarkably vary in case of pathological conditions. The intestinal bacteria perform important metabolic functions: (a) digestion of non-digestible carbohydrates, (b) production of short-chain fatty acids representing an energy source for bacteria and intestinal epithelial cells and regulating the sensitivity to insulin, (c) acidification of the intestinal lumen limiting the formation of endogenous mutagens such as putrescins and nitrosable amines, (d) physiological maintenance of the intestinal motility, (e) production of vitamins of group B (pantothenic acid, pyridoxine, and riboflavin) and biotin, (f) participation in the transformation and re-adsorption of bile, and (g) synthesis of amino acids. The microbiota can be seen as a tuned metabolic "organ" of our physiology [24]. It also performs protective functions and increases the barrier effect increasing the production of mucin and zoludine, a component of the tight junctions allowing the intestinal epithelium to perform a protective barrier function.

Nutrition is an acceptable intervention opportunity which plays a key role in many aspects of health. Food imbalances are the main determinants of chronic diseases, including cardiovascular disease, obesity, diabetes, and cancer. Many epidemiological and experimental data show that suboptimal early nutrition can have consequences for health even several decades later, supporting the hypothesis that epigenetic mechanisms form the link between nutritional imbalances and disease risk [25]. Of course, diet is one of the factors that most affects the variability of genetic expression since, in addition to a direct biochemical action of nutrients, it determines the composition of the microbiota, especially the intestinal one. However, it is only one of the complex modulators of health that has been studied under an exposome approach, including external and internal factors. Accordingly, the microbiota represents a dialogue interface between the environment and the host.

The microbiota affects host health by regulating epigenetic mechanisms such as host microRNAs (small non-coding RNAs), chromatin dynamics, and histone modifications [26] as well as DNA methylation [27].

In pregnant women an association was revealed between bacterial predominance and epigenetic profile. In particular, in mothers in which *Firmicutes* bacteria were dominant, methylation profile analysis carried out in blood samples found 568 hypermethylated genes and 254 hypomethylated genes, some of which are associated with the risk of cardiovascular disease, lipid metabolism, obesity, and inflammatory response [28]. In mice, microbial intestinal colonization of the mother may alter epigenetic signatures of the gut establishing an inflammatory environment predisposing to the delivery of premature infants. The same study analyzed intestinal bacteria in mice at 2 weeks of life showing that 16S RNA sequencing conditioned early microbiota colonization leading to differential bacterial colonization at different taxonomic levels [29].

The microbiota amplifies our adaptive capacity as it changes quickly in relation to the environment and protects us from environmental changes. Microbiota colonization by pathogenic bacteria such as *Helicobacter pylori* and *Klebsiella* sp. influences the methylation patterns of the host. Individuals with *Helicobacter pylori* infection display very high methylation levels in several CpG islands in the gastric mucosa, this finding indicating that the infection alters DNA methylation [30]. Different studies have shown that changes in the gut bacterial composition can alter methylation and inhibit histone deacetylases [31].

The microbiota metabolites influence activity of epigenetic enzymes. For example, butyrate, a metabolite produced in case of dysbiosis, inhibits histone deacetylases increasing the expression of the FOXP3 gene through the acetylation of histone H3 in its promoter [27,32]. Environmental exposure during the first years of life can induce persistent alterations in the epigenome thus leading to an increased risk of obesity later in life. This also means that it is feasible to predict the risk of obesity of an individual at a young age by analyzing their intestinal microbiota. This prediction is the prerequisite for targeted prevention strategies modifying unfavorable epigenomic and microbiota profiles, starting from the lifestyle of the pregnant woman and then continuing during adulthood and ageing [33].

3. Air Pollution Can Modify the Intestinal Microbiota

The development of techniques based on the sequencing of the 16S subunit of ribosomal RNA, allowing the detection of "living" and "non-living" bacteria, has facilitated the identification of the metagenome, that is the complex superorganism consisting of the microbiota and the host genome [34]. This ecosystem, in which billions of bacteria coexist and interact with the host organism, is capable of (a) regulating many systemic functions; (b) contributing to the state of health; (c) playing a role in gastrointestinal diseases (irritable colon, chronic inflammatory colitis, diverticulitis, colon cancer); and (d) playing a role in systemic diseases (allergies, obesity, metabolic syndrome, type 2 diabetes, atherosclerosis) [35].

Air pollution seems to be able to modify the composition and the function of the human gut microbiome even if the mechanism of action is not yet clearly understood. A recent study reported that inhalation for 24 h of high levels of ozone gas was associated with *Bacteroides caecimuris increase* in gut microbiota and alteration of multiple gene pathways in the microbiome. Conversely, exposure to high nitrogen oxide was associated with *Firmicutes* increase in gut microbiota [36].

The percent of variation in gut bacterial composition that was explained by exposure to air pollution was up to 11.2% for ozone, thus identifying this pollutant as able to alter the human gut microbiota [37]. A significant association between exposure to air pollutants and gut microbiome alterations was reported in young adults residing in Southern California, identifying inhalation of ozone gas as an important pollutant that may alter the human gut microbiome [37]. They found that 128 bacterial species were associated with inhalation of ozone gas, and four and five bacterial species were associated with inhalation of nitrogen oxides. Various atmospheric pollutants have been associated with modifications of gut microbiota in humans. A positive correlation was shown between the abundance of the *Micrococcus* and *Actinobacteria* and exposure to high levels of polycyclic aromatic hydrocarbons (PAHs) such as dibenzo (a, h) anthracene and indeno (1,2,3-cd) pyrene. Accordingly, PAH exposure may disturb metabolic pathways (such as metabolism of purine, pyrimidine, lipid, and folate) through imbalance of commensal microbiota. Two studies have shown that exposure to nitrogen oxide near roadways correlated to an increase in gut bacteria associated with obesity and altered metabolism [38]. A recent population-based epidemiological study found that the gut microbiota partially mediates the effect of fine particulate matter (PM) on the risk of developing type 2 diabetes [7]. Studies suggested that air pollutants can adversely affect the gastrointestinal tract [39], where ultrafine particles can reach the intestine through inhalation and diffusion from the terminal alveoli into the systemic circulation or through the ingestion of inhaled particles after mucociliary clearance from the airways to the oropharynx [39–41]. Once in the gut, PM components can alter the composition and the function of the gut microbiota selecting the growth of specific bacteria [42–44]. PM 2.5 and inhaled ozone gas have been shown to have extrapulmonary effects that can alter the hypothalamic–pituitary–adrenal axis through vagal nerve activation [45] or effects on the hippocampus [46] thus increasing the levels of catecholamines and steroid hormones. Recent studies revealed a link between PM and gastrointestinal diseases including appendicitis [47] and colorectal cancer [48]. In PM-exposed mice, increases of gut microbiota diversity in the small bowel, colon, and feces and alterations of the gut microbiota composition along the gastrointestinal tract have been reported [49]. Experimental studies have indicated that alterations in the gut microbiota play a role in the pathway of diabetes induction resulting from particulate matter pollution with aerodynamic diameters <2.5 µm (PM 2.5 was positively associated with the risks of impaired fasting glucose (IFG) and type 2 diabetes and negatively associated with alpha diversity indices of the gut microbiota [50] (Figure 1, Table 1).

Table 1. An overview of studies focused on associations between particulate matter, gut, and lung microbiota alteration.

Particulate Matter	Microbiota	References
PM2.5 exposure in mice	Lung/intestinal damage and systemic inflammatory reactions	[51]
Inhaled diesel PM2.5 in mice	Alteration of gut microbiota diversity and community	[7]
PM can be indirectly deposited in oropharynx via mucociliary clearance and upon swallowing of saliva and mucus	Alteration of the GI epithelium and gut microbiome	[49]
Antibiotics, air pollutants, lifestyle, diet, breast feeding	Mucosal inflammation	[52]
Particulate matter, nitrogen oxides, and ozone	Alteration of the gut microbiota with risk of obesity and type 2 diabetes	[53]
Traffic-related air pollution	Gut microbial taxa and fasting glucose levels	[38]
Polycyclic aromatic hydrocarbons (PAHs)	Modulation of endocrine signaling pathways in gut microbiota	[54]
Particulate matter (PM)	PM-induced neutrophilia	[55]
Air pollution	Increased risk of metabolic dysfunction in obese individuals	[56]
Particulate matter including diesel exhaust particles	At relevant doses, changes the composition and function of the gut microbiota	[57]
Particulate matter	Promote Pseudomonas aeruginosa infection	[50]
Particulate matter	multiple gastrointestinal symptoms in patients with COVID-19 and progression with special emphasis on the lung–gut axis	[58]

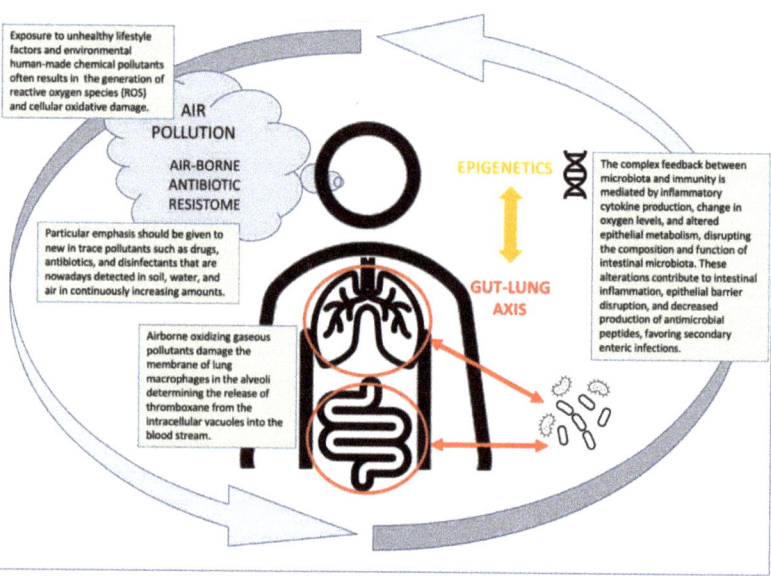

Figure 1. How the environment affects the lung–gut axis of microbiota.

4. The Lung–Gut Axis and the Influence of the Microbiota on the Immune System

Intestinal microbiota modifications can modulate disease outcomes in the gut but also in distant organs as demonstrated in animal models by experimentally transferring of dysbiotic microbiota [53,54,59,60].

The communication between the gut and other organs and tissues is mainly mediated by microbial metabolites and immunity modulation [61]

Gut and lung microbiota are different, both in terms of abundance and in terms of composition, even if there are some structural and functional similarities between lung and gut epithelium [62]. The different composition is due to the existing differences in oxygen availability. One of the most relevant similarities is the ability to interact with the immune system in conjunction with associated lymphoid tissue [63].

The lungs have a large surface area with high environmental exposure. In healthy lungs, microbial DNA was detected. Microorganisms probably reached the lungs from the oral cavity through microaspiration, as the taxonomic profiles of the two sites were quite similar. Comparing the two profiles, the lung microbiota had a decreased abundance of *Prevotella* spp. and an enrichment of Enterobacteriaceae, *Ralstonia* spp., and *Haemophilus* spp. with respect to the oral cavity microbiota [64].

The lung microbiota differential genera in healthy individuals with respect to COPD and lung cancer patients are mainly *Moraxella, Haemophilus, Streptococcus, Pseudomonas, Staphylococci, Veillonella, Enterobacter, Escherichia*, and *Megasphaera* [65]

A lower lung microbiota alpha diversity was observed in subjects with a higher exposition to air pollutants [38]. Moreover, variance in both the respiratory microbiota [66] and gut microbiota [67] was observed also in relation to air pollution exposure.

The gut microbiota metabolites can reach distant organs including both the lungs and particularly protected organs such as the brain [68]. Promising research frontiers include psychobiotics development as a complementary treatment for depression or other mental illness and personalized care protocols considering the genetic and microbiome patient characteristics for example in chemotherapy treatment [69]. Alterations in the microbiota can also modulate host behaviors such as social activity, stress, and anxiety-related responses that are linked to diverse neuropsychiatric disorders [70]. Indeed, some researchers demonstrated that manipulation of the microbiota in either antibiotic-treated or germ-free adult mice results in significant deficits in fear extinction learning [71,72]. After birth, the microbiota strictly influences the host's immune system maturation. A range of hypotheses exist for disease pathogenic pathways [64] such as for T1DM [71–73] and (Bowel Inflammatory Disease) IBD [74]. All such models include an altered stimulation of the host immune system by the microbiota [75].

The complex feedback between microbiota and immunity is mediated by inflammatory cytokine production, change in oxygen levels, and altered epithelial metabolism, disrupting the composition and function of intestinal microbiota. These alterations contribute to intestinal inflammation, epithelial barrier disruption, and decreased production of antimicrobial peptides, favoring secondary enteric infections.

Recent evidence on the respiratory diseases showed that gut dysbiosis due to viral respiratory infection also results in diminished production of microbial associated protective molecular patterns including toll-like receptor and microbial metabolites such as SCFAs, thus reducing antibacterial pulmonary immunity. Such lung–gut interconnections might be particularly relevant during SARS-CoV-2 infection [76], especially when associated with other weakening of the lung defenses due to high level of air pollutants [77]. However, the experimental data are fast increasing on lung–gut interaction, and one of the main questions is how to clear a causation or an association relationship, also considering the role of the air pollution exposure of the host.

CO_2, SO_2, and other toxic gases and airborne particulate matter (PM) constitute a universal danger to exposed organisms. Correlations of long-term exposure to air pollution and mortality have been addressed in different studies worldwide [78]. The existence of an association between long term exposure to fine PM and an increased risk of cardiovascular and lung disease, as well as lung cancer, has been established [79] Air pollution is also associated with gastrointestinal disorders and inflammatory bowel diseases [80]. Where inhaled particles are deposited in the respiratory system depends on their size. Most of the larger particles are sequestered in the upper airways such as trachea and large bronchi [81]. Smaller size particles, particularly PM 2.5 or less, can reach the bronchioles and alveolar spaces where they are phagocytosed by alveolar macrophages [49]. Particles sequestered in macrophages and directly in the mucus layer in lower airways are subsequently transported up to the oropharynx and then swallowed into the gastrointestinal tract [82]. PM can also be ingested directly by consumption of food and water contaminated by PM [36,41,74,75,83]. It has been estimated that 10^{12}–10^{14} particles are ingested per day by an individual on a Western diet [84]. Treatment of gut epithelial cells with PM caused increased production of mitochondrial reactive oxygen species (ROS), release of inflammatory cytokines, and induced apoptosis of colonocytes [37]. Several studies suggested that smoking suppresses the innate immune response to bacteria through the direct inhibition of bacterial sensing patterns such as the recognition of lipopolysaccharides by the TLR4/MD-2 receptor. Smokers with active Crohn's disease were reported to have a clinically relevant dysbiosis of the gut microbiota [85]. In mice, high-fat and fiber-deprived diets change the composition of intestinal microbiota and damage the intestinal barrier through increased intestinal permeability, reduced thickness of the mucous layer, abnormalities of tight junction proteins of the epithelial barrier, and low-grade intestinal inflammation [41]. A variety of environmental factors, such as diet and PM exposure can influence H_2S regulation and function. Epigenetics also have a role in H_2S regulation. In addition, new research into the role of gut microbiota in the development of hypertension has highlighted the need to further explore these microorganisms and how they influence the levels of H_2S throughout the body affecting the microbiota [41].

In bronchoalveolar lavage cells, tobacco smoke exposure increased the activity of inflammatory pathways by inducing continuous active demethylation processes [86].

Exposure of human macrophages to cigarette smoke extract also promoted pro-inflammatory cytokine release by activation of the NF-κB pathway and concomitant post-translational modifications of HDACs [87].

5. Metagenomics Approaches to Study Microbial Communities

Metagenomics is a set of research techniques, comprising many related approaches and methods, to understand the genetic composition and activities of microbial communities so complex that they can only be sampled, never completely characterized. The use of new high-throughput technologies is driving microbiology from an approach predominantly focused on the study of single species in pure laboratory culture into a new era focused on the characterization of whole microbial communities. Metagenomics involves the characterization of the genomes in these microbial communities, as well as their corresponding messenger RNA, protein, and metabolic products. Thus, metagenomics combines the power of genomics, bioinformatics, and systems biology to analyze the genomes of many organisms simultaneously. Particularly, in metagenomics studies, DNA is extracted directly from all the microbes living in a particular environment, and the mixed DNA sample is analyzed, using different high-throughput DNA sequencing approaches and computational methods, in order to create a plethora of metagenomic library/datasets that contain the genomes of all the microbes found in that environment [88]. This can be used to analyze the microbial diversity, population structure, evolutionary relationship, functional activity, and the relationship between community and environment [89] and is one of the best technological innovations to improve bioremediation strategies. Metagenomic datasets from different microbial ecosystems can also be compared to uncover the traits that are important to each ecosystem [90]. Metagenomics can address several potential prospects in different areas ranging from life and biomedical sciences to environmental biotechnologies, agriculture, and microbial forensics. Furthermore, metagenomics has most frequently been utilized to study the microbial communities capable of degrading hydrocarbon and thus establishing new mitigation approaches for polluted environment [91].

In 2007, the National Institutes of Health (NIH) launched the Human Microbiome Project (HMP) in order to study and characterize the microbiome and the factors that influence the distribution and evolution of the microbiota. The project aims to identify new diagnostic biomarkers for health applications and a deeper understanding of the nutritional requirements of humans to drive new recommendations for food production, distribution, and consumption [92].

Over the past decade, numerous technologies have been developed for analyzing microbial community structure and functions. In traditional techniques, cultivation-based methodologies and phenotypic characterization were used to describe the diversity of microorganisms in the studied samples. Although amplicon sequencing, as the PCR-based 16S rRNA analysis, is the most widely used method for characterizing the diversity of microbiota, these methods, also referred to as metataxonomic, have some limitations. For example, novel or highly diverged microbes are difficult to study using this approach since sequencing is limited to the analysis of taxa for which taxonomically informative genetic markers are known. In any case metataxonomic methods, requiring sequences from a single gene, provide a cost-effective means to identify a wide range of organisms. Limitations of this approach have been addressed by the development of metagenomic analysis that uses sequencing, and now high-throughput sequencing and microarray technologies—"open-format" and "closed-format" detection technologies, respectively—combined with high-performance computational tools, to provide information on the species composition of a microbiome [15]. In recent years, next generation sequencing technology has been used to rapidly and efficiently profile whole microbial communities in various samples, revolutionizing genome research because of its capability to produce a large quantity of sequence data in a relatively short period of time [93]. Shotgun metagenomic sequencing, a relatively new and powerful sequencing approach that uses the random sequencing of all genomic content of a microbiome, allows researchers to measure all genes in all organisms present in the community of the study sample, overcoming many of the limitations of amplicon sequencing. Shotgun metagenomics also provides a means to study unculturable microorganisms and to study biological functions encoded in the genomes of the organisms that make up the community [94]. In a recent study, results obtained by the metataxonomic approach and metagenomics were compared to investigate their reliability for bacteria profiling. The results showed that 16S rRNA gene sequencing detects only part of the gut microbiota community revealed by shotgun sequencing, and interestingly, the less abundant genera detected only by shotgun sequencing are biologically meaningful [95]. However, targeted and shotgun sequencing of DNA cannot distinguish between expressed and nonexpresser genes in a given environment. Thus, new meta-transcriptomic sequencing approaches have provided insight into microbial community functions and activities from diverse habitats in understanding how a microbial community responds over time to its changing environmental conditions [96].

6. Environmental Antibiotic Pollution and Microbiota: Implication for Public Health

Antimicrobial resistance (AMR) is one of the top 10 global public health threats facing humanity that requires urgent multisectoral action to achieve the Sustainable Development Goals (SDGs). AMR occurs naturally, and antimicrobial resistant organisms and antimicrobial resistant genes (ARG) are found in humans, animals, food, plants, and in the environment, including water, soil, and air [15]. However, one of the most reported consequences of the widespread overuse and inappropriate usage of antibiotics is the increased frequency of bacteria harboring ARGs in different environments, now referred to as "antibiotic resistance pollution" [97]. Since ARGs may cause consequences for human health, understanding their occurrence would be of great public health interest and value. New technologies such as next generation sequencing and metagenomics approaches allow the real-time monitoring of antimicrobial resistant organisms and ARGs in the environment and have the potential to detect microbial reservoirs and transmission routes [98] in order to prevent the increase and the spread of AMR with consequences for human health. Recently, due to an emerging public health concern, airborne ARGs carried by antimicrobial resistant organisms found in urban air have received more attention. Interestingly, it has been reported that the quantity of ARGs inhaled via airborne fine particulate matter (PM 2.5) was equivalent to that ingested via water intake [99]. A recent article reports results of a global metagenomic map of urban microbiomes and antimicrobial resistance in 60 cities across the world identifying 4246 known species of urban microorganisms, a set of 31 species distinct from human commensal organisms and an irregular distribution of AMR genes across cities that could be the result of different levels of antibiotic usage or reflect the background microbiome in different places in the world [100]. A global survey of ARG abundance in air conducted across 19 world cities demonstrated that urban air had been polluted by several ARGs and that different cities are challenged with health risks due to airborne ARG exposure [101]. The study of Hu et al., using publicly available metagenome sequences characterized the diversity and abundance of ARGs in the PM during a severe smog event in Beijing and revealed that both the abundance and diversity of airborne ARGs were higher in smog days than in non-smog days [102]. In another recent study using a high-throughput sequencing approach, profiles of ARGs were obtained from PM2.5 and PM10 sampled in four seasons for one year from a general hospital, the urban community near the hospital, and the nearest suburban community in China. In total, 643 ARG subtypes belonging to 22 different ARG types were identified. The hospital exhibited higher ARG abundance and was more closely associated with clinically important pathogens than the nearby communities [103]. In conclusion, the availability of environmental microbiome and ARG characterization and of metagenomic maps could provide the opportunity to generate significant evidence on the impact of environmental antibiotic pollution and microbiota on human health and give tools to public health authorities to assess risk, map outbreaks, and predict epidemiological risks and trends [104]. Understanding and fighting antibiotic resistance pollution using a "One Health Approach", in which multiple sectors—public health, animal health, plant health, and the environment—work together to achieve better public health outcomes, may aid in creating more societal engagement and ultimately more efficient policies to evaluate direct risks of transmission posed by certain contaminated environments [105] (Figure 2).

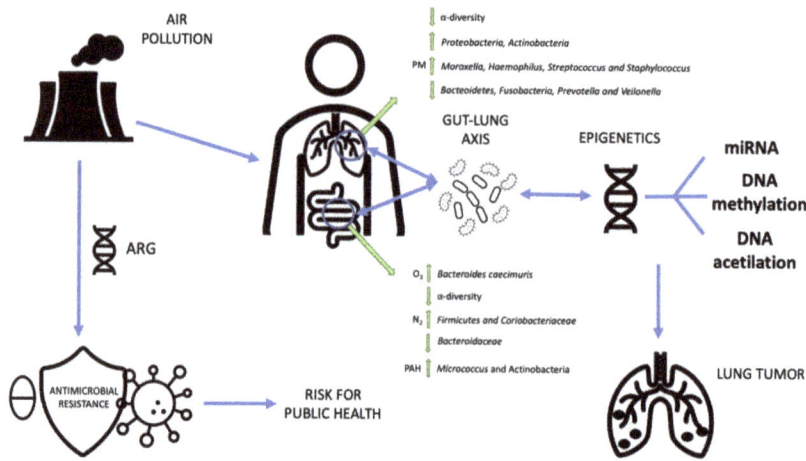

Figure 2. Bidirectional communication between the lung and gut microbiota. The impact of environmental pollution, including the airborne resistome, on human lung health is influenced by the lung–gut axis microbiome and epigenetic regulation. The green arrows represent the microorganisms that change after exposure to air pollution [31–57].

7. Conclusions

The microbiota is considered a "system" that carries out various vital functions in our bodies. Many factors are involved in the normal functioning of this organ system of the body which leads to microbial dysbiosis. This not only alters the composition of microbial communities but also leads to alteration in normal physiological functioning associated with normal microflora. Alteration in the composition and function of the gut microbiota has a direct effect on human health and plays an important role in the occurrence of several diseases.

In this review, we discuss various host and environmental factors that significantly influence the biodiversity of microbiota. There is evidence suggesting that respiratory infections not only alter the lung microbiome but also promote signals of infection from the lungs to the gut with consequent alterations in the gut microbiome [106]. During a respiratory infection, bacteria and immune cells can translocate across lung epithelial cells and reach the gastrointestinal tract via lymphatic or blood circulation to activate local intestinal immunity. The microbiome of the lung and the gut have been implicated in environmentally determined diseases. The symbiosis between the microbiota and its mammalian host encompasses multiple relationships [107]. The capacity of a given microbe, including those composing the microbiota, to trigger or promote disease is highly contextual, and some microbes can shift from mutualist to commensal to parasite according to the state of activation of the host, coinfection, or localization [108]. These results demonstrate the level of communication between the gut and the lungs in response to alterations in the intestinal microbiota and intestinal permeability. The lung–gut axis is a two-way system that involves interactions between the respective microbiota and immune cells. There has been growing evidence of host–microbe and microbe–microbe interactions that shape immune responses in respiratory diseases and the development of subsequent effects in the gut. Environmental insults induce these imbalances but environ-mental exposure has also been identified to protect against allergies, foster in particular microbiome diversity, and contribute significantly to barrier organ functioning. Pollutants induce oxidative stress and inflammation, genomic and epigenetic alterations, mitochondrial dysfunction, altered intercellular communication, and altered microbiome communities. Taken together, they provide a framework for understanding how environmental insults, even at relatively low concentrations, can manifest chronic diseases. Advances in biomedical technologies will elucidate the complex interplay of environmental insults down to the single cell level. There is an important potential for harnessing the understanding of the links between environmental insults and health to propose individualized prevention and treatment strategies. As reviewed herein, experimental studies to date provide evidence that exposure to environmental pollutants triggers alteration of the human microbiome. Still pending is the possibility of preventing, or at least attenuating, these alterations by preventive approaches such as diet modification, dietary integration, oral administration of probiotics, and fecal transplant. Further studies are required to evaluate whether or not these approaches may represent a new strategy in protecting the human organism form environmental pollutants.

The variability of experimental conditions combined with the presence of mixtures of emerging contaminants as well as the epigenetic effects constitute the main challenges to be overcome for prioritization of "One Health" environmental pollutants.

Author Contributions: Conceptualization, Sections 1–3, and Abstract: A.P.; Section 4 D.T. writing—original draft preparation, writing—review and editing; Sections 5 and 6: M.B. and A.A. All authors: editing; coordination assembly and homogenization: A.P. and A.I. Supervision: A.P., D.T. and A.I., Figure draft preparation, editing collaboration and writing the draft: E.F. All authors have read and agreed to the published version of the manuscript.

Funding: This research received no external funding.

Conflicts of Interest: The authors declare no conflict of interest.

References

1. Marchesi, J.R.; Ravel, J. The vocabulary of microbiome research: A proposal. *Microbiome* **2015**, *30*, 31. [CrossRef] [PubMed]
2. Budden, K.F.; Shukla, S.D.; Rehman, S.F.; Bowerman, K.L.; Keely, S.; Hugenholtz, P.; Armstrong-James, D.P.H.; Adcock, I.M.; Chotirmall, S.; Chung, K.F.; et al. Functional effects of the microbiota in chronic respiratory disease. *Lancet Respir Med.* **2019**, *7*, 907–920. [CrossRef]
3. Hu, J.; Bao, Y.; Zhu, Y.; Osman, R.; Shen, M.; Zhang, Z.; Wang, L.; Cao, S.; Li, L.; Wu, Q. The Preliminary Study on the Association Between PAHs and Air Pollutants and Microbiota Diversity. *Arch Environ. Contam. Toxicol* **2020**, *79*, 321–332. [CrossRef] [PubMed]
4. Adar, S.D.; Huffnagle, G.B.; Curtis, J.L. The respiratory microbiome: An underappreciated player in the human response to inhaled pollutants? *Ann Epidemiol.* **2016**, *26*, 355–359. [CrossRef]
5. Maier, K.L.; Alessandrini, F.; Beck-Speier, I.; Josef Hofer, T.P.; Diabaté, S.; Bitterle, E.; Stöger, T.; Jakob, T.; Behrendt, H.; Horsch, M.; et al. Health effects of ambient particulate matter—Biological mechanisms and inflammatory responses to in vitro and in vivo particle exposures. *Inhal. Toxicol.* **2008**, *20*, 319–337. [CrossRef] [PubMed]
6. Conti, P.; Allegretta, M.; Williams, T.W.; Cifone, M.G.; Alesse, E.; Reale, M.; Boidi, E.; Dempsey, R.A. Enhanced thromboxane synthesis and vacuolization in human polymorphonuclear leucocytes induced by human lymphokine containing supernatants. *Clin Rheumatol.* **1985**, *4*, 410–419. [CrossRef] [PubMed]
7. Liu, T.; Chen, X.; Xu, Y.; Wu, W.; Tang, W.; Chen, Z.; Ji, G.; Peng, J.; Jiang, Q.; Xiao, J.; et al. Gut microbiota partially mediates the effects of fine particulate matter on type 2 diabetes: Evidence from a population-based epidemiological study. *Environ. Int.* **2019**, *130*, 104882. [CrossRef] [PubMed]
8. Cani, P.D. Human gut microbiome: Hopes, threats and promises. *Gut* **2018**, *67*, 1716–1725. [CrossRef]
9. Koppel, N.; Maini Rekdal, V.; Balskus, E.P. Chemical transformation of xenobiotics by the human gut microbiota. *Science* **2017**, *356*, eaag2770. [CrossRef]
10. Levin, B.J.; Huang, Y.Y.; Peck, S.C.; Wei, Y.; Martínez-Del Campo, A.; Marks, J.A.; Franzosa, E.A.; Huttenhower, C.; Balskus, E.P. A prominent glycyl radical enzyme in human gut microbiomes metabolizes *trans*-4-hydroxy-l-proline. *Science* **2017**, *355*, eaai8386. [CrossRef]
11. Mah, J.H.; Park, Y.K.; Jin, Y.H.; Lee, J.H.; Hwang, H.J. Bacterial Production and Control of Biogenic Amines in Asian Fermented Soybean Foods. *Foods* **2019**, *8*, 85. [CrossRef] [PubMed]
12. Elgamal, Z.; Singh, P.; Geraghty, P. The Upper Airway Microbiota, Environmental Exposures, Inflammation, and Disease. *Medicina* **2021**, *57*, 823. [CrossRef]
13. Gruzieva, O.; Xu, C.J.; Yousefi, P.; Relton, C.; Merid, S.K.; Breton, C.V.; Gao, L.; Volk, H.E.; Feinberg, J.I.; Ladd-Acosta, C.; et al. Prenatal Particulate Air Pollution and DNA Methylation in Newborns: An Epigenome-Wide Meta-Analysis. *Environ Health Perspect.* **2019**, *127*, 57012. [CrossRef] [PubMed]
14. Zhou, J.; He, Z.; Yang, Y.; Deng, Y.; Tringe, S.G.; Alvarez-Cohen, L. High-throughput metagenomic technologies for complex microbial community analysis: Open and closed formats. *mBio* **2015**, *6*, e02288-14. [CrossRef] [PubMed]
15. Al-Gubory, K.H. Environmental pollutants and lifestyle factors induce oxidative stress and poor prenatal development. *Reprod Biomed Online* **2014**, *29*. [CrossRef]
16. De Steenhuijsen Piters, W.A.; Sanders, E.A.; Bogaert, D. The role of the local microbial ecosystem in respiratory health and disease. *Philos. Trans. R. Soc. Lond. B Biol. Sci.* **2015**, *370*, 20140294. [CrossRef] [PubMed]
17. Hanada, S.; Pirzadeh, M.; Carver, K.Y.; Deng, J.C. Respiratory Viral Infection-Induced Microbiome Alterations and Secondary Bacterial Pneumonia. *Front. Immunol.* **2018**, *9*, 2640. [CrossRef]
18. Teo, S.M.; Mok, D.; Pham, K.; Kusel, M.; Serralha, M.; Troy, N.; Holt, B.J.; Hales, B.J.; Walker, M.L.; Hollams, E.; et al. The infant nasopharyngeal microbiome impacts severity of lower respiratory infection and risk of asthma development. *Cell Host Microbe.* **2015**, *17*, 704–715. [CrossRef]
19. Sharma, N.S.; Vestal, G.; Wille, K.; Patel, K.N.; Cheng, F.; Tipparaju, S.; Tousif, S.; Banday, M.M.; Xu, X.; Wilson, L.; et al. Differences in airway microbiome and metabolome of single lung transplant recipients. *Respir. Res.* **2020**, *21*, 104. [CrossRef]
20. Saenen, N.D.; Martens, D.S.; Neven, K.Y.; Alfano, R.; Bové, H.; Janssen, B.G.; Roels, H.A.; Plusquin, M.; Vrijens, K.; Nawrot, T.S. Air pollution-induced placental alterations: An interplay of oxidative stress, epigenetics, and the aging phenotype? *Clin. Epigenet.* **2019**, *11*, 124. [CrossRef]
21. Zhang, Y.J.; Li, S.; Gan, R.Y.; Zhou, T.; Xu, D.P.; Li, H.B. Impacts of gut bacteria on human health and diseases. *Int. J. Mol. Sci.* **2015**, *12*, 7493–7519. [CrossRef]
22. Hugon, P.; Dufour, J.C.; Colson, P.; Fournier, P.E.; Sallah, K.; Raoult, D. A comprehensive repertoire of prokaryotic species identified in human beings. *Lancet Infect. Dis.* **2015**, *10*, 1211–1219. [CrossRef]
23. Alcon-Giner, C.; Caim, S.; Mitra, S.; Ketskemety, J.; Wegmann, U.; Wain, J.; Belteki, G.; Clarke, P.; Hall, L.J. Optimisation of 16S rRNA gut microbiota profiling of extremely low birth weight infants. *BMC Genom.* **2017**, *18*, 841. [CrossRef] [PubMed]
24. Bäckhed, F.; Ding, H.; Wang, T.; Hooper, L.V.; Koh, G.Y.; Nagy, A.; Semenkovich, C.F.; Gordon, J.I. The gut microbiota as an environmental factor that regulates fat storage. *Proc. Natl. Acad. Sci. USA* **2004**, *44*, 15718–15723. [CrossRef]
25. Wu, G.D.; Chen, J.; Hoffmann, C. Linking long-term dietary patterns with gut microbial enterotypes. *Science* **2011**, *334*, 105–108. [CrossRef]
26. Li, K.; Liu, Y.; Cao, H.; Zhang, Y.; Gu, Z.; Liu, X.; Yu, A.; Kaphle, P.; Dickerson, K.E.; Ni, M.; et al. Interrogation of enhancer function by enhancer-targeting CRISPR epigenetic editing. *Nat. Commun.* **2020**, *11*, 485. [CrossRef] [PubMed]

27. Ansari, I.; Raddatz, G.; Gutekunst, J.; Ridnik, M.; Cohen, D.; Abu-Remaileh, M.; Tuganbaev, T.; Shapiro, H.; Pikarsky, E.; Elinav, E.; et al. The microbiota programs DNA methylation to control intestinal homeostasis and inflammation. *Nat. Microbiol.* **2020**, *5*, 610–619. [CrossRef] [PubMed]
28. Kumar, H.; Salminen, S.; Verhagen, H.; Rowland, I.; Heimbach, J.; Bañares, S.; Young, T.; Nomoto, K.; Lalonde, M. Novel probiotics and prebiotics: Road to the market. *Curr. Opin. Biotechnol.* **2015**, *32*, 99–103. [CrossRef]
29. Cortese, R.; Lu, L.; Yu, Y.; Ruden, D.; Claud, E.C. Epigenome-Microbiome crosstalk: A potential new paradigm influencing neonatal susceptibility to disease. *Epigenetics* **2016**, *11*, 205–215. [CrossRef]
30. Pero, R.; Angrisano, T.; Brancaccio, M.; Falanga, A.; Lombardi, L.; Natale, F.; Laneri, S.; Lombardo, B.; Galdiero, S.; Scudiero, O. Beta-defensins and analogs in Helicobacter pylori infections: mRNA expression levels, DNA methylation, and antibacterial activity. *PLoS ONE* **2019**, *14*, e0222295. [CrossRef] [PubMed]
31. Arpaia, N.; Campbell, C.; Fan, X.; Dikiy, S.; van der Veeken, J.; de Roos, P.; Liu, H.; Cross, J.R.; Pfeffer, K.; Coffer, P.J.; et al. Metabolites produced by commensal bacteria promote peripheral regulatory T-cell generation. *Nature* **2013**, *504*, 451–455. [CrossRef]
32. Kogut, M.H.; Lee, A.; Santin, E. Microbiome and pathogen interaction with the immune system. *Poult. Sci.* **2020**, *99*, 1906–1913. [CrossRef]
33. Goldenberg, R.L.; Hauth, J.C.; Andrews, W.W. Intrauterine infection and preterm delivery. *N. Engl. J. Med.* **2000**, *20*, 1500–1507. [CrossRef]
34. Guarner, F. Role of intestinal flora in health and disease. *Nutr. Hosp.* **2007**, *22*, 14–19.
35. Sekirov, I.; Gill, N.; Jogova, M.; Tam, N.; Robertson, M.; de Llanos, R.; Li, Y.; Finlay, B.B. Salmonella SPI-1-mediated neutrophil recruitment during enteric colitis is associated with reduction and alteration in intestinal microbiota. *Gut Microbes* **2010**, *1*, 30–41. [CrossRef]
36. Mutlu, E.A.; Engen, P.A.; Soberanes, S. Particulate matter air pollution causes oxidant-mediated increase in gut permeability in mice. *Part. Fibre Toxicol.* **2011**, *8*, 19. [CrossRef] [PubMed]
37. Fouladi, F.; Bailey, M.J.; Patterson, W.B.; Sioda, M.; Blakley, I.C.; Fodor, A.A.; Jones, R.B.; Chen, Z.; Kim, J.S.; Lurmann, F.; et al. Air pollution exposure is associated with the gut microbiome as revealed by shotgun metagenomic sequencing. *Environ. Int.* **2020**, *138*, 105604. [CrossRef]
38. Alderete, T.L.; Jones, R.B.; Chen, Z.; Kim, J.S.; Habre, R.; Lurmann, F.; Gilliland, F.D.; Goran, M.I. Exposure to traffic-related air pollution and the composition of the gut microbiota in overweight and obese adolescents. *Environ. Res.* **2018**, *161*, 472–478. [CrossRef] [PubMed]
39. Beamish, L.A.; Osornio-Vargas, A.R.; Wine, E.J. Air pollution: An environmental factor contributing to intestinal disease. *Crohns Colitis* **2011**, *5*, 279–286. [CrossRef] [PubMed]
40. Elder, A.; Oberdörster, G. Translocation and effects of ultrafine particles outside of the lung. *Clin. Occup. Environ. Med.* **2006**, *5*, 785–796.
41. Salim, S.Y.; Kaplan, G.G.; Madsen, K.L. Air pollution effects on the gut microbiota: A link between exposure and inflammatory disease. *Gut Microbes* **2014**, *5*, 215–219. [CrossRef] [PubMed]
42. Jia, W.; Rajani, C.A. The Influence of Gut Microbial Metabolism on the Development and Progression of Non-alcoholic Fatty Liver Disease. *Exp. Med. Biol.* **2018**, *1061*, 95–110.
43. Li, K.J.; Chen, Z.L.; Huang, Y.; Zhang, R.; Luan, X.Q.; Lei, T.T. Dysbiosis of lower respiratory tract microbiome are associated with inflammation and microbial function variety. *Respir Res.* **2019**, *20*, 272. [CrossRef]
44. Yasuyuki, M.; Kunihiro, K.; Kurissery, S.; Kanavillil, N.; Sato, Y.; Kikuchi, Y. Antibacterial properties of nine pure metals: A laboratory study using Staphylococcus aureus and Escherichia coli. *Biofouling* **2010**, *26*, 851–858. [CrossRef]
45. Gackière, F.; Saliba, L.; Baude, A.; Bosler, O.; Strube, C. Ozone inhalation activates stress-responsive regions of the CNS. *J. Neurochem.* **2011**, *117*, 961–972. [CrossRef]
46. Thomson, E.M.J. Air Pollution, Stress, and Allostatic Load: Linking Systemic and Central Nervous System Impacts. *Alzheimers Dis.* **2019**, *69*, 597–614. [CrossRef] [PubMed]
47. Kaplan, G.G.; Hubbard, J.; Korzenik, J.; Sands, B.E.; Panaccione, R.; Ghosh, S. The inflammatory bowel diseases and ambient air pollution: A novel association. *Am. J. Gastroenterol.* **2010**, *105*, 2412–2419. [CrossRef]
48. López-Abente, G.; García-Pérez, J.; Fernández-Navarro, P.; Boldo, E.; Ramis, R. Colorectal cancer mortality and industrial pollution in Spain. *BMC Public Health* **2012**, *12*, 589. [CrossRef] [PubMed]
49. Mutlu, E.A.; Comba, I.Y.; Cho, T.; Engen, P.A.; Yazıcı, C.; Soberanes, S.; Hamanaka, R.B.; Niğdelioğlu, R.; Meliton, A.Y.; Ghio, A.J.; et al. Inhalational exposure to particulate matter air pollution alters the composition of the gut microbiome. *Environ. Pollut.* **2018**, *240*, 817–830. [CrossRef] [PubMed]
50. Ran, Z.; An, Y.; Zhou, J.; Yang, J.; Zhang, Y.; Yang, J.; Wang, L.; Li, X.; Lu, D.; Zhon, J.; et al. Subchronic exposure to concentrated ambient PM2.5 perturbs gut and lung microbiota as well as metabolic profiles in mice. *Environ. Pollut.* **2021**, *272*, 115987. [CrossRef]
51. Liu, Y.; Wang, T.; Si, B.; Du, H.; Liu, Y.; Waqas, A.; Huang, S.; Zhao, G.; Chen, S.; Xu, A. Intratracheally instilled diesel PM$_{2.5}$ significantly altered the structure and composition of indigenous murine gut microbiota. *Ecotoxicol. Environ. Saf.* **2021**, *210*, 111903. [CrossRef]

52. Curciarello, R.; Canziani, K.E.; Docena, G.H.; Muglia, C.I. Contribution of Non-immune Cells to Activation and Modulation of the Intestinal Inflammation. *Front Immunol.* **2019**, *10*, 647. [CrossRef]
53. Bailey, J.M.; Noopur, N.; Naik, N.N.; Laura, E.; Wild, E.L.; Patterson, B.W.; Alderete, L.T. Exposure to air pollutants and the gut microbiota: A potential link between exposure, obesity, and type 2 diabetes. *Gut Microbes* **2020**, *11*, 1188–1202. [CrossRef]
54. Vari, H.K.; Roslund, M.I.; Oikarinen, S.; Nurminen, N.; Puhakka, R.; Parajuli, A.; Grönroos, M.; Siter, N.; Laitinen, O.H.; Hyöty, H.; et al. ADELE research group. Associations between land cover categories, gaseous PAH levels in ambient air and endocrine signaling predicted from gut bacterial metagenome of the elderly. *Chemosphere* **2021**, *265*, 128965. [CrossRef] [PubMed]
55. Yang, C.; Kwon, D.I.; Kim, M.; Im, S.H.; Lee, Y.J. Commensal Microbiome Expands Tγδ17 Cells in the Lung and Promotes Particulate Matter-Induced Acute Neutrophilia. *Front Immunol.* **2021**, *12*, 645741. [CrossRef]
56. Yang, K. Ultrafine particles altered gut microbial population and metabolic profiles in a sex-specific manner in an obese mouse. *Sci. Rep.* **2021**, *25*, 6906. [CrossRef]
57. Van den Brule, S.; Rappe, M.; Ambroise, J.; Bouzin, C.; Dessy, C.; Paquot, A.; Muccioli, G.G.; Lison, D. Diesel exhaust particles alter the profile and function of the gut microbiota upon subchronic oral administration in mice. *Part. Fibre Toxicol.* **2021**, *18*, 7. [CrossRef] [PubMed]
58. Crawford, S.M.; Nordgren, M.T.; McCole, F.D. Every breath you take: Impacts of environmental dust exposure on intestinal barrier function—From the gut-lung axis to COVID-19. *Am. J. Physiol. Gastrointest. Liver Physiol.* **2021**, *320*, G586–G600. [CrossRef]
59. Gilbert, J.A.; Blaser, M.J.; Caporaso, J.G.; Jansson, J.K.; Lynch, S.V.; Knight, R. Current understanding of the human microbiome. *Nat. Med.* **2018**, *24*, 392–400. [CrossRef] [PubMed]
60. Maruvada, P.; Leone, V.; Kaplan, L.M.; Chang, E.B. The Human Microbiome and Obesity: Moving beyond Associations. *Cell Host Microbe* **2017**, *22*, 589–599. [CrossRef] [PubMed]
61. Yang, K.L.; Lejeune, A.; Scher, G.C.J.; Koralov, S.B. Microbial-derived antigens and metabolites in spondyloarthritis. *Semin. Immunopathol.* **2021**, *43*, 163–172. [CrossRef]
62. Woodby, B.; Schiavone, M.L.; Pambianchi, E.; Mastaloudis, A.; Hester, S.N.; Wood, S.M.; Pecorelli, A.; Valacchi, A. Particulate matter decreases intestinal barrier-associated proteins levels in 3D human intestinal model. *Int. J. Environ. Res. Public Health* **2020**, *17*, 3234. [CrossRef]
63. Alemao, C.A.; Budden, K.F.; Gomez, H.M.; Rehman, S.F.; Marshall, J.E.; Shukla, S.D.; Donovan, C.; Forster, S.C.; Yang, I.A.; Keely, S.; et al. Impact of diet and the bacterial microbiome on the mucous barrier and immune disorders. *Allergy* **2021**, *76*, 714–734. [CrossRef]
64. Xue, Y.; Chu, J.; Li, Y.; Kong, X. The influence of air pollution on respiratory microbiome: A link to respiratory disease. *Toxicol. Lett.* **2020**, *334*, 14–20. [CrossRef]
65. Mariani, J.; Favero, C.; Spinazzè, A.; Cavallo, D.M.; Carugno, M.; Motta, V.; Bonzini, M.; Cattaneo, A.; Pesatori, A.C.; Bollati, V. Short-term particulate matter exposure influences nasal microbiota in a population of healthy subjects. *Environ. Res.* **2018**, *162*, 119–126. [CrossRef] [PubMed]
66. Vignal, C.; Guilloteau, E.; Gower-Rousseau, C.; Body-Malapel, M. Review article: Epidemiological and animal evidence for the role of air pollution in intestinal diseases. *Sci. Total Environ.* **2021**, *757*, 143718. [CrossRef] [PubMed]
67. Morais, L.H.; Schreiber, H.L.; Mazmanian, S.K. The gut microbiota–brain axis in behaviour and brain disorders. *Nat. Rev. Microbiol.* **2021**, *19*, 241–255. [CrossRef] [PubMed]
68. Misra, S.; Mohanty, D. Psychobiotics: A new approach for treating mental illness? *Crit. Rev. Food Sci. Nutr.* **2019**, *59*, 1230–1236. [CrossRef] [PubMed]
69. Cammarota, G.; Ianiro, G.; Ahern, A.; Carbone, C.; Temko, A.; Claesson, M.J.; Gasbarrini, A.; Tortora, G. Gut microbiome, big data and machine learning to promote precision medicine for cancer. *Nat. Rev. Gastroenterol. Hepatol.* **2020**, *17*, 635–648. [CrossRef]
70. Chu, C.; Murdock, M.H.; Jing, D.; Won, T.H.; Chung, H.; Kressel, A.M.; Tsaava, T.; Addorisio, M.E.; Putzel, G.G.; Zhou, L.; et al. The microbiota regulate neuronal function and fear extinction learning. *Nature* **2019**, *574*, 543–548. [CrossRef] [PubMed]
71. Siljander, H.; Honkanen, J.; Knip, M. Microbiome and type 1 diabetes. *EBioMedicine* **2019**, *46*, 512–521. [CrossRef]
72. Kamada, N.; Seo, S.U.; Chen, G.Y.; Núñez, G. Role of the gut microbiota in immunity and inflammatory disease. *Nat. Rev. Immunol.* **2013**, *13*, 321–335. [CrossRef]
73. Zununi Vahed, S.; Moghaddas Sani, H.; Rahbar Saadat, Y.; Barzegari, A.; Omidi, Y. Type 1 diabetes: Through the lens of human genome and metagenome interplay. *Biomed. Pharmacother.* **2018**, *104*, 332–342. [CrossRef]
74. Sencio, V.; Machado, M.G.; Trottein, F. The lung-gut axis during viral respiratory infections: The impact of gut dysbiosis on secondary disease outcomes. *Mucosal. Immunol.* **2021**, *14*, 296–304. [CrossRef] [PubMed]
75. Brunekreef, B.; Downward, G.; Forastiere, F.; Gehring, U.; Heederik, D.J.J.; Hoek, G.; Koopmans, M.P.G.; Smith, L.A.M.; Vermeulen, R.C.H. Air Pollution and COVID-19. *Eur. Parliam.* **2021**, *2*, 317–328.
76. Franklin, B.A.; Brook, R.; Arden Pope, C., III. Air pollution and cardiovascular disease. *Curr. Probl. Cardiol.* **2015**, *40*, 207–238. [CrossRef]
77. Hamra, G.B.; Guha, N.; Cohen, A.; Laden, F.; Raaschou-Nielsen, O.; Samet, J.M. Outdoor particulate matter exposure and lung cancer. *Environ. Health Perspect.* **2014**, *122*, 906–911. [CrossRef] [PubMed]
78. Kreyling, W.G.; Semmler, M.; Möller, W. Dosimetry and toxicology of ultrafine particles. *J. Aerosol Med.* **2004**, *17*, 140–152. [CrossRef]

79. Kreyling, W.G.; Dirscherl, P.; Ferron, G.A.; Heilmann, P.; Josten, M.; Miaskowski, U.; DNeuner, M.; Reitmeir, P.; Ruprecht, L.; Schumann, G.; et al. Health effects of sulfur-related environmental air pollution. III. Nonspecific respiratory defense capacities. *Inhal Toxicol.* **1999**, *11*, 391–422.
80. Semmler-Behnke, M.; Takenaka, S.; Fertsch, S.; Wenk, A.; Seitz, J.; Mayer, P.; Oberdörster, G.; Kreyling, W.G. Efficient elimination of inhaled nanoparticles from the alveolar region: Evidence for interstitial uptake and subsequent reentrainment onto airways epithelium. *Environ. Health Perspect.* **2007**, *115*, 728–733. [CrossRef]
81. De Brouwere, K.; Buekers, J.; Cornelis, C.; Schlekat, C.E.; Oller, A.R. Assessment of indirect human exposure to environmental sources of nickel: Oral exposure and risk characterization for systemic effects. *Sci. Total Environ.* **2012**, *419*, 25–36. [CrossRef]
82. Tilly-Kiesi, M.; Schaefer, E.J.; Knudsen, P.; Welty, F.K.; Dolnikowski, G.G.; Taskinen, M.R.; Lichtenstein, A.H. Lipoprotein metabolism in sujects with hepatic lipase deficiency. *Metabolism* **2004**, *53*, 520–525. [CrossRef] [PubMed]
83. Benjamin, J.L.; Hedin, C.R.H.; Koutsoumpas, A.; Ng, S.C.; McCarthy, N.E.; Prescott, N.J.; Pessoa-Lopes, P.; Mathew, C.G.; Sanderson, J.; Hart, A.L.; et al. Smokers with active Crohn's disease have a clinically relevant dysbiosis of the gastrointestinal microbiota. *Inflamm. Bowel Dis.* **2012**, *18*, 1092–1100. [CrossRef] [PubMed]
84. Schroeder, B.O.; Birchenough, G.M.H.; Ståhlman, M.; Arike, L.; Johansson, M.E.V.; Hansson, G.C.; Bäckhed, F. Bifidobacteria or Fiber Protects against Diet-Induced Microbiota-Mediated Colonic Mucus Deterioration. *Cell Host Microbe* **2018**, *23*, 27–40. [CrossRef] [PubMed]
85. Ostrakhovitch, E.A.; Tabibzadeh, S. Homocysteine in Chronic Kidney Disease. *Adv. Clin. Chem.* **2015**, *72*, 77–106. [PubMed]
86. Ringh, M.V.; Hagemann-Jensen, M.; Needhamsen, M.; Kular, L.; Breeze, C.E.; Sjöholm, L.K.; Slavec, L.; Kullberg, J.; Wahlström, J.; Grunewald, J.; et al. Tobacco smoking induces changes in true DNA methylation, hydroxymethylation and gene expression in bronchoalveolar lavage cells. *BioMedicine* **2019**, *46*, 290–304. [CrossRef]
87. Yang, S.R.; Chida, A.S.; Bauter, M.R.; Shafiq, N.; Seweryniak, K.; Maggirwar, S.B.; Kilty, I.; Rahman, I. Cigarette smoke induces proinflammatory cytokine release by activation of NF-kappaB and posttranslational modifications of histone deacetylase in macrophages. *Am. J. Physiol. Lung Cell Mol. Physiol.* **2006**, *291*, L46–L57. [CrossRef]
88. The Committee on Metagenomics. *The New Science of Metagenomics: Revealing the Secrets of Our Microbial Planet*; The National Academies Press: Washington, DC, USA, 2007.
89. Li, M.; Wen, J. Recent progress in the application of omics technologies in the study of bio-mining microorganisms from extreme environments. *Microb. Cell Fact.* **2021**, *20*, 178. [CrossRef]
90. Tringe, S.G.; von Mering, C.; Kobayashi, A.; Salamov, A.A.; Chen, K.; Chang, H.W.; Podar, M.; Short, J.M.; Mathur, E.J.; Detter, J.C.; et al. Comparative metagenomics of microbial communities. *Science* **2005**, *308*, 554–557. [CrossRef]
91. Gaur, V.K.; Gupta, S.; Pandey, A. Evolution in mitigation approaches for petroleum oil-polluted environment: Recent advances and future directions. *Environ. Sci. Pollut. Res. Int.* **2021**. [CrossRef]
92. Turnbaugh, P.J.; Ley, R.E.; Hamady, M.; Fraser-Liggett, C.M.; Knight, R.; Gordon, J.I. The human microbiome project. *Nature* **2007**, *449*, 804–810. [CrossRef]
93. Wani, G.A.; Khan, M.A.; Dar, M.A.; Shah, M.A.; Reshi, Z.A. Next Generation High Throughput Sequencing to Assess Microbial Communities: An Application Based on Water Quality. *Bull. Environ. Contam. Toxicol.* **2021**, *106*, 727–733. [CrossRef] [PubMed]
94. Young, R.B.; Marcelino, V.R.; Chonwerawong, M.; Gulliver, E.L.; Forster, S.C. Key Technologies for Progressing Discovery of Microbiome-Based Medicines. *Front. Microbiol.* **2021**, *12*, 685935. [CrossRef]
95. Durazzi, F.; Sala, C.; Castellani, G.; Manfreda, G.; Remondini, D.; De Cesare, A. Comparison between 16S rRNA and shotgun sequencing data for the taxonomic characterization of the gut microbiota. *Sci Rep.* **2021**, *11*, 3030. [CrossRef]
96. Shakya, M.; Lo, C.C.; Chain, P.S.G. Advances and Challenges in Metatranscriptomic Analysis. *Front. Genet.* **2019**, *10*, 904. [CrossRef] [PubMed]
97. World Health Organization. Antimicrobial Resistance. Available online: https://www.who.int/news-room/fact-sheets/detail/antimicrobial-resistance (accessed on 29 September 2021).
98. Martínez, J.L. Antibiotics and antibiotic resistance genes in natural environments. *Science* **2008**, *321*, 365–367. [CrossRef]
99. Zhu, Y.G.; Gillings, M.; Simonet, P.; Stekel, D.; Banwart, S.; Penuelas, J. Microbial mass movements. *Science* **2017**, *357*, 1099–1100. [CrossRef]
100. Xie, J.; Jin, L.; He, T.; Chen, B.; Luo, X.; Feng, B.; Huang, W.; Li, J.; Fu, P.; Li, X. Bacteria and Antibiotic Resistance Genes (ARGs) in PM2.5 from China: Implications for Human Exposure. *Environ. Sci. Technol.* **2019**, *52*, 963–972. [CrossRef]
101. Danko, D.; Bezdan, D.; Afshin, E.E.; Ahsanuddin, S.; Bhattacharya, C.; Butler, D.J.; Chng, K.R.; Donnellan, D.; Hecht, J.; Jackson, K.; et al. International MetaSUB Consortium. A global metagenomic map of urban microbiomes and antimicrobial resistance. *Cell* **2021**, *184*, 3376–3393.e17. [CrossRef] [PubMed]
102. Li, J.; Cao, J.; Zhu, Y.G.; Chen, Q.L.; Shen, F.; Wu, Y.; Xu, S.; Fan, H.; Da, G.; Huang, R.J.; et al. Global Survey of Antibiotic Resistance Genes in Air. *Environ. Sci. Technol.* **2018**, *52*, 10975–10984. [CrossRef]
103. Hu, J.; Zhao, F.; Zhang, X.X.; Li, K.; Li, C.; Ye, L.; Li, M. Metagenomic profiling of ARGs in airborne particulate matters during a severe smog event. *Sci. Total Environ.* **2018**, *615*, 1332–1340. [CrossRef]
104. He, P.; Wu, Y.; Huang, W.; Wu, X.; Lv, J.; Liu, P.; Bu, L.; Bai, Z.; Chen, S.; Feng, W.; et al. Characteristics of and variation in airborne ARGs among urban hospitals and adjacent urban and suburban communities: A metagenomic approach. *Environ. Int.* **2020**, *139*, 105625. [CrossRef] [PubMed]

105. Kraemer, S.A.; Ramachandran, A.; Perron, G.G. Antibiotic Pollution in the Environment: From Microbial Ecology to Public Policy. *Microorganisms* **2019**, *7*, 180. [CrossRef] [PubMed]
106. Enaud, R.; Prevel, R.; Ciarlo, E.; Beaufils, F.; Wieërs, G.; Guery, B.; Delhaes, L. The gut-lung axis in health and respiratory diseases: A place for inter-organ and inter-kingdom crosstalks. *Front. Cell Infect. Microbiol.* **2020**, *10*, 9. [CrossRef]
107. Zhao, Y.; Liu, Y.; Li, S.; Peng, Z.; Liu, X.; Chen, J.; Zheng, X. Role of lung and gut microbiota on lung cancer pathogenesis. *J. Cancer Res. Clin. Oncol.* **2021**, *14*, 2177–2186. [CrossRef]
108. Belkaid, Y.; Hand, T.W. Role of the microbiota in immunity and inflammation. *Cell* **2014**, *157*, 121–141. [CrossRef] [PubMed]

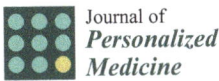

Article

Diagnostic and Prognostic Value of Three microRNAs in Environmental Asbestiform Fibers-Associated Malignant Mesothelioma

Veronica Filetti [1,†], Carla Loreto [1,†], Luca Falzone [2], Claudia Lombardo [3], Emanuele Cannizzaro [4], Sergio Castorina [3], Caterina Ledda [5,*] and Venerando Rapisarda [5]

1. Human Anatomy and Histology, Department of Biomedical and Biotechnology Sciences, University of Catania, 95123 Catania, Italy; verofiletti@gmail.com (V.F.); carla.loreto@unict.it (C.L.)
2. Epidemiology Unit, IRCCS Istituto Nazionale Tumori "Fondazione G. Pascale", 80131 Naples, Italy; l.falzone@istitutotumori.na.it
3. Human Anatomy, Department of Medical and Surgical Sciences and Advanced Technologies, University of Catania, 95123 Catania, Italy; claudia.lombardo@unict.it (C.L.); sergio.castorina@unict.it (S.C.)
4. Occupational Medicine, Department of Sciences for Health Promotion and Mother and Child Care, University of Palermo, 90128 Palermo, Italy; emanuele.cannizzaro@unipa.it
5. Occupational Medicine, Department of Clinical and Experimental Medicine, University of Catania, Via Santa Sofia 87, 95123 Catania, Italy; vrapisarda@unict.it
* Correspondence: cledda@unict.it
† These authors contributed equally to this research.

Abstract: Fluoro-edenite (FE) is an asbestiform fiber identified in Biancavilla (Sicily, Italy). Environmental exposure to FE has been associated with a higher incidence of malignant mesothelioma (MM). The present study aimed to validate the predicted diagnostic significance of hsa-miR-323a-3p, hsa-miR-101-3p, and hsa-miR-20b-5p on a subset of MM patients exposed to FE and matched with healthy controls. For this purpose, MM tissues vs. nonmalignant pleura tissues were analyzed through droplet digital PCR (ddPCR) to evaluate differences in the expression levels of the selected miRNAs and their MM diagnostic potential. In addition, further computational analysis has been performed to establish the correlation of these miRNAs with the available online asbestos exposure data and clinic-pathological parameters to verify the potential role of these miRNAs as prognostic tools. ddPCR results showed that the three analyzed miRNAs were significantly down-regulated in MM cases vs. controls. Receiver operating characteristic (ROC) analysis revealed high specificity and sensitivity rates for both hsa-miR-323a-3p and hsa-miR-20b-5p, which thus acquire a diagnostic value for MM. In silico results showed a potential prognostic role of hsa-miR-101-3p due to a significant association of its higher expression and increased overall survival (OS) of MM patients.

Keywords: fluoro-edenite; asbestos; malignant mesothelioma; microRNA; diagnosis; prognosis

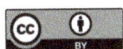

1. Introduction

The types of minerals forming fibers that have been used commercially and that are known by the term "asbestos" include serpentine (chrysotile) and fibrous amphiboles cummingtonite-grunerite (amosite asbestos), actinolite, anthophyllite, riebeckite (crocidolite asbestos), anthracite, and tremolite [1,2]. Such fibers represent an environmental health problem as chronic exposure to these minerals has been associated with respiratory diseases, including cancer [3,4].

Additionally, exposure to several other types of mineral particles found in the natural environment and termed "naturally occurring asbestos" (NOA) such as fibers of the minerals erionite, winchite, magnesio-riebeckite, Libby asbestos, richterite, antigorite, and fluoro-edenite (FE) have also been associated with malignant mesothelioma (MM) [1,2].

FE is a calcium amphibole of transparent and intense yellow color [5]. This silicate has several properties similar to the asbestos group [6,7]; in particular, it presents the same morphological and compositional aspect of the two fibrous phases tremolite and actinolite [2]. However, the peculiar feature of Biancavilla FE is its composition, characterized by high aluminum, fluorine, and sodium contents, compared with other known oncogenic minerals [8].

The International Agency of Research on Cancer (IARC) classified the FE fibers as carcinogenic to humans [9]. FE fibers effects similar to those already reported after exposure to asbestos fibers have been shown by several epidemiological studies [10–17]. Several studies have reported an increased incidence of malignant neoplasms affecting the pleura, the peritoneum, and the lung, after chronic inhalation of FE fibers [18–20]. All data suggest that FE fibers exposure is caused by environmental contamination and it is not due to specific occupational tasks [18]. The environmental exposure estimate is responsible for 10.8% of MM cases in Italy [21]. Material from the quarry of Monte Calvario (Biancavilla, Italy) has been used for about 50 years for local construction [10,12,22], and none of the residents diagnosed for MM had been significantly exposed to asbestos during their occupational activities [23].

Local inflammation in the lung and pleura is among the most recognized toxic effects of FE fibers exposure predisposing the individuals to MM development [24,25]. At present, MM is still considered a lethal cancer characterized by a considerable period of latency ($\geq$30–60 years) [26] and late diagnosis that determines bad prognosis and quality of life and unresponsiveness to presently available treatments [27]. To date, there are no diagnostic tools with high sensitivity and specificity that can be used to perform an early diagnosis of MM in asymptomatic people. Many biomarkers have been proposed for the screening and diagnosis of MM in exposed subjects [28–32]. The unique Food and Drug Administration (FDA)-approved biomarker for MM is mesothelin [33–35], but its poor sensitivity limits the diagnosis of MM [36]. In this context, several studies demonstrated how miRNAs may be used as effective biomarkers of environmental contamination and exposure to toxic substances [37,38]. Furthermore, recent studies demonstrated that microRNAs (miRNAs) play an important role in MM biology and they have the potential to be considered as good non-invasive diagnostic and prognostic biomarkers and therapeutic targets for cancer [39–41]. In particular, Micolucci and colleagues [42] propose an early diagnosis of MM or a tool to monitor the therapy sensitivity through the expression levels analysis of several MM-associated miRNAs designated as "mesomiRs" [42,43].

This study aimed to evaluate the expression levels of a set of miRNAs previously identified and already validated in MM cellular models [44] to confirm their potential use as diagnostic biomarkers for MM. In this study, for the first time, hsa-miR-323a-3p, hsa-miR-101-3p, and hsa-miR-20b-5p have been analyzed in FE-mediated MM tissues vs. nonmalignant pleura tissues. Furthermore, an in silico analysis has been performed to evaluate the prognostic and therapeutic role of these three miRNAs. With this research work, we would contribute to basic biomarkers research, and we hope to transfer these results to clinical practice.

2. Materials and Methods

2.1. Patients and Samples Collection

Tissue specimens of ten cases of malignant mesothelioma and eight cases of healthy pleural mesothelium were retrospectively analyzed. Formalin-fixed and paraffin-embedded (FFPE) tissue specimens were obtained from the biobank of the Section of Anatomic Pathology, Department Gian Filippo Ingrassia, University of Catania. The exclusion criteria adopted in the choice of the cases were the following: (i) it was not possible to obtain additional slides from FFPE blocks for the analysis; (ii) no representative neoplastic tissue was contained in FFPE blocks. No written informed consent was necessary because of the retrospective nature of the study; the study protocols conformed to the ethical regulations of the Helsinki Declaration.

The cohort of patients of Biancavilla with FE-mediated MM was composed of six men and four women (mean age: 68.4 $\pm$ 13.9 years; age range: 50–93 years). Agreeing to the

World Health Organization (WHO) criteria, six cases were histologically classified as epithelioid, three were classified as biphasic subtypes, and one was classified as sarcomatoid [21]. The cohort of control cases was composed of eight men (mean age: 44 ± 25.5 years; age range: 15–76 years). These patients did not live in Biancavilla, and they did not show oncological pathologies but pulmonary emphysema (n = 3) and pleurisy (n = 5). Data including MM cases and controls are summarized in Table 1.

Table 1. Features of the fluoro-edenite (FE)-related malignant mesothelioma (MM) cases and controls.

	Age Range (Years)	Mean Age (Years)	Gender	Pathologies	Pathological Subtype	Survival Time Range (Days)	Mean Survival Time (Days)
Cases (n = 10)	50–93	68.4 ± 13.9	60% men, 40% women	100% malignant mesothelioma	60% epithelioid, 10% sarcomatoid, 30% biphasic	45–1800	579 ± 525
Controls (n = 8)	15–76	44 ± 25.5	100% men	37.5% pulmonary emphysema, 62.5% pleurisy			

Freshly cut sections of FFPE tissue, each with a thickness of 20 µm, were obtained using a rotary microtome. Two sections for each sample were collected and stored at room temperature.

2.2. RNA Isolation and RT

Total RNA containing small non-coding RNA was extracted from FFPE tissue using a miRNeasy FFPE Kit (QIAGEN; Hilden, Germany) according to the manufacturer's recommended protocol (miRNeasy FFPE Handbook 01/2020). The RNA extraction and quantification were performed as previously described [44]. All samples were then stored at −80 °C until use. The purified RNA was reverse transcribed into cDNA as previously described [44].

2.3. Droplet Digital PCR

As previously described, a customized droplet digital PCR (ddPCR) assay was used to amplify hsa-miR-323a-3p, hsa-miR-101-3p, and hsa-miR-20b-5p [45]. The reaction mixture was made by combining ddPCR Supermix for probes (no dUTP) (cat. n. 1,863,010—Bio-Rad Laboratories), TaqMan Advanced miRNA Assays specific for each miRNA (cat. no. 477863, 477804, 477,853—Thermo Fisher Scientific), a miR-Amp cDNA sample and PCR water. The cartridge was loaded with 20 microliters of PCR reaction and 70 µL of Droplet Generation Oil (cat. no. 1,863,005—Bio-Rad Laboratories) in appropriate wells, and then Droplet Generator QX200 was used to generate droplets. Subsequently, the generated droplets were amplified using a C 1000 Touch Thermal Cycler (Bio-Rad Laboratories) at the cycling conditions previously described [44]. A non-template control (NTC) was inserted for each probe.

After the amplification, the droplets were read using a QX200 Droplet Reader (Bio-Rad Laboratories). Finally, the absolute quantification of targets was performed using QuantaSoft software, version 1.7.4 (QuantaSoft, Prague, Czech Republic), as previously described [44,46].

2.4. In Silico Analysis

To clarify the role of hsa-miR-323a-3p, hsa-miR-101-3p, and hsa-miR-20b-5p in MM, different computational tools were used.

By consulting the Catalogue of Somatic Mutation In Cancer (COSMIC) (http://cancer.sanger.ac.uk/cosmic (accessed on 20 September 2021) it was possible to identify the 20 most mutated genes that are known to be involved in MM development and therefore have a dysregulated expression. The selection was performed using the search term "Malignant Mesothelioma" including the terms "Pleura" in tissue selection and "Mesothelioma" in histology selection.

Subsequently, using the bioinformatics prediction tool microRNA Data Integration Portal (mirDIP version 4.1.11.2, Database version 4.1.0.3, November 2020) (http://ophid.utoronto.ca/mirDIP, accessed on 20 September 2021) [47,48], the interaction levels between the miRNA previously identified via computational analysis and the main genes mutated and altered in MM were evaluated.

Furthermore, the clinical implication of the three analyzed miRNAs was assessed through the clinic-pathological data and the miRNA expression profiles analysis contained in The Cancer Genome Atlas Mesothelioma (TCGA-MESO) database and downloaded using the online exploration tool UCSC Xena Browser (https://xenabrowser.net/, accessed on 21 September 2021) [49]. In particular, the TCGA database was used to verify if the three miRNAs here analyzed were dysregulated in MM according to asbestos exposure, tumor stage, and patient survival. A total of 17 MM patient-related datasets were found containing a total of 87 MM samples (35 exposed to asbestos, 49 not exposed to asbestos, 3 excluded due to lack of useful information). The datasets contained the expression levels of 1,964 different miRNAs, but we focused on hsa-miR-323a-3p, hsa-miR-101-3p, and hsa-miR-20b-5p for further investigation.

2.5. Statistical Analysis

The Shapiro-Wilk normality test was applied for the calculation of the distribution of hsa-miR-323a-3p, hsa-miR-101-3p, and hsa-miR-20b-5p expression levels observed with ddPCR and deposited on the TCGA-MESO database. The Mann-Whitney test was utilized for the comparison between miRNAs expression of MM samples and healthy controls. Receiver operating characteristic (ROC) curves were obtained to evaluate the specificity and sensitivity of the analyzed miRNAs. An unpaired Student t-test and one-way ANOVA test were used for assessing the statistical differences existing between the expression levels of hsa-miR-323a-3p, hsa-miR-101-3p, and hsa-miR-20b-5p reported in the TCGA-MESO database according to the asbestos exposure and the MM tumor stages, respectively. Cancer-specific survival analysis was performed using the Kaplan-Meier method, and for comparison of the survival curves, the Mantel-Cox log-rank test was used.

A value of $p < 0.05$ was considered statistically significant. The graphs were plotted using Prism for Windows version 7.00 (Graphpad Software; San Diego, CA, USA), and data were represented as the mean with SD.

3. Results

3.1. Evaluation of miRNA Expression Profiling Using ddPCR

The expression of hsa-miR-323a-3p, hsa-miR-101-3p, and hsa-miR-20b-5p was examined in MM tissues and relative controls of healthy pleural mesothelium.

The Shapiro-Wilk normality test showed that the expression levels of the three miRNAs analyzed in MM cases and healthy controls differed significantly from a normal distribution.

The comparison between tumor and normal tissues showed a different expression of the three miRNAs analyzed in MM and healthy controls. The expression levels of hsa-miR-323a-3p, hsa-miR-101-3p, and hsa-miR-20b-5p in MM cases were significantly lower compared to controls (Figure 1; Supplementary Figure S1). There was a statistically significant trend of down-regulation observed for the three selected miRNAs analyzed in MM cases vs. controls.

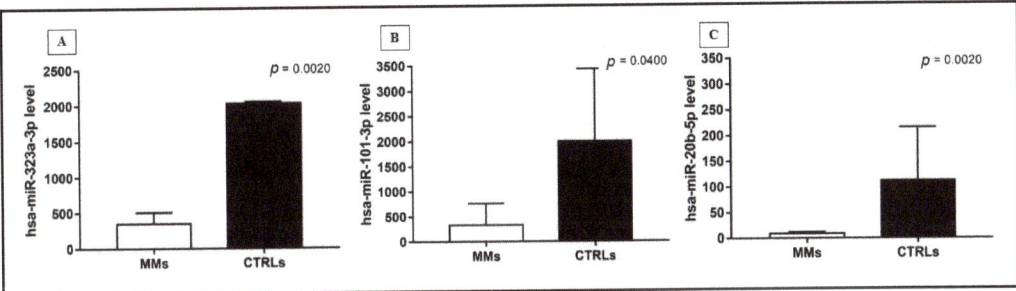

Figure 1. MiRNAs expression, reported as number of copies/uL of reaction, in MM cases and healthy controls, through the Mann-Whitney test, according to: (**A**) hsa-miR-323a-3p, (**B**) hsa-miR-101-3p, (**C**) hsa-miR-20b-5p. Data were represented as the mean with SD.

To evaluate the sensitivity and specificity of these miRNAs and their role as novel, promising diagnostic biomarkers for MM, ROC (receiver operating characteristic) curves were calculated (Figure 2). ROC analysis revealed high specificity and sensitivity rates for both hsa-miR-323a-3p and hsa-miR-20b-5p. In particular, the sensitivity and specificity for hsa-miR-323a-3p and hsa-miR-20b-5p were 100% and 100% (AUC (area under the curve) = 1). For hsa-miR-101-3p the sensitivity was 100% and the specificity was 40% (AUC = 0.8625). However, the AUCs of all analyzed miRNAs were statistically significant ($p < 0.05$).

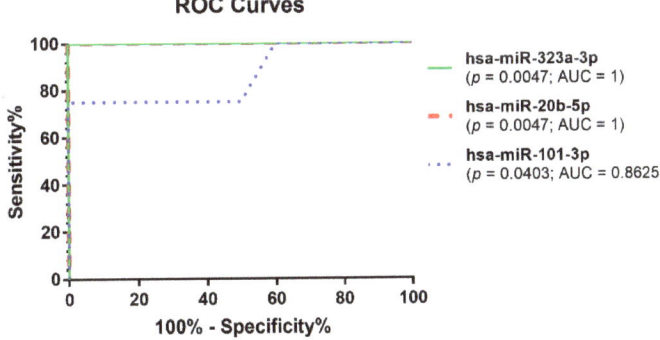

Figure 2. ROC curves demonstrated the diagnostic value of hsa-miR-323a-3p (100% sensitivity and 100% specificity), hsa-miR-20b-5p (100% sensitivity and 100% specificity), and hsa-miR-101-3p (100% sensitivity and 40% specificity).

3.2. In Silico Interaction between miRNAs and Main Genes Involved in Malignant Mesothelioma

Gene target analysis performed using the bioinformatics tool mirDIP showed the level of interaction of the three computationally identified miRNAs with the main altered or mutated gene in MM.

We took into account 20 different genes obtained from COSMIC and the mirDIP analysis revealed that the three evaluated miRNAs were able to interact with all genes involved in MM with high levels of intensity. These genes were: BAP1 (24%), NF2 (18%), TP53 (12%), SETD2 (7%), LATS2 (5%), FBXW7 (2%), DDX3X (3%), EGFR (1%), SF3B1 (2%), PBRM1 (2%), KRAS (1%), PIK3CA (1%), CTNNB1 (1%), CREBBP (2%), NSD1 (2%), ZFHX3 (2%), APC (1%), LATS1 (2%), LRP1B (2%), BRAF (1%). In particular, for each miRNA the intensity of interaction was reported to be from medium to very high specificity. All miRNAs showed very high and high interaction levels with at least 50% of the genes analyzed, suggesting a potential role of these miRNAs in the development of MM. According to this analysis, hsa-miR-20b-5p showed very high and high interaction levels with 85% of the genes mutated in MM. The genes linked with higher levels of intensity by miRNAs were found to be PBRM1 and ZFHX3, which showed in all cases very high levels of interaction. In addition, the KRAS gene showed very high levels of interaction with hsa-miR-323a-3p and hsa-miR-20b-5p and high levels of interaction with hsa-miR-101-3p. In opposition, the genes associated with medium levels of intensity for all miRNAs were found to be BAP1 and BRAF. None of the genes analyzed showed low levels of interaction intensity with the miRNAs evaluated (Figure 3).

Top 20 genes	miRNAs	Intensity of interaction		Medium	High	Very High
BAP1	hsa-miR-323a-3p	Medium	hsa-miR-323a-3p	50%	30%	20%
BAP1	hsa-miR-101-3p	Medium	hsa-miR-101-3p	45%	25%	30%
BAP1	hsa-miR-20b-5p	Medium	hsa-miR-20b-5p	15%	45%	40%
NF2	hsa-miR-323a-3p	Medium				
NF2	hsa-miR-101-3p	Medium				
NF2	hsa-miR-20b-5p	High				
TP53	hsa-miR-323a-3p	Medium				
TP53	hsa-miR-101-3p	Medium				
TP53	hsa-miR-20b-5p	High				
SETD2	hsa-miR-323a-3p	High				
SETD2	hsa-miR-101-3p	High				
SETD2	hsa-miR-20b-5p	Very High				
LATS2	hsa-miR-323a-3p	High				
LATS2	hsa-miR-101-3p	Medium				
LATS2	hsa-miR-20b-5p	High				
FBXW7	hsa-miR-323a-3p	Medium				
FBXW7	hsa-miR-101-3p	Very High				
FBXW7	hsa-miR-20b-5p	Very High				
DDX3X	hsa-miR-323a-3p	Very High				
DDX3X	hsa-miR-101-3p	Very High				
DDX3X	hsa-miR-20b-5p	High				
EGFR	hsa-miR-323a-3p	Medium				
EGFR	hsa-miR-101-3p	High				
EGFR	hsa-miR-20b-5p	Very High				
SF3B1	hsa-miR-323a-3p	High				
SF3B1	hsa-miR-101-3p	High				
SF3B1	hsa-miR-20b-5p	Medium				
PBRM1	hsa-miR-323a-3p	Very High				
PBRM1	hsa-miR-101-3p	Very High				
PBRM1	hsa-miR-20b-5p	Very High				
KRAS	hsa-miR-323a-3p	Very High				
KRAS	hsa-miR-101-3p	High				
KRAS	hsa-miR-20b-5p	Very High				
PIK3CA	hsa-miR-323a-3p	High				
PIK3CA	hsa-miR-101-3p	Medium				
PIK3CA	hsa-miR-20b-5p	High				
CTNNB1	hsa-miR-323a-3p	Medium				
CTNNB1	hsa-miR-101-3p	High				
CTNNB1	hsa-miR-20b-5p	High				
CREBBP	hsa-miR-323a-3p	High				
CREBBP	hsa-miR-101-3p	Medium				
CREBBP	hsa-miR-20b-5p	High				
NSD1	hsa-miR-323a-3p	Medium				
NSD1	hsa-miR-101-3p	Very High				
NSD1	hsa-miR-20b-5p	High				
ZFHX3	hsa-miR-323a-3p	Very High				
ZFHX3	hsa-miR-101-3p	Very High				
ZFHX3	hsa-miR-20b-5p	Very High				
APC	hsa-miR-323a-3p	Medium				
APC	hsa-miR-101-3p	Very High				
APC	hsa-miR-20b-5p	Very High				
LATS1	hsa-miR-323a-3p	Medium				
LATS1	hsa-miR-101-3p	Medium				
LATS1	hsa-miR-20b-5p	High				
LRP1B	hsa-miR-323a-3p	High				
LRP1B	hsa-miR-101-3p	Medium				
LRP1B	hsa-miR-20b-5p	Very High				
BRAF	hsa-miR-323a-3p	Medium				
BRAF	hsa-miR-101-3p	Medium				
BRAF	hsa-miR-20b-5p	Medium				

Figure 3. Interaction between selected miRNAs and main altered genes in MM via mirDIP gene target analysis. For each miRNA the level of interaction with the 20 genes involved in MM is reported. The intensity of interaction is highlighted with a color scale ranging from yellow (medium interaction) to red (very high interaction).

According to this analysis, these three miRNAs can target and modulate both tumor suppressor and oncogene genes playing a potentially key role in tumor cell development.

3.3. In Silico Interaction between miRNAs and Asbestos Exposure, Tumor Stage, and Patient Survival

The Shapiro-Wilk normality test showed that the expression levels of the three miRNAs contained in the TCGA-MESO database have a normal distribution.

The analysis of miRNAs expression levels according to the asbestos exposure data contained in the TCGA-MESO database revealed that the expression levels of hsa-miR-323a-3p, hsa-miR-101-3p, and hsa-miR-20b-5p did not change significantly in MM patients exposed and not exposed to asbestos fibers (Figure 4).

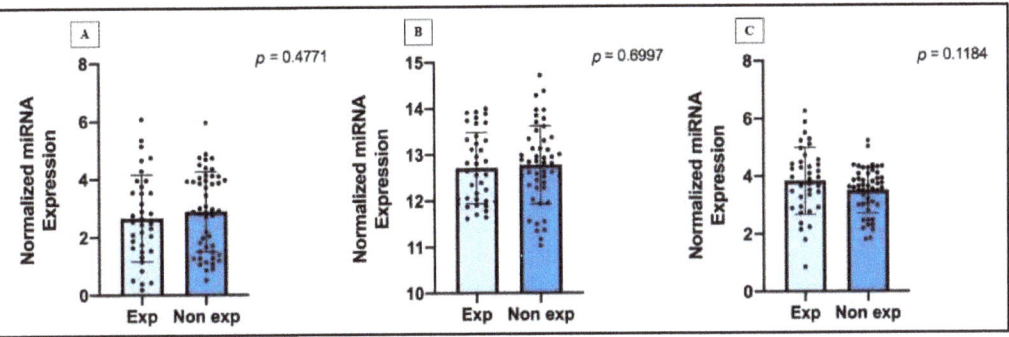

Figure 4. Normalized miRNAs expression in MM cases exposed and non-exposed to asbestos, through unpaired Student t-test, according to: (**A**) hsa-miR-323a-3p, (**B**) hsa-miR-101-3p, (**C**) hsa-miR-20b-5p. Data are represented as the mean with SD.

The analysis of miRNAs expression levels according to the clinic-pathological data contained in the TCGA-MESO database showed that the expression levels of hsa-miR-323a-3p, hsa-miR-101-3p, and hsa-miR-20b-5p did not change significantly in MM patients with different tumor stages (Figure 5).

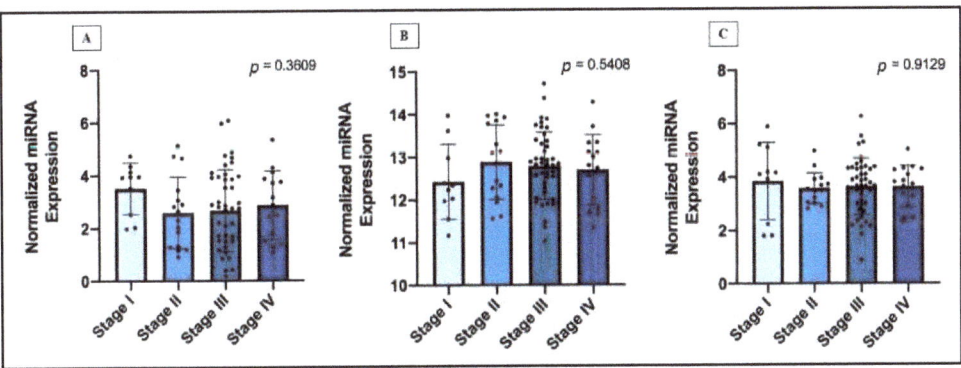

Figure 5. Normalized miRNAs expression in different MM stages, through one-way ANOVA test, according to: (**A**) hsa-miR-323a-3p, (**B**) hsa-miR-101-3p, (**C**) hsa-miR-20b-5p. Data represented as the mean with SD.

Finally, considering the median overall survival (OS), the disease-specific survival (DSS), and the progression-free interval (PFI) between high and low miRNAs expression, significance for hsa-miR-101-3p ($p < 0.0001$) was shown. In particular, there was an association of high hsa-miR-101-3p expression and increased OS time (Figure 6A),

DSS time (Figure 6B), and PFI time (Figure 6C). On the contrary, hsa-miR-323a-3p and hsa-miR-20b-5p did not show significant results in MM patients' survival.

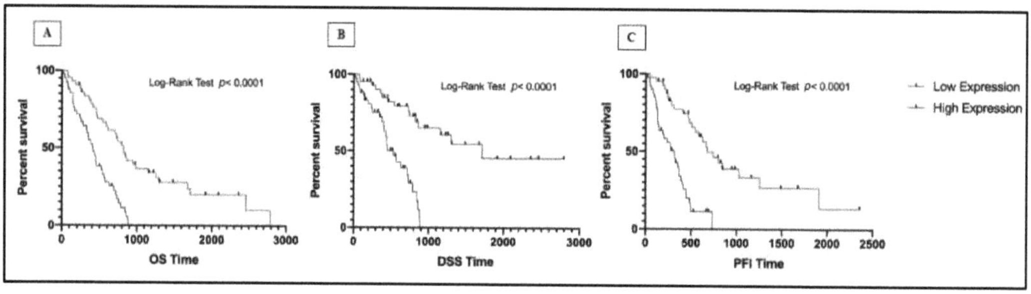

Figure 6. Kaplan-Meier survival curve of hsa-miR-101-3p expression in MM patients according to: (**A**) OS time; (**B**) DSS time; (**C**) PFI time.

4. Discussion

In this study, for the first time, hsa-miR-323a-3p, hsa-miR-101-3p, and hsa-miR-20b-5p have been analyzed in MM tissues vs. nonmalignant pleura tissues. All tested miRNAs in MM tissue showed a down-regulation compared to controls.

The translational data obtained for hsa-miR-101-3p in the present study were totally in accordance with our previous computational study which showed a significant down-regulation in MM samples compared to controls [44]. Furthermore, this miRNA showed a prognostic value for MM because the in silico analyses performed here demonstrated a significant association between hsa-miR-101-3p high expression levels and increased OS. In line with our research, a study by Ramírez-Salazar et al. [50] demonstrated that the targets of the down-regulated hsa-miR-101-3p in MM were significantly enriched in pathways in cancer, including the signaling molecule mitogen-activated protein kinase 1 (MAPK1), the transcription factor v-ets erythroblastosis virus E26 oncogene homolog 1 (ETS1), and the mesenchymal transition-associated molecule frizzled class receptor 4 (FZD4). Multiple down-regulated miRNAs targeted multiple common oncogenic genes, as their reduced expression could increase the expression of these genes and consequently promote tumorigenesis [50]. This explains why an increase in hsa-miR-101-3p levels increases the survival of MM patients, in which the high expression of hsa-miR-101-3p decreases the expression of these oncogenic genes and consequently counteracts tumorigenesis. Interestingly, although hsa-miR-20b-5p showed higher interaction levels with the most altered genes in MM, the expression levels of this miRNA were not associated with the overall survival or progression-free survival of patients. This phenomenon may be related to the multiple binding activities of miRNAs exerted towards different genes. Our results may support the hypothesis that miRNAs reach their biological impact by targeting multiple genes with similar biological effects. Therefore, although hsa-miR-20b-5p showed high levels of interaction with the genes analyzed, hsa-miR-101-3p can activate a more complex network of genes involved in the progression of tumors and the survival of patients, as demonstrated in other studies [50–53].

Of note, all the miRNAs previously identified and here validated in human samples have already been associated with the development of different tumors, including breast cancer, glioblastoma multiform, lymphomas, etc. [54–56].

It is noteworthy that the results obtained for hsa-miR-323a-3p and hsa-miR-20b-5p were opposite to those obtained in our previous in silico and in vitro analysis, however, for these miRNAs ROC analysis revealed high sensitivity and specificity in correctly distinguishing MM and normal samples.

The computational analysis performed to further establish the functional role of these three miRNAs in MM pathogenesis has shown that these miRNAs can target and modulate both tumor suppressor and oncogene genes playing a potentially key role in tumor cell development. In particular, the genes targeted with higher levels of interaction by the selected miRNAs were PBRM1, ZFHX3, and KRAS. The alteration of the expression levels of PBRM1 was associated with the development of both renal cell carcinoma and MM [57]. Recent evidence suggests that PBRM1 genomic alterations are strongly associated with neoantigen production and responsiveness to immune checkpoint inhibitors (ICIs), therefore, the analysis of the expression levels and gene mutation affecting this gene may be predictive for the therapeutic choice in MM. ZFHX3, named also *ATBF1*, has been widely associated with the development of lung cancer when dysregulated. In addition, the analysis of ZFHX3 is also a positive prognostic biomarker for patients treated with ICIs [58]. Similarly, other studies have demonstrated the predictive role of *KRAS* alteration for the treatment of lung cancer [59]. In addition, a recent study also established an important role of KRAS mutation in the development of MM [60].

Several studies have tried to identify novel diagnostic biomarkers for the management of MM patients, however, the currently available diagnostic strategies, mainly based on the evaluation of tumor biomarkers such as calretinin, cytokeratin 5, podoplanin, mesothelin, osteopontin, hyaluronic acid, fibulin-3 [28], vascular endothelium growth factor [30], aquaporin-1 [29], high mobility group box 1 [31], and macroH2A.1 [32], often fail to correctly diagnose MM due to the low rates of sensitivity and specificity of these biomarkers.

To date, liquid biopsy is emerging as a helpful tool for non-invasive diagnosis, screening, prognosis, and stratification of cancer patients [61–63] and to characterize tumor heterogeneity [64]. The literature already proposes an early diagnosis of MM through the expression levels analysis of several "mesomiRs" [42]. Circulating miRNA-126-3p, miRNA-625-3p, and miRNA-103a-3p in blood paired with mesothelin and fibulin-3 have been suggested as potential diagnostic biomarkers of MM [42]. This approach could avoid the histopathological and immunohistochemistry techniques used as the standard for the late diagnosis of pleural biopsies [21]. It could be particularly helpful to study and subsequently use a combination of several proteins and molecular markers to improve diagnostic accuracy.

For this purpose, droplet digital PCR (ddPCR) investigations as well as in silico analysis were performed to assess the functional role of the selected miRNAs and their predictive value for MM patients' diagnosis and prognosis.

Our results indicated that by increasing the number of samples these miRNAs should be further evaluated not just as diagnostic tools, but additionally as prognostic predictors. Thus, their potential as therapeutic targets could be explored by assessing their molecular role. Another key task will be the validation of their targets and regulators, which would clarify how miRNAs induce or suppress critical pathways involved in the carcinogenesis triggered by carcinogenic fibers exposure.

5. Conclusions

Our goal is the validation of these results in a subset of patients chronically exposed to FE using liquid biopsy, to provide a minimally invasive screening tool for the secondary prevention of MM. Early detection of circulating tumor biomarkers and tumor DNA represents one of the most promising strategies to enhance the survival of cancer patients by increasing treatment efficiency [63,64]. Besides these preliminary data, further studies will be designed for the validation of "mesomiRs" with diagnostic potential, alone or in combination with other protein biomarkers, to test their clinical role in high-risk individuals. Certainly, a limitation of the work is the low number of samples available and the reliance on the diagnostic values (sensitivity and specificity) of miRNAs based on the obtained ROC curves until the evaluation on the independent test sample. It would also be interesting to have available a cohort of subjects exposed to FE fibers but in the absence of tumors. This comparison could highlight any similarities or epigenetic differences not only between oncological and non-oncological subjects but also between those exposed to carcinogenic fibers and those not. Moreover, further basic research studies should be aimed at investigating the molecular pathways that are regulated by aberrantly expressed miRNAs.

Supplementary Materials: The following are available online at https://www.mdpi.com/article/10.3390/jpm11111205/s1, Figure S1: ddPCR amplification signals obtained for NTC sample, MM sample and control sample for the three investigated miRNAs.

Author Contributions: V.F.: conceptualization, data curation, formal analysis, investigation, methodology, project administration, software, validation, visualization, roles/writing—original draft, writing—review and editing; C.L. (Carla Loreto): conceptualization, funding acquisition, resources, visualization, supervision, writing—review and editing; L.F.: conceptualization, data curation, formal analysis, investigation, methodology, software, validation, visualization, writing—review and editing; C.L. (Claudia Lombardo): visualization, supervision; E.C.: visualization, supervision; S.C.: visualization, supervision; C.L. (Caterina Ledda): conceptualization, funding acquisition, resources, visualization, supervision; V.R.: conceptualization, funding acquisition, resources, visualization, supervision. All authors have read and agreed to the published version of the manuscript.

Funding: This research received no external funding.

Institutional Review Board Statement: The study was conducted according to the guidelines of the Declaration of Helsinki and approved by Ethics Committee of University Hospital of Catania no. 768/2014.

Informed Consent Statement: Informed consent was obtained from family members of all subjects involved in the study.

Conflicts of Interest: The authors declare no conflict of interest.

References

1. Baumann, F.; Ambrosi, J.-P.; Carbone, M. Asbestos is not just asbestos: An unrecognised health hazard. *Lancet Oncol.* **2013**, *14*, 576–578. [CrossRef]
2. Filetti, V.; Vitale, E.; Broggi, G.; Hagnäs, M.P.; Candido, S.; Spina, A.; Lombardo, C. Update of in vitro, in vivo and ex vivo fluoro-edenite effects on malignant mesothelioma: A systematic review. *Biomed. Rep.* **2020**, *13*, 60. [CrossRef]
3. Rapisarda, V.; Salemi, R.; Marconi, A.; Loreto, C.; Graziano, A.C.E.; Cardile, V.; Basile, M.S.; Candido, S.; Falzone, L.; Spandidos, D.A.; et al. Fluoro-edenite induces fibulin-3 overexpression in non-malignant human mesothelial cells. *Oncol. Lett.* **2016**, *12*, 3363–3367. [CrossRef]
4. Falzone, L.; Marconi, A.; Loreto, C.; Franco, S.; Spandidos, D.A.; Libra, M. Occupational exposure to carcinogens: Benzene, pesticides and fibers. *Mol. Med. Rep.* **2016**, *14*, 4467–4474. [CrossRef]
5. Soffritti, M.; Minardi, F.; Bua, L.; Degli Esposti, D.; Belpoggi, F. First experimental evidence of peritoneal and pleural mesotheliomas induced by fluoro-edenite fibres present in Etnean volcanic material from Biancavilla (Sicily, Italy). *Eur. J. Oncol.* **2004**, *9*, 169–175.
6. Comba, P.; Gianfagna, A.; Paoletti, L. Pleural Mesothelioma Cases in Biancavilla are Related to a New Fluoro-Edenite Fibrous Amphibole. *Arch. Environ. Health Int. J.* **2003**, *58*, 229–232. [CrossRef] [PubMed]
7. Biggeri, A.; Pasetto, R.; Belli, S.; Bruno, C.; Di Maria, G.; Mastrantonio, M.; Trinca, S.; Uccelli, R.; Comba, P. Mortality from chronic obstructive pulmonary disease and pleural mesothelioma in an area contamined by natural fibre (fluoro-edenite). *Scand. J. Work Environ. Health* **2004**, *30*, 249–252. [CrossRef] [PubMed]
8. Gianfagna, A.; Ballirano, P.; Bellatreccia, F.; Bruni, B.; Paoletti, L.; Oberti, R. Characterization of amphibole fibres linked to mesothelioma in the area of Biancavilla, Eastern Sicily, Italy. *Miner. Mag.* **2003**, *67*, 1221–1229. [CrossRef]
9. Grosse, Y.; Loomis, D.; Guyton, K.Z.; Lauby-Secretan, B.; El Ghissassi, F.; Bouvard, V.; Benbrahim-Tallaa, L.; Guha, N.; Scoccianti, C.; Mattock, H.; et al. Carcinogenicity of fluoro-edenite, silicon carbide fibres and whiskers, and carbon nanotubes. *Lancet Oncol.* **2014**, *15*, 1427–1428. [CrossRef]
10. Ledda, C.; Loreto, C.; Matera, S.; Massimino, N.; Cannizzaro, E.; Musumeci, A.; Migliore, M.; Fenga, C.; Pomara, C.; Rapisarda, V. Early effects of fluoro-edenite: Correlation between IL-18 serum levels and pleural and parenchymal abnormalities. *Future Oncol.* **2016**, *12*, 59–62. [CrossRef]
11. Ledda, C.; Rapisarda, V. Malignant Pleural Mesothelioma: The Need to Move from Research to Clinical Practice. *Arch. Med Res.* **2016**, *47*, 407. [CrossRef]
12. Ledda, C.; Pomara, C.; Bracci, M.; Mangano, D.; Ricceri, V.; Musumeci, A.; Ferrante, M.; Musumeci, G.; Loreto, C.; Fenga, C.; et al. Natural carcinogenic fiber and pleural plaques assessment in a general population: A cross-sectional study. *Environ. Res.* **2016**, *150*, 23–29. [CrossRef] [PubMed]

13. Ledda, C.; Loreto, C.; Pomara, C.; Rapisarda, G.; Fiore, M.; Ferrante, M.; Bracci, M.; Santarelli, L.; Fenga, C.; Rapisarda, V. Sheep lymph-nodes as a biological indicator of environmental exposure to fluoro-edenite. *Environ. Res.* **2016**, *147*, 97–101. [CrossRef] [PubMed]
14. Ledda, C.; Costa, C.; Matera, S.; Puglisi, B.; Costanzo, V.; Bracci, M.; Fenga, C.; Rapisarda, V.; Loreto, C. Immuno-modulatory effects in workers exposed to naturally occurring asbestos fibers. *Mol. Med. Rep.* **2017**, *15*, 3372–3378. [CrossRef]
15. Ledda, C.; Caltabiano, R.; Loreto, C.; Cinà, D.; Senia, P.; Musumeci, A.; Ricceri, V.; Pomara, C.; Rapisarda, V. Prevalence of anti-nuclear autoantibodies in subjects exposed to natural asbestiform fibers: A cross-sectional study. *J. Immunotoxicol.* **2017**, *15*, 24–28. [CrossRef]
16. Martinez, G.; Loreto, C.; Rapisarda, V.; Musumeci, G.; Valentino, M.; Carnazza, M.L. Effects of exposure to fluo-ro-edenite fibre pollution on the respiratory system: An in vivo model. *Histol. Histopathol.* **2006**, *21*, 595–601. [PubMed]
17. Rapisarda, V.; Loreto, C.; Castorina, S.; Romano, G.; Garozzo, S.F.; Musumeci, A.; Migliore, M.; Avola, R.; Cinà, D.; Pomara, C.; et al. Occupational exposure to fluoro-edenite and prevalence of anti-nuclear autoantibodies. *Future Oncol.* **2018**, *14*, 59–62. [CrossRef]
18. Paoletti, L.; Batisti, D.; Bruno, C.; Di Paola, M.; Gianfagna, A.; Mastrantonio, M.; Nesti, M.; Comba, P. Unusually High Incidence of Malignant Pleural Mesothelioma in a Town of Eastern Sicily: An Epidemiological and Environmental Study. *Arch. Environ. Health Int. J.* **2000**, *55*, 392–398. [CrossRef]
19. Di Paola, M.; Mastrantonio, M.; Carboni, M.; Belli, S.; Grignoli, M.; Comba, P.; Nesti, M. Mortality from malignant pleural neoplasms in Italy in the years 1988–1992. *Rapporti ISTISAN* **1996**, *96*, 1–30.
20. Fazzo, L.; De Santis, M.; Minelli, G.; Bruno, C.; Zona, A.; Marinaccio, A.; Conti, S.; Comba, P. Pleural mesothelioma mortality and asbestos exposure mapping in Italy. *Am. J. Ind. Med.* **2011**, *55*, 11–24. [CrossRef] [PubMed]
21. Salle, F.G.; Churg, A.; Roggli, V.; Travis, W.D. The 2015 World Health Organization Classification of Tumors of the Pleura: Advances since the 2004 Classification. *J. Thorac. Oncol.* **2016**, *11*, 142–154. [CrossRef]
22. Rapisarda, V.; Ledda, C.; Ricceri, V.; Arena, F.; Musumeci, A.; Marconi, A.; Fago, L.; Bracci, M.; Santarelli, L.; Ferrante, M. Detection of pleural plaques in workers exposed to inhalation of natural fluoro-edenite fibres. *Oncol. Lett.* **2015**, *9*, 2046–2052. [CrossRef] [PubMed]
23. Traviglione, S.; Bruni, B.; Falzano, L.; Paoletti, L.; Fiorentini, C. Effects of the new-identified amphibole fluoro-edenite in lung epithelial cells. *Toxicol. In Vitro* **2003**, *17*, 547–552. [CrossRef]
24. Ledda, C.; Lombardo, C.; Tendi, E.A.; Hagnäs, M.; Paravizzini, G.; Filetti, V.; Rapisarda, V. Pathway of Inflammation due to Asbestos Fiber "Fluoro-edenite" Exposure: An Update. *Curr. Respir. Med. Rev.* **2020**, *16*, 73–75. [CrossRef]
25. Loreto, C.; Caltabiano, R.; Graziano, A.C.E.; Castorina, S.; Lombardo, C.; Filetti, V.; Vitale, E.; Rapisarda, G.; Cardile, V.; Ledda, C.; et al. Defense and protection mechanisms in lung exposed to asbestiform fiber: The role of macrophage migration inhibitory factor and heme oxygenase-1. *Eur. J. Histochem.* **2020**, *64*, 3073. [CrossRef]
26. Yang, H.; Testa, J.R.; Carbone, M. Mesothelioma epidemiology, carcinogenesis, and pathogenesis. *Curr. Treat. Options Oncol.* **2008**, *9*, 147–157. [CrossRef] [PubMed]
27. Micolucci, L.; Rippo, M.R.; Olivieri, F.; Procopio, A.D. Progress of research on microRNAs with diagnostic value in asbestos exposure: A call for method standardization. *Biosci. Trends* **2017**, *11*, 105–109. [CrossRef]
28. Caltabiano, R.; Loreto, C.; Vitale, E.; Matera, S.; Miozzi, E.; Migliore, M.; Angelico, G.; Tumino, R.; Ledda, C.; Rapisarda, V. Fibulin-3 immunoexpression in malignant mesothelioma due to fluoro-edenite: A preliminary report. *Future Oncol.* **2018**, *14*, 53–57. [CrossRef]
29. Angelico, G.; Caltabiano, R.; Loreto, C.; Ieni, A.; Tuccari, G.; Ledda, C.; Rapisarda, V. Immunohistochemical Expression of Aquaporin-1 in Fluoro-Edenite-Induced Malignant Mesothelioma: A Preliminary Report. *Int. J. Mol. Sci.* **2018**, *19*, 685. [CrossRef]
30. Arnold, D.T.; Maskell, N.A. Biomarkers in mesothelioma. *Ann. Clin. Biochem. Int. J. Lab. Med.* **2017**, *55*, 49–58. [CrossRef]
31. Wu, T.; Zhang, W.; Yang, G.; Li, H.; Chen, Q.; Song, R.; Zhao, L. HMGB1 overexpression as a prognostic factor for survival in cancer: A meta-analysis and systematic review. *Oncotarget* **2016**, *7*, 50417–50427. [CrossRef]
32. Loreto, C.; Lombardo, C.; Caltabiano, R.; Ledda, C.; Hagnäs, M.; Filetti, V.; Rapisarda, V. An in vivo immunohisto-chemical study on MacroH2A.1 in lung and lymph-node tissues exposed to an asbestiform fiber. *Curr. Mol. Med.* **2020**, *20*, 653–660. [CrossRef]
33. Chen, Z.; Gaudino, G.; Pass, H.I.; Carbone, M.; Yang, H. Diagnostic and prognostic biomarkers for malignant meso-thelioma: An update. *Transl. Lung Cancer Res.* **2017**, *6*, 259–269. [CrossRef]
34. Creaney, J.; Sneddon, S.; Dick, I.M.; Dare, H.; Boudville, N.; Musk, A.W.; Skates, S.J.; Robinson, B.W. Comparison of the diagnostic accuracy of the MSLN gene products, mesothelin and megakaryocyte potentiating factor, as biomarkers for meso-thelioma in pleural effusions and serum. *Dis. Markers* **2013**, *35*, 119–127. [CrossRef]
35. Creaney, J.; Dick, I.M.; Meniawy, T.; Leong, S.L.; Leon, J.S.; Demelker, Y.; Segal, A.; Musk, A.W.; Lee, Y.C.G.; Skates, S.J.; et al. Comparison of fibulin-3 and mesothelin as markers in malignant mesothelioma. *Thorax* **2014**, *69*, 895–902. [CrossRef] [PubMed]
36. Cui, A.; Jin, X.-G.; Zhai, K.; Tong, Z.-H.; Shi, H.-Z. Diagnostic values of soluble mesothelin-related peptides for malignant pleural mesothelioma: Updated meta-analysis. *BMJ Open* **2014**, *4*, e004145. [CrossRef]
37. Polo, A.; Crispo, A.; Cerino, P.; Falzone, L.; Candido, S.; Giudice, A.; De Petro, G.; Ciliberto, G.; Montella, M.; Budillon, A.; et al. Environment and bladder cancer: Molecular analysis by interaction networks. *Oncotarget* **2017**, *8*, 65240–65252. [CrossRef] [PubMed]

38. Vrijens, K.; Bollati, V.; Nawrot, T.S. MicroRNAs as Potential Signatures of Environmental Exposure or Effect: A Systematic Review. *Environ. Health Perspect.* **2015**, *123*, 399–411. [CrossRef] [PubMed]
39. Reid, G. MicroRNAs in mesothelioma: From tumour suppressors and biomarkers to therapeutic targets. *J. Thorac. Dis.* **2015**, *7*, 1031–1040.
40. Falzone, L.; Scola, L.; Zanghì, A.; Biondi, A.; Di Cataldo, A.; Libra, M.; Candido, S. Integrated analysis of colorectal cancer microRNA datasets: Identification of microRNAs associated with tumor development. *Aging* **2018**, *10*, 1000–1014. [CrossRef]
41. Falzone, L.; Lupo, G.; La Rosa, G.R.M.; Crimi, S.; Anfuso, C.D.; Salemi, R.; Rapisarda, E.; Libra, M.; Candido, S. Identification of Novel MicroRNAs and Their Diagnostic and Prognostic Significance in Oral Cancer. *Cancers* **2019**, *11*, 610. [CrossRef]
42. Micolucci, L.; Akhtar, M.M.; Olivieri, F.; Rippo, M.R.; Procopio, A.D. Diagnostic value of microRNAs in asbestos ex-posure and malignant mesothelioma: Systematic review and qualitative meta-analysis. *Oncotarget* **2016**, *7*, 58606–58637. [CrossRef] [PubMed]
43. Ledda, C.; Senia, P.; Rapisarda, V. Biomarkers for Early Diagnosis and Prognosis of Malignant Pleural Mesothelioma: The Quest Goes on. *Cancers* **2018**, *10*, 203. [CrossRef]
44. Filetti, V.; Falzone, L.; Rapisarda, V.; Caltabiano, R.; Graziano, A.C.E.; Ledda, C.; Loreto, C. Modulation of microRNA expression levels after naturally occurring asbestiform fibers exposure as a diagnostic biomarker of mesothelial neoplastic transformation. *Ecotoxicol. Environ. Saf.* **2020**, *198*, 110640. [CrossRef] [PubMed]
45. Crimi, S.; Falzone, L.; Gattuso, G.; Grillo, C.M.; Candido, S.; Bianchi, A.; Libra, M. Droplet Digital PCR Analysis of Liquid Biopsy Samples Unveils the Diagnostic Role of hsa-miR-133a-3p and hsa-miR-375-3p in Oral Cancer. *Biology* **2020**, *9*, 379. [CrossRef] [PubMed]
46. Salemi, R.; Falzone, L.; Madonna, G.; Polesel, J.; Cinà, D.; Mallardo, D.; Ascierto, P.A.; Libra, M.; Candido, S. MMP-9 as a Candidate Marker of Response to BRAF Inhibitors in Melanoma Patients with BRAFV600E Mutation Detected in Circulating-Free DNA. *Front. Pharmacol.* **2018**, *9*, 856. [CrossRef]
47. Shirdel, E.A.; Xie, W.; Mak, T.W.; Jurisica, I. NAViGaTing the Micronome—Using Multiple MicroRNA Prediction Databases to Identify Signalling Pathway-Associated MicroRNAs. *PLoS ONE* **2011**, *6*, e17429. [CrossRef]
48. Tokar, T.; Pastrello, C.; Rossos, A.E.M.; Abovsky, M.; Hauschild, A.-C.; Tsay, M.; Lu, R.; Jurisica, I. mirDIP 4.1—integrative database of human microRNA target predictions. *Nucleic Acids Res.* **2018**, *46*, D360–D370. [CrossRef]
49. Goldman, M.J.; Craft, B.; Hastie, M.; Repečka, K.; McDade, F.; Kamath, A.; Banerjee, A.; Luo, Y.; Rogers, D.; Brooks, A.N.; et al. Visualizing and interpreting cancer genomics data via the Xena platform. *Nat. Biotechnol.* **2020**, *38*, 675–678. [CrossRef]
50. Ramírez-Salazar, E.G.; Salinas-Silva, L.C.; Vázquez-Manríquez, M.E.; Gayosso-Gómez, L.V.; Negrete-Garcia, M.C.; Ramírez-Rodriguez, S.L.; Chávez, R.; Zenteno, E.; Santillán, P.; Kelly-García, J.; et al. Analysis of microRNA expression signatures in malignant pleural mesothelioma, pleural inflammation, and atypical mesothelial hyperplasia reveals common predictive tumorigenesis-related targets. *Exp. Mol. Pathol.* **2014**, *97*, 375–385. [CrossRef]
51. Lu, H.M.; Yi, W.W.; Ma, Y.S.; Wu, W.; Yu, F.; Fan, H.W.; Lv, Z.W.; Yang, H.Q.; Chang, Z.Y.; Zhang, C.; et al. Prognostic implications of decreased microRNA-101-3p expression in patients with non-small cell lung cancer. *Oncol. Lett.* **2018**, *16*, 7048–7056. [CrossRef]
52. Yao, Z.-S.; Li, C.; Liang, D.; Jiang, X.-B.; Tang, J.-J.; Ye, L.-Q.; Yuan, K.; Ren, H.; Yang, Z.-D.; Jin, D.-X.; et al. Diagnostic and prognostic implications of serum miR-101 in osteosarcoma. *Cancer Biomark.* **2018**, *22*, 127–133. [CrossRef]
53. Hu, J.; Wu, C.; Zhao, X.; Liu, C. The prognostic value of decreased miR-101 in various cancers: A meta-analysis of 12 studies. *OncoTargets Ther.* **2017**, *10*, 3709–3718. [CrossRef]
54. Falzone, L.; Grimaldi, M.; Celentano, E.; Augustin, L.S.A.; Libra, M. Identification of Modulated MicroRNAs Associated with Breast Cancer, Diet, and Physical Activity. *Cancers* **2020**, *12*, 2555. [CrossRef]
55. Candido, S.; Lupo, G.; Pennisi, M.; Basile, M.S.; Anfuso, C.D.; Petralia, M.C.; Gattuso, G.; Vivarelli, S.; Spandidos, D.A.; Libra, M.; et al. The analysis of miRNA expression profiling datasets reveals inverse microRNA patterns in glioblastoma and Alzheimer's disease. *Oncol. Rep.* **2019**, *42*, 911–922. [CrossRef]
56. Hafsi, S.; Candido, S.; Maestro, R.; Falzone, L.; Soua, Z.; Bonavida, B.; Spandidos, D.A.; Libra, M. Correlation between the overexpression of Yin Yang 1 and the expression levels of miRNAs in Burkitt's lymphoma: A computational study. *Oncol. Lett.* **2016**, *11*, 1021–1025. [CrossRef]
57. Ross, J.S.; Gay, L.M.; Sokol, E.; Elvin, J.A.; Vergilio, J.-A.; Suh, J.; Ramkissoon, S.H.; Daniel, S.; Severson, E.A.; Killian, J.K.; et al. PBRM1 genomic alterations in mesothelioma: Potential predictor of immunotherapy efficacy. *J. Clin. Oncol.* **2018**, *36*, 8562. [CrossRef]
58. Zhang, J.; Zhou, N.; Lin, A.; Luo, P.; Chen, X.; Deng, H.; Kang, S.; Guo, L.; Zhu, W.; Zhang, J. ZFHX3 mutation as a protective biomarker for immune checkpoint blockade in non-small cell lung cancer. *Cancer Immunol. Immunother.* **2021**, *70*, 137–151. [CrossRef] [PubMed]
59. Kim, J.H.; Kim, H.S.; Kim, B.J. Prognostic value of KRAS mutation in advanced non-small-cell lung cancer treated with immune checkpoint inhibitors: A meta-analysis and review. *Oncotarget* **2017**, *8*, 48248–48252. [CrossRef] [PubMed]
60. Marazioti, A.; Blanquart, C.; Krontira, A.C.; Pepe, M.A.A.; Hackl, C.M.; Iliopoulou, M.; Lamort, A.S.; Koch, I.; Lindner, M.; Hatz, R.A.; et al. KRAS signalling in malignant pleural mesothelioma. *bioRxiv* **2020**.
61. Cavallari, I.; Urso, L.; Sharova, E.; Pasello, G.; Ciminale, V. Liquid Biopsy in Malignant Pleural Mesothelioma: State of the Art, Pitfalls, and Perspectives. *Front. Oncol.* **2019**, *9*, 740. [CrossRef] [PubMed]

62. Sato, H.; Soh, J.; Aoe, K.; Fujimoto, N.; Tanaka, S.; Namba, K.; Torigoe, H.; Shien, K.; Yamamoto, H.; Tomida, S.; et al. Droplet digital PCR as a novel system for the detection of microRNA-34b/c methylation in circulating DNA in malignant pleural mesothelioma. *Int. J. Oncol.* **2019**, *54*, 2139–2148. [CrossRef] [PubMed]
63. Tuaeva, N.O.; Falzone, L.; Porozov, Y.B.; Nosyrev, A.E.; Trukhan, V.M.; Kovatsi, L.; Spandidos, D.A.; Drakoulis, N.; Kalogeraki, A.; Mamoulakis, C.; et al. Translational Application of Circulating DNA in Oncology: Review of the Last Decades Achievements. *Cells* **2019**, *8*, 1251. [CrossRef] [PubMed]
64. Tomasetti, M.; Amati, M.; Neuzil, J.; Santarelli, L. Circulating epigenetic biomarkers in lung malignancies: From early diagnosis to therapy. *Lung Cancer* **2017**, *107*, 65–72. [CrossRef]

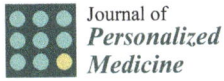

Article

Extracellular Vesicle Enriched miR-625-3p Is Associated with Survival of Malignant Mesothelioma Patients

Katja Goričar [1,†], Marija Holcar [1,†], Nina Mavec [1], Viljem Kovač [2,3], Metka Lenassi [1] and Vita Dolžan [1,*]

1. Institute of Biochemistry and Molecular Genetics, Faculty of Medicine, University of Ljubljana, Vrazov trg 2, 1000 Ljubljana, Slovenia; katja.goricar@mf.uni-lj.si (K.G.); marija.holcar@mf.uni-lj.si (M.H.); nina.mavec@yahoo.com (N.M.); metka.lenassi@mf.uni-lj.si (M.L.)
2. Institute of Oncology Ljubljana, Zaloška 2, 1000 Ljubljana, Slovenia; vkovac@onko-i.si
3. Faculty of Medicine, University of Ljubljana, Vrazov trg 2, 1000 Ljubljana, Slovenia
* Correspondence: vita.dolzan@mf.uni-lj.si; Tel.: +386-1-543-76
† Authors contributed equally.

Abstract: Malignant mesothelioma (MM) is characterized by poor prognosis and short survival. Extracellular vesicles (EVs) are membrane-bound particles released from cells into various body fluids, and their molecular composition reflects the characteristics of the origin cell. Blood EVs or their miRNA cargo might serve as new minimally invasive biomarkers that would enable earlier detection of MM or treatment outcome prediction. Our aim was to evaluate miRNAs enriched in serum EVs as potential prognostic biomarkers in MM patients in a pilot longitudinal study. EVs were isolated from serum samples obtained before and after treatment using ultracentrifugation on 20% sucrose cushion. Serum EV-enriched miR-103-3p, miR-126-3p and miR-625-3p were quantified using qPCR. After treatment, expression of miR-625-3p and miR-126-3p significantly increased in MM patients with poor treatment outcome ($p = 0.012$ and $p = 0.036$, respectively). A relative increase in miR-625-3p expression after treatment for more than 3.2% was associated with shorter progression-free survival (7.5 vs. 19.4 months, HR = 3.92, 95% CI = 1.20–12.80, $p = 0.024$) and overall survival (12.5 vs. 49.1 months, HR = 5.45, 95% CI = 1.06–28.11, $p = 0.043$) of MM patients. Bioinformatic analysis showed enrichment of 33 miR-625-3p targets in eight biological pathways. Serum EV-enriched miR-625-3p could therefore serve as a prognostic biomarker in MM and could contribute to a more personalized treatment.

Keywords: mesothelioma; extracellular vesicles; miR-625; prognosis

1. Introduction

Malignant mesothelioma (MM) is a rare aggressive malignancy of the pleura or the peritoneum that is mostly associated with exposure to asbestos [1]. Even though asbestos use has been banned in most countries, MM incidence is still rising due to a long latency period between asbestos exposure and development of MM [2]. As MM symptoms are often non-specific, diagnosis is usually made when the disease is already in the advanced stages [3]. MM is therefore characterized by poor prognosis and short survival [1,4].

MM treatment is often multimodal and includes chemotherapy, surgery, and radiation. Even though implementation of chemotherapy increased survival of MM patients, outcome is still limited [1,5,6]. Standard chemotherapy includes treatment with a combination of pemetrexed and cisplatin [7], and comparable results were shown for treatment with a combination of gemcitabine and cisplatin [1,8–10]. New treatment options based on immunotherapy or targeted treatment are currently extensively investigated in clinical trials (reviewed in [11–13]). Just recently, the combination of nivolumab and ipilimumab was approved by the U.S. Food and Drug Administration as a first-line treatment for unresectable pleural MM [14].

Several studies have tried to identify biomarkers that could improve the outcome of MM patients, mostly focusing on biomarkers for early diagnosis of MM. The best known MM biomarker is mesothelin; cell-surface glycoprotein increased in both tumor tissue and serum of MM patients [15–18]. Osteopontin and fibulin-3 were often proposed as additional MM biomarkers [18–21]. *MSLN* genetic variability also affects mesothelin levels and accounting for genetic factors can improve predictive ability of mesothelin [22–25]. On the other hand, fewer studies focused on identifying prognostic biomarkers in MM that would be able to predict treatment outcome. For example, increased mesothelin was associated with worse survival in a meta-analysis [26]. We have also identified several other pharmacogenetic biomarkers in drug transport, metabolism and target genes as well as DNA repair pathways that could help to predict response to chemotherapy based on clinical-pharmacogenetic models [27]. However, current biomarkers alone have limited sensitivity or specificity, preventing their widespread implementation in clinical practice [28]. The search for appropriate minimally invasive diagnostic and prognostic biomarkers in MM therefore continues, with studies focusing on composite biomarkers or new types of biomarkers.

MicroRNAs (miRNAs), endogenous, small, non-coding RNA sequences, which help to regulate gene expression at the post-transcriptional level, are emerging as important novel circulating biomarkers in cancer and other diseases [3]. In MM, several studies investigated miRNA expression in tumor tissue, blood cells, plasma or serum, pleural effusions or cell lines, and a number of miRNAs were implicated in MM pathogenesis and diagnosis (reviewed in [3,29,30]). Among them, miR-103-3p, miR-126-3p, and miR-625-3p were identified as suitable biomarkers in multiple studies [30–42]. In MM patients, miR-103-3p and miR-126 were downregulated compared to asbestos-exposed or healthy controls [30–41], while miR-625-3p was upregulated [30,42]. Some of the studies also suggested that a combination of a few miRNAs or their combination with mesothelin could serve as a better diagnostic biomarker [32,34,39,40]. On the other hand, the role of miRNAs in MM prognosis is not well established. So far, miR-126-3p expression was associated with shorter survival of MM patients in a few studies, alone or in combination with other miRNAs [35,41]. Additionally, increased circulating miR-625-3p expression after chemotherapy was associated with disease progression [43].

Recent studies have shown that miRNAs secreted by cells of primary tumors and metastatic sites into biofluids are often encapsulated within extracellular vesicles (EVs). EVs are phospholipid bilayer enclosed spherical nanoparticles, secreted by all cells investigated so far and reflecting their (patho)physiological state [44]. They can accumulate signals of disease or distress in form of nucleic acids, proteins, lipids and different metabolites and transport them to distant sites throughout the body. EVs are very heterogeneous in their biogenesis, release pathways, size, morphology, cargo and biophysical characteristics, and can be subdivided into exosomes, microvesicles and apoptotic bodies [45]. Their cargo is protected from degradation in the extracellular space and can be co-enriched from biofluids with EVs [46,47]. Changes in EV concentration or size as well as cargo composition were observed in different cancer types [48–50]. EVs or their cargo, e.g., miRNA, could therefore be used in liquid biopsy as diagnostic or prognostic cancer biomarkers, to assess disease progression, treatment response or resistance [51]. EV-miRNA cargo specifically has been shown to be actively involved in the regulation of diverse targets in recipient cells, among others regulating disease progression, metastasis and even sensitivity to specific drugs [52–54].

In MM, EVs secreted from cell lines were already shown to be enriched with proteins involved in different cellular pathways, including signalling, response to stress, angiogenesis, and metastasis [28,55,56]. Additionally, asbestos exposure modified EV cargo leading to gene expression changes in mesothelial cells [57]. However, only a few studies investigated EV-miRNA in MM to date [30,58,59]. The most abundant EV-bound miRNAs in MM were reported to be tumor suppressors [59]. EV-miR-103a-3p and miR-30e-3p were reported as candidate diagnostic markers in MM [58]. A meta-analysis of diagnostic value of miRNA in asbestos exposure and MM reported in the miRandola database found EVs-linked miR-126-3p and miR-103a-3p to be downregulated, while miR-625-3p, miR-29c-5p and miR-92a-3p were upregulated in MM [30].

MiRNAs miR-103-3p, miR-126-3p, and miR-625-3p were proposed as circulating diagnostic MM biomarkers in several studies and were previously also detected in EVs [58,60]. On the other hand, the prognostic role of EV-miRNA is largely unexplored. Therefore, the aim of the present pilot study was to evaluate serum EV-enriched miRNAs miR-103a-3p, miR-126-3p, and miR-625-3p as potential minimally invasive biomarkers of treatment outcome in patients with MM in a longitudinal setting.

2. Materials and Methods

2.1. Patients

We performed a pilot longitudinal study that included MM patients with pleural or peritoneal mesothelioma treated with chemotherapy at the Institute of Oncology Ljubljana in the period between 1 February 2009 and 31 July 2016. The diagnosis of pleural or peritoneal MM was established by thoracoscopy or laparoscopy, respectively. For all patients, MM diagnosis was confirmed histologically by an experienced pathologist. MM stage was determined according to the TNM staging system for pleural MM, while performance status was evaluated according to the Eastern Cooperative Oncology Group (ECOG) scores. Demographic and clinical data were obtained from medical records or assessed during a clinical interview. Written informed consent was obtained for all patients. The study was approved by the Slovenian Ethics Committee for Research in Medicine (41/02/09) and was carried out according to the Declaration of Helsinki.

Inclusion criteria were treatment in the specified period and availability of longitudinal samples. Among MM patients treated in this period, we selected 10 patients with poor treatment outcome and 10 patients with good treatment outcome based on overall survival (OS): patients with poor treatment outcome had OS of less than 15 months (10 patients), while patients with good treatment outcome had OS of more than 20 months (10 patients).

Serum samples of 20 MM patients were collected at two time points: at diagnosis and after completion of chemotherapy. Blood was sampled on the day of the last chemotherapy cycle, unless disease progression occurred before the last cycle. Serum samples were prepared within 4 h after blood sampling, aliquoted and stored at $-20\ °C$. In total, 40 samples were evaluated.

2.2. Isolation of Small EVs with Sucrose Cushion Ultracentrifugation (sUC)

We used the established sUC method for enrichment of small EVs [61]. In short, sera aliquots were first defrosted on ice and centrifuged at $10,000 \times g$ for 20 min at $4\ °C$ to remove any large extracellular particles. Next, 2 mL of 20% sucrose (sucrose (Merck Millipore, Burlington, MA, USA) in Dulbecco's phosphate-buffered saline (dPBS, Sigma-Aldrich, St. Louis, MO, USA) was pipetted in polypropylene tubes (Beckman Coulter, Brea, CA, USA) and overlaid with diluted serum (1 mL of serum, mixed with 8.5 mL of particle-free dPBS). Samples were ultracentrifuged at $100,000 \times g$ for 135 min at $4\ °C$ (MLA-55 rotor, Beckman Coulter, USA) and supernatant was aspirated from the tubes and walls of the tubes dried by low-lint highly absorbent paper. Finally, the pellet containing isolated EVs was fully resuspended in 200 µL of dPBS, mixed with 800 µL Tri-reagent (Sigma-Aldrich, USA), and stored at $-20\ °C$.

2.3. Extraction of miRNA and Transcription to cDNA

Before miRNA extraction, 1 mL aliquots of frozen serum small EV-enriched samples, mixed with Tri-reagent, were defrosted on ice. 1 µL of MS2 RNA carrier (final concentration 0.8 µg/µL; Roche, Basel, Switzerland), 1 µL of spike-in (exogenous control, ath-miR-159a, final concentration 0.4 fM; Applied Biosystems, Waltham, MA, USA), and 200 µL of chloroform (Sigma-Aldrich, USA) were added to the samples and thoroughly mixed [61]. MiRNA was extracted using the miRNeasy Mini Kit (Qiagen, Hilden, Germany), according to the manufacturers' instructions, with following adaptations of the protocol: (I) addition of extra 500 µL of RNase/DNase-free water and subsequent chloroform extraction after the first removal of aqueous phase from the chloroform-sample mixture, and (II) elution of miRNA from the column into DNA low binding tubes (Eppendorf, Hamburg, Germany) by two successive additions of 25 µL of RNase/DNase free water and centrifugations (15,000× g, 30 s). Samples of extracted miRNA were stored at −20 °C until batch reverse transcription of total isolated miRNA to cDNA for all samples. For this, TaqMan™ Advanced miRNA cDNA Synthesis Kit (Applied Biosystems, USA) was used, following the manufacturer's instructions. cDNA samples were stored at −20 °C.

2.4. Quantitative Polymerase Chain Reaction (qPCR)

qPCR for miRNA expression analysis was performed using the TaqMan™ Advanced MicroRNA assays (Applied Biosystems, USA) on QuantStudio™ 7 Flex Real-Time PCR System (Applied Biosystems, USA). The analysis was performed using QuantStudio Software (Applied Biosystems, USA) and the miRNA levels were expressed as cycle threshold (Ct). Ct of spike-in (ath-miR-159a) was analyzed to evaluate the efficiency of miRNA isolation as well as transcription to cDNA, to exclude deviating samples according to the manufacturer's instructions. All of the samples were also tested for hemolysis by analyzing miR-23a-3p and miR-451a expression. $\Delta Ct((miR\text{-}23a\text{-}3p)-(miR\text{-}451a)) \geq 7$ indicated hemolysis and led to exclusion of the sample from further analysis [62]. In addition to three miRNAs of interest (miR-103a-3p, miR-126-3p, miR-625-3p), two control miRNAs with reportedly stable expression in plasma or serum (let-7i-5p and miR-425-5p) [63,64] were analyzed. Expression of miRNAs of interest was normalized to the average expression of control miRNAs let-7i-5p and miR-425-5p. The relative expression of miRNAs was calculated as $2^{-\Delta Ct}$. Temporal changes in miRNA expression were assessed using relative change, defined as the difference of miRNA expression after treatment and at diagnosis, divided by its value at diagnosis.

2.5. Bioinformatic Analysis of miR-625-3p Targets

Experimentally validated miR-625-3p targets were obtained using miRTarBase (2020 update) [65]. Interaction network predicting the relationship between miR-625-3p target genes and genes correlating with target genes was obtained using GeneMania based on automatically selected weighting method [66]. We used gProfiler for functional enrichment analysis based on Gene Ontology (GO), Kyoto Encyclopedia of Genes and Genomes (KEGG), Reactome, and WikiPathways as well as Transfac, miRTarBase, Human Protein Atlas, CORUM, and Human Phenotype Ontology databases [67]. To account for multiple comparisons, multiple testing correction based on g:SCS algorithm was used.

2.6. Statistical Analysis

Continuous variables were described using median and interquartile range (25–75%), and categorical variables were described using frequencies. For continuous dependent variables, the nonparametric Mann–Whitney test was used to compare the distribution among different groups, while Fisher's exact test was used to compare the distribution of categorical variables. For related samples, the nonparametric Wilcoxon signed-rank test was used for comparison of continuous variables in different time points. For the differentiation between MM patients with poor and good treatment outcome, a receiver operating characteristic (ROC) curve analysis was used to determine the specificity, sensitivity and area under the curve (AUC). Cutoff values were selected as values with the highest sum of specificity and sensitivity.

In survival analysis, progression-free survival (PFS) was defined as the time from diagnosis to the day of documented disease progression or death from any cause, and OS was defined as the time from diagnosis to death from any cause. Patients without progression or death at the time of the analysis were censored at the date of the last follow-up. Kaplan–Meier analysis was used to calculate median survival or follow-up time. Univariable and multivariable Cox regression was used to calculate the hazard ratios (HR) and the 95% confidence intervals (CIs). Clinical variables used for adjustment in multivariable survival analysis were selected using stepwise forward conditional selection.

All statistical analyses were carried out by IBM SPSS Statistics version 21.0 (IBM Corporation, Armonk, NY, USA). All statistical tests were two-sided and the level of significance was set at 0.05.

3. Results

3.1. Patient Characteristics

The final study group consisted of 18 MM patients. Two patients were excluded from the analysis because their samples obtained at diagnosis did not pass the quality control for spike-in and/or hemolysis levels. Patients' clinical characteristics are presented in Table 1. Among them, 8 (44.4%) patients had poor treatment outcome, while 10 (55.6%) patients had good treatment outcome. In total, 17 (94.4%) patients had pleural and 1 (5.6%) patient had peritoneal MM. The median follow-up time was 30.8 months. The relative change of miRNA expression during treatment was only evaluated in 17 patients (8 (47.1%) patients with poor and 9 (52.9%) with good outcome), as one sample obtained at the end of chemotherapy was excluded due to hemolysis.

Table 1. Clinical characteristics of malignant mesothelioma patients ($n = 18$).

Characteristic	Category/Unit	n (%)
Gender	Male	10 (55.6)
	Female	8 (44.4)
Age	Years, Median (25–75%)	68.5 (59.8–72.5)
Stage	I	4 (22.2)
	II	2 (11.1)
	III	8 (44.4)
	IV	3 (16.7)
	Peritoneal	1 (5.6)
Histological type	Epithelioid	12 (66.7)
	Biphasic	3 (16.7)
	Sarcomatoid	3 (16.7)
ECOG performance status	0	4 (22.2)
	1	8 (44.4)
	2	6 (33.3)
Asbestos exposure	Not exposed	5 (27.8)
	Exposed	13 (72.2)
Smoking	Non-smokers	11 (61.1)
	Smokers	7 (38.9)
CRP	mg/L, Median (25–75%)	15.5 (2.8–46.5)
Chemotherapy	Gemcitabine + cisplatin	12 (66.7)
	Pemetrexed + cisplatin	6 (33.3)
PFS	Months, Median (25–75%)	14.1 (7.2–20.2)
OS	Months, Median (25–75%)	27.3 (12.5–29.4)
Follow-up time	Months, Median (25–75%)	30.8 (23.4–30.8)

CRP: C-reactive protein; ECOG: Eastern Cooperative Oncology Group; EV: extracellular vesicles; OS: overall survival; PFS: progression-free survival.

Among all MM patients, 12 (66.7%) were treated with gemcitabine and cisplatin doublet chemotherapy, while 6 (33.3%) received pemetrexed and cisplatin doublet chemotherapy. There were no significant differences in treatment outcome between both chemotherapy regimens ($p = 0.638$).

3.2. Comparison of Serum EV-Enriched miRNA Expression at Diagnosis and after Treatment

First, we evaluated if the expression of target serum EV-enriched miRNAs changes after treatment with chemotherapy in MM patients (Table 2, Figure S1). The expression of EV-enriched miR-126-3p increased after treatment in 12 (70.6%) patients ($p = 0.035$, Table 2, Figure S1c). Expression of EV-enriched miR-625-3p and miR-103a-3p did not differ significantly after treatment (Figure S1a,b, respectively).

Table 2. Comparison of expression of serum EV-enriched miRNAs at diagnosis and after treatment in malignant mesothelioma patients.

	miRNA	At Diagnosis Relative Expression Median (25–75%)	After Treatment Relative Expression Median (25–75%)	p
All patients ($n = 17$)	miR-625-3p	0.05 (0.01–0.13)	0.07 (0.03–0.15)	0.227
	miR-103a-3p	0.40 (0.34–0.47)	0.39 (0.32–0.48)	0.981
	miR-126-3p	45.73 (38.30–74.96)	68.05 (46.17–101.77)	0.035
Poor outcome ($n = 8$)	miR-625-3p	0.06 (0.02–0.13)	0.11 (0.08–0.21)	0.012
	miR-103a-3p	0.39 (0.28–0.42)	0.37 (0.28–0.48)	0.889
	miR-126-3p	55.01 (038.03–72.06)	78.81 (55.58–140.34)	0.036
Good outcome ($n = 9$)	miR-625-3p	0.04 (0.01–0.14)	0.04 (0.01–0.05)	0.173
	miR-103a-3p	0.43 (0.34–0.50)	0.40 (0.33–0.51)	0.953
	miR-126-3p	44.46 (38.76–77.33)	51.51 (37.69–94.09)	0.374

EV: extracellular vesicles.

When patients were stratified according to outcome, the expression of EV-enriched miR-625-3p and miR-126-3p was significantly increased after treatment in patients with poor outcome ($p = 0.012$ and $p = 0.036$, respectively, Table 2). Expression of EV-enriched miR-625-3p increased after treatment in all 8 patients with poor outcome, while EV-enriched miR-126-3p expression increased in 6 (75.0%) patients with poor outcome (Figure S1d,f, respectively). On the other hand, no differences between miRNA expression at diagnosis and after treatment were observed in patients with good outcome (Table 2).

3.3. Differentiation between MM Patients with Poor and Good Treatment Outcome Based on Serum EV-Enriched miRNA Expression

There were no significant differences in the expression of serum EV-enriched miRNAs collected at diagnosis between MM patients with poor and good treatment outcome (Table 3). On the other hand, a relative change in EV-enriched miR-625-3p expression over time could discriminate between patients with poor and good treatment outcome. After treatment, miR-625-3p expression increased in patients with poor outcome (median 85.2%) and decreased in patients with good outcome (median −17.5%), and the difference was statistically significant ($p = 0.036$). AUC for miR-625-3p was 0.806 (0.588–1.000) ($p = 0.034$). At the cutoff value of 3.2% with the highest sum of specificity and sensitivity, sensitivity was 0.667 and specificity was 1.000. Relative change of EV-enriched miR-103a-3p or miR-126-3p expression after treatment was not associated with treatment outcome (Table 3). The relative change of EV-enriched miRNA expression did not differ between different chemotherapy regimens ($p = 0.884$ for miR-625-3p, $p = 0.733$ for miR-103a-3p, and $p = 0.525$ for miR-126-3p).

Table 3. Expression of serum EV-enriched miRNAs and treatment outcome of malignant mesothelioma patients and ROC curve analysis.

	miRNA	Poor Outcome Median (25–75%)	Good Outcome Median (25–75%)	p	AUC (95% CI)	p	Cutoff	Sensitivity	Specificity
At diagnosis ($n = 18$)	miR-625-3p	0.06 (0.02–0.13)	0.05 (0.01–0.13)	0.897	0.556 (0.273–0.838)	0.700	0.01	0.333	0.875
	miR-103a-3p	0.39 (0.28–0.42)	0.45 (0.36–0.54)	0.146	0.681 (0.414–0.947)	0.211	0.47	0.444	1.000
	miR-126-3p	55.01 (38.03–72.06)	45.09 (39.81–76.49)	0.965	0.514 (0.221–0.807)	0.923	46.28	0.667	0.925
Change (%) ($n = 17$)	miR-625-3p	85.2 (25.8–565.9)	−17.5 (−82.8–150.6)	0.036	0.806 (0.588–1.000)	0.034	3.2	0.667	1.000
	miR-103a-3p	1.6 (-13.9–25.2)	−10.5 (−29.8–37.1)	0.888	0.528 (0.242–0.814)	0.847	−16.7	0.333	0.875
	miR-126-3p	16.1 (1.7–175.97)	20.7 (−24.8–86.8)	0.606	0.583 (0.297–0.869)	0.564	−8.7	0.333	1.000

AUC: area under the curve; CI: confidence interval; EV: extracellular vesicles; ROC: receiver operating characteristic.

3.4. Survival Analysis

For MM patients with poor outcome, median PFS was 6.9 (5.8–7.5) months and median OS was 10.0 (7.7–12.5) months. For MM patients with good outcome, median PFS was 19.4 (14.9–23.2) months and median OS was 29.4 (27.3–49.1) months. Among clinical characteristics, higher C-reactive protein (CRP) level was an important predictor of shorter OS (HR = 1.01, 95% CI = 1.00–1.04, p = 0.029) and was therefore used for adjustment in multivariable analyses. The chemotherapy regimen was not a significant predictor of OS (HR = 0.21, 95% CI = 0.03–1.67, p = 0.141).

Serum EV-enriched miRNA expression at diagnosis was not associated with survival of MM patients (Table S1). On the other hand, a higher relative change in miR-625-3p was associated with both worse PFS (HR = 1.02, 95% CI = 1.00–1.04, p = 0.044) and worse OS (HR = 1.02, 95% CI = 1.00–1.05, p = 0.045). The association remained significant after adjustment for clinical variables in multivariable analysis (PFS: HR = 1.02, 95% CI = 1.00–1.04, p = 0.046; OS: HR = 1.03, 95% CI = 1.00–1.05, p = 0.042; Table S1). EV-enriched miR-103a-3p or miR-126-3p was not associated with survival of MM patients.

Patients were then stratified according to cutoff values obtained from comparison between patients with poor and good outcome (Table 3), and the association with PFS and OS was assessed (Table 4). A relative increase in EV-enriched miR-625-3p expression after treatment for more than 3.2% was associated with significantly shorter PFS (7.5 compared to 19.4 months, Figure 1a). The difference was significant both in univariable analysis (HR = 3.92, 95% CI = 1.20–12.80, p = 0.024) and after adjustment for CRP levels at diagnosis (HR = 4.13, 95% CI = 1.25–13.65, p = 0.020). Similarly, a relative increase in miR-625-3p expression after treatment for more than 3.2% was associated with significantly shorter OS (12.5 vs. 49.1 months, Figure 1b). The difference was again significant both in univariable analysis (HR = 5.45, 95% CI = 1.06–28.11, p = 0.043) and after adjustment for CRP levels at diagnosis (HR = 6.32, 95% CI = 1.18–33.99, p = 0.032).

Table 4. Relative change in expression of serum EV-enriched miRNAs and progression-free survival (PFS) and overall survival (OS) of malignant mesothelioma patients.

miRNA	PFS						OS					
	<Cutoff Months, Median (25–75%)	>Cutoff Months, Median (25–75%)	HR (95% CI)	p	HR (95% CI)$_{adj}$	P$_{adj}$	<Cutoff Months, Median (25–75%)	>Cutoff Months, Median (25–75%)	HR (95% CI)	p	HR (95% CI)$_{adj}$	P$_{adj}$
miR-625-3p	19.4 (14.9–23.2)	7.5 (6.4–14.7)	3.92 (1.2–12.8)	0.024	4.13 (1.25–13.65)	0.020	49.1 (27.3–49.1)	12.5 (9.1–28.3)	5.45 (1.06–28.11)	0.043	6.32 (1.18–33.99)	0.032
miR-103a-3p	14.9 (5.8–17.1)	14.1 (7.2–19.4)	1.84 (0.52–6.56)	0.348	1.76 (0.47–6.56)	0.403	27.3 (5.8–49.1)	25.7 (10.6–28.3)	1.50 (0.30–7.37)	0.621	1.35 (0.26–6.95)	0.716
miR-126-3p	19.4 (14.9–23.2)	8.5 (6.9–17.1)	1.89 (0.53–6.76)	0.327	2.90 (0.71–11.89)	0.140	27.3 (27.3–27.3)	25.7 (10.6–49.1)	2.40 (0.29–19.60)	0.416	7.77 (0.72–84.17)	0.092

adj: adjusted for C-reactive protein levels at diagnosis. CI: confidence interval; EV: extracellular vesicles; HR: hazard ratio.

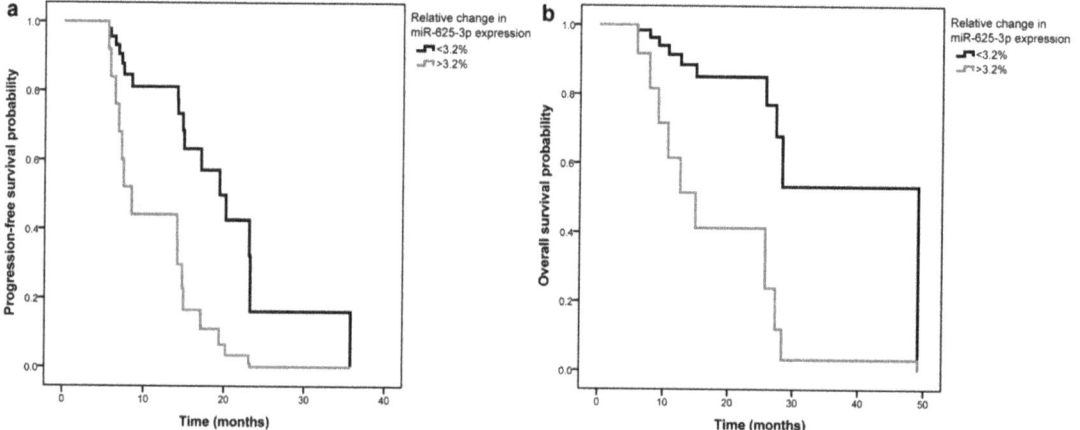

Figure 1. Relative change in serum EV-enriched miR-625-3p expression and progression free survival (a) and overall survival (b) of malignant mesothelioma patients. EV: extracellular vesicles.

3.5. Bioinformatic Analysis of miR-625-3p Targets

miRTarBase listed 33 experimentally confirmed miR-625-3p targets. Only one of them, mitogen-activated protein kinase kinase 6 (MAP2K6), was experimentally confirmed using reporter assay, Western blot and qPCR, while other targets were only confirmed using next-generation sequencing.

Using GeneMania, we evaluated co-expression, physical interactions, co-localization, genetic interactions, shared protein domains, and predicted interactions of miR-625-3p target genes. Interaction network revealed several associations between miR-625-3p target genes, as well as 20 additional interacting genes (Figure 2a).

A gProfiler analysis showed that the identified miR-625-3p target genes were significantly associated not only with miR-625-3p but also with five other miRNAs, especially miR-1295b-3p (Figure 2b). After GO and KEGG enrichment analysis of miR-625-3p target genes, eight GO (seven biological pathways and one molecular function) and two KEGG terms were enriched in this gene set. The most significant pathway after enrichment was PD-L1 expression and PD-1 checkpoint pathway in cancer (KEGG:05235). The most significant GO biological process terms were regulation of cell communication (GO:0010646) and regulation of signal transduction (GO:0009966). The only significant GO molecular function term was insulin-like growth factor II binding (GO:0031995). Additionally, two WikiPathways were also enriched among miR-625-3p target genes. Based on Transfac data, BEN transcription factor binding motif was significantly enriched in our data set. A detailed description of all significant pathways and processes and their significance level is represented in Figure 2b.

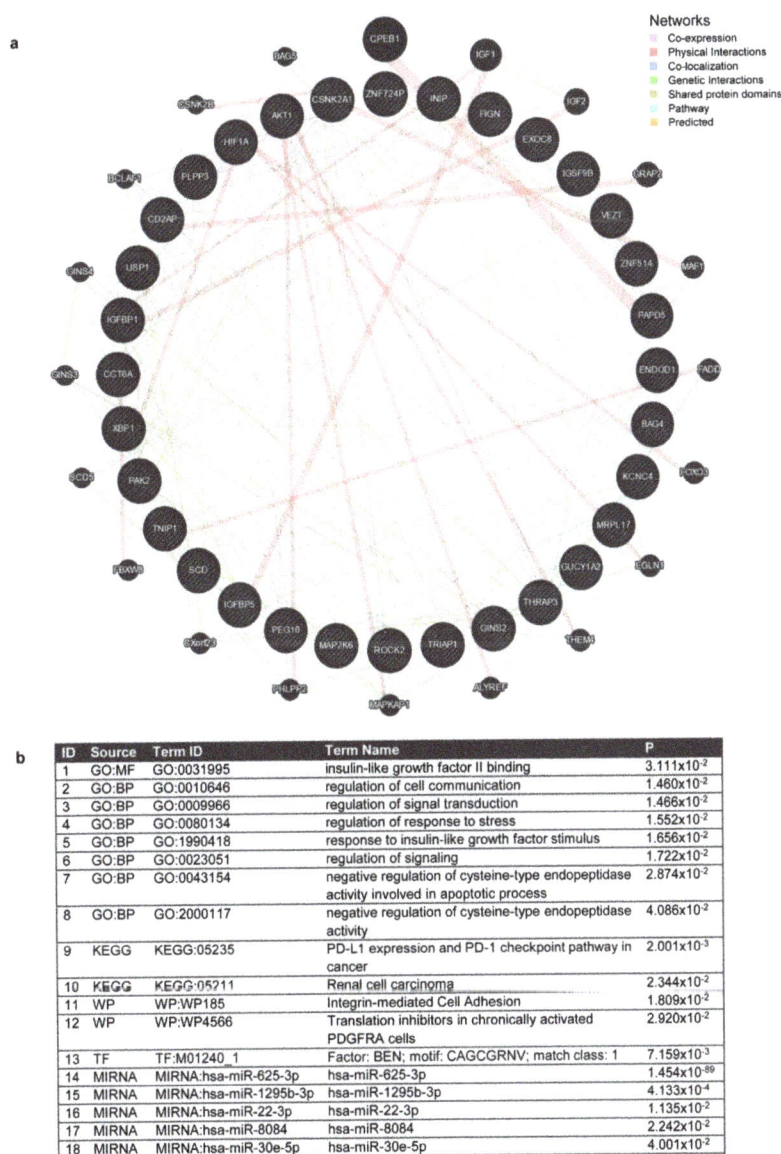

ID	Source	Term ID	Term Name	P
1	GO:MF	GO:0031995	insulin-like growth factor II binding	3.111×10^{-2}
2	GO:BP	GO:0010646	regulation of cell communication	1.460×10^{-2}
3	GO:BP	GO:0009966	regulation of signal transduction	1.466×10^{-2}
4	GO:BP	GO:0080134	regulation of response to stress	1.552×10^{-2}
5	GO:BP	GO:1990418	response to insulin-like growth factor stimulus	1.656×10^{-2}
6	GO:BP	GO:0023051	regulation of signaling	1.722×10^{-2}
7	GO:BP	GO:0043154	negative regulation of cysteine-type endopeptidase activity involved in apoptotic process	2.874×10^{-2}
8	GO:BP	GO:2000117	negative regulation of cysteine-type endopeptidase activity	4.086×10^{-2}
9	KEGG	KEGG:05235	PD-L1 expression and PD-1 checkpoint pathway in cancer	2.001×10^{-3}
10	KEGG	KEGG:05211	Renal cell carcinoma	2.344×10^{-2}
11	WP	WP:WP185	Integrin-mediated Cell Adhesion	1.809×10^{-2}
12	WP	WP:WP4566	Translation inhibitors in chronically activated PDGFRA cells	2.920×10^{-2}
13	TF	TF:M01240_1	Factor: BEN; motif: CAGCGRNV; match class: 1	7.159×10^{-3}
14	MIRNA	MIRNA:hsa-miR-625-3p	hsa-miR-625-3p	1.454×10^{-89}
15	MIRNA	MIRNA:hsa-miR-1295b-3p	hsa-miR-1295b-3p	4.133×10^{-4}
16	MIRNA	MIRNA:hsa-miR-22-3p	hsa-miR-22-3p	1.135×10^{-2}
17	MIRNA	MIRNA:hsa-miR-8084	hsa-miR-8084	2.242×10^{-2}
18	MIRNA	MIRNA:hsa-miR-30e-5p	hsa-miR-30e-5p	4.001×10^{-2}
19	MIRNA	MIRNA:hsa-miR-4307	hsa-miR-4307	4.442×10^{-2}

Figure 2. (**a**) Experimentally confirmed miR-625-3p targets and their interactions based on co-expression, physical interactions, co-localization, genetic interactions, shared protein domains, and predicted interactions. MiR-625-3p target genes are presented in the inner circle, while the outer circle shows other associated genes based on GeneMania analysis. Target gene *c7orf65* was not included in GeneMania. (**b**) gProfiler pathway enrichment analysis: biological processes and pathways linked to miR-625-3p target genes, term names, codes and significance level. BP: biological process; GO: gene ontology; KEGG: Kyoto Encyclopedia of Genes and Genomes; MF: molecular function; TF: transcription factor; WP: WikiPathways.

4. Discussion

In the present pilot longitudinal study, we investigated expression of candidate miRNAs enriched in serum small EVs as potential prognostic biomarkers in MM. After treatment with platinum-based chemotherapy, expression of serum EV-enriched miR-625-3p and miR-126-3p significantly increased only in MM patients with poor treatment outcome. A relative increase in EV-enriched miR-625-3p expression after treatment was associated with significantly shorter survival and could be used as a prognostic biomarker in MM.

The most important result of our study is the association of serum EV-enriched miR-625-3p with treatment outcome and survival of MM patients. Expression of serum EV-enriched miR-625-3p significantly increased after treatment with platinum-based chemotherapy in MM patients with poor treatment outcome, while a nonsignificant decrease was observed in MM patients with good outcome. Relative change in serum EV-enriched miR-625-3p expression over time could discriminate between patients with poor and good treatment outcome with high specificity. If serum EV-enriched miR-625-3p expression after treatment increased for more than 3.2%, MM patients had significantly shorter PFS and OS, even after adjustment for clinical parameters. In previous studies, circulating plasma miR-625-3p was generally upregulated in MM compared to healthy controls, but the results are conflicting [30,34,42]. In the only study evaluating EVs in MM, no differences in miR-625-3p expression were observed compared to controls, while its prognostic potential was not assessed [58]. In a longitudinal study that investigated plasma miR-625-3p in MM before and after cisplatin-based chemotherapy, expression increased in patients with progressive disease [43], which is consistent with our results. The combination of increased miR-625-3p and decreased long noncoding RNA (lncRNA) GAS5 expression could distinguish between patients with good or poor outcome, even though only GAS5 was associated with overall survival [43]. In concordance with our results, increased tumor miR-625-3p expression was associated with worse response to oxaliplatin and oxaliplatin resistance in colorectal cancer [68,69], emphasizing the association between miR-625-3p and response to platinum compounds. Additionally, increased tumor miR-625-3p expression was also significantly associated with tumor relapse in esophageal small cell carcinoma [70]. High tumor miR-625-3p expression was observed in thyroid and clear cell renal cell carcinoma [71,72]. Increased miR-625-3p expression was associated with poor prognosis, tumor proliferation, migration or invasion in various cancers [71–73].

Despite strong evidence that miR-625-3p may be associated with unfavorable prognosis, miR-625 was also observed to be downregulated in serum, plasma or tissue in some cancer types; however, most of these studies did not specify whether they investigated the expression of miR-625-3p or miR-625-5p [74–77]. Decreased miR-625 expression was associated with shorter survival of esophageal squamous cell carcinoma [74], and its expression increased in non-small cell lung cancer after surgery and in acute lymphoblastic leukemia in remission [75,77]. Some studies also suggested miR-625 might suppress cell proliferation, migration and invasion, and identified a number of different miR-625 target genes [78–81]. Based on data from miRTarBase, these target genes were associated with miR-625-5p, suggesting these studies were investigating miR-625-5p and that there are important differences in the biological roles of these two miRNAs as they might regulate different pathways or be differentially regulated themselves. For example, different lncRNAs were identified as potential regulators of miR-625-3p or miR-625-5p expression [43,81,82]. Additionally, several isoforms of miR-625-3p with potentially differential expression were reported, but their role is not yet established [43].

We therefore tried to further elucidate the role of miR-625-3p using bioinformatic analysis. According to the miRTarBase database, 33 miR-625-3p targets were experimentally confirmed, and the interaction network revealed several interactions between them as well as some common interacting genes. However, *MAP2K6* was the only target confirmed with strong evidence. Mitogen-activated protein kinase kinase MAP2K6 is involved in p38 phosphorylation in response to stress and thus affects apoptosis and cell cycle [69]. Intrachromosomal rearrangements of this gene were previously observed in MM [83].

MAP2K6 was identified as a direct mediator of miR-625-3p associated oxaliplatin resistance in colorectal cancer [69], and it was proposed that miR-625-3p and *MAP2K6* could even be used to guide treatment selection [84]. Evaluation of *MAP2K6* expression would therefore also be of great interest in MM.

A number of other miR-625-3p target genes identified by bioinformatic analysis were previously implicated in MM or in response to asbestos, further confirming this miRNA might play an important role. For example, asbestos exposure was associated with modified expression of THRAP3 and PEG10 [85], XBP1 [86], TNIP1 and PLPP3 [87]. AKT1 and its signalling pathway were implicated in various processes in MM, including resistance to cisplatin [88]. ROCK2 was overexpressed in MM tumor tissue and implicated in the Hippo signalling pathway [89]. Additionally, HIF1A and hypoxia were also associated with MM, for example, with proliferation and inflammation as well as histological type [90].

Pathway enrichment analysis showed miR-625-3p target genes are involved in several different processes. In GO analysis, seven biological process terms were enriched, most significantly regulation of cell communication and regulation of signal transduction, while insulin-like growth factor II binding was the only significant molecular function term. Insulin-like growth factor II mRNA-binding protein 3 was already proposed as a biomarker for distinguishing between MM and benign mesothelial proliferations [91]. Identified miR-625-3p target genes were associated with five additional miRNAs, especially miR-1295b-3p; however, not much is known about this miRNA.

Interestingly, among two significant KEGG pathways, the most significant was PD-L1 expression and PD-1 checkpoint pathway in cancer. Immune checkpoint proteins programmed cell death protein (PD-1) and programmed cell death 1 ligand 1 (PD-L1) were extensively investigated in MM in the past few years due to their potential as targets in immunotherapy [11–13]. However, there is great interindividual variability in response to anti-PD-1 and anti-PD-L1 treatment, and the success of treatment with a single immune checkpoint inhibitor is limited [12]. Tumor PD-L1 expression is not a sufficient biomarker for identification of MM patients that could benefit from immunotherapy, and novel biomarkers are needed [12,13]. Importantly, PD-L1 expression was also identified in EVs [28], and EVs could therefore be a potential additional biomarker guiding immunotherapy personalization. Further studies investigating PD-L1 in EVs, also in combination with EV-enriched miR-625-3p, are therefore needed.

In our study, we also evaluated the potential biomarker role of EV-enriched miR-126-3p and miR-103-3p. Expression of EV-enriched miR-126-3p significantly increased only in MM patients with poor treatment outcome. However, the relative expression change after treatment was not associated with outcome or survival. Multiple studies identified miR-126-3p as a standalone or composite diagnostic biomarker that can discriminate between MM patients and controls, both in serum or plasma and in tissue samples [30,33–41], suggesting this miRNA has an important role in MM pathogenesis. Studies show that miR-126 plays a role in the regulation of mitochondrial metabolism, and is associated with oxidative stress, hypoxia and autophagy pathways [92,93]. However, miR-126-3p was not a suitable screening biomarker for early detection of MM in prediagnostic plasma samples [94]. Serum or tissue miR-126-3p expression was previously associated with shorter survival of MM patients [35,41], but this association was not confirmed in all studies [36,37]. Interestingly, miR-126 might be involved in cell communication, as exosomal transfer of miR-126 was associated with anti-tumor response and angiogenesis in MM cell lines [60]. On the other hand, EV-miR-126-3p expression did not differ among MM patients and controls [58]. Further studies focusing on change of miR-126-3p expression after treatment are therefore needed to better evaluate miR-126-3p as a prognostic biomarker in MM.

Serum EV-enriched miR-103-3p was not a good prognostic biomarker in MM in our study. So far, studies have shown miR-103-3p is downregulated, especially in cellular fraction of peripheral blood samples in MM patients compared to asbestos-exposed controls and was proposed as a diagnostic biomarker, standalone or in combination with mesothelin [30–33]. However, it did not enable early detection of MM in prediagnostic plasma samples [94]. In plasma EVs, miR-103-3p was downregulated compared to asbestos-exposed controls and the combination of miR-103a-3p and miR-30e-3p was the best diagnostic marker [58]. Patients with higher expression of EV-miR-103-3p tended to have longer overall survival, but the difference was not statistically significant [58]. However, expression change after treatment was not evaluated. Other studies did not investigate miR-103-3p as a potential prognostic biomarker in MM.

The vast majority of previous studies investigated circulating miRNAs, while we focused on miRNAs enriched in EVs. Previous studies suggested that miRNA in cancer-derived EVs might be a more suitable biomarker than circulating miRNAs, as EVs protect miRNAs from degradation. Additionally, EVs may be enriched with miRNAs reflecting their origin cell that are therefore more specific [95]. Furthermore, since miRNAs are often present in serum at very low concentrations, their EV-related enrichment in the sample can also improve sensitivity. On the other hand, enrichment of EVs from serum samples introduces an additional step in the miRNA-extraction protocol, which could present a drawback in larger studies or in clinical practice. Standardized methods for EV and miRNA extraction and the use of appropriate exogenous and endogenous controls for quality control and normalization are also needed to enable direct comparison between studies. Many different approaches for normalization of miRNA expression were previously proposed; however, there is still no universally accepted method of normalization for EVs-miRNAs, which can contribute to differences between studies [41,96–98]. It is also important to point out that our study did not focus exclusively on vesicle-enclosed miRNA, as miRNAs can also bind to the surface of EVs and we did not treat samples of isolated EVs with RNAse A prior to RNA extraction.

The main limitation of our study is the small sample size however, it was designed as a proof-of-concept study. Due to the strict inclusion criteria and quality-control exclusion criteria, we were nevertheless able to identify the most differentially expressed serum EV-enriched miRNAs. Furthermore, one of the key advantages of our study was its longitudinal design that enabled measurement of temporal changes in EV-miRNA expression after treatment. Still, studies including more MM patients are needed to validate our results and evaluate the usefulness of EV-enriched miR-625-3p in practical use in treatment prognosis in MM. Another limitation of our study is that no data on *BAP1* mutation status or other germline mutations were available. Inherited loss-of-function mutations in DNA repair genes or other tumor suppressor genes, especially *BAP1*, were associated with increased MM risk, but also improved survival, particularly following platinum-based chemotherapy [99–101]. In the future, evaluation of the combined effect of EV-enriched miRNA and germline mutations on survival could enable identification of better prognostic biomarkers. Additionally, even though previous studies showed that miRNAs miR-126-3p and miR-625-3p expression is deregulated in MM tumor tissue [33,35–38,40,42], studies evaluating EVs derived from MM tumor tissue are lacking. Further larger studies on EVs in MM, focusing also on biomarker combinations, are therefore needed to confirm our results.

5. Conclusions

Biological fluids are an ideal source for liquid biopsies, a complementary tool to traditional tissue biopsies that may aid in early disease discovery, monitoring of disease progression or success of the treatment [102,103]. Peripheral circulating venous blood is an easily accessible body fluid and still the most widely used source for biomarkers of a variety of the diseases, including different cancers [102,104,105]. However, differences in results and study design currently limit the translation of miRNA biomarkers to clinical practice. Our results and the results of other studies suggest EVs should also be considered as potential diagnostic or prognostic biomarkers in MM, especially in patients receiving platinum-based chemotherapy. Monitoring EV-enriched miR-625-3p expression might contribute to the prediction of treatment outcome and selection of therapy in MM patients, especially for subsequent lines of systemic treatment. For MM patients with predicted poor treatment outcome with platinum-based chemotherapy, novel systemic treatment approaches might be implemented sooner, while additional surgical treatment might be used for MM patients with predicted good treatment outcome. Additionally, EVs could in the future also be used in novel treatment approaches, for example, modulating miRNA expression [59,106].

In conclusion, serum EV-enriched miR-625-3p was associated with treatment outcome and survival of MM patients in our proof-of-concept study and might serve as a prognostic biomarker. EVs or their cargo might therefore contribute to a more personalized treatment that could improve the prognosis of MM patients.

Supplementary Materials: The following are available online at https://www.mdpi.com/article/10.3390/jpm11101014/s1, Figure S1: Comparison of expression of serum EV-enriched miRNAs at diagnosis and after treatment in each malignant mesothelioma patient in the whole study group (a: miR-625-3p, b: miR-103a-3p, c: miR-126-3p; dark blue: increased expression, light blue: decreased expression) and in each patient with poor treatment outcome (d: miR-625-3p, e: miR-103a-3p, f: miR-126-3p; dark green: increased expression, light green: decreased expression), Table S1: Expression of serum EV-enriched miRNAs and progression-free survival (PFS) and overall survival (OS) of malignant mesothelioma patients.

Author Contributions: Conceptualization, M.L. and V.D.; methodology, K.G., M.H., M.L. and V.D.; validation, K.G., M.H. and N.M.; formal analysis, K.G.; investigation, K.G., M.H., N.M. and V.K.; resources, V.K., M.L. and V.D.; writing—original draft preparation, K.G. and M.H.; writing—review and editing, K.G., M.H., N.M., V.K., M.L. and V.D.; visualization, K.G., M.H., N.M. and M.L.; supervision, V.K., M.L. and V.D.; project administration, K.G. and M.H.; funding acquisition, M.L. and V.D. All authors have read and agreed to the published version of the manuscript.

Funding: This study was funded by the Javna Agencija za Raziskovalno Dejavnost RS (Eng. Slovenian Research Agency) (ARRS), research grants P1-0170, L3-8203, L3-2622, and J3-9255.

Institutional Review Board Statement: The study was conducted according to the guidelines of the Declaration of Helsinki and approved by the Republic of Slovenia National Medical Ethics Committee (41/02/09, 07.03.2009).

Informed Consent Statement: Informed consent was obtained from all subjects involved in the study.

Data Availability Statement: All the data are presented within the article and in Supplementary Materials. Any additional information is available on request from the corresponding author.

Conflicts of Interest: The authors declare no conflict of interest. The funders had no role in the design of the study; in the collection, analyses, or interpretation of data; in the writing of the manuscript, or in the decision to publish the results.

References

1. Kovac, V.; Zwitter, M.; Zagar, T. Improved survival after introduction of chemotherapy for malignant pleural mesothelioma in Slovenia. Population-based survey of 444 patients. *Radiol. Oncol.* **2012**, *46*, 136–144. [CrossRef]
2. Chapman, S.J.; Cookson, W.O.; Musk, A.W.; Lee, Y.C. Benign asbestos pleural diseases. *Curr. Opin. Pulm. Med.* **2003**, *9*, 266–271. [CrossRef] [PubMed]
3. Lo Russo, G.; Tessari, A.; Capece, M.; Galli, G.; de Braud, F.; Garassino, M.C.; Palmieri, D. MicroRNAs for the diagnosis and management of malignant pleural mesothelioma: A literature review. *Front. Oncol.* **2018**, *8*, 650. [CrossRef]
4. Johnen, G.; Gawrych, K.; Raiko, I.; Casjens, S.; Pesch, B.; Weber, D.G.; Taeger, D.; Lehnert, M.; Kollmeier, J.; Bauer, T.; et al. Calretinin as a blood-based biomarker for mesothelioma. *BMC Cancer* **2017**, *17*, 386. [CrossRef] [PubMed]
5. Damhuis, R.A.; Schroten, C.; Burgers, J.A. Population-based survival for malignant mesothelioma after introduction of novel chemotherapy. *Eur. Respir. J.* **2012**, *40*, 185–189. [CrossRef]
6. Helland, A.; Solberg, S.; Brustugun, O.T. Incidence and survival of malignant pleural mesothelioma in Norway: A population-based study of 1686 cases. *J. Thorac. Oncol.* **2012**, *7*, 1858–1861. [CrossRef]
7. Vogelzang, N.J.; Rusthoven, J.J.; Symanowski, J.; Denham, C.; Kaukel, E.; Ruffie, P.; Gatzemeier, U.; Boyer, M.; Emri, S.; Manegold, C.; et al. Phase III study of pemetrexed in combination with cisplatin versus cisplatin alone in patients with malignant pleural mesothelioma. *J. Clin. Oncol.* **2003**, *21*, 2636–2644. [CrossRef]
8. Kovac, V.; Zwitter, M.; Rajer, M.; Marin, A.; Debeljak, A.; Smrdel, U.; Vrankar, M. A phase II trial of low-dose gemcitabine in a prolonged infusion and cisplatin for malignant pleural mesothelioma. *Anticancer Drugs* **2012**, *23*, 230–238. [CrossRef] [PubMed]
9. Lee, C.W.; Murray, N.; Anderson, H.; Rao, S.C.; Bishop, W. Outcomes with first-line platinum-based combination chemotherapy for malignant pleural mesothelioma: A review of practice in British Columbia. *Lung Cancer* **2009**, *64*, 308–313. [CrossRef]

10. Ak, G.; Metintas, S.; Akarsu, M.; Metintas, M. The effectiveness and safety of platinum-based pemetrexed and platinum-based gemcitabine treatment in patients with malignant pleural mesothelioma. *BMC Cancer* **2015**, *15*, 510. [CrossRef] [PubMed]
11. Gray, S.G.; Mutti, L. Immunotherapy for mesothelioma: A critical review of current clinical trials and future perspectives. *Transl. Lung Cancer Res.* **2020**, *9*, S100–S119. [CrossRef]
12. De Gooijer, C.J.; Borm, F.J.; Scherpereel, A.; Baas, P. Immunotherapy in malignant pleural mesothelioma. *Front. Oncol.* **2020**, *10*, 187. [CrossRef]
13. Cantini, L.; Hassan, R.; Sterman, D.H.; Aerts, J. Emerging treatments for malignant pleural mesothelioma: Where are we heading? *Front. Oncol.* **2020**, *10*, 343. [CrossRef]
14. Baas, P.; Scherpereel, A.; Nowak, A.K.; Fujimoto, N.; Peters, S.; Tsao, A.S.; Mansfield, A.S.; Popat, S.; Jahan, T.; Antonia, S.; et al. First-line nivolumab plus ipilimumab in unresectable malignant pleural mesothelioma (CheckMate 743): A multicentre, randomised, open-label, phase 3 trial. *Lancet* **2021**, *397*, 375–386. [CrossRef]
15. Creaney, J.; Olsen, N.J.; Brims, F.; Dick, I.M.; Musk, A.W.; de Klerk, N.H.; Skates, S.J.; Robinson, B.W. Serum mesothelin for early detection of asbestos-induced cancer malignant mesothelioma. *Cancer Epidemiol. Biomark. Prev.* **2010**, *19*, 2238–2246. [CrossRef]
16. Hollevoet, K.; Reitsma, J.B.; Creaney, J.; Grigoriu, B.D.; Robinson, B.W.; Scherpereel, A.; Cristaudo, A.; Pass, H.I.; Nackaerts, K.; Rodriguez Portal, J.A.; et al. Serum mesothelin for diagnosing malignant pleural mesothelioma: An individual patient data meta-analysis. *J. Clin. Oncol.* **2012**, *30*, 1541–1549. [CrossRef]
17. Hollevoet, K.; van Cleemput, J.; Thimpont, J.; de Vuyst, P.; Bosquee, L.; Nackaerts, K.; Germonpre, P.; Vansteelandt, S.; Kishi, Y.; Delanghe, J.R.; et al. Serial measurements of mesothelioma serum biomarkers in asbestos-exposed individuals: A prospective longitudinal cohort study. *J. Thorac. Oncol.* **2011**, *6*, 889–895. [CrossRef] [PubMed]
18. Gillezeau, C.; van Gerwen, M.; Ramos, J.; Liu, B.; Flores, R.; Taioli, E. Biomarkers for malignant pleural mesothelioma: A meta-analysis. *Carcinogenesis* **2019**, *40*, 1320–1331. [CrossRef]
19. Foddis, R.; Bonotti, A.; Landi, S.; Fallahi, P.; Guglielmi, G.; Cristaudo, A. Biomarkers in the prevention and follow-up of workers exposed to asbestos. *J. Thorac. Dis.* **2018**, *10*, S360–S368. [CrossRef] [PubMed]
20. Cristaudo, A.; Bonotti, A.; Guglielmi, G.; Fallahi, P.; Foddis, R. Serum mesothelin and other biomarkers: What have we learned in the last decade? *J. Thorac. Dis.* **2018**, *10*, S353–S359. [CrossRef] [PubMed]
21. Cavallari, I.; Urso, L.; Sharova, E.; Pasello, G.; Ciminale, V. Liquid biopsy in malignant pleural mesothelioma: State of the art, pitfalls, and perspectives. *Front. Oncol.* **2019**, *9*, 740. [CrossRef] [PubMed]
22. Cristaudo, A.; Foddis, R.; Bonotti, A.; Simonini, S.; Vivaldi, A.; Guglielmi, G.; Bruno, R.; Gemignani, F.; Landi, S. Two novel polymorphisms in 5′ flanking region of the mesothelin gene are associated with soluble mesothelin-related peptide (SMRP) levels. *Int. J. Biol. Markers* **2011**, *26*, 117–123. [CrossRef]
23. Garritano, S.; de Santi, C.; Silvestri, R.; Melaiu, O.; Cipollini, M.; Barone, E.; Lucchi, M.; Barale, R.; Mutti, L.; Gemignani, F.; et al. A common polymorphism within MSLN affects miR-611 binding site and soluble mesothelin levels in healthy people. *J. Thorac. Oncol.* **2014**, *9*, 1662–1668. [CrossRef]
24. De Santi, C.; Pucci, P.; Bonotti, A.; Melaiu, O.; Cipollini, M.; Silvestri, R.; Vymetalkova, V.; Barone, E.; Paolicchi, E.; Corrado, A.; et al. Mesothelin promoter variants are associated with increased soluble mesothelin-related peptide levels in asbestos-exposed individuals. *Occup. Environ. Med.* **2017**, *74*, 456–463. [CrossRef] [PubMed]
25. Goricar, K.; Kovac, V.; Dodic-Fikfak, M.; Dolzan, V.; Franko, A. Evaluation of soluble mesothelin-related peptides and MSLN genetic variability in asbestos-related diseases. *Radiol. Oncol.* **2020**, *54*, 86–95. [CrossRef]
26. Tian, L.; Zeng, R.; Wang, X.; Shen, C.; Lai, Y.; Wang, M.; Che, G. Prognostic significance of soluble mesothelin in malignant pleural mesothelioma: A meta-analysis. *Oncotarget* **2017**, *8*, 46425–46435. [CrossRef]
27. Goricar, K.; Kovac, V.; Dolzan, V. Clinical-pharmacogenetic models for personalized cancer treatment: Application to malignant mesothelioma. *Sci. Rep.* **2017**, *7*, 46537. [CrossRef]
28. Ahmadzada, T.; Kao, S.; Reid, G.; Clarke, S.; Grau, G.E.; Hosseini-Beheshti, E. Extracellular vesicles as biomarkers in malignant pleural mesothelioma: A review. *Crit. Rev. Oncol. Hematol.* **2020**, *150*, 102949. [CrossRef]
29. Tomasetti, M.; Gaetani, S.; Monaco, F.; Neuzil, J.; Santarelli, L. Epigenetic regulation of miRNA expression in malignant mesothelioma: miRNAs as biomarkers of early diagnosis and therapy. *Front. Oncol.* **2019**, *9*, 1293. [CrossRef]
30. Micolucci, L.; Akhtar, M.M.; Olivieri, F.; Rippo, M.R.; Procopio, A.D. Diagnostic value of microRNAs in asbestos exposure and malignant mesothelioma: Systematic review and qualitative meta-analysis. *Oncotarget* **2016**, *7*, 58606–58637. [CrossRef] [PubMed]
31. Weber, D.G.; Johnen, G.; Bryk, O.; Jöckel, K.H.; Brüning, T. Identification of miRNA-103 in the cellular fraction of human peripheral blood as a potential biomarker for malignant mesothelioma—A pilot study. *PLoS ONE* **2012**, *7*, e30221. [CrossRef] [PubMed]
32. Weber, D.G.; Casjens, S.; Johnen, G.; Bryk, O.; Raiko, I.; Pesch, B.; Kollmeier, J.; Bauer, T.T.; Brüning, T. Combination of MiR-103a-3p and mesothelin improves the biomarker performance of malignant mesothelioma diagnosis. *PLoS ONE* **2014**, *9*, e114483. [CrossRef]
33. Cappellesso, R.; Nicolè, L.; Caroccia, B.; Guzzardo, V.; Ventura, L.; Fassan, M.; Fassina, A. Young investigator challenge: MicroRNA-21/MicroRNA-126 profiling as a novel tool for the diagnosis of malignant mesothelioma in pleural effusion cytology. *Cancer Cytopathol.* **2016**, *124*, 28–37. [CrossRef] [PubMed]

34. Weber, D.G.; Gawrych, K.; Casjens, S.; Brik, A.; Lehnert, M.; Taeger, D.; Pesch, B.; Kollmeier, J.; Bauer, T.T.; Johnen, G.; et al. Circulating miR-132-3p as a Candidate Diagnostic Biomarker for Malignant Mesothelioma. *Dis. Markers* **2017**, *2017*, 9280170. [CrossRef] [PubMed]
35. Andersen, M.; Grauslund, M.; Ravn, J.; Sørensen, J.B.; Andersen, C.B.; Santoni-Rugiu, E. Diagnostic potential of miR-126, miR-143, miR-145, and miR-652 in malignant pleural mesothelioma. *J. Mol. Diagn.* **2014**, *16*, 418–430. [CrossRef]
36. De Santi, C.; Melaiu, O.; Bonotti, A.; Cascione, L.; di Leva, G.; Foddis, R.; Cristaudo, A.; Lucchi, M.; Mora, M.; Truini, A.; et al. Deregulation of miRNAs in malignant pleural mesothelioma is associated with prognosis and suggests an alteration of cell metabolism. *Sci. Rep.* **2017**, *7*, 3140. [CrossRef]
37. Mozzoni, P.; Ampollini, L.; Goldoni, M.; Alinovi, R.; Tiseo, M.; Gnetti, L.; Carbognani, P.; Rusca, M.; Mutti, A.; Percesepe, A.; et al. MicroRNA expression in malignant pleural mesothelioma and asbestosis: A pilot study. *Dis. Markers* **2017**, *2017*, 9645940. [CrossRef]
38. Santarelli, L.; Gaetani, S.; Monaco, F.; Bracci, M.; Valentino, M.; Amati, M.; Rubini, C.; Sabbatini, A.; Pasquini, E.; Zanotta, N.; et al. Four-miRNA signature to identify asbestos-related lung malignancies. *Cancer Epidemiol. Biomark. Prev.* **2019**, *28*, 119–126. [CrossRef]
39. Santarelli, L.; Staffolani, S.; Strafella, E.; Nocchi, L.; Manzella, N.; Grossi, P.; Bracci, M.; Pignotti, E.; Alleva, R.; Borghi, B.; et al. Combined circulating epigenetic markers to improve mesothelin performance in the diagnosis of malignant mesothelioma. *Lung Cancer* **2015**, *90*, 457–464. [CrossRef]
40. Santarelli, L.; Strafella, E.; Staffolani, S.; Amati, M.; Emanuelli, M.; Sartini, D.; Pozzi, V.; Carbonari, D.; Bracci, M.; Pignotti, E.; et al. Association of MiR-126 with soluble mesothelin-related peptides, a marker for malignant mesothelioma. *PLoS ONE* **2011**, *6*, e18232. [CrossRef]
41. Tomasetti, M.; Staffolani, S.; Nocchi, L.; Neuzil, J.; Strafella, E.; Manzella, N.; Mariotti, L.; Bracci, M.; Valentino, M.; Amati, M.; et al. Clinical significance of circulating miR-126 quantification in malignant mesothelioma patients. *Clin. Biochem.* **2012**, *45*, 575–581. [CrossRef]
42. Kirschner, M.B.; Cheng, Y.Y.; Badrian, B.; Kao, S.C.; Creaney, J.; Edelman, J.J.; Armstrong, N.J.; Vallely, M.P.; Musk, A.W.; Robinson, B.W.; et al. Increased circulating miR-625-3p: A potential biomarker for patients with malignant pleural mesothelioma. *J. Thorac. Oncol.* **2012**, *7*, 1184–1191. [CrossRef] [PubMed]
43. Kresoja-Rakic, J.; Szpechcinski, A.; Kirschner, M.B.; Ronner, M.; Minatel, B.; Martinez, V.D.; Lam, W.L.; Weder, W.; Stahel, R.; Früh, M.; et al. miR-625-3p and lncRNA GAS5 in liquid biopsies for predicting the outcome of malignant pleural mesothelioma patients treated with neo-adjuvant chemotherapy and surgery. *Non-coding RNA* **2019**, *5*, 41. [CrossRef] [PubMed]
44. Karimi, N.; Cvjetkovic, A.; Jang, S.C.; Crescitelli, R.; Hosseinpour Feizi, M.A.; Nieuwland, R.; Lotvall, J.; Lasser, C. Detailed analysis of the plasma extracellular vesicle proteome after separation from lipoproteins. *Cell. Mol. Life Sci.* **2018**, *75*, 2873–2886. [CrossRef]
45. Zaborowski, M.P.; Balaj, L.; Breakefield, X.O.; Lai, C.P. Extracellular vesicles: Composition, biological relevance, and methods of study. *Bioscience* **2015**, *65*, 783–797. [CrossRef]
46. Chen, J.; Xu, Y.; Wang, X.; Liu, D.; Yang, F.; Zhu, X.; Lu, Y.; Xing, W. Rapid and efficient isolation and detection of extracellular vesicles from plasma for lung cancer diagnosis. *Lab Chip* **2019**, *19*, 432–443. [CrossRef]
47. Mateescu, B.; Kowal, E.J.; van Balkom, B.W.; Bartel, S.; Bhattacharyya, S.N.; Buzas, E.I.; Buck, A.H.; de Candia, P.; Chow, F.W.; Das, S.; et al. Obstacles and opportunities in the functional analysis of extracellular vesicle RNA—An ISEV position paper. *J. Extracell. Vesicles* **2017**, *6*, 1286095. [CrossRef] [PubMed]
48. Huang, K.; Fang, C.; Yi, K.; Liu, X.; Qi, H.; Tan, Y.; Zhou, J.; Li, Y.; Liu, M.; Zhang, Y.; et al. The role of PTRF/Cavin1 as a biomarker in both glioma and serum exosomes. *Theranostics* **2018**, *8*, 1540–1557. [CrossRef] [PubMed]
49. Navarro, A.; Molins, L.; Marrades, R.M.; Moises, J.; Viñolas, N.; Morales, S.; Canals, J.; Castellano, J.J.; Ramírez, J.; Monzo, M. Exosome analysis in tumor-draining pulmonary vein identifies NSCLC patients with higher risk of relapse after curative surgery. *Cancers* **2019**, *11*, 249. [CrossRef]
50. Silva, J.; Garcia, V.; Rodriguez, M.; Compte, M.; Cisneros, E.; Veguillas, P.; Garcia, J.M.; Dominguez, G.; Campos-Martin, Y.; Cuevas, J.; et al. Analysis of exosome release and its prognostic value in human colorectal cancer. *Genes Chromosomes Cancer* **2012**, *51*, 409–418. [CrossRef] [PubMed]
51. Vasconcelos, M.H.; Caires, H.R.; Ābols, A.; Xavier, C.P.R.; Linē, A. Extracellular vesicles as a novel source of biomarkers in liquid biopsies for monitoring cancer progression and drug resistance. *Drug Resist. Updates* **2019**, *47*, 100647. [CrossRef] [PubMed]
52. Chang, W.H.; Cerione, R.A.; Antonyak, M.A. Extracellular vesicles and their roles in cancer progression. *Methods Mol. Biol.* **2021**, *2174*, 143–170. [CrossRef]
53. Chiam, K.; Mayne, G.C.; Wang, T.; Watson, D.I.; Irvine, T.S.; Bright, T.; Smith, L.T.; Ball, I.A.; Bowen, J.M.; Keefe, D.M.; et al. Serum outperforms plasma in small extracellular vesicle microRNA biomarker studies of adenocarcinoma of the esophagus. *World J. Gastroenterol.* **2020**, *26*, 2570–2583. [CrossRef]
54. Grange, C.; Brossa, A.; Bussolati, B. Extracellular vesicles and carried miRNAs in the progression of renal cell carcinoma. *Int. J. Mol. Sci.* **2019**, *20*, 1832. [CrossRef] [PubMed]
55. Greening, D.W.; Ji, H.; Chen, M.; Robinson, B.W.; Dick, I.M.; Creaney, J.; Simpson, R.J. Secreted primary human malignant mesothelioma exosome signature reflects oncogenic cargo. *Sci. Rep.* **2016**, *6*, 32643. [CrossRef] [PubMed]

56. Creaney, J.; Dick, I.M.; Leon, J.S.; Robinson, B.W. A proteomic analysis of the malignant mesothelioma secretome using iTRAQ. *Cancer Genom. Proteom.* **2017**, *14*, 103–117. [CrossRef]
57. Munson, P.; Lam, Y.W.; Dragon, J.; MacPherson, M.; Shukla, A. Exosomes from asbestos-exposed cells modulate gene expression in mesothelial cells. *FASEB J.* **2018**, *32*, 4328–4342. [CrossRef]
58. Cavalleri, T.; Angelici, L.; Favero, C.; Dioni, L.; Mensi, C.; Bareggi, C.; Palleschi, A.; Rimessi, A.; Consonni, D.; Bordini, L.; et al. Plasmatic extracellular vesicle microRNAs in malignant pleural mesothelioma and asbestos-exposed subjects suggest a 2-miRNA signature as potential biomarker of disease. *PLoS ONE* **2017**, *12*, e0176680. [CrossRef]
59. Munson, P.B.; Hall, E.M.; Farina, N.H.; Pass, H.I.; Shukla, A. Exosomal miR-16-5p as a target for malignant mesothelioma. *Sci. Rep.* **2019**, *9*, 11688. [CrossRef]
60. Monaco, F.; Gaetani, S.; Alessandrini, F.; Tagliabracci, A.; Bracci, M.; Valentino, M.; Neuzil, J.; Amati, M.; Bovenzi, M.; Tomasetti, M.; et al. Exosomal transfer of miR-126 promotes the anti-tumour response in malignant mesothelioma: Role of miR-126 in cancer-stroma communication. *Cancer Lett.* **2019**, *463*, 27–36. [CrossRef]
61. Holcar, M.; Ferdin, J.; Sitar, S.; Tušek-Žnidarič, M.; Dolžan, V.; Plemenitaš, A.; Žagar, E.; Lenassi, M. Enrichment of plasma extracellular vesicles for reliable quantification of their size and concentration for biomarker discovery. *Sci. Rep.* **2020**, *10*, 21346. [CrossRef]
62. Blondal, T.; Jensby Nielsen, S.; Baker, A.; Andreasen, D.; Mouritzen, P.; Wrang Teilum, M.; Dahlsveen, I.K. Assessing sample and miRNA profile quality in serum and plasma or other biofluids. *Methods* **2013**, *59*, S1–S6. [CrossRef] [PubMed]
63. Donati, S.; Ciuffi, S.; Brandi, M.L. Human circulating miRNAs real-time qRT-PCR-based analysis: An Overview of endogenous reference genes used for data normalization. *Int. J. Mol. Sci.* **2019**, *20*, 4353. [CrossRef] [PubMed]
64. Shen, J.; Wang, Q.; Gurvich, I.; Remotti, H.; Santella, R.M. Evaluating normalization approaches for the better identification of aberrant microRNAs associated with hepatocellular carcinoma. *Hepatoma Res.* **2016**, *2*, 305–315. [CrossRef]
65. Huang, H.Y.; Lin, Y.C.; Li, J.; Huang, K.Y.; Shrestha, S.; Hong, H.C.; Tang, Y.; Chen, Y.G.; Jin, C.N.; Yu, Y.; et al. miRTarBase 2020: Updates to the experimentally validated microRNA-target interaction database. *Nucleic Acids Res.* **2020**, *48*, D148–D154. [CrossRef]
66. Warde-Farley, D.; Donaldson, S.L.; Comes, O.; Zuberi, K.; Badrawi, R.; Chao, P.; Franz, M.; Grouios, C.; Kazi, F.; Lopes, C.T.; et al. The GeneMANIA prediction server: Biological network integration for gene prioritization and predicting gene function. *Nucleic Acids Res.* **2010**, *38*, W214–W220. [CrossRef]
67. Raudvere, U.; Kolberg, L.; Kuzmin, I.; Arak, T.; Adler, P.; Peterson, H.; Vilo, J.G. Profiler: A web server for functional enrichment analysis and conversions of gene lists (2019 update). *Nucleic Acids Res.* **2019**, *47*, W191–W198. [CrossRef]
68. Rasmussen, M.H.; Jensen, N.F.; Tarpgaard, L.S.; Qvortrup, C.; Rømer, M.U.; Stenvang, J.; Hansen, T.P.; Christensen, L.L.; Lindebjerg, J.; Hansen, F.; et al. High expression of microRNA-625-3p is associated with poor response to first-line oxaliplatin based treatment of metastatic colorectal cancer. *Mol. Oncol.* **2013**, *7*, 637–646. [CrossRef] [PubMed]
69. Rasmussen, M.H.; Lyskjær, I.; Jersie-Christensen, R.R.; Tarpgaard, L.S.; Primdal-Bengtson, B.; Nielsen, M.M.; Pedersen, J.S.; Hansen, T.P.; Hansen, F.; Olsen, J.V.; et al. miR-625-3p regulates oxaliplatin resistance by targeting MAP2K6-p38 signalling in human colorectal adenocarcinoma cells. *Nat. Commun.* **2016**, *7*, 12436. [CrossRef] [PubMed]
70. Okumura, T.; Shimada, Y.; Omura, T.; Hirano, K.; Nagata, T.; Tsukada, K. MicroRNA profiles to predict postoperative prognosis in patients with small cell carcinoma of the esophagus. *Anticancer Res.* **2015**, *35*, 719–727.
71. Fang, L.; Kong, D.; Xu, W. MicroRNA-625-3p promotes the proliferation, migration and invasion of thyroid cancer cells by up-regulating astrocyte elevated gene 1. *Biomed. Pharmacother.* **2018**, *102*, 203–211. [CrossRef]
72. Zhao, L.; Liu, K.; Pan, X.; Quan, J.; Zhou, L.; Li, Z.; Lin, C.; Xu, J.; Xu, W.; Guan, X.; et al. miR-625-3p promotes migration and invasion and reduces apoptosis of clear cell renal cell carcinoma. *Am. J. Transl. Res.* **2019**, *11*, 6475–6486.
73. Zheng, H.; Ma, R.; Wang, Q.; Zhang, P.; Li, D.; Wang, Q.; Wang, J.; Li, H.; Liu, H.; Wang, Z. MiR-625-3p promotes cell migration and invasion via inhibition of SCAI in colorectal carcinoma cells. *Oncotarget* **2015**, *6*, 27805–27815. [CrossRef]
74. Li, C.; Li, D.C.; Che, S.S.; Ma, K.; Wang, Y.J.; Xia, L.H.; Dai, X.M.; Zhang, G.T.; Shen, Y.; Jiao, W.J.; et al. The decreased expression of miR-625 predicts poor prognosis of esophageal squamous cell carcinoma. *Int. J. Clin. Exp. Med.* **2015**, *8*, 9560–9564. [PubMed]
75. Roth, C.; Stückrath, I.; Pantel, K.; Izbicki, J.R.; Tachezy, M.; Schwarzenbach, H. Low levels of cell-free circulating miR-361-3p and miR-625* as blood-based markers for discriminating malignant from benign lung tumors. *PLoS ONE* **2012**, *7*, e38248. [CrossRef] [PubMed]
76. Lou, X.; Qi, X.; Zhang, Y.; Long, H.; Yang, J. Decreased expression of microRNA-625 is associated with tumor metastasis and poor prognosis in patients with colorectal cancer. *J. Surg. Oncol.* **2013**, *108*, 230–235. [CrossRef] [PubMed]
77. Jiang, Q.; Lu, X.; Huang, P.; Gao, C.; Zhao, X.; Xing, T.; Li, G.; Bao, S.; Zheng, H. Expression of miR-652-3p and effect on apoptosis and drug sensitivity in pediatric acute lymphoblastic leukemia. *BioMed Res. Int.* **2018**, *2018*, 5724686. [CrossRef]
78. Zhou, X.; Zhang, C.Z.; Lu, S.X.; Chen, G.G.; Li, L.Z.; Liu, L.L.; Yi, C.; Fu, J.; Hu, W.; Wen, J.M.; et al. miR-625 suppresses tumour migration and invasion by targeting IGF2BP1 in hepatocellular carcinoma. *Oncogene* **2015**, *34*, 965–977. [CrossRef]
79. Fang, W.; Fan, Y.; Fa, Z.; Xu, J.; Yu, H.; Li, P.; Gu, J. microRNA-625 inhibits tumorigenicity by suppressing proliferation, migration and invasion in malignant melanoma. *Oncotarget* **2017**, *8*, 13253–13263. [CrossRef] [PubMed]
80. Wang, M.; Li, C.; Nie, H.; Lv, X.; Qu, Y.; Yu, B.; Su, L.; Li, J.; Chen, X.; Ju, J.; et al. Down-regulated miR-625 suppresses invasion and metastasis of gastric cancer by targeting ILK. *FEBS Lett.* **2012**, *586*, 2382–2388. [CrossRef] [PubMed]

81. Zhao, F.; Fang, T.; Liu, H.; Wang, S. Long non-coding RNA MALAT1 promotes cell proliferation, migration and invasion in cervical cancer by targeting miR-625-5p and AKT2. *Panminerva Med.* **2020**. [CrossRef]
82. Chen, Z.; Wu, H.; Zhang, Z.; Li, G.; Liu, B. LINC00511 accelerated the process of gastric cancer by targeting miR-625-5p/NFIX axis. *Cancer Cell Int.* **2019**, *19*, 351. [CrossRef]
83. Bueno, R.; de Rienzo, A.; Dong, L.; Gordon, G.J.; Hercus, C.F.; Richards, W.G.; Jensen, R.V.; Anwar, A.; Maulik, G.; Chirieac, L.R.; et al. Second generation sequencing of the mesothelioma tumor genome. *PLoS ONE* **2010**, *5*, e10612. [CrossRef]
84. Lyskjær, I.; Rasmussen, M.H.; Andersen, C.L. Putting a brake on stress signaling: miR-625-3p as a biomarker for choice of therapy in colorectal cancer. *Epigenomics* **2016**, *8*, 1449–1452. [CrossRef] [PubMed]
85. Nymark, P.; Lindholm, P.M.; Korpela, M.V.; Lahti, L.; Ruosaari, S.; Kaski, S.; Hollmén, J.; Anttila, S.; Kinnula, V.L.; Knuutila, S. Gene expression profiles in asbestos-exposed epithelial and mesothelial lung cell lines. *BMC Genom.* **2007**, *8*, 62. [CrossRef] [PubMed]
86. Kamp, D.W.; Liu, G.; Cheresh, P.; Kim, S.J.; Mueller, A.; Lam, A.P.; Trejo, H.; Williams, D.; Tulasiram, S.; Baker, M.; et al. Asbestos-induced alveolar epithelial cell apoptosis. The role of endoplasmic reticulum stress response. *Am. J. Respir. Cell Mol. Biol.* **2013**, *49*, 892–901. [CrossRef]
87. Qi, F.; Okimoto, G.; Jube, S.; Napolitano, A.; Pass, H.I.; Laczko, R.; Demay, R.M.; Khan, G.; Tiirikainen, M.; Rinaudo, C.; et al. Continuous exposure to chrysotile asbestos can cause transformation of human mesothelial cells via HMGB1 and TNF-α signaling. *Am. J. Pathol.* **2013**, *183*, 1654–1666. [CrossRef]
88. Borchert, S.; Suckrau, P.M.; Wessolly, M.; Mairinger, E.; Hegedus, B.; Hager, T.; Herold, T.; Eberhardt, W.E.E.; Wohlschlaeger, J.; Aigner, C.; et al. Screening of pleural mesothelioma cell lines for kinase activity may identify new mechanisms of therapy resistance in patients receiving platin-based chemotherapy. *J. Oncol.* **2019**, *2019*, 2902985. [CrossRef]
89. Zhang, W.Q.; Dai, Y.Y.; Hsu, P.C.; Wang, H.; Cheng, L.; Yang, Y.L.; Wang, Y.C.; Xu, Z.D.; Liu, S.; Chan, G.; et al. Targeting YAP in malignant pleural mesothelioma. *J. Cell. Mol. Med.* **2017**, *21*, 2663–2676. [CrossRef]
90. Pasello, G.; Urso, L.; Mencoboni, M.; Grosso, F.; Ceresoli, G.L.; Lunardi, F.; Vuljan, S.E.; Bertorelle, R.; Sacchetto, V.; Ciminale, V.; et al. MDM2 and HIF1alpha expression levels in different histologic subtypes of malignant pleural mesothelioma: Correlation with pathological and clinical data. *Oncotarget* **2015**, *6*, 42053–42066. [CrossRef] [PubMed]
91. Chang, S.; Oh, M.H.; Ji, S.Y.; Han, J.; Kim, T.J.; Eom, M.; Kwon, K.Y.; Ha, S.Y.; Choi, Y.D.; Lee, C.H.; et al. Practical utility of insulin-like growth factor II mRNA-binding protein 3, glucose transporter 1, and epithelial membrane antigen for distinguishing malignant mesotheliomas from benign mesothelial proliferations. *Pathol. Int.* **2014**, *64*, 607–612. [CrossRef]
92. Tomasetti, M.; Nocchi, L.; Staffolani, S.; Manzella, N.; Amati, M.; Goodwin, J.; Kluckova, K.; Nguyen, M.; Strafella, E.; Bajzikova, M.; et al. MicroRNA-126 suppresses mesothelioma malignancy by targeting IRS1 and interfering with the mitochondrial function. *Antioxid. Redox Signal.* **2014**, *21*, 2109–2125. [CrossRef] [PubMed]
93. Tomasetti, M.; Monaco, F.; Manzella, N.; Rohlena, J.; Rohlenova, K.; Staffolani, S.; Gaetani, S.; Ciarapica, V.; Amati, M.; Bracci, M.; et al. MicroRNA-126 induces autophagy by altering cell metabolism in malignant mesothelioma. *Oncotarget* **2016**, *7*, 36338–36352. [CrossRef] [PubMed]
94. Weber, D.G.; Brik, A.; Casjens, S.; Burek, K.; Lehnert, M.; Pesch, B.; Taeger, D.; Brüning, T.; Johnen, G. Are circulating microRNAs suitable for the early detection of malignant mesothelioma? Results from a nested case-control study. *BMC Res. Notes* **2019**, *12*, 77. [CrossRef]
95. Endzelinš, E.; Berger, A.; Melne, V.; Bajo-Santos, C.; Soboļevska, K.; Ābols, A.; Rodriguez, M.; Šantare, D.; Rudņickiha, A.; Lietuvietis, V.; et al. Detection of circulating miRNAs: Comparative analysis of extracellular vesicle-incorporated miRNAs and cell-free miRNAs in whole plasma of prostate cancer patients. *BMC Cancer* **2017**, *17*, 730. [CrossRef]
96. Dai, Y.; Cao, Y.; Kohler, J.; Lu, A.; Xu, S.; Wang, H. Unbiased RNA-Seq-driven identification and validation of reference genes for quantitative RT-PCR analyses of pooled cancer exosomes. *BMC Genom.* **2021**, *22*, 27. [CrossRef]
97. Gouin, K.; Peck, K.; Antes, T.; Johnson, J.L.; Li, C.; Vaturi, S.D.; Middleton, R.; de Couto, G.; Walravens, A.S.; Rodriguez-Borlado, L.; et al. A comprehensive method for identification of suitable reference genes in extracellular vesicles. *J. Extracell. Vesicles* **2017**, *6*, 1347019. [CrossRef]
98. Grimolizzi, F.; Monaco, F.; Leoni, F.; Bracci, M.; Staffolani, S.; Bersaglieri, C.; Gaetani, S.; Valentino, M.; Amati, M.; Rubini, C.; et al. Exosomal miR-126 as a circulating biomarker in non-small-cell lung cancer regulating cancer progression. *Sci. Rep.* **2017**, *7*, 15277. [CrossRef] [PubMed]
99. Hassan, R.; Morrow, B.; Thomas, A.; Walsh, T.; Lee, M.K.; Gulsuner, S.; Gadiraju, M.; Panou, V.; Gao, S.; Mian, I.; et al. Inherited predisposition to malignant mesothelioma and overall survival following platinum chemotherapy. *Proc. Natl. Acad. Sci. USA* **2019**, *116*, 9008–9013. [CrossRef] [PubMed]
100. Baumann, F.; Flores, E.; Napolitano, A.; Kanodia, S.; Taioli, E.; Pass, H.; Yang, H.; Carbone, M. Mesothelioma patients with germline BAP1 mutations have 7-fold improved long-term survival. *Carcinogenesis* **2015**, *36*, 76–81. [CrossRef]
101. Carbone, M.; Adusumilli, P.S.; Alexander, H.R., Jr.; Baas, P.; Bardelli, F.; Bononi, A.; Bueno, R.; Felley-Bosco, E.; Galateau-Salle, F.; Jablons, D.; et al. Mesothelioma: Scientific clues for prevention, diagnosis, and therapy. *CA Cancer J. Clin.* **2019**, *69*, 402–429. [CrossRef]
102. Bracht, J.W.P.; Mayo-de-Las-Casas, C.; Berenguer, J.; Karachaliou, N.; Rosell, R. The present and future of liquid biopsies in non-small cell lung cancer: Combining four biosources for diagnosis, prognosis, prediction, and disease monitoring. *Curr. Oncol. Rep.* **2018**, *20*, 70. [CrossRef]

103. Morrison, G.J.; Goldkorn, A. Development and Application of liquid biopsies in metastatic prostate cancer. *Curr. Oncol. Rep.* **2018**, *20*, 35. [CrossRef]
104. Gonzalez, E.; Falcon-Perez, J.M. Cell-derived extracellular vesicles as a platform to identify low-invasive disease biomarkers. *Expert Rev. Mol. Diagn.* **2015**, *15*, 907–923. [CrossRef] [PubMed]
105. Witwer, K.W.; Buzas, E.I.; Bemis, L.T.; Bora, A.; Lasser, C.; Lotvall, J.; Nolte-'t Hoen, E.N.; Piper, M.G.; Sivaraman, S.; Skog, J.; et al. Standardization of sample collection, isolation and analysis methods in extracellular vesicle research. *J. Extracell. Vesicles* **2013**, *2*, 20360. [CrossRef] [PubMed]
106. Reid, G.; Johnson, T.G.; van Zandwijk, N. Manipulating microRNAs for the Treatment of Malignant Pleural Mesothelioma: Past, Present and Future. *Front. Oncol.* **2020**, *10*, 105. [CrossRef] [PubMed]

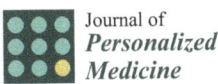

Article

Identification by MicroRNA Analysis of Environmental Risk Factors Bearing Pathogenic Relevance in Non-Smoker Lung Cancer

Alberto Izzotti [1,2], Gabriela Coronel Vargas [3], Alessandra Pulliero [3], Simona Coco [4], Cristina Colarossi [5], Giuseppina Blanco [5], Antonella Agodi [6], Martina Barchitta [6], Andrea Maugeri [6], CT-ME-EN Cancer Registry Workers [7,†], Gea Oliveri Conti [6,*], Margherita Ferrante [6,7] and Salvatore Sciacca [5]

1. Department of Experimental Medicine, University of Genoa, 16132 Genoa, Italy; izzotti@unige.it
2. UOC Mutagenesis and Cancer Prevention, IRCCS San Martino Hospital, 16132 Genova, Italy
3. Department of Health Sciences, University of Genoa, 16132 Genoa, Italy; gabrielafernanda.coronelvargas@edu.unige.it (G.C.V.); alessandra.pulliero@unige.it (A.P.)
4. Lung Cancer Unit, IRCCS Ospedale Policlinico San Martino, 16132 Genova, Italy; simona.coco@hsanmartino.it
5. Mediterranean Oncological Institute (IOM), 95029 Catania, Italy; cristina.colarossi@grupposamed.com (C.C.); giusi.blanco@grupposamed.com (G.B.); sciacca@unict.it (S.S.)
6. Department of Medical and Surgical Sciences and Advanced Technologies "G.F. Ingrassia", University of Catania, 95123 Catania, Italy; agodia@unict.it (A.A.); martina.barchitta@unict.it (M.B.); andrea.maugeri@unict.it (A.M.); marfer@unict.it (M.F.)
7. Catania, Messina, Enna Cancer Registry, Via S. Sofia 87, 95123 Catania, Italy; segreteria.rti@policlinico.unict.it
* Correspondence: olivericonti@unict.it; Tel.: +39-095-378-2133; Fax: +39-095-378-2177
† The contacts of authors from CT-ME-EN Cancer Registry are provided in Acknowledgments: Andrea Benedetto, Marine Castaing, Alessia Di Prima, Paolo Fidelbo, Antonella Ippolito, Eleonora Irato, Anna Leone, Fiorella Paderni, Paola Pesce, Alessandra Savasta, Carlo Sciacchitano, Antonietta Torrisi, Antonina Torrisi, Massimo Varvarà.

Abstract: MicroRNA and DNA adduct biomarkers may be used to identify the contribution of environmental pollution to some types of cancers. The aim of this study was to use integrated DNA adducts and microRNAs analyses to study retrospectively the contribution of exposures to environmental carcinogens to lung cancer in 64 non-smokers living in Sicily and Catania city near to the Etna volcano. MicroRNAs were extracted from cancer lung biopsies, and from the surrounding lung normal tissue. The expression of 2549 human microRNAs was analyzed by microarray. Benzo(a)Pyrene-DNA adducts levels were analyzed in the patients' blood by HPLC—fluorescence detection. Correlations between tetrols and environmental exposures were calculated using Pearson coefficients and regression variable plots. Compared with the healthy tissue, 273 microRNAs were downregulated in lung cancer. Tetrols levels were inversely related both with the distance from Etna and years since smoking cessation, but they were not significantly correlated to environmental exposures. The analysis of the microRNA environmental signatures indicates the contribution of environmental factors to the analyzed lung cancers in the following decreasing rank: (a) car traffic, (b) passive smoke, (c) radon, and (d) volcano ashes. These results provide evidence that microRNA analysis can be used to retrospectively investigate the contribution of environmental factors in human lung cancer occurring in non-smokers.

Keywords: no-smokers lung cancer; microRNA; DNA adducts; environmental risk factors

1. Introduction

The lung epithelium undergoes a series of morphological changes before becoming invasive, such as hyperplasia, metaplasia, and finally dysplasia and in situ carcinoma. The two main types of lung cancer are small and non-small cell lung cancer (NSCLC), accounting for 80% to 85% of all cases. The three most common histological forms of

NSCLC are epidermoid or squamous cell carcinoma, large cell carcinoma, and adenoma; among them, adenocarcinoma accounts for 40% of all lung cancer cases. [1] Environmental factors, including smoking, diet, and environmental carcinogens, are important in the pathogenesis of cancers through epigenetic modifications.

Interestingly, some miRNAs are dysregulated in NSCLC, which may be indicative of disease status or therapeutic outcome. [2]. It is nowadays well established that environmental pollutants alter the microRNA machinery, a situation resulting in adaptive effects in the case of short-term exposures and adverse effects in the case of long-term exposure [3]. MicroRNAs (miRNAs) are little non-coding RNA molecules that have different regulatory roles in cell differentiation, proliferation, and survival. miRNAs can inhibit complementary mRNA targets, regulating translation through RNA degradation, and are found to be dysregulated in numerous diseases, including cancer, frequently altered owing to mutations or transcriptional changes of the enzymes that regulate miRNA biogenesis [4]. However, approximately 25% of lung cancer cases worldwide, mainly adenocarcinoma, cannot be attributed to tobacco smoking; lung cancer in never smokers is the seventh leading cause of cancer deaths worldwide [5]. According to clinical experience, a different epidemiology and natural history are observed between lung cancers in never smokers and those in smokers [6], suggesting that lung cancer in never smokers is a "different" disease, with a specific etiology and molecular differences. A still unsolved problem is the evaluation of the environmental contribution to lung cancer in non-smokers. Concerning the use of miRNAs as biomarkers for lung cancer, it has been noticed that miR-146a-5p, miR-324-5p, miR-223-3p, and miR-223-5p may regulate cancer-associated gene expression, as they are down expressed in the normal bronchial airways of smokers with lung cancer [7]. Our previous research addresses the identification of a reliable cluster of miRNAs to be used as early cancer predictors, considering the high heterogeneity of lung cancer patients. Differences between miRNA profiles based on gender have being suggested in animal models of adenoma-free and adenoma bearing mice exposed to mainstream cigarette smoking [8]. Moreover, the early diagnosis of lung cancers using miR-33a-5p and miR-128-3p signatures has being proposed, as they are linked to tumor suppression processes. [9] Different response to air pollutants as particulate matter, ultrafine particles, nitrogen oxides, black carbon, and carbon oxides (CO and CO_2) may be related to a different expression of miR-92a-3p, miR-484, and miR-186-5p, linking traffic-related exposure to disease risk [10]. It is known that microRNA and other molecular alterations (oncogene mutations, DNA adducts, transcriptional silencing activation, and proteosome alteration) induced by environmental pollution are quite specific, as each pollutant preferentially alters the expression of a cluster of identifiable molecular fingerprints [11]. This issue has been explored in a peculiar environmental situation characterized by the presence of an active volcano (Etna) near to the analyzed population (Sicily, Italy). Indeed, volcanic dust from Etna has been related to a higher risk of pleural mesothelioma, thyroid cancer [12], and other non-malignant respiratory diseases [13], as well as having a possible pathogenic role in the epidemiology of amyotrophic lateral sclerosis [14] and neurodegenerative diseases [15]. Etna's volcanic dust is also a vector of atmospheric pollutants, such as polycyclic aromatic hydrocarbons and particulates rich on mercury [16]. Furthermore, in a recent study, the surface reactivity of ash from Etna's activity was characterized and, although most of the released elements are below the Italian legal limits, a few inorganic elements (B, Cd, Ni, and As) are released in a higher level than permitted, with possible negative consequence for human health [17]. miR-19a, miR-30e, miR-335, and miR451a in peripheral blood have been suggested as potential biomarkers of radon radiation damage [18]. To the best of our knowledge, the correlation between volcanic ash exposure and miRNA alterations has never been explored.

To ascertain whether or not there was an association between the cancer-related pattern of microRNA alteration induced by passive smoke exposure, airborne car traffic pollution, volcano ash, and radon exposure, we herein present a retrospective study to investigate the correlation between miRNAs expression and DNA adducts in lung cancer tissue and healthy tissue in non- and former-smokers in order to shed light on the differential contribution of environmental factors to the lung carcinogenesis process. The aim of this paper is to use integrated DNA adducts and miRNA analyses in order to shed light on the differential contribution of environmental factors to lung carcinogenesis in non-smokers.

The presented approach integrates both molecular biomarkers (DNA adducts) and post-transcriptional regulation analysis (miRNAs expression in lung tissue) in order to shed light on the differential contribution of environmental factors to lung carcinogenesis in non- and former-smokers, ranking each environmental risk factor, mainly including passive smoke, car traffic pollution, volcano ashes, and radon. The presented approach can contribute to prioritize public health intervention for the primary prevention of lung cancer in non-smokers.

2. Materials and Methods

2.1. Patient's Recruitment and Sampling

Patient recruitment was carried out in four hospitals of Catania (University Hospital "G. Rodolico, San Marco"; "Garibaldi-Nesima" Hospital; "Cannizzaro" Hospital; and "Morgagni" Clinic) and "San Vincenzo" Hospital of Taormina (Messina province). The study protocol was performed according to the Declaration of Helsinki and was approved by the Ethic Committee Catania 1 (n. 11,778 released on 17 March 2015) and Ethic Committee Catania 2 (346/C.E. released on 28 May 2015), respectively.

The criteria used for the patient enrolment was as follows: over 18 years of age, have lung cancer for which surgery treatment has been indicated, have been non-smokers or former smokers for at least 5 years, and have signed the written informed consent. No restriction was made regarding the sex of patients or the morphology of the reported neoplastic lesions. Both the neoplastic and healthy tissue samples were taken from the same patient and the tissue samples were obtained directly from the pathological anatomies of the hospitals involved in the project. Instead, the blood samples were collected by the thoracic surgery units of the hospitals. The interviews were carried out directly in the thoracic surgery wards by the cancer registry doctors involved in the study. A total of 64 patients were finally enrolled. All of the patients lived near the Etna volcano (average 56 km away, min 13 km away, and max 152 km away), their average age was 69.02 years old (min 43 years old and max 84 years old), 34.4% were female, and 20.3% of patients died within three years after the biopsy. A total of 15 subjects had never smoked, while 20 were former smokers for more than 20 years, 13 for 11 to 19 years, and 9 for 10 to 5 years, and the smoking habits data was missed for 14 patients. Data were collected by trained personnel using a semi-structured questionnaire to obtain information on the sociodemographic and lifestyle data, including smoke history, nutrition, home characteristic, and home location (for Radon and urban traffic pollution exposure evaluation) (Figure 1).

2.2. Lung Biopsies Collection

Lung biopsy specimens ($n = 64$) were collected at the onset of disease from patients who were diagnosed with lung cancer between 2015 and 2018, and were referred to the Catania, Messina, Enna Cancer Registry, Italy. The study was approved by Ethics committee—informed consent was obtained by "G. Rodolico—San Marco" University Hospital. All patients were classified as cases according to the 2021 ICD-10-CM Diagnosis Code C34.90. microRNA were comparatively evaluated in the cancer and surrounding normal tissue, as identified by intra-surgery histopathological analysis.

2.3. miRNA Extraction

The total RNA was extracted from the lung biopsies using a standardized protocol that combined a phenol/guanidine-based lysis of samples and silica-membrane-based purification. In brief, 30 mg of the starting material was first disrupted and homogenized in 700 μL of the QIAzol Lysis Reagent, using the TissueRuptor II (Qiagen, Milan, Italy) for 20–40 s. Next, the total RNA was purified from the homogenate using the miRNeasy

Mini Kit (Qiagen, Milan, Italy), as described by the manufacturer's protocol. Purification of RNA was automated on the QIAcube instrument (Qiagen, Milan, Italy).

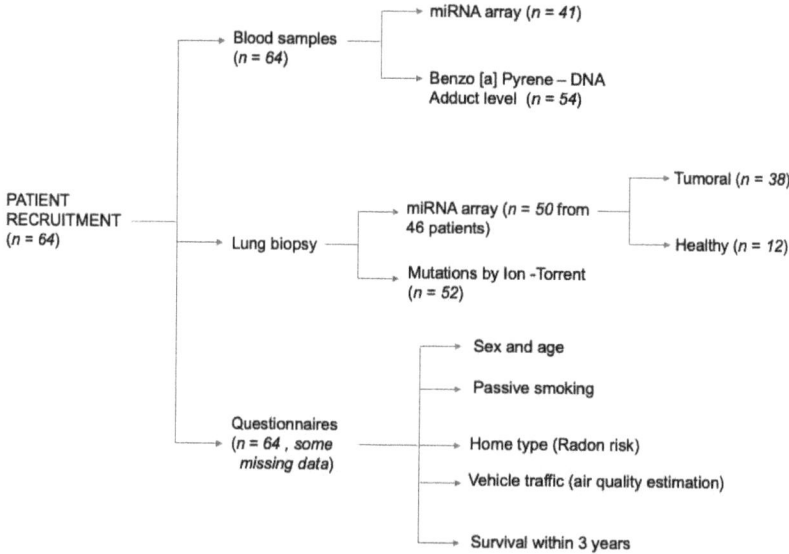

Figure 1. Patients enrolled-characteristics and sample sizes of analytical determinations carried out.

2.4. miRNA-Microarray and Bioinformatic Analyses

The miRNA expression profiling was carried out with the Agilent platform following the miRNA Microarray protocol v.3.1.1 (Agilent Technologies, Santa Clara, CA, USA). Briefly, 50 ng of total RNA, containing miRNAs and Spike-in controls underwent dephosphorylation and a labelling step with Cyanine 3-pCp. The Cy3-labeled RNA was then purified using a Micro Bio-Spin P-6 Gel Column (Bio-Rad Laboratories, Inc., Hercules, CA, USA) and hybridized on Human miRNA microarray slide 8 × 60 K (Agilent Technologies; including 2549 miRNAs, miRBase 21.0) at 55 °C for 20 h. After washing, the slides were scanned with a G2565CA scanner (Agilent Technologies) and the images were extracted by Feature Extraction software v.10 (Agilent Technologies). The microarray raw data were previously deposited in the Gene Expression Omnibus (http://www.ncbi.nlm.nih.gov/geo/; accessed on 8 March 2021, GEO accession number GSE169587, ID: 200169587) for a previous study from the same authors [4].

The bioinformatic analyses of the microarray data were performed with GeneSpring software (GeneSpring Multi-Omic Analysis version 14.9 Build 11,939 by Agilent Technologies). For each specimen, the intensities of the replicated spots on each array were log transformed and averaged. All the lung-tissue-miRNA raw data files from the Agilent Technologies Microarray Scanner System G2565CA were imported to GeneSpring using miRNA analysis type, Technology 70156_v21_0, without baseline transformation. Data processing was performed by 3D principal component analysis (PCA) scores and Hierarchical Clustering.

Comparisons between sets of data were done by evaluating the fold variations. A volcano plot t-test analysis for all the miRNA entities between the averaged tumoral and healthy tissues was run, using fold change ≥ 2 and p-value ≤ 0.05, without multiple test corrections as the threshold values.

miRNAs related to five different environmental exposures (Environmental Exposure miRNA Signature) were determined analysing lung cancer related miRNAs comparatively in exposed vs. non-exposed subjects. Environmental exposures were determined for each patient using the questionnaires information according to (a) passive smoking at home,

(b) passive smoking at work, (c) vehicle traffic at home, (d) distance (km) from the Etna volcano, and (e) radon risk according to home type.

To understand the relationship between environmental exposure signatures and their biological significance in lung cancer tissues, a target detection for each environmental exposure signature was done using the TargetScan prediction database. This database was chosen as it is the most updated database, and the number of target genes are reported for different cut-offs. The most interesting genes targeted by environmental exposure miRNA signatures that are potentially related with each environmental exposure were identified.

After the target detection, a prediction model was build using a Neural Network class prediction algorithm for each Environmental Exposure miRNA Signature to test the overall accuracy prediction for the chosen miRNAs.

2.5. Validation of Microarray Results by qPCR Analysis

Microarray results for let-7a and miR-15 were further validated by qPCR on a subset of 20 patients for which enough RNA was still available. These miRNAs were selected because of their relevance lung carcinogenesis. The total RNA (10 ng) was reverse transcribed using miR-specific stem-loop RT primers (TaqMan MicroRNA Assays; Applied Biosystems, Thermo-Fisher) and components of the High Capacity cDNA Reverse Transcription kit (Life Technologies) according to the manufacturer's protocols.

The expression levels of individual miRNAs were detected by subsequent RQ-PCR using TaqMan MicroRNA assays (Life Technologies) and a Rotor Gene 3000 PCR System Corbett (Qiagen) using standard thermal cycling conditions in accordance with manufacturer recommendations. The PCR reactions were performed in triplicate in final volumes of 30 µL, including inter-assay controls (IAC) in order to account for variations between runs. RT-PCR (TaqMan MicroRNA Assays; Applied Biosystems, Thermo-Fisher) was used to quantify the expression of let-7a and miR-15 according to the manufacturer's instructions. To normalize the data for quantifying miRNAs, the universal small nuclear RNU38B (RNU38B Assay ID 001004; Applied Biosystems) as an endogenous control was used.

2.6. Benzo[a]Pyrene-DNA Adduct Levels in Human White Blood Cells

Hydrolyzed BPDE adducts or Tetrol I-1 and Tetrol II-2 were analyzed in lymphocyte DNA through the modified High-Performance Liquid Chromatography–Fluorescence (HPLC–FL) method described by Alexandrov et al. [19] and Oliveri Conti et al. [20].

Briefly, lymphocytes were separated from whole blood samples using HISTOPAQUE-1077 (Sigma-Aldrich Chemie Gmbh, Munich, Germany). The lymphocyte DNA was extracted using the DNeasy Blood and Tissue kit according to customer's procedure (Qiagen, Milan, Italy).

Hence, DNA was subjected to a procedure of hydrolysis and purification, and Tetrols were quantified according to the methodology of Oliveri Conti et al. [20]. HCl, also if hypergrade certified, can contain traces of fluorescent active contaminants that could interfere with the peak detection of the studied analytes and reduce analytical sensitivity of the method.

To avoid this important bias in the sample preparative phase, all of the HCl impurities visibly reactive to the FL detector were deleted by chemical purification [20]. To improve the sensibility of detection, Thermo Scientific™ PEEK Capillary Tubing (0.005 in) was used. The extracted and purified DNA was dissolved in 1 mL of water and analyzed in a Varian Pro Star System HPLC using a TOSOH (C18 RP 25 × 0.46 cm, 5 µm) column with the following elution program: 15 min with 20% water/acetonitrile of equilibrium phase, 5 min with 20% water/acetonitrile and 60 min to acetonitrile (100%) (slop of 1) and, finally 10 min to 100% acetonitrile.

An isocratic program (0.85 mL/min) was used, and the FL detector (FLD) was programmed to 344 nm (ext.) and 388 nm (em.) for the excitation and emission wavelengths, respectively. The sensitivity of the FLD was fixed to a high modality. The wavelength of

UV−VIS detector (UV) was set at 238 nm, permitting the dual detection of both Tetrols (I-1 and II-2).

The chromatographic system was calibrated using external certified pure standards of Tetrol I-1 and Tetrol II-2 (purity 99.0%) (Chemical Carcinogen Reference Standard Repository, Kansas City, MO, USA).

Recoveries were 94% and 82% for Tetrol I-1 and Tetrol II-2, respectively. The processing of reagent blank disclosed no trace of Tetrol I-1 and Tetrol II-2. The linearities (R^2) obtained of FLD were 0.9980 and 0.9990 for Tetrol I-1 and Tetrol II-2, respectively. For UV, the Rs^2 were 0.9850 e 0.9803 for Tetrol I-1 and Tetrol II-2, respectively. MDL were 2.0 pg/mL and 3.1 pg/mL for Tetrol I-1 and Tetrol II-2, respectively. The validated method permitted detecting Tetrol I-1 and Tetrol II-2 in a minimum of 3μg of extracted DNA.

2.7. Statistical Analysis

The statistical significance of the differences between groups was evaluated by ANOVA, followed by Student's *t*-test for unpaired data. *p*-values lower than 0.05 were regarded as statistically significant. Correlations (i.e., Pearson coefficients and regression variable plots) between Benzo[a]Pyrene-DNA adducts and the different environmental exposures were calculated with IBM SPSS statistics (Version 22).

3. Results

3.1. Comparison of miRNA Profile between Healthy and Cancer Tissue in Lung

The scatter plot analysis of the miRNA-arrays comparing healthy and lung cancer tissues presents a general trend toward down regulation in cancer tissue, as indicated by the slope of the black regression line (Figure 2a). The volcano plot analysis highlighted a list of 273 miRNAs that were altered more than two folds and above the statistical significantly threshold ($p < 0.05$) in cancer vs. healthy tissue. Of these miRNAs, 222 were down-regulated (blue dots) and 51 were up-regulated (red dots) (Figure 2b). This group represents the Lung Cancer Related miRNAs. This list is reported in the supplementary material (Supplementary Table S1) and includes well established oncogenic miRNAs, such as an extensive downregulation of the whole let-7 miRNA family and of the miR-34 family, an established effector of p53.

The lung cancer related miRNAs downregulation trend was well distinguishable between the cancer and healthy tissue, as also indicated by the hierarchical cluster analysis (Figure 3a), where healthy tissue profiles (yellow bar) were clustered in the upper part of the hierarchical tree separately from cancer tissue profiles (blue bar). Colour range indicates lung cancer related miRNAs' intensity signal.

In the principal component analysis of variance (Figure 3b), healthy tissue samples (yellow dots) were mainly clustered in the lower left part of the 3D space. Instead, cancer tissue samples (blue dots) were mainly located in the upper right part of the 3D space.

The most significant predicted target genes for each of the lung cancer related miRNAs were identified using the TOP-Go Bioconductor R package and REVIGO online tool. The tree map of the most representative biological processes for lung cancer related miRNAs is reported in (Supplementary Figure S1). The most representative biological processes were as follows: regulation of RNA splicing, tissue migration, monosaccharide transmembrane transport, protein modification by small protein conjugation or removal, and cellular protein-containing complex assembly.

qPCR analyses performed for let-7a confirmed the downregulation of this miRNAs in cancer vs. healthy lung tissues of the same patient (Figure 4).

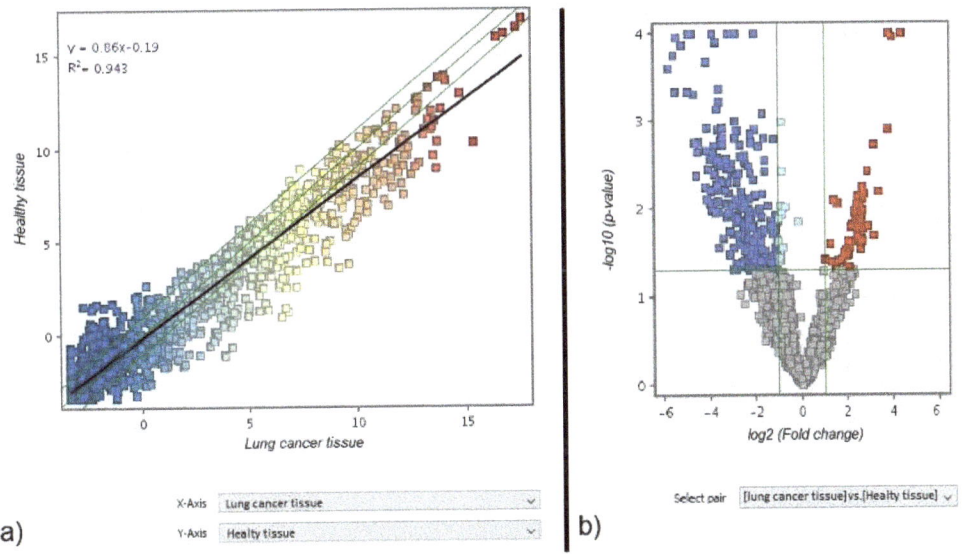

Figure 2. (**a**) Scatter plot analysis comparing miRNA expression (dots) according to their level of expression in healthy (vertical axis) vs. cancer (horizontal axis) tissues of the examined patients. The miRNA colour reflects the signal intensity (red is high, yellow is intermediate, and blue is low). The diagonal green lines indicate the two-fold variation interval. The best-fit regression line is reported in black. Its slope towards the horizontal axis reflects the overall downregulation of miRNA expression in cancer compared with healthy lung tissue. (**b**) Volcano plot analysis identifying miRNAs with an altered expression above two-fold (horizontal axis) and above the statistical significance threshold ($p < 0.05$) (vertical axis) in cancer vs. healthy lung tissue, either downregulated (blue) or upregulated (red).

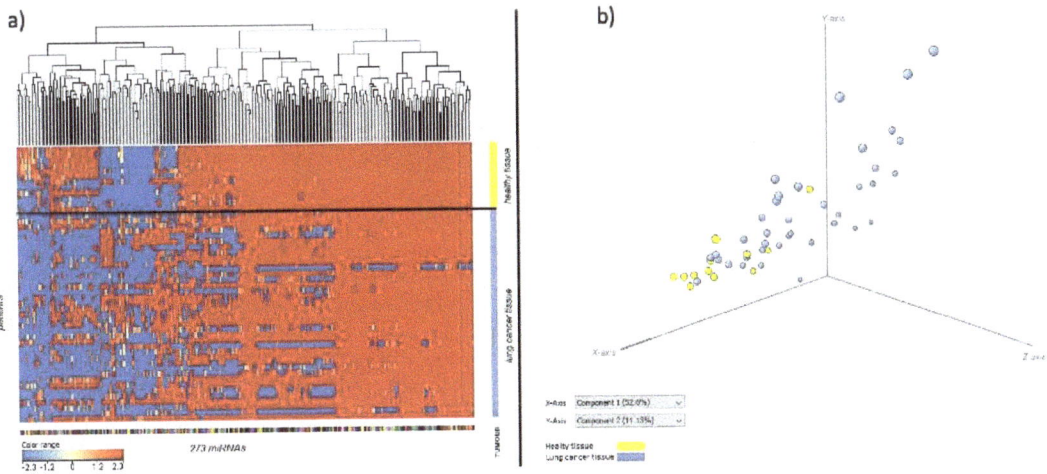

Figure 3. (**a**) Clustering hierarchical analysis reporting the expression of the 273 lung cancer related miRNAs in healthy tissue (vertical axis, yellow bar) and lung cancer tissue (vertical axis, blue bar) in the 50 samples tested (horizontal lines). (**b**) Principal component analysis of variance identifying the samples from healthy tissues (yellow dots) and cancer tissues (blue dots) according to the variance of the expression of the 273 lung cancer related miRNAs. dots size = principal component analysis score.

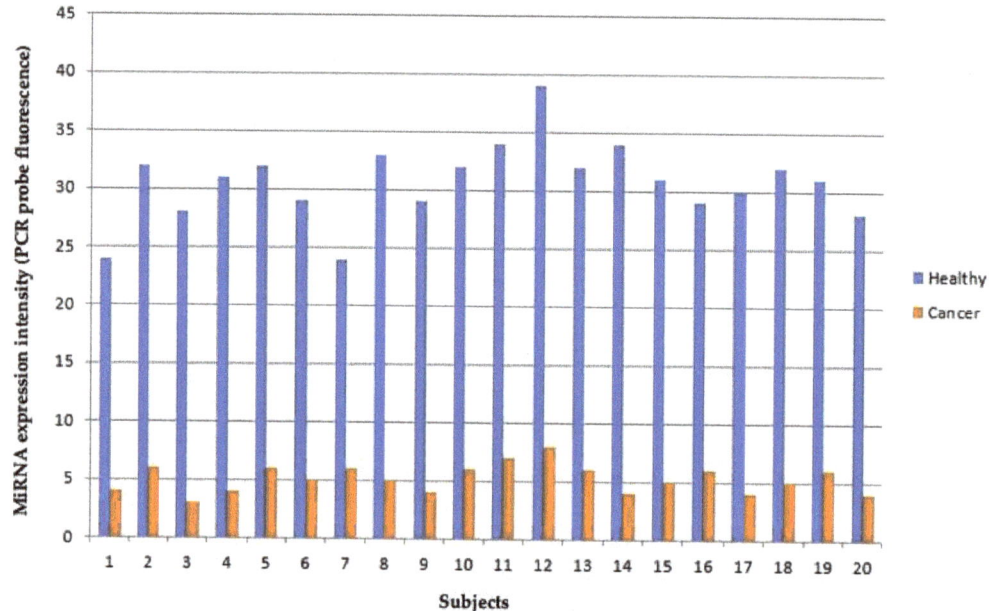

Figure 4. Let-7a expression in healthy (blue) vs. cancer (red) lung tissue as evaluated by qPCR in 20 patients (x-axis). miRNA expression intensity is expressed in fluorescent units (y-axis).

On an average, Let-7a expression was down-regulated in cancer vs. healthy tissues by 6.2 ± 1.4 fold as evaluated by qPCR, and 7.4 ± 2.2 fold as evaluated by microarray.

3.2. miRNA Profile Was Related with Cancer Histotype

The miRNA expression was different between small cell lung cancer (SCLC) and NSCLC, as shown by the scatter plot analysis (Figure 5a). The volcano plot analysis indicated that 26 out of the 273 cancer related miRNAs were differentially expressed between SCLC and NSCL (Figure 5b). Of these miRNAs, 25 were up-regulated in NSCLC compared with SCLC and one was down-regulated. The identity of these 26 miRNAs permitted distinguishing between these two main cancer histotypes, and is reported in the supplementary material (Supplementary Table S2).

3.3. B(a)P-DNA Adducts and Environmental Exposures

The ANOVA analysis did not detect a statistically significant difference between the B(a)P-DNA adducts levels under different environmental exposures, including passive smoking at home, passive smoking at work, radon risk related to home type, and vehicle traffic at home (Figure 6). The linear regression analysis showed that the level of B(a)P-DNA adducts in the lymphocytes was inversely related with the distance from the Etna volcano (Figure 6e) and years since smoking cessation (Figure 6f).

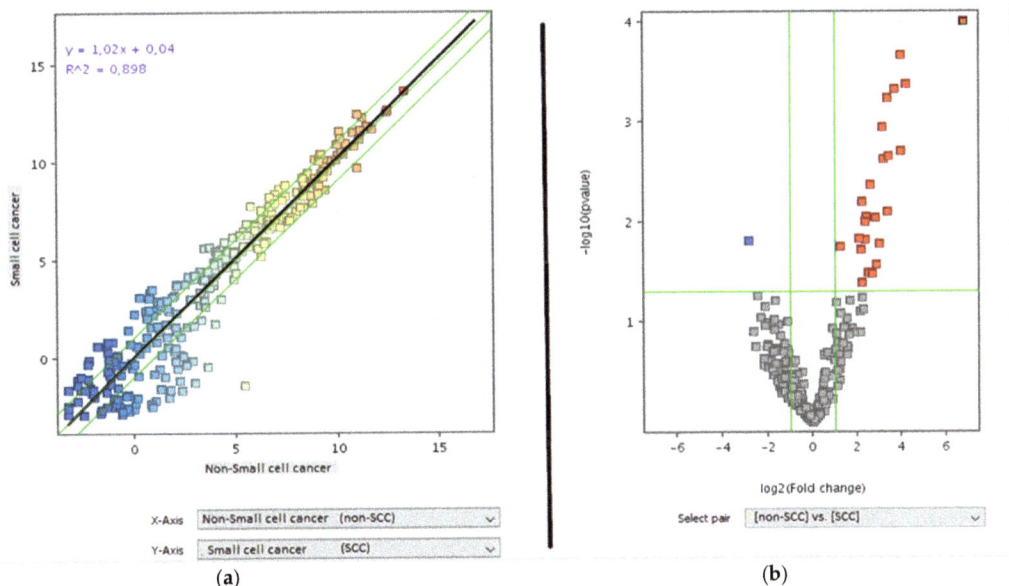

Figure 5. (a) Scatter plot analysis comparing miRNA expressions (dots) according to their level of expression in SCLC (vertical axis) vs. NSCLC (horizontal axis). miRNA color reflects the level of expression (red is high, yellow is intermediate, and blue is low). The diagonal lines indicate the two-fold variation interval. (b) Volcano plot analysis identifying miRNAs whose expression was altered more than two-fold (horizontal axis) and above the statistical significance threshold ($p < 0.05$) (vertical axis) in SCLC vs. NSCLC cancer downregulated (blue) or upregulated (red).

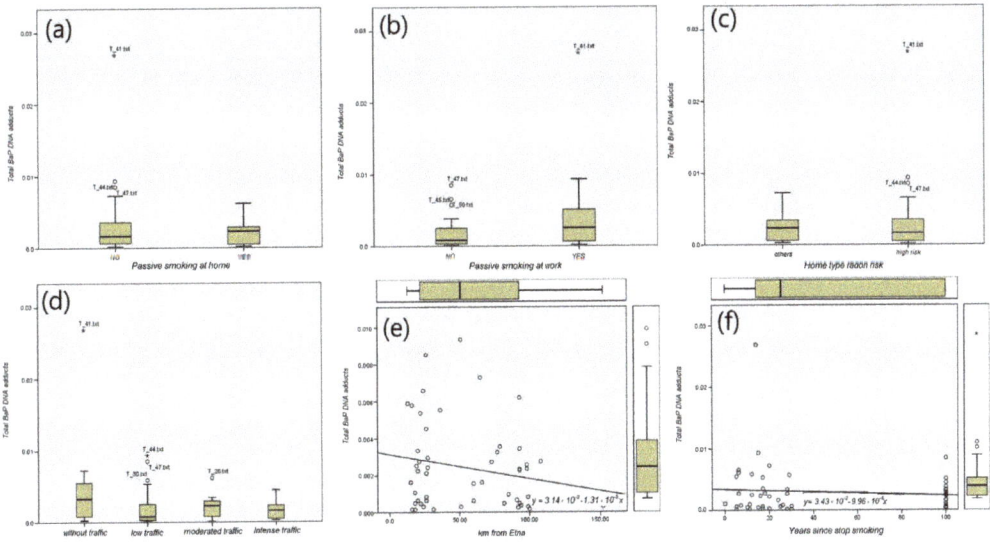

Figure 6. Box plot analysis for total BaP DNA adducts in: (a) passive smoking at home, (b) passive smoking at work, (c) radon risk home type, (d) vehicle traffic at home, and linear regression for (e) distance from the Etna volcano, and (f) years since smoking cessation.

3.4. Contribution of Environmental Exposures to Lung Carcinogenesis as Inferred from miRNA Profiling

Five miRNA signatures were obtained comparing the miRNA expression in the tumoral lung tissue between patients undergoing a low or high exposure for each one of the environmental exposures. The cancer related miRNAs included in each miRNA environmental signature were used to run a volcano plot analysis (FC ≥ 2, $p \leq 0.05$). These environmental signatures were further integrated with the established miRNA, as linked with the specific exposure from the available literature.

The number of miRNAs composing each environmental signature was as follows: (a) passive smoke at home, $n = 8$; (b) passive smoke at work, $n = 1$; (c) vehicle traffic, $n = 53$; (d), distance from the Etna volcano, $n = 21$; and (e) radon risk, $n = 19$. The volcanos plot analyses comparing miRNA expression in the lungs between unexposed vs. exposed subjects for each environmental signature are reported in Figure 7.

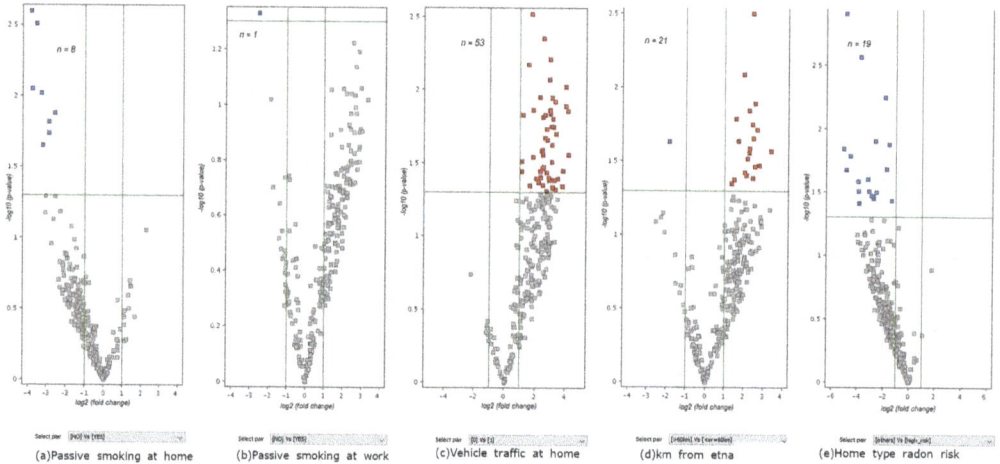

Figure 7. *t*-test volcano plot analyses identifying the miRNA environmental signatures (among the 273 lung cancer related miRNAs).

Accurate questionnaire data were available for 38 out of the 50 patients for whom the microRNA microarray data were collected. A volcano plot *t*-test using each EES was run to identify the altered miRNAs per patient.

Environmental exposure miRNA signatures were compared by Venn diagram analysis, with the miRNAs composing the individual cancer-related signature of each patient. This approach was used to identify the relative contribution of the environmental risk factors to cancer development in each patient (Figure 8).

The number of patients with a higher number of differentially regulated miRNAs than the median value for each environmental risk factor was as follows: (a) 38 for passive smoke, (b) 38 for vehicle traffic, (c) 21 for distance from the Etna volcano, and (d) 13 for radon risk

The targeted genes for each environmental exposure signature were analyzed. The number of target genes for each signature and different *p*-values cut-off are summarized in Table 1.

Most of the genes targeted by the environmental exposure miRNA signatures with statistical significance are also expressed in the lung tissue. The gene RIF (gene reference into function) and RPKM (reads per kilobase of transcript, per million mapped reads) values in the lung tissue for each targeted gene were found using the NCBI gene database (https://www.ncbi.nlm.nih.gov/gene) accessed on 11 December 2021. These findings are reported in Table 2.

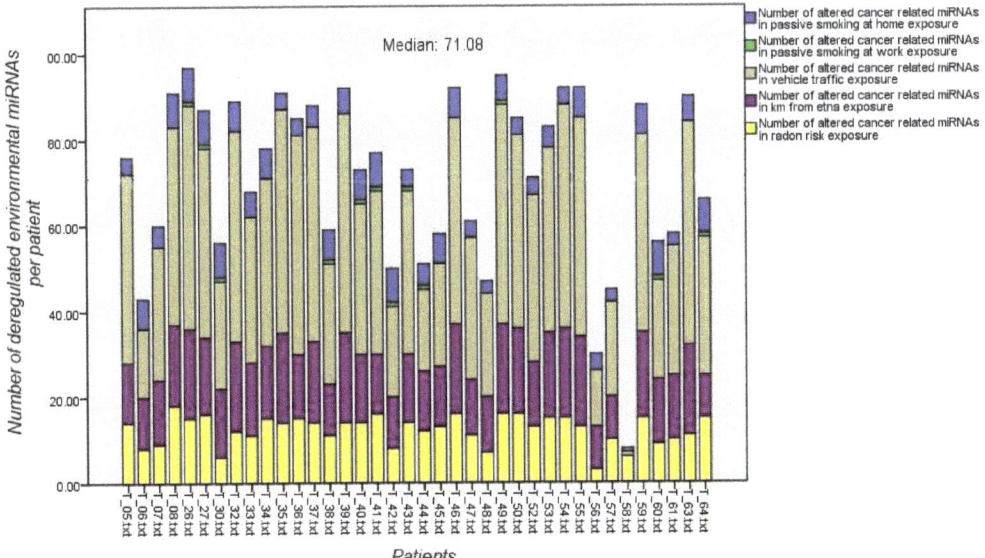

Figure 8. Number of altered environmental exposure miRNAs (*y*-axes, color codes) per patient (*x*-axes). Median of the summation of each environmental exposure miRNA signature are shown as horizontal colored lines. Patients having environmental risk factors above the median value underwent lung cancer contribution by this risk factor.

Table 1. Number of predicted target genes (Targetscan database) according to each environmental exposure with a *p*-value cut off.

Environmental Exposure Signature	Number of Predicted Target Genes by *p*-Value Cut Off				
	0.05	0.01	0.005	0.001	0.0001
Passive smoking at home (n = 8)	8726	8726	8726	6	1
Passive smoking at work (n = 1)	1796	3	0	0	0
Vehicle traffic at home (n = 53)	16,132	16,132	16,132	16,132	7
Home distance from the Etna volcano (n = 21)	14,662	14,662	14,662	20	4
Home type radon risk (n = 19)	13,762	13,762	15	0	0

The most significant targeted genes for each signature are summarized in Table 2.

Table 2. Most significative gene target detection per environmental exposure miRNA signature by *p*-value cut-off.

Environmental Exposure Signature	*p*-Value	Genes	Gene Name
Passive smoking at home (n = 8)	0.001	PTX4	pentraxin 4
		NAXD	NAD(P)HX dehydratase
		MAPK3	mitogen-activated protein kinase 3
		VPS16	core subunit of CORVET and HOPS complexes
		CACNA1S	calcium voltage-gated channel subunit alpha1 S
		SHARPIN	SHANK associated RH domain interactor
Passive smoking at work (n = 1)	0.01	HBG2	hemoglobin subunit gamma 2
		RNASE12	ribonuclease A family member 12
		IFT88	intraflagellar transport 88

Table 2. Cont.

Environmental Exposure Signature	p-Value	Genes	Gene Name
Vehicle traffic at home (n = 53)	0.0001	LEFTY1 RTTN THYN1 CASKIN1 SERPING1 OGFOD2 PKDCC	left-right determination factor 1 Rotatin thymocyte nuclear protein 1 CASK interacting protein 1 serpin family G member 1 2-oxoglutarate and iron dependent oxygenase domain containing 2 protein kinase domain containing, cytoplasmic
Home distance from the Etna volcano (n = 21)	0.001	ARHGEF33 COX17 RAI2 KIF12 COL26A1 RMDN2 GADD45A DTNA HTRA4 TAS2R30 STRN3 BRINP3 EYS JAG2 HSD17B12 NIN NAA35 ZNF37A GLT8D2 DDX59	Rho guanine nucleotide exchange factor 33 COX17 retinoic acid induced 2 kinesin family member 12 collagen type XXVI alpha 1 chain regulator of microtubule dynamics 2 growth arrest and DNA damage inducible alpha dystrobrevin alpha HtrA serine peptidase 4 taste 2 receptor member 30 striatin 3 BMP/retinoic acid inducible neural specific 3 eyes shut homolog jagged canonical Notch ligand 2 hydroxysteroid 17-beta dehydrogenase 12 Ninein N-alpha-acetyltransferase 35, NatC auxiliary subunit zinc finger protein 37° glycosyltransferase 8 domain containing 2 DEAD-box helicase 59
Home type radon risk (n = 19)	0.005	CNPY3 SUB1 CLTC ZNF280A ALS2CR12 TMEM139 BTBD3 WDR7 RAB15 KRT84 MAZ ATAD2B PSPH PGBD1 BEX2	canopy FGF signaling regulator 3 SUB1 regulator of transcription clathrin heavy chain zinc finger protein 280° (or FLACC1) flagellum associated containing coiled-coil domains 1 transmembrane protein 139 BTB domain containing 3 WD repeat domain 7 member RAS oncogene family keratin 84 MYC associated zinc finger protein ATPase family AAA domain containing 2B phosphoserine phosphatase piggyBac transposable element derived 1 brain expressed X-linked 2

3.5. Evaluation of Environmental Exposure miRNA Signatures Efficacy by Neural Network Analysis

GeneSpring 14.9 was used to build a prediction model to validate the accuracy of each of the environmental exposure signatures. The network was tested in tumoral tissue. The accuracy of the environmental signature increased compared with the number of miRNAs included, as follows: (a) remarkably, for passive smoking at home, distance from the Etna volcano, and home type radon risk; (b) slightly for vehicle traffic and distance from the Etna volcano; and (c) remained equal for passive smoking at work (Table 3).

Table 3. Results of the neural network class prediction for each environmental exposure miRNA signature.

Environmental Exposure (Number of miRNA Entities)	Score of All miRNAs Prediction Overall Accuracy ($n = 2570$)	Environmental Exposure miRNA Signatures Prediction Overall Accuracy Score
Passive smoking at home ($n = 8$)	0.73	0.96 (+0.23)
Passive smoking at work ($n = 1$)	0.68	0.68 (+0)
Vehicle traffic at home ($n = 53$)	0.77	0.81 (+0.04)
Home distance from the Etna volcano ($n = 21$)	0.60	0.82 (+0.22)
Home type radon risk ($n = 19$)	0.83	0.96 (+0.13)

3.6. Environmental Exposure miRNA Signatures and B(a)P-DNA Adduct Levels

The weight of different exposures to lung cancer were profiled by analyzing the B(a)P-DNA adduct levels in the lymphocytes and miRNAs profiles in lung cancer together. For this purpose, we ranked the four exposures on the basis of the number of altered miRNAs. Correlation tests (Pearson and Spearman's Rho) were run to evaluate whether or not B[a]P-DNA adducts were related with environmental exposure miRNA signatures. The B[a]P-DNA adduct levels were correlated only with the passive smoking miRNA signature (p-value = 0.049) (Table 4).

Table 4. Correlation between EESs miRNA and B(a)P-DNA adduct levels. (*) Statistical significance $p < 0.05$.

		Vehicle Traffic at Home	Distance from Etna Volcano	Radon Risk	Passive Smoking
Correlation Test RRSs and B[a]P-DNA adducts. Pearson (for parametric) or Spearman's Rho (for non parametric)	Correlation Coefficient	0.54 (Parametric)	0.48 (Non-Parametric)	0.25 (Parametric)	0.34 * (Parametric)
	p-value	0.76	0.79	0.16	0.049

* Statistical significance $p < 0.05$.

4. Discussion and Conclusions

Our results provide evidence that miRNAs are massively deregulated in lung cancer compared with the surrounding normal tissue. This finding is in line with other studies [21]. A major problem in using miRNA analysis for lung cancer prediction and early diagnosis is the reproducibility of the results and the invasiveness of the biopsy approach. Our cancer related miRNAs signature at least in part overlaps with the most common lung cancer miRNA-related signatures found in the literature. Indeed, 27 miRNAs were included in our cancer related signature and also in other cancer miRNA-related signatures found in literature [22]. The miRNAs downregulated in lung cancer tissue included established anti-oncogenic miRNA such as let-7, miR-30, miR-34, and miR-140. The comparison of DNA adducts and miRNA expression provided evidence that post-transcriptional alteration is massive in lung cancer, while DNA adducts alteration of an environmental origin is detectable, but only at a very low level. DNA adducts are a hallmark of the environmental contribution to the analyzed cancers, with particular reference to environmental sources of polycyclic aromatic hydrocarbons derived from combustion, such as car traffic and passive smoke. However, BaP-DNA adducts are poor predictors of cancer because (a) they can be removed by DNA repair [23], (b) the resulting mutation can be silenced thus not having phenotypical or functional consequences, and (c) the bearing cell can be removed by apoptosis. Conversely, miRNA alterations are necessary to develop lung cancer. These alterations are initially adaptive, aimed at activating defensive processes counteracting the damage induced by environmental pollutants such as DNA repair, mutation silencing, and apoptosis. However, whenever the environmental exposure lasts for decades, microRNA alterations become irreversible and commit cells to the occurrence of lung cancer environmental risk factors, inducing specific alterations in the microRNA machinery depending on the specificity of the environmental pollutant involved [3–11]. Accordingly, microRNA alteration is more predictive of lung cancer occurrence than genomic alterations. Indeed, microRNAs have been proposed as a tool for the early diagnosis of cancer or to identify subjects at a high risk for cancer development needing to undergo personalized cancer screening with a high frequency and sensitivity.

The negative correlation observed between the adduct level and some environmental exposures (i.e., traffic and volcano distance) is in line with the results previously published by other research groups reporting that populations undergoing long-term exposure to environmental pollution develop resistance mechanisms [24]. These events are referred to as adaptive events triggered by heterogeneous exposures [25].

The biological function of miRNAs identified as lung cancer contributors in environmental signatures reflect the pivotal role of the damage to the microRNA machinery during the carcinogenesis process. These events have been previously analyzed in detail during lung carcinogenesis in mice [8,26].

The results presented herein provide evidence that miRNA alteration in lung cancer results from exposure to environmental factors. This situation results in miRNA failure to control pivotal defensive mechanisms against cancer, mainly including oncogene suppression, cell adhesion and differentiation maintenance, cell cycle blockage, DNA and protein repair, intracellular signaling, and apoptosis.

The obtained results provide evidence that miRNA signatures may be used to identify the comparative contribution of environmental factors to lung carcinogenesis in humans. According to our environmental exposure miRNA signatures results, the contribution of the analysed environmental factors was, in decreasing order, car traffic, passive smoke, volcano, and radon. These results may be useful for stakeholders to prioritize public health intervention for the primary prevention of lung cancer in non-smokers. Indeed, it is commonly thought that the contribution of volcano ash is the main public health problem in Catania, one of the few cities in the world to be directly exposed to volcano emissions located in its near proximity. However, the obtained results indicate that the main public health problem in this town is the car traffic. Accordingly, preventive measures, such as the substitution of old with new cars characterized by low emission rates, are urgently required. In the second rank, there is passive smoke, which is a problem to be faced by stronger information campaigns and other measures (such as the increase of cigarettes price), which appears to be urgent in a country (i.e., Italy) still having the prevalence of 13 million of smokers out of a total population of 60 million.

In conclusion, the results presented herein provide more evidence that the analyses of epigenetic components may be used to face public health issues related with cancer prevention [27], with particular reference to the identification of the environmental risk factors to be prevented.

Supplementary Materials: The following are available online at https://www.mdpi.com/article/10.3390/jpm11070666/s1, Figure S1: Revigo TreeMap of GO-BP analysis. Most significant BPs are classified by colour with BPs subset, Table S1: *Cancer Related miRNAs*, Table S2: Significant altered miRNAs.

Author Contributions: Conceptualization, A.I. and S.S.; methodology, A.I., G.C.V., S.S. and A.P.; CT-ME-EN Cancer Registry Authors, G.O.C., M.F. and A.A.; validation, G.O.C., A.P., G.C.V., S.C. and M.B.; investigation, Cancer Registry Authors, G.O.C., M.B., A.M., C.C. and G.B.; resources, S.S. and M.F.; data curation, G.O.C., A.P., G.C.V. and A.I.; writing—original draft preparation, A.I., G.C.V., A.P. and G.O.C.; writing—review and editing, all authors; visualization, all authors; supervision, A.I. and M.F.; project administration, A.I. and S.S.; funding acquisition, S.S. All authors have read and agreed to the published version of the manuscript.

Funding: This research was supported by Regional CT-ME-EN-Cancer Register fund-2015, and partially by the Italian Association for Cancer Research (AIRC, IG2017-20699 to A.I.) and the Italian Association for Cancer Research (AIRC, IG2017-20699 to A.I.).

Institutional Review Board Statement: The study was conducted according to the guidelines of the Declaration of Helsinki and approved by the Institutional Review Board Ethics Committees (n. 11778 released on 17 March 2015. and 346/C.E. released on 28 May 2015).

Informed Consent Statement: Informed consent was obtained from all subjects involved in the study.

Data Availability Statement: The datasets used and/or analyzed during the current study are available from the corresponding author on reasonable request.

Acknowledgments: We would like to thank all co-authors including the staff from CT-ME-EN Cancer Registry Group for their contribution: Andrea Benedetto (andrea.benedetto@registrotumoriintegrato.it) Marine Castaing (marinecastaing@hotmail.com), Alessia Di Prima (alessia26d@gmail.com), Paolo Fidelbo (paolo.fidelbo@gmail.com), Antonella Ippolito (antonellaippolito81@gmail.com), Eleonora Irato (eleonorairato@hotmail.it), Anna Leone (annaleone76@yahoo.it), Fiorella Paderni (fpaderni@gmail.com), Paola Pesce (paolapesce@tiscali.it), Alessandra Savasta (alessandrasavasta@virgilio.it), Carlo Sciacchitano (carlo@carlosciacchitano.it), Antonietta Torrisi (torrisidora@gmail.com), Antonina Torrisi (torrisinina@gmail.com), Massimo Varvarà (max.varvara@libero.it), Carmelo Viscosi (ettore.viscosi@gmail.com).

Conflicts of Interest: The authors declare no conflict of interest.

References

1. Travis, W.D.; Brambilla, E.; Burke, A.P.; Marx, A.; Nicholson, A.G. Introduction to the 2015 World Health Organization classification of tumors of the lung, pleura, thymus, and heart. *J. Thorac. Oncol.* **2015**, *10*, 1240–1242. [CrossRef]
2. Kumar, M.S.; Lu, J.; Mercer, K.L.; Golub, T.R.; Jacks, T. Impaired microRNA processing enhances cellular transformation and tumorigenesis. *Nat. Genet.* **2007**, *39*, 673–677. [CrossRef] [PubMed]
3. Izzotti, A.; Cartiglia, C.; Longobardi, M.; Larghero, P.; De Flora, S. Dose responsiveness and persistence of microRNA alterations induced by cigarette smoke in mice. *Mutat. Res. Fundam. Mol. Mech. Mutagen.* **2011**, *717*, 9–16. [CrossRef] [PubMed]
4. Rupaimoole, R.; Slack, F.J. MicroRNA therapeutics: Towards a new era for the management of cancer and other diseases. *Nat. Rev. Drug Discov.* **2017**, *16*, 203–222. [CrossRef] [PubMed]
5. Bray, F.; Ferlay, J.; Soerjomataram, I.; Siegel, R.L.; Torre, L.A.; Jemal, A. CA Global cancer statistics 2018: GLOBOCAN estimates of incidence and mortality worldwide for 36 cancers in 185 countries. *Cancer J. Clin.* **2018**, *68*, 394–424. [CrossRef]
6. Sun, S.; Schiller, J.H.; Gazdar, A.F. Lung cancer in never smokers—A different disease. *Nat. Rev. Cancer* **2007**, *7*, 778–790. [CrossRef]
7. Pavel, A.B.; Campbell, J.D.; Liu, G.; Elashoff, D.; Dubinett, S.; Smith, K. Alterations in Bronchial Airway miRNA Expression for Lung Cancer Detection. *Cancer Prev. Res.* **2017**, *10*, 651–659. [CrossRef] [PubMed]
8. Izzotti, A.; Balansky, R.; Ganchev, G.; Iltcheva, M.; Longobardi, M.; Pulliero, A.; Geretto, M.; Micale, R.T.; La Maestra, S.; Miller, M.S.; et al. Blood and lung microRNAs as biomarkers of pulmonary tumorigenesis in cigarette smoke-exposed mice. *Oncotarget* **2016**, *7*, 51. [CrossRef]
9. Pan, J.; Zhou, C.; Zhao, X.; He, J.; Tian, H.; Shen, W. A two-miRNA signature (miR-33a-5p and miR-128-3p) in whole blood as potential biomarker for early diagnosis of lung cancer. *Sci. Rep.* **2018**, *12*, 8. [CrossRef]
10. Espín-Pérez, A.; Krauskopf, J.; Chadeau-Hyam, M.; van Veldhoven, K.; Chung, F.; Cullinan, P. Short-term transcriptome and microRNAs responses to exposure to different air pollutants in two population studies. *Environ. Pollut.* **2018**, *242*, 182–190. [CrossRef] [PubMed]
11. Ceccaroli, C.; Pulliero, A.; Geretto, M.; Izzotti, A. Molecular fingerprints of environmental carcinogens in human cancer. *J. Environ. Sci. Health* **2015**, *33*, 188–228. [CrossRef]
12. Boffetta, P.; Memeo, L.; Giuffrida, D.; Ferrante, M.; Sciacca, S. Exposure to emissions from Mount Etna (Sicily, Italy) and incidence of thyroid cancer: A geographic analysis. *Sci. Rep.* **2020**, *10*, 21298. [CrossRef]
13. Bruno, C.; Combra, P.; Zona, A. Adverse Health Effects of Fluoro-Edenitic Fibers: Epidemiological Evidence and Public Health Priorities. *Ann. N. Y. Acad. Sci.* **2006**, *1076*, 778–783. [CrossRef] [PubMed]
14. Nicoletti, A.; Vasta, R.; Venti, V.; Mostile, G.; Lo Fermo, S.; Patti, F. The epidemiology of amyotrophic lateral sclerosis in the Mount Etna region: A possible pathogenic role of volcanogenic metals. *Eur. J. Neurol.* **2016**, *23*, 964–972. [CrossRef]
15. Giacoppo, S.; Galuppo, M.; Calabrò, R.S.; D'Aleo, G.; Marra, A.; Sessa, E. Heavy Metals and Neurodegenerative Diseases: An Observational Study. *Biol. Trace Elem. Res.* **2014**, *161*, 151–160. [CrossRef]
16. Stracquadanio, M.; Dinelli, E.; Trombini, C. Role of volcanic dust in the atmospheric transport and deposition of polycyclic aromatic hydrocarbons and mercury. *J. Environ. Monit.* **2003**, *5*, 984. [CrossRef] [PubMed]
17. Barone, G.; De Giudici, G.; Gimeno, D.; Lanzafame, G.; Podda, F.; Cannas, C.; Giuffrida, A.; Barchitta, M.; Agodi, A.; Mazzoleni, P. Surface reactivity of Etna volcanic ash and evaluation of health risks. *Sci. Total Environ.* **2020**, 143248. [CrossRef] [PubMed]

18. Sun, L.; Pan, Y.; Wang, X.; Gao, G.; Wu, L.; Piao, C. Screening for Potential Biomarkers in Peripheral Blood From Miners Exposed to Radon Radiation. *Dose-Response* **2020**, *18*. [CrossRef]
19. Alexandrov, K.; Rojas, M.; Geneste, O.; Castegnaro, M.; Camus, A.M.; Petruzzelli, S.; Giuntini, C.; Bartsch, H. An improved fluorometric assay for dosimetry of benzo(a)pyrene diol-epoxide-DNA adducts in smokers' lung: Comparisons with total bulky adducts and aryl hydrocarbon hydroxylase activity. *Cancer Res.* **1992**, *52*, 6248–6253.
20. Oliveri Conti, G.; Calogero, A.E.; Giacone, F.; Fiore, M.; Barchitta, M.; Agodi, A.; Ferrante, M. B(a)P adduct levels and fertility: A cross sectional study in a Sicilian population. *Mol. Med. Rep.* **2017**, *15*, 3398–3404. [CrossRef]
21. Joshi, P. MicroRNA in lung cancer. *World J. Methodol.* **2014**, *4*, 59–72. [CrossRef] [PubMed]
22. Izzotti, A.; Carozzo, S.; Pulliero, A.; Zhabayeva, D.; Ravetti, J.L.; Bersimbaev, R. Extracellular MicroRNA in liquid biopsy: Applicability in cancer diagnosis and prevention. *Am. J. Cancer Res.* **2016**, *6*, 1461–1493.
23. Duan, Y.; Huang, S.; Yang, J.; Niu, P.; Gong, Z.; Liu, X. HspA1A facilitates DNA repair in human bronchial epithelial cells exposed to Benzo[a]pyrene and interacts with casein kinase 2. Cell Stress and Chaperones. *Springer Sci. Bus. Media* **2013**, *19*, 271–279. [CrossRef]
24. Rossnerova, A.; Pokorna, M.; Svecova, V.; Sram, R.J.; Topinka, J.; Zölzer, F.; Rossner, P., Jr. Adaptation of the human population to the environment: Current knowledge, clues from Czech cytogenetic and "omics" biomonitoring studies and possible mechanisms. *Mutat. Res.* **2017**, *773*, 188–203. [CrossRef]
25. Rossnerova, A.; Izzotti, A.; Pulliero, A.; Bast, A.; Rattan, S.; Rossner, P. The molecular mechanisms of adaptive response related to environmental stress. *Int. J. Mol. Sci.* **2020**, *21*, 7053. [CrossRef] [PubMed]
26. Izzotti, A.; Longobardi, M.G.; La Maestra, S.; Micale, R.T.; Pulliero, A.; Camoirano, A.; Geretto, M.; D'Agostini, F.; Balansky, R.; Miller, M.S.; et al. Release of microRNAs into body fluids form ten organs in mice exposed to cig-arette smoke. *Theranostics* **2018**, *8*, 2147–2160. [CrossRef] [PubMed]
27. Ferrante, M.; Cristaldi, A.; Oliveri Conti, G. Oncogenic Role of miRNA in Environmental Exposure to Plasticizers: A Systematic Review. *J. Pers. Med.* **2021**, *11*, 500. [CrossRef] [PubMed]

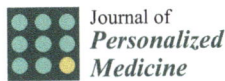

Review

Oncogenic Role of miRNA in Environmental Exposure to Plasticizers: A Systematic Review

Margherita Ferrante [1,2,*], Antonio Cristaldi [1] and Gea Oliveri Conti [1]

[1] Department of Medical, Surgical Sciences and Advanced Technologies "G.F. Ingrassia", University of Catania, 95123 Catania, Italy; antonio.cristaldi@unict.it (A.C.); olivericonti@unict.it (G.O.C.)
[2] Catania, Messina, Enna Cancer Registry, Via S. Sofia 87, 95123 Catania, Italy
* Correspondence: marfer@unict.it; Tel.: +39-095-378-2181; Fax: +39-095-378-2177

Abstract: The daily environmental exposure of humans to plasticizers may adversely affect human health, representing a global issue. The altered expression of microRNAs (miRNAs) plays an important pathogenic role in exposure to plasticizers. This systematic review summarizes recent findings showing the modified expression of miRNAs in cancer due to exposure to plasticizers. Following the Preferred Reporting Items for Systematic Reviews and Meta-Analyses (PRISMA) methodology, we performed a systematic review of the literature published in the past 10 years, focusing on the relationship between plasticizer exposure and the expression of miRNAs related to cancer. Starting with 535 records, 17 articles were included. The results support the hypothesis that exposure to plasticizers causes changes in or the deregulation of a number of oncogenic miRNAs and show that the interaction of plasticizers with several redundant miRNAs, such as let-7f, let-7g, miR-125b, miR-134, miR-146a, miR-22, miR-192, miR-222, miR-26a, miR-26b, miR-27b, miR-296, miR-324, miR-335, miR-122, miR-23b, miR-200, miR-29a, and miR-21, might induce deep alterations. These genotoxic and oncogenic responses can eventually lead to abnormal cell signaling pathways and metabolic changes that participate in many overlapping cellular processes, and the evaluation of miRNA-level changes can be a useful target for the toxicological assessment of environmental pollutants, including plastic additives and plasticizers.

Keywords: plasticizers; cancer; microRNA; in vitro study; PRISMA

1. Introduction

The continuous daily environmental exposure of humans to different chemicals may adversely affect human health, thus representing a global issue [1–11]. In the last decade especially, ecological and epidemiological studies have focused on the presence of plastics and their additives in food and the environment [6,12–14].

Plasticizers are added to plastics to increase their flexibility, durability, and pliability. A large broad of molecules are used by the polymer industry, including phthalates, bisphenolates, flame retardants, metals, parabens, polychlorinated biphenyls, tributyltin, organophosphate esters, etc.

Among the plasticizers, phthalates, are the most widely used in polyvinyl chloride (PVC), polyethylene terephthalate (PET), polyvinyl acetate (PVA), and polyethylene (PE). Phthalates can be found in toys, personal care products, food packages, paints, pharmaceuticals and drugs, medical devices, catheters, blood transfusion devices, cosmetics, and PVC products for home furnishing such as PVC films for floors or household accessories [12,15,16].

Bisphenol A (BPA), another plasticizer, is the major component in the manufacture of epoxy and polycarbonate plastics and flame retardants. The uses of BPA include coatings for PVC water pipe walls, plastic bottles for water, baby bottles, food packaging, receipt inks, cosmetics, plastic toys, etc. BPA has drawn attention from public health and governmental agencies due to its widespread use. Also, BPA exerts genotoxic and carcinogenic activities due to the similarity of its chemical structure that resembles that of diethylstilbestrol, an accredited human carcinogen [17,18]. Plasticizer exposure has been reported as a reproductive and developmental toxicant and carcinogen [19,20].

Plasticizers have been associated with hormone-sensitive cancers such as breast, prostate, endometrial, ovarian, testicular and thyroid cancers, but also with non-hormonally sensitive cancers such as cervical and lung cancers, osteosarcoma, and meningioma [21].

Based on the evidence that is already available, several countries regulated some plasticizers, especially in food and human consume products. Some laws and limits are formulated under which certain plasticizers are permitted to be used in the plastics industry, for instance, the USA Consumer Product Safety Improvement Act (CPSIA) [22], the Proposition 65 list of California State (PROP65) [23], the European Commission Regulation (EC) no. 372/2007 of 2 April 2007 [24], etc.

However, the Chang and Flow study [25] showed that also subchronic exposures to DEHP and DiNP in adulthood lead both to immediate and long-term reproductive consequences in female mice.

The altered expression of microRNAs (miRNAs) represents an epigenetic mechanism that exerts an important pathogenic role linked to exposure to environmental pollutants with several pathological outcomes, including cancer promotion and development [26–28]. These miRNAs are very-short RNA, ranging from 19 to 25 nucleotides in size, that regulate the post-transcriptional silencing of target genes. A single miRNA can target hundreds of mRNAs and influence the expression of a large number of genes often involved in several important functional pathways [26]. The miRNAs are differentially regulated in various types of cancer, including ovarian, liver, gastric, pancreatic, esophageal, colorectal, breast, and lung cancers [29].

An emerging hypothesis explores the supposed coordination between miRNA-mediated gene control and splicing events in gene regulatory networks [27]. Several studies suggest that the maturation of miRNAs may depend on splicing factors [30]. However, microRNA modification results in carcinogenesis only when other molecular changes occur simultaneously, such as suppression of the inhibition of the expression of mutated oncogenes, the formation of microRNA adducts, p53-microRNA interconnections, and alterations of the *Dicer* function [26].

Due to the considerable stability of miRNAs, they are measurable both in blood and tissues and are therefore eligible as potential biomarkers for several non-communicable diseases, including cancer [29].

This systematic review summarizes recent findings showing the aberrant expression of miRNAs in cancer due to plasticizer exposure. We further discuss the challenges in environmental-miRNA research because this approach can be key for understanding the mechanism of cancer pathophysiology but also for early screening and/or personalized cancer therapy.

2. Materials and Methods

A brief critical review of scientific papers from the last ten years selected using the PubMed, Scopus, and Web of Science databases was carried out. The "Preferred Reporting Items for Systematic Reviews and Meta-Analysis" (PRISMA) methodology was applied in this study.

To assess the influence of plasticizer exposure on the expression of miRNAs in humans, all original articles published from 1 January 2010 to 29 December 2020 were selected based on the following criteria:

- the articles are original,
- articles report on plasticizer or plasticizer exposure,
- articles report on miRNAs analysis and identification,
- articles have correct scientific methodology,
- articles include the identification of miRNAs for cancers of all target organs.

We searched the databases for controlled randomized studies, cohort studies, case–control studies, case reports, and in vitro studies. Only original articles written in English were collected for the PRISMA review.

We excluded papers that did not include original data such as informative reviews, commentaries, and editorials. Systematic reviews and meta-analyses were not eligible, but their references were screened for recovery of eligible studies missing in the databases.

Two investigators (A.C. and G.O.C.) screened all citations for potentially eligible studies and extracted data independently. Disagreements were adjudicated by a third investigator (M.F.).

The research was conducted using keywords including "Plasticizers and microRNA", "Plasticizers and oncogenic microRNA", "additives of plastic and miRNA cancer", "endocrine disrupting chemicals and miRNA cancer", "BPA and miRNA cancer", "di-n-butyl phthalate and miRNA cancer", "DBP and miRNA cancer", "monobutyl phthalate and miRNA cancer", "MBP and miRNA cancer", "Organophoshorus flame retardants and miRNA cancer", "flame retardants and miRNA cancer", "di(2-ethylhexyl) phthalate and miRNA cancer", "DEHP and miRNA cancer", "mono-(2-ethylhexyl) phthalate and miRNA cancer", "MEHP and miRNA cancer", "methylparaben and miRNA cancer", "parabens and miRNA cancer", "phthalates and miRNA cancer", "environmental phenols and miRNA cancer", "organophosphate esters and miRNA cancer", "Tributyltin and miRNA cancer", "PCBs and microRNAs cancer", "butylbenzyl phthalate and miRNA cancer", "PVC and miRNA cancer".

We also used combinations of the keywords, such as "Plasticizers and oncogenic effects" and "Plasticizers and microRNA changes".

All eligible studies were evaluated as eligible using a modified Newcastle Ottawa scale (rating system to score each study) [4].

3. Results

3.1. Literature Inclusion Criteria

Our initial search produced 477 potential references (Figure 1) from databases and 58 references from other sources.

Starting with 535 records, we identified in the first phase 322 records after the deletion of 213 duplicates. In addition, via evaluation of the title and abstract, we screened 57 records. Of these, 40 records were excluded due to the absence of some criteria of eligibility (reporting on miRNAs or indications, evidence about exposure to plasticizers, cancer tissue or cells analysis reporting, correct sample size, in vivo or in vitro study, statistical analysis of data, analysis of plasticizers in biological tissues) as listed in Figure 1. Finally, we included 17 studies in the systematic review. These studies used various approaches or study designs, but all focused on the effects of exposure to plasticizers on outcomes defined as "oncogenic miRNA identification and their down or upregulation description".

3.2. Summary of Literature Included

Figure 1 describes the findings of the performed collection and screening procedures.

We included the following studies, in chronological order: Tilghman et al., 2012 [31], Meng et al., 2013 [32], Li et al., 2014 [33], Kim et al., 2015 [34], Buñay et al., 2017 [35], Chang et al., 2017 [36], Chou et al., 2017 [37], Hui et al., 2018 [38], Wu et al., 2018 [39], Yin et al., 2018 [40], Scarano et al., 2019 [41]; Wang et al., 2019 [42], Zhu et al., 2019 [43], Cui et al., 2019 [44], Chorley et al., 2020 [45]; Duan et al., 2020 [46], and Zota et al., 2020 [47].

All the studies are in vitro cell studies on rats, mice, or human cancer cell lines. Several plasticizers were studied through controlled in vitro exposure as reported in Table 1.

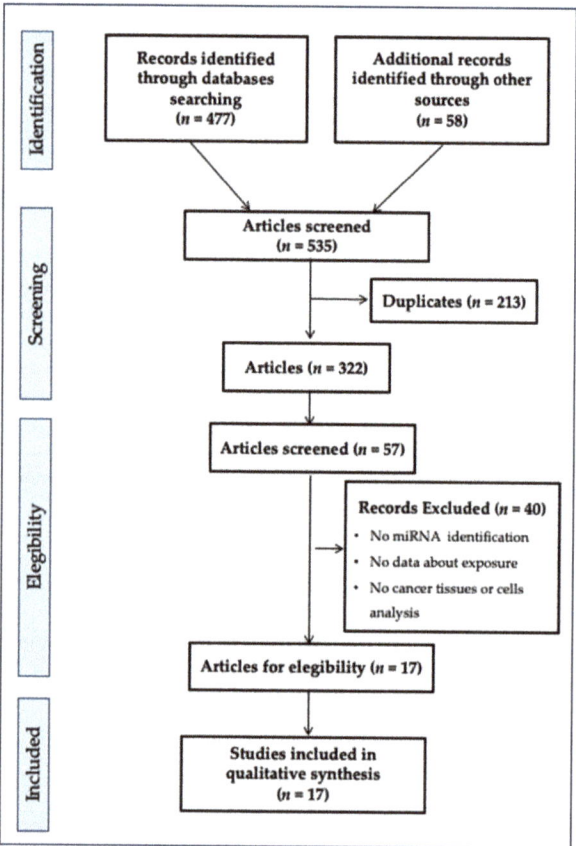

Figure 1. PRISMA flow diagram.

Table 1. The included studies and their results [++].

Study	In Vitro/Vivo	Plasticizer	miRNA	Expression	Reference No.
Wu et al., 2018	^ MCF-7 ^ MDA-MB-231	BBP	miR-19a	Up	[39]
			miR-19b	Up	
Zhu et al., 2019	π LNCaP and PC-3cells	BBP	miR-34a	Down	[43]
Duan et al., 2020	β AML U937, Raji, and HL-60 cell lines.	BBP	miR-15b-5p	Down	[45]
Chou et al., 2017	** RL95–2 cell line	BPA	miR-182	NE	[37]
			miR-107	Up	
			miR-203	Up	
			miR-205	Up	
			miR-103a	Up	
			miR-200c	Up	
			miR-141	Up	
			miR-221	Up	
			Let-7a-5p	Up	
			miR-193b	Up	
			miR-423	Up	
			miR-513	Down	
			miR-149	Down	
			miR-765	Down	

Table 1. Cont.

Study	In Vitro/Vivo	Plasticizer	miRNA	Expression	Reference No.
Tilghman et al., 2012	ˆ MCF-7 cell line	BPA	miR-21	Down	[31]
			let-7g	Down	
			let-7c	Down	
			miR-923	Down	
			let-7f	Down	
			miR-15b	Down	
			miR-27b	Down	
			miR-26b	Down	
			miR-342-3p	Down	
			miR-638	Up	
			miR-663	Up	
			miR-1915	Up	
			miR-93	Up	
			miR-320a	Up	
			miR-1308	Up	
			miR-1275	Up	
			miR-222	Up	
			miR-149	Up	
	ρ MCF-7F cells		miR-21	Up	
Meng et al., 2013	$ BEL-7402 cells	BPA	miR-21	Down [a]/Up [b]	[32]
	ˆ MCF-7 cells		miR-21	Down [a]/Up [b]	
Li et al., 2014	ˆ MCF-7 cell line	BPA	miR-19°	Up	[33]
			miR-19b	Up	
Kim et al., 2015	° HepG2 cell line	BPA	miR-22	Up	[34]
Chou et al., 2017	** RL95–2 cell line	BPA	miR-107	Up	[37]
			miR-203	Up	
			miR-205	Up	
			miR-103a	Up	
			miR-200c	Up	
			miR-141	Up	
			miR-221	Up	
			Let-7a-5p	Up	
			miR-193b	Up	
			miR-423	Up	
			miR-513	Down	
			miR-149	Down	
			miR-765	Down	
Hui et al., 2018	§ SKOV3 and § A2780 cell lines	BPA	miR-21-5p	Up	[38]
			miR-222-3p	Up	
Yin et al., 2018	Juvenile rat Sertoli cells	MBP	miR-199a-3p	Up	[40]
			miR-301b-3p	Up	
			miR-3584-5p	Up	
Chang et al., 2017	* AS52 CHO cells inoculated in mouse	MEHP	miR-let-7a	Down	[36]
			miR-125b-5p	Down	
			miR-130a-3p	Down	
			miR-27a-3p	Down	
			miR-25-3p	Down	
			miR-92a-3p	Down	
Wang et al., 2019	In vivo Σ OSCC cells/subcutaneously injected in mice	MEHP	miR-27b-5p	Down	[48]
			miR-372-5p	Down	
Buñay et al., 2017	In vivo Adult mice	Cocktail (DEHP, DBP, BBP, NP, OP)	miR20b-5p	Down	[35]
			miR-1291	Down	
Cui et al., 2019	+ HA HDEC, + CRL-2586 OEMA	Cocktail MEHP, DEHP, DCHP and BBP	miR-655 [(BBP)]	Down	[44]
			miR-182	NE	

Table 1. Cont.

Study	In Vitro/Vivo	Plasticizer	miRNA	Expression	Reference No.
Scarano et al., 2019	In vivo Pregnant rat exposure/Ventral prostate tissues from puppies	Cocktail DEHP, DEP, DBP, DiBP, BBzP, DiNP	miR-30d-5p	Up	[41]
			miR-30b-5p	Up	
			miR-141-3p	Up	
			miR-30d-3p	Up	
			mir-184	Up	
Chorley et al., 2020	In vivo Serum and liver tissue of mice	Cocktail DEHP BBP and DNOP	miR-182–5p (DEHP)	Up	[46]
			miR-378a–3p (DEHP)	Up	
			miR-125a–5p	Up	
Zota et al., 2020 (FORGE) study	In vivo Human Fibroid and myometrium tissue—Uterine Leiomyoma	Cocktail ΣDEHP and ΣAA phthalates	miR-10a-5p	Up	[47]
	Myometrium		miR-10a-3p	Up	
	Myometrium		miR-140-3p	Up	
	Myometrium		miR-144-5p	Up	
	Myometrium		miR-150-5p	Up	
	Myometrium		miR-205-5p	Up	
	Myometrium		miR-27a-5p	Up	
	Myometrium		miR-29b-2-5p	Up	
	Myometrium		miR-29c-5p	Up	
	Myometrium		miR-451a	Up	
	Myometrium		miR-95-3p	Up	
	Fibroid		miR-135a-5p	Up	
	Fibroid		miR-135b-5p	Up	
	Fibroid		miR-137-3p	Up	
	Fibroid		miR-302b-3p	Up	
	Fibroid		miR-335-3p	Up	
	Fibroid		miR-34a-5p	Up	
	Fibroid		miR-34a-3p	Up	
	Fibroid		miR-34b-5p	Up	
	Fibroid		miR-34c-5p	Up	
	Fibroid		miR-483-5p	Up	
	Fibroid		miR-488-3p	Up	
	Fibroid		miR-488-5p	Up	
	Fibroid		miR-508-3p	Up	
	Fibroid		miR-577	Up	
	Fibroid		miR-592	Up	
	Fibroid		miR-651-5p	Up	
	Fibroid		miR-885-5p	Up	
	Fibroid		miR-9-3p	Up	

[++] List of studies are organized according to chronological order in subgroup on the type of plasticizer/cocktail of plasticizers alphabetical basis basis. * AS52-mutant cell (ASMC) clones; ** Human endometrial cancer cell line; [+] Human Hemangioma cells; [β] Acute myeloid leukemia; [§] Human ovarian cancer cell lines; [ˆ] Human breast cancer cells; [ρ] (ERα-negative and estrogen-resistant); NE: no effect; UP: upregulated, Down: downregulated, [°] Human hepatocellular carcinoma; [Σ] Human oral squamous cell carcinoma; [π] Human prostate cancer cells; [$] cancer cells; [a] ($10^{-4}$ or 10^{-5} M); [b] (10^{-6} to 10^{-11} M); Mono-ethylhexyl phthalate (MEHP); Bis (2-ethylhexyl) phthalate (DEHP); diethyl-phthalate (DEP); dibutyl phthalate (DBP); di-isobutyl-phthalate (DiBP), butylbenzyl-phthalate (BBzP); di-isononyl-phthalate (DiNP); benzyl butyl phthalate (BBP); 4-nonylphenol (NP); 4-tert-octylphenol (OP); di-noctyl phthalate (DNOP); Tris (1,3-dichloro-2-propyl) phosphate (TDCIPP) = organophosphate flame retardants. Observational Research on Genes and the Environment (FORGE) study; ΣDEHP = Sum of 21 phthalates and metabolites; ΣAA phthalates = Sum of 31 antiandrogenic phthalate metabolites.

Human endometrial, hemangioma, acute myeloid leukemia, ovarian, breast, hepatocellular, oral squamous, and prostate cancer cells lines were evaluated.

3.3. Detailed Overview of the Literature Included

3.3.1. In Vitro Studies

Tilghman et al. (2012) [31] studied the effects of BPA (10 μM) and DDT (10 μM) on miRNA regulation and expression levels in hormone-responsive human breast cancer cells. The MCF-7 breast cancer cell line showed that both pollutants increased the expression of *ER* receptor target genes, including the progesterone receptor, bcl-2, and trefoil factor. The revealed miRNAs (27) were outlined in the exposed cells (miR-21, miR-638, miR-663, miR-1915, let-7g, let-7c, miR-923, miR-93, miR-320a, miR-1308, let-7f, miR-15b, miR-1275, miR-27b, miR-222, miR-193a-5p, miR-16, miR-26b, miR-149, miR-92a, miR-99b, miR-92b, miR-342-3p), of which several were upregulated and downregulated according to Table 1.

Several genes were differentially regulated by the compounds. For example, *Jun* and *Fas* genes were increased approximately 1.8- and 1.5-fold by BPA, but were relatively unchanged by DDT. The onco-miR-21 is an estrogen-regulated miRNA that plays an important role in breast cancer. In this study, miR-21 expression was downregulated by BPA, and several members of the let-7 family (let-7a, let-7b, let-7c, let-7d, let-7e and let-7f), were downregulated ($p < 0.05$) by all treatments. In contrast, miR-638 ($p < 0.005$), miR-663 ($p < 0.005$), and miR-1915 ($p < 0.005$) were upregulated by BPA and DDT.

Chou et al. (2017) [37] investigated the role of BPA exposure in the disruption of miRNA regulation and whether the related gene expression is decisive for carcinogenic progression. This study was carried out using human endometrial cancer RL95-2 cells and treatment with low to moderate BPA concentrations (10, 10^3, and 10^5 nM).

Chou and colleagues reported that BPA exposure reduced miR-149 expression, downregulating the DNA repair gene *ARF6* (ADP ribosylation factor 6) and tumor protein p53 (*TP53*) and upregulating *CCNE2* (cyclin E2). The results of the study also showed that BPA was able to increase miR-107 to suppress hedgehog signaling factors, acting as a suppressor of fused homologs (*SUFU*) and GLI family zinc finger 3 (*GLI3*) and providing proof of the potential epigenetic mechanism of BPA exposure on endometrial carcinogenesis risk. In fact, miR107, miR149, miR200c, miR203, miR205, and miR765 changed the expression of some genes (*TP53, JUN, LAMB4, CCCDC6, PRKCA, STAT1, SUFU, CXCL8, DVL1, GLI3, CRK, LAMC1, MAPK1, MAPK9*) involved in the cancer pathway, recording a significant fold change of $N > 2.0$ compared to the control.

This study permitted the discovery and identification of five relevant pathways for potential BPA-induced endometrial cancer progression, including the cancer pathway, hedgehog pathway, cell cycle, adherens junction, and MAPK signaling pathway. In addition, *TP53, GLI3, CCNE2, CRK, KIF23, SAMD2, CCDC6, FZD3, ARF6, MAPK9, SUFU, PRC1, MDM2, SMAD4, DVL1, EGLN1, JUN, MYC, LAMC1, PRKACA*, and *STAT1* were genes that overlapped and were expressed significantly differently in these five pathways.

Meng et al. (2013) [32] developed an miRNA biosensor and applied this novel tool to detect miRNA-21 extracted from human hepatocarcinoma BEL-7402 cells and human mastocarcinoma MCF-7 cells and their expression under in vitro exposure to BPA. Normal human hepatic L-02 cells, BEL-7402 cells, and MCF-7 cells were incubated with 100 μM BPA at the same concentration for three and five days, respectively. The expression profiles of miRNA-21 in BEL-7402 and MCF-7 became 1.415-fold and 1.468-fold higher than that of normal L-02 cells, respectively, showing that the miRNA expression levels of cancer cells were upregulated compared to normal cells.

Li et al. (2014) [33] studied how microRNAs are involved in curcumin-mediated protection from BPA-associated induced effects on a breast cancer MCF-7 cell line. The MCF-7 cell line was exposed to BPA for 4 days. The results showed that BPA exhibited estrogenic activity by increasing the proliferation of estrogen-receptor-positive MCF-7 human breast cancer cells and promoting the transition of the cells from the G1 to S phase. Curcumin was able to inhibit the proliferative effects of BPA on MCF-7 cells. In addition, the BPA-induced upregulation of oncogenic miR-19a and miR-19b and the dysregulated expression of miR-19-related downstream proteins, including *PTEN, p-AKT, p-MDM2, p53*, and proliferating cell nuclear antigen, were sufficiently reversed by curcumin. Furthermore, Li and colleagues highlighted the important role of miR-19 in BPA-mediated MCF-7 cell proliferation, suggesting for the first time that curcumin modulates the miR-19/*PTEN*/*AKT*/*p53* axis to exhibit its protective effects against BPA-associated breast cancer.

Kim et al. (2015) [34] used HepG2 cells that are widely used as a model system for studies of liver metabolism and genotoxicity. In particular, the authors determined the role of BPA exposure in the epigenetically affected expression of miR-22. The authors found methylated Chr17:1565786-1565940 regions (promoter sites for miR-22) in the normal samples, but unmethylated ones in samples exposed to BPA. Kim et al. identified seven differentially expressed miRNAs, including miR-22, in the BPA-exposed sample vs. the control. Notably, in samples exposed to BPA, miR-22 showed a 3.38-fold upregulation compared to normal samples. The study results highlight the regulation of miR-22 expression via hypomethylation of the promoter region due to BPA exposure.

Hui et al. (2018) [38] focused on BPA and ovarian cancer. This study was performed using in vitro exposure to BPA (10 or 100 nM) or 0.1% DMSO for 24 h using human ovarian adenocarcinoma SKOV3 cells, and then, the global gene expression profile was determined via high-throughput RNA sequencing. Transcriptomic analysis revealed 94 different expression genes related to tumorigenesis and metastasis.

The authors revealed the upregulation of miR-21-5p and miR-222-3p, also reporting that BPA (10 and 100 nM) increased migration and invasion as well as induced epithelial to mesenchymal transitions in SKOV3 and A2780 cells. Accordingly, doses of BPA found in the environment are capable of activating the regular Wnt signaling pathway. This study analyzed the possible mechanisms underlying the effects of BPA on ovarian cancer. Environmentally relevant doses of BPA modulated the gene expression profile and promoted the progress of epithelial to mesenchymal transition via the canonical Wnt signaling pathway of ovarian cancer.

Wu et al. (2018) [39] showed that BBP induced the proliferation of both ER(+) MCF-7 and ER(−) MDA-MB-231 breast cancer cells. This was proven by the increased cell viability, the transition of the cell cycle from the G1 to the S phase, the upregulation of *PCNA* and *Cyclin D1*, and the downregulation of *p21*. Moreover, BBP modulated the expression of the oncogenic miR-19a/b and *PTEN/AKT/p21* axis, revealing that miR-19 plays a crucial role in the promoting effect of BBP on breast cancer cells via the targeting of PTEN 3'UTR. These findings provide an important tool for targeted cancer intervention.

Zhu et al. (2019) [43] investigated the role of BBP in the cell proliferation of prostate cancer cells. Human prostate cancer LNCaP and PC-3 cell lines were exposed to low doses (0, 10^{-4}, 10^{-5}, 10^{-6}, 10^{-7} and 10^{-8} mol/L) of BBP for 6 days. Zhu's results showed that 10^{-6} and 10^{-7} mol/L BBP increased the expression of *cyclinD1* and *PCNA*, decreased *p21* expression, and induced cell growth in both LNCaP and PC-3 cells vs. the control group. Furthermore, the authors found that BBP significantly downregulated the expression of miR-34a, along with upregulating miR-34a target gene *c-Myc*. Via cell transfection of an miR-34a mimic and inhibitor, the authors demonstrated that, in prostate cancer cells, the BBP trigger promoted cell proliferation mediated through the miR-34a/c-myc axis.

Duan et al. (2020) [45] also studied the effects of BBP on human acute monocytic leukemia AML U937 (isolated from the histiocytic lymph), Raji (lymphoblast Burkitt's lymph), and HL-60 (a promyelocytic cell line) cell lines, and normal blood cells. BBP doses of 10^{-9} and 10^{-4} M were used for investigating the potential effect of BBP on the malignancy of AML cells. Instead for carrying out a mechanistic study, a dose of 10^{-8} M was used. The authors examined the effects of BBP on the proliferation of AMLU937, Raji, and HL-60 cell lines. Moreover, the authors verified BBP's perturbation of treated U937 cells against the efficacy of chemotherapy using a double-exposure with increasing concentrations of daunorubicin or cytarabine with or without 10^{-8} M BBP.

The results revealed that (10^{-8} M) BBP can induce the proliferation and reduce the chemotherapy sensitivity of acute monocytic leukemia cells. *PDK1*, *PDK2*, *PDK3*, *PDK4*, *PDP2*, and *PDPR* genes can regulate the glucose metabolism and glycolysis of cancer cells. In fact, cancer cells are characterized by high rates of glycolysis. The pyruvate dehydrogenase kinase (*PDK*) supports these energetic needs and also favors apoptosis resistance. Duan showed that BBP increased the expression of *PDK4* and *PDP2* in U937 cells, while in Raji cells, BBP only increased the expression of *PDK4*. This study confirmed that BBP can decrease the expression of miR-15b-5p, while it had no effect on miR-182 in both U937 and Raji cells. The overexpression of miR-15b-5p can abolish the BBP-induced mRNA and protein expression of *PDK4* in U937 cells. Furthermore, the inhibitor of miR-15b-5p can increase the mRNA and protein expression of *PDK4* in U937 cells.

Duan's results suggested that the downregulation of miR-15b-5p was involved in BBP-induced *PDK* and demonstrated that BBP can increase the mRNA stability of *PDK4* via the downregulation of miR-15b-5p.

Hence, BBP had no effect on the transcription and protein stability of *PDK4*; however, it significantly increased the mRNA stability of *PDK4*.

In Yin et al. (2018) [41], the global alterations of miRNA and mRNA expression in juvenile rat Sertoli cells (SCs) treated with 0.1 mM MBP were evaluated. Yin's results revealed that miR-3584-5p and miR-301b-3p were upregulated and their common target gene, Dexamethasone-induced Ras-related protein 1 (*Rasd1*), was downregulated. SC proliferation induced by low MBP concentration in vitro could be mediated by *Rasd1* regulation of the *ERK1/2* signaling pathway. These results represent a possible avenue to apply personalized medicine screening and therapy in testicular tumors induced by exogenous chemicals.

Cui et al. (2019) [44] studied the potential influence of MEHP, DEHP, DCHP, and BBP on the progression of hemangioma, one of the most common tumors of infancy. This in vitro study was carried out using hemangioma cells. The authors found that 100 nM of BBP can significantly trigger the migration and invasion of hemangioma cells, also inducing the overexpression of *Zeb1*, a powerful transcription factor for cell migration and invasion, via miR-655 suppression or downregulation. As 100 nM of BBP might also be found in human tissues, the potential health risks of BBP, particularly for oncologic HA patients, should be given more attention.

3.3.2. In Vivo Studies

Buñay et al. (2017) [35] studied the consequences of chronic exposure to a mixture of phthalates and alkylphenols for the testes of male mice and in particular, reported changes in the expression patterns of miRNA/isomiRs, which act as regulators of gene expression in the testes. Additionally, damage to the testis and changes in the genes responsible for encoding proteins involved in the biogenesis, processing, editing, stability, or degradation of miRNAs were assessed. Buñay et al. carried out a case-control exposure study on a mix of phthalates and alkylphenols using adult male mice.

The exposed mice showed the degeneration of seminiferous tubules and hypertrophy/hyperplasia in Leydig cells and also an increase in exfoliation of germ cells of seminiferous tubules that close the lumen or showed fully closed tubules. Regarding mRNA levels, the authors report that the miRNAs of *Star* and *Cyp17a1* and *Sp1* and *Cyp11a1* were upregulated and downregulated, respectively. Instead, no significant differences in *Hsd3b1* mRNA expression were detected.

The authors quantified the mRNA expression levels of genes encoding proteins that are involved in pri-miRNA processing (*Drosha*), nuclear export (*Xpo5*), stability/degradation (*Lin28*, *Zcchc11*, *Zcchc6*, and *Snd1*), editing (*Adar*) and processing of pre-miRNAs (*Dicer*, *Ago2*).

A significant increase in the mRNA levels of *Drosha*, *Adar*, and *Zcchc11* in the testes of exposed mice was found compared to control mice, contrary to *Zcchc6*, *Dicer*, *Xpo5*, *Ago2*, *Lin28b*, and *Snd1*, which showed no differences.

miR20b-5p and miR-1291, which are implicated in cancer, and miR-3085-3p, implicated in inflammation, were all downregulated. miR-1291 targets DNA methyltransferases (*Dnmt3a*, *Dnmt3b*) that are involved in (de novo) histone methylation, genomic imprinting, X-chromosome inactivation, and testicular germ cell tumors due to exposure to alkylphenols. In addition, *Ccnd2*, *Ccnd1*, and *Raf1* are targets of the downregulated miR-15b-5p in exposed mice, and these targets are implicated in cancer and cell cycle regulation. Hence, this study suggests that the downregulation of sncRNAs through miR-1291 related to exposure to plasticizer mixtures might promote changes in the DNA methylation pattern, causing the epigenetic transmission of several diseases, including cancer.

In Chang et al. (2017) [36], the role of MEHP-induced reactive oxygen species (ROS) for genotoxicity was explained. Mono-ethylhexyl phthalate (MEHP) is a metabolite of DEPH. The toxicity of MEHP is more potent than that of DEPH. Chang's study provided evidence of the carcinogenicity of MEHP in Chinese hamster AA8, UV5, and EM9 ovary cells, as well as its ability to induce epigenetic modifications.

The cell lines were exposed to 0, 10, 25, and 50 mM MEHP. However, at 50 mM MEHP, all the cells died. The protection was not significant at 25 mM MEHP, and, even after exposure to a lower dose of MEHP (1 mM), the PARP-1-KD cells had a higher level of single-strand breaks. The subsequent *gpt* gene sequencing used to analyze the mutation points on the genes of AS52 mutant cells (ASMC) showed that 90% of all mutations were single-base pair substitutions, especially G:C to A:T mutations. Independent AS52-mutant cell clones were collected and used to perform sequential in vivo xenograft tumorigenic studies, and 4 of 20 clones had aggressive tumor growth. The study also showed that miR-let-7a and miR-125b has been downregulated in ASMC, which might raise oncogenic MYC and RAS levels and promote the activation of the *ErbB* pathway. The mutagenic pathway of MEHP can probably be triggered via the generation of ROS, causing base excision damage and resulting in carcinogenicity.

Wang et al. (2019) [48] sought to evaluate the capability of MEHP to promote the proliferation of oral cancer through an in vitro/in vivo study using human oral squamous carcinoma (OSCC) (human OSCC SCC-4, SCC-9, and SCC-25) cells and cell nuclear antigen (PCNA). SCC-4 cancer cells (2×10^6 per mouse) were diluted in 100 µL of normal medium and a researcher injected these subcutaneously into the left flank of each mouse to obtain OSCC cancer xenografts. When the tumor grew to 100 mm^3, the mice of the MEHPs group were treated with MEHP (4 mg per kg, body weight) via intratumoral injection four times every three days. Tumor volume was measured every three days and, at the end of the experiment, mice were sacrificed and the xenograft tumors were removed to measure the expression of miRNAs and proteins.

The authors supported their hypothesis with results that showed the proliferation of oral cancer via MEHP through the downregulation of miR-27b-5p and miR-372-5p. In addition, MEHP induced the expression of *c-Myc*, which can suppress the transcription of miR-27b-5p in OSCC cells. Therefore, Wang's study showed that MEHP can promote the growth and progression of OSCC via the downregulation of miR-27b-5p and miR-372-5p.

Scarano et al. (2019) [41] studied the genome-wide levels of mRNAs to determine if perinatal exposure to a phthalate mixture in pregnant rats was capable of modifying gene expression during the prostate development of the filial generation. The study sought to determine the epigenetic role of these pollutants in prostate cancer.

Pregnant female Sprague Dawley rats were exposed daily (from gestational day 10 to postnatal day 21) to a mixture of phthalate by gavage and were suppressed after. Four groups were established—a control group exposed only to corn oil; (T1) 20 mg of the mixture (20 mg/kg/day); (T2) 200 mg of the mixture (200 mg/kg/day); and (T3) 200 mg of the mixture (200 mg/kg/day). The cocktail contained DEHP, DEP, DBP, DiBP, BBzP, and DiNP. The two lower doses mimicked daily human exposure levels based on the amount of DEHP, and the higher dose was selected to compare our results with those of similar phthalate studies. Rats from groups T1 to T3 received the respective doses of the phthalate cocktail prepared with 21% DEHP, 35% DEP, 15% DBP, 8% DiBP, 5% BBzP, and 15% DiNP. After birth, the number of F1 offspring per litter was reduced to 8 (at a 1:1 ratio between males and females whenever possible), and litters with fewer than six pups were suppressed.

miRNAs in the treated groups versus the control were upregulated in T1 vs. C and in T2 vs. C. miR-141-3p was exclusively upregulated in the T1 vs. C group, whereas other miRNAs, such as miR-30d-5p, were deregulated in both groups with weak but significant alterations in gene expression. miRNA-184 was upregulated in all treatment groups vs. C. Among the possible targets for miR-141-3p (53 targets), 51 were downregulated. The MiRNAs differentially expressed in the prostate tissue of these exposed animals were elicited in Table 1. Scarano's study, based on the evaluation of miRNAs and histopathological and immunostaining analyses, support the hypothesis of the epigenetic role of phthalate in prostate oncogenesis.

Chorley et al. (2020) [46] measured liver and blood miRNAs in male B6C3F1 mice exposed both to a known chemical activator of the peroxisome proliferator-activated receptor alpha (PPARα) and DEHP, respectively, for 7 and 28 days at concentrations of 0, 750, 1500, 3000, and 6000 ppm through oral exposure (feed). The PPARα pathway is a common target of several environmental chemicals. At the highest DEHP dose tested, 61 miRNAs were altered after 7 days, and 171 miRNAs after 28 days of exposure, with 48 overlapping miRNAs. Analysis of the 48 common miRNAs indicated the enrichment in PPARα–related targets and other pathways related to liver injury and cancer. The experiment was repeated using mmu-miRs-182-5p and -378a-3p analysis for DEHP, as well as di-n-octyl phthalate (DNOP) and n-butyl benzyl phthalate (BBP), two other related phthalates with weaker PPARα activity.

The results showed that the deregulatory potency of DEHP was superior to DNOP and BBP, and mmu-miRs-125a-5p, -182-5p, -20a-5p, and -378a-3p showed a clear dose relation linked to the PPARα pathway. These findings also highlight the putative miRNA biomarkers, as well as the stratified chemical potency of plasticizers and environmental pollutants in general.

Zota et al. (2020) [47] conducted the only human study included in this review. The Fibroids Observational Research on Genes and the Environment (FORGE) study involved 45 women living in Washington, DC, from 2014–2017. Eligible women were nonpregnant, pre-menopausal, English-speaking, and ≥18 years of age. The authors quantified the expression levels of 754 miRNAs in fibroid tumor samples and analyzed spot urine samples for phthalate metabolites collected from women undergoing surgery for fibroid treatment.

Associations between the miRNA levels in fibroids and phthalate biomarkers were also evaluated using a linear regression adjusted for age, race/ethnicity, and body mass index (BMI), and all the statistical tests were adjusted for multiple comparisons.

Fibroid tissues were collected during hysterectomy or myomectomy procedures. For patients with multiple fibroids, only the largest fibroid was sampled.

In addition, the evaluation of single metabolites was carried out, including diethyl phthalate (DEP), monoethyl phthalate (MEP), di-n-butyl phthalate (DnBP), mono-n-butyl phthalate (MnBP), mono-hydroxybutyl phthalate (MHBP), diisobutyl phthalate (DiBP), monoisobutyl phthalate (MiBP), mono-hydroxyisobutyl phthalate (MHiBP), butylbenzyl phthalate (BBzP), monobenzyl phthalate (MBzP), DnOP, mono(3-carboxypropyl) phthalate (MCPP), diisononyl phthalate (DiNP), monocarboxyoctyl phthalate (MCOP), diisodecyl phthalate (DiDP), monocarboxynonyl phthalate (MCNP), di(2-ethylhexyl) phthalate (DEHP), mono(2-ethylhexyl) phthalate (MEHP), mono(2-ethyl-5-hydroxyhexyl) phthalate (MEHHP), mono(2-ethyl-5-oxohexyl) phthalate (MEOHP), and mono(2-ethyl-5-carboxypentyl) phthalate (MECPP). The authors also calculated two summary measures, the molar sum of DEHP metabolites (ΣDEHP)21 and a potency-weighted sum of antiandrogenic phthalate metabolites (ΣAA phthalates).

The fibroid characteristics were similar across racial/ethnic groups. Phthalate exposure was ubiquitous in the enrolled woman, but nine phthalate metabolites were detected in >90% of participants. However, MEP levels were significantly higher in Black women. The enrolled women were Black (62%), overweight or obese (76%), privately insured (64%), and undergoing a myomectomy (58%). Compared with White/Latina women, Black women were more likely to be obese, publicly insured, and undergoing hysterectomy. The miRNA profiles detected were surprising with respect to social determinants.

A total of 35 miRNAs were underexpressed, and 39 miRNAs were overexpressed in fibroids rather than myometrium. Also, the expression of miR-10a-5p, miR-10a-3p, miR-140-3p, miR-144-5p, miR-150-5p, miR-205-5p, miR-27a-5p, miR-29b-2-5p, miR-29c-5p, miR-451a, and miR-95-3p was three-fold greater in myometrium; while expressions of miR-135a-5p, miR-135b-5p, miR-137-3p, miR-302b-3p, miR-335-3p, miR-34a-5p, miR-34a-3p, miR-34b-5p, miR-34c-5p, miR-483-5p, miR-488-3p, miR-488-5p, miR-508-3p, miR-577, miR-592, miR-651-5p, miR-885-5p, and miR-9-3pthese miRNAs were three-fold greater in fibroids.

The authors found 285 significant associations between phthalate biomarkers and miRNAs ($p < 0.05$), 34 of which were significant at $p < 0.005$.

After adjusting for multiple testing, we found two miRNAs associated with phthalate biomarkers—MHBP, associated with an increase in miR-10a-5p of 0.76 (95% CI = (0.40, 1.11)), and MEHHP, associated with miR-577 ($\beta = 1.06$, 95% CI = (0.53, 1.59)). Eight phthalate-miRNA associations varied significantly between White/Latina and Black women, and among these, there was an association between MBzP and miR-494-3p. Also, among white/Latina women, there were associations between MCPP and miR-337-5p; MBzP and miR-1227-3p; MEP and miR-645; MEP and miR-564; MEP and miR-374-5p; MEHP and miR-128-3p; and MEHP and miR-337-3p. Ten miRNAs were significantly associated with phthalate biomarkers either in the main analysis or in racial groups (miR-10a-5p, miR-577 miR-494-3p, miR-337-5p, miR-1227-3p, miR-645, miR-564, miR-374a-5p, miR-128-3p, miR-337-3p).

Zota et al. identified 923 mRNA targets that were experimentally observed or highly predicted targets of the 10 miRNAs, but 3 miRNAs (miR-10a-5p, miR-128-3p, miR-494-3p) were significantly associated with multiple fibroid-related processes, including angiogenesis, apoptosis, the proliferation of connective tissues, cell viability, tumorigenesis of the reproductive tract, and smooth muscle tumors.

miR-10a, miR-150, miR-29b, miR-29c, and miR-451 were underexpressed, and miR-34a was overexpressed in fibroids. The authors reported that miR-10a-5p expression in particular is associated with concentrations of MHBP, an oxidative metabolite of DnBP which is found in some personal care products, demonstrating that the epigenome is sensitive to interactions between chemical and non-chemical stressors, but also to social determinants that can influence a wide range of physical and social environmental exposures altering the biological response to environmental pollutants. On the basis of these results, the lack of human studies needs to be addressed urgently.

4. Discussion and Conclusions

The epigenetic effects of environmental chemicals such as plasticizers, including BPA and phthalates, on DNA methylation, as well as the expression of miRNAs, have substantiated our knowledge about the etiology of chronic diseases in humans, such as cancer. Evidence from in vitro and in vivo models has proved that epigenetic modifications due to exposure to common environmental pollutants can induce alterations in gene expression that may persist throughout life, increasing susceptibility to cancer. Epigenetics can affect the gene expression profiles of various organs and tissues. Among the phthalates, BPA, DEHP, MEHP, DBP, BBP, and MBP were found to cause 1232 and 265 interactions with the same genes and proteins, respectively.

This systematic review shows that miRNA-based diagnostic models can predict several targets of cancerous organs targets in humans with high accuracy. Also, the evidence regarding the carcinogenicity of several plasticizers was further supported by expression studies, permitting the future use of specific miRNA as valuable predictor or screening method for early diagnosis biomarkers as showed by Meng et al. study [32].

The use of profiling of miRNA as screening test through the high-throughput omic methods (microarrays and real-time quantitative PCR or qPCR, as well as real time PCR and next-generation sequencing) should be improved and applied in molecular early diagnosis to identify novel oncogenes, mechanisms, and/or pathways in which a stimuli, whether genetic or environmental, exerts a change on cell physiology to an oncological status.

Although the use of miRNAs is currently applied as a basic science tool, the overall miRNA's gene expression is moving from research laboratories to the large-scale clinical trials for the validation of a new diagnostic tool or for allowing clinical states to be determined in diseases such as cancer or other miRNA-diseases or altered gene expression related diseases. The use of miRNAs, as non-invasive tool of early diagnosis, need to be implemented in the clinical approach and miRNAs may be promising and effective candidates in the development of highly sensitive, noninvasive biomarkers for tumors screening prevention.

The miRNA-level changes can be useful for the toxicological assessment of several environmental pollutants, including plastic additives and plasticizers.

In this review, we showed that the interaction of plasticizers with several redundant miRNAs such as let-7f, let-7g, miR-125b, miR-134, miR-146a, miR-22, miR-192, miR-222, miR-26a, miR-26b, miR-27b, miR-296, miR-324, miR-335, miR-122, miR-23b, miR-200, miR-29a, and miR-21 might induce deep alterations in miRNA-mediated regulation and functions. These genotoxic and oncogenic responses can eventually lead to abnormal cell signaling pathways and metabolisms that participate in many intercrossed or overlapped cellular processes.

BPA induces the hypomethylation of histone promoter regions, indicating methylation changes as one of the possible mechanisms of BPA-induced adverse effects on carcinogenesis. BPA is also involved in the downregulation of gene repair ARF6 (involved in cell differentiation, apoptosis, and cell regulation), *TP53* (a tumor suppressor gene also referred to as the "Guardian of the Genome"), and over-regulates *CCNE2*, which is able to interact with *CDKN1A* and *CDKN1B* proteins, and with *CDK3*. The aberrant expression of *CCNE2* is a cause of cancer [48].

Phthalates downregulated the activity of some miRNAs (see Tab.1) implicated in cell cycle regulation and cancer. Additionally, the activation and overexpression of *ErbB*, *PPARα* pathways, the generation of ROS, and the overexpression of *Zeb1* (a transcription factor involved in cell migration and invasion) resulted from phthalate exposure.

It is important to note that the machinery by which plasticizers alter the epigenetic assets of cells require further study to elucidate the biology and biochemistry relatively to epigenetic alterations but also to disease-associated epigenetic alterations. A better understanding of these mechanisms will lead to better prediction of the health effects of plasticizers, allowing more targeted, easy, and appropriate disease-prevention and therapy strategies [49,50].

The lack of human studies needs to be addressed. Experimental evidence will permit the proposal of dedicated epidemiological studies to evaluate the real effects of plasticizers on human health, especially for cancer derived by microplastics and their plasticizers that are yet to be properly studied by oncologists yet.

Author Contributions: Conceptualization, M.F. and G.O.C.; Methodology, G.O.C.; Validation, M.F., A.C. and G.O.C.; Formal analysis, M.F., A.C. and G.O.C.; Investigation, M.F. and G.O.C.; Resources, M.F.; Data curation, A.C. and G.O.C.; Writing—original draft preparation, M.F. and G.O.C.; Writing—review and editing, M.F. and G.O.C.; Visualization, M.F., A.C. and G.O.C.; Supervision, M.F. All authors have read and agreed to the published version of the manuscript.

Funding: This research received no external funding.

Conflicts of Interest: The authors declare no conflict of interest.

References

1. Filippini, T.; Heck, J.E.; Malagoli, C.; Del Giovane, C.; Vinceti, M. A Review and Meta-Analysis of Outdoor Air Pollution and Risk of Childhood Leukemia. *J. Environ. Sci. Health Part C* **2015**, *33*, 36–66. [CrossRef]
2. Conti, G.O.; Calogero, A.E.; Giacone, F.; Fiore, M.; Barchitta, M.; Agodi, A.; Ferrante, M. B(a)P adduct levels and fertility: A cross-sectional study in a Sicilian population. *Mol. Med. Rep.* **2017**, *15*, 3398–3404. [CrossRef] [PubMed]
3. Rapisarda, V.; Loreto, C.; Ledda, C.; Musumeci, G.; Bracci, M.; Santarelli, L.; Renis, M.; Ferrante, M.; Cardile, V. Cytotoxicity, oxidative stress and genotoxicity induced by glass fibers on human alveolar epithelial cell line A549. *Toxicol. Vitr.* **2015**, *29*, 551–557. [CrossRef] [PubMed]

4. Signorelli, S.S.; Conti, G.O.; Zanobetti, A.; Baccarelli, A.; Fiore, M.; Ferrante, M. Effect of particulate matter-bound metals exposure on prothrombotic biomarkers: A systematic review. *Environ. Res.* **2019**, *177*, 108573. [CrossRef] [PubMed]
5. De Domenico, E.; Mauceri, A.R.; Giordano, D.; Maisano, M.; Gioffrè, G.; Natalotto, A.; D'Agata, A.; Ferrante, M.; Brundo, M.V.; Fasulo, S. Effects of "in vivo" exposure to toxic sediments on juveniles of sea bass (Dicentrarchus labrax). *Aquat. Toxicol.* **2011**, *105*, 688–697. [CrossRef]
6. Cristaldi, A.; Fiore, M.; Zuccarello, P.; Conti, G.O.; Grasso, A.; Nicolosi, I.; Copat, C.; Ferrante, M. Efficiency of Wastewater Treatment Plants (WWTPs) for Microplastic Removal: A Systematic Review. *Int. J. Environ. Res. Public Health* **2020**, *17*, 8014. [CrossRef]
7. Filippini, T.; Tesauro, M.; Fiore, M.; Malagoli, C.; Consonni, M.; Violi, F.; Iacuzio, L.; Arcolin, E.; Conti, G.O.; Cristaldi, A.; et al. Environmental and Occupational Risk Factors of Amyotrophic Lateral Sclerosis: A Population-Based Case-Control Study. *Int. J. Environ. Res. Public Health* **2020**, *17*, 2882. [CrossRef]
8. Capolongo, S.; Rebecchi, A.; Dettori, M.; Appolloni, L.; Azara, A.; Buffoli, M.; Capasso, L.; Casuccio, A.; Conti, G.O.; D'Amico, A.; et al. Healthy Design and Urban Planning Strategies, Actions, and Policy to Achieve Salutogenic Cities. *Int. J. Environ. Res. Public* **2018**, *15*, 2698. [CrossRef]
9. Ledda, C.; Loreto, C.; Zammit, C.; Marconi, A.; Fago, L.; Matera, S.; Costanzo, V.; Sanzà, G.F.; Palmucci, S.; Ferrante, M.; et al. Non-infective occupational risk factors for hepatocellular carcinoma: A review. *Mol. Med. Rep.* **2016**, *15*, 511–533. [CrossRef]
10. Ferrante, M.; Zanghì, G.; Cristaldi, A.; Copat, C.; Grasso, A.; Fiore, M.; Signorelli, S.S.; Zuccarello, P.; Conti, G.O. PAHs in seafood from the Mediterranean Sea: An exposure risk assessment. *Food Chem. Toxicol.* **2018**, *115*, 385–390. [CrossRef]
11. Conte, F.; Copat, C.; Longo, S.; Conti, G.O.; Grasso, A.; Arena, G.; Dimartino, A.; Brundo, M.V.; Ferrante, M. Polycyclic aromatic hydrocarbons in Haliotis tuberculata (Linnaeus, 1758) (Mollusca, Gastropoda): Considerations on food safety and source investigation. *Food Chem. Toxicol.* **2016**, *94*, 57–63. [CrossRef] [PubMed]
12. Zuccarello, P.; Ferrante, M.; Cristaldi, A.; Copat, C.; Grasso, A.; Sangregorio, D.; Fiore, M.; Conti, G.O. Exposure to microplastics (<10 µm) associated to plastic bottles mineral water consumption: The first quantitative study. *Water Res.* **2019**, *157*, 365–371. [CrossRef] [PubMed]
13. Conti, G.O.; Ferrante, M.; Banni, M.; Favara, C.; Nicolosi, I.; Cristaldi, A.; Fiore, M.; Zuccarello, P. Micro- and nano-plastics in edible fruit and vegetables. The first diet risks assessment for the general population. *Environ. Res.* **2020**, *187*, 109677. [CrossRef]
14. Fiore, M.; Conti, G.O.; Caltabiano, R.; Buffone, A.; Zuccarello, P.; Cormaci, L.; Cannizzaro, M.A.; Ferrante, M. Role of Emerging Environmental Risk Factors in Thyroid Cancer: A Brief Review. *Int. J. Environ. Res. Public Health* **2019**, *16*, 1185. [CrossRef] [PubMed]
15. Li, J.-H.; Ko, Y.-C. Plasticizer incident and its health effects in Taiwan. *Kaohsiung J. Med Sci.* **2012**, *28*, S17–S21. [CrossRef] [PubMed]
16. Giuliani, A.; Zuccarini, M.; Cichelli, A.; Khan, H.; Reale, M. Critical Review on the Presence of Phthalates in Food and Evidence of Their Biological Impact. *Int. J. Environ. Res. Public Health* **2020**, *17*, 5655. [CrossRef] [PubMed]
17. Farahani, M.; Rezaei-Tavirani, M.; Arjmand, B. A systematic review of microRNA expression studies with exposure to bisphenol A. *J. Appl. Toxicol.* **2021**, *41*, 4–19. [CrossRef]
18. Izzotti, A.; Kanitz, S.; D'Agostini, F.; Camoirano, A.; De Flora, S. Formation of adducts by bisphenol A, an endocrine disruptor, in DNA in vitro and in liver and mammary tissue of mice. *Mutat. Res. Toxicol. Environ. Mutagen.* **2009**, *679*, 28–32. [CrossRef]
19. Annex_11_Report_from_Lowell_Center.pdf. Available online: https://ec.europa.eu/environment/aarhus/pdf/35/Annex_11_report_from_Lowell_Center.pdf (accessed on 13 April 2021).
20. Hafezi, S.A. The Endocrine Disruptor Bisphenol A (BPA) Exerts a Wide Range of Effects in Carcinogenesis and Response to Therapy. *Curr. Mol. Pharmacol.* **2019**, *12*, 230–238. [CrossRef]
21. Emfietzoglou, R.; Spyrou, N.; Mantzoros, C.S.; Dalamaga, M. Could the endocrine disruptor bisphenol-A be implicated in the pathogenesis of oral and oropharyngeal cancer? Metabolic considerations and future directions. *Metabolism* **2019**, *91*, 61–69. [CrossRef]
22. Available online: https://www.cpsc.gov/Regulations-Laws--Standards/Statutes/The-Consumer-Product-Safety-Improvement-Act (accessed on 25 May 2021).
23. Available online: https://oehha.ca.gov/proposition-65 (accessed on 25 May 2021).
24. Available online: https://eur-lex.europa.eu/LexUriServ/LexUriServ.do?uri=OJ:L:2007:092:0009:0012:EN:PDF (accessed on 25 May 2021).
25. Chiang, C.; Flaws, J.A. Subchronic Exposure to Di(2-ethylhexyl) Phthalate and Diisononyl Phthalate During Adulthood Has Immediate and Long-Term Reproductive Consequences in Female Mice. *Toxicol. Sci.* **2019**, *168*, 620–631. [CrossRef] [PubMed]
26. Izzotti, A.; Pulliero, A. The effects of environmental chemical carcinogens on the microRNA machinery. *Int. J. Hyg. Environ. Health* **2014**, *217*, 601–627. [CrossRef]
27. Ferrante, M. Environment and Neurodegenerative Diseases: An Update on miRNA Role. *MicroRNA* **2017**, *6*, 157–165. [CrossRef]
28. Singh, S.; Li, S.S. Epigenetic effects of environmental chemicals bisphenol A and phthalates. *Int. J. Mol. Sci.* **2012**, *13*, 10143–10153. [CrossRef] [PubMed]
29. Asakura, K.; Kadota, T.; Matsuzaki, J.; Yoshida, Y.; Yamamoto, Y.; Nakagawa, K.; Takizawa, S.; Aoki, Y.; Nakamura, E.; Miura, J.; et al. A miRNA-based diagnostic model predicts resectable lung cancer in humans with high accuracy. *Commun. Biol.* **2020**, *3*, 1–9. [CrossRef]

30. Catalanotto, C.; Cogoni, C.; Zardo, G. MicroRNA in Control of Gene Expression: An Overview of Nuclear Functions. *Int. J. Mol. Sci.* **2016**, *17*, 1712. [CrossRef]
31. Tilghman, S.L.; Bratton, M.; Segar, H.C.; Martin, E.C.; Rhodes, L.; Li, M.; McLachlan, J.A.; Wiese, T.E.; Nephew, K.P.; Burow, M.E. Endocrine Disruptor Regulation of MicroRNA Expression in Breast Carcinoma Cells. *PLoS ONE* **2012**, *7*, e32754. [CrossRef] [PubMed]
32. Meng, X.; Zhou, Y.; Liang, Q.; Qu, X.; Yang, Q.; Yin, H.; Ai, S. Electrochemical determination of microRNA-21 based on bio bar code and hemin/G-quadruplet DNAenzyme. *Analyst* **2013**, *138*, 3409–3415. [CrossRef] [PubMed]
33. Li, X.; Xie, W.; Xie, C.; Huang, C.; Zhu, J.; Liang, Z.; Deng, F.; Zhu, M.; Zhu, W.; Wu, R.; et al. Curcumin Modulates miR-19/PTEN/AKT/p53 Axis to Suppress Bisphenol A-induced MCF-7 Breast Cancer Cell Proliferation. *Phytother. Res.* **2014**, *28*, 1553–1560. [CrossRef] [PubMed]
34. Kim, S.J.; Yu, S.-Y.; Yoon, H.-J.; Lee, S.Y.; Youn, J.-P.; Hwang, S.Y. Epigenetic Regulation of miR-22 in a BPA-exposed Human Hepatoma Cell. *BioChip J.* **2015**, *9*, 76–84. [CrossRef]
35. Buñay, J.; Larriba, E.; Moreno, R.D.; Del Mazo, J. Chronic low-dose exposure to a mixture of environmental endocrine disruptors induces microRNAs/isomiRs deregulation in mouse concomitant with intratesticular estradiol reduction. *Sci. Rep.* **2017**, *7*, 1–16. [CrossRef]
36. Chang, Y.-J.; Tseng, C.-Y.; Lin, P.-Y.; Chuang, Y.-C.; Chao, M.-W. Acute exposure to DEHP metabolite, MEHP cause genotoxicity, mutagenesis and carcinogenicity in mammalian Chinese hamster ovary cells. *Carcinogenesis* **2017**, *38*, 336–345. [CrossRef]
37. Chou, W.-C.; Lee, P.-H.; Tan, Y.-Y.; Lin, H.-C.; Yang, C.-W.; Chen, K.-H.; Chuang, C.-Y. An integrative transcriptomic analysis reveals bisphenol A exposure-induced dysregulation of microRNA expression in human endometrial cells. *Toxicol. Vitr.* **2017**, *41*, 133–142. [CrossRef] [PubMed]
38. Hui, L.; Li, H.; Lu, G.; Chen, Z.; Sun, W.; Shi, Y.; Fu, Z.; Huang, B.; Zhu, X.; Lu, W.; et al. Low Dose of Bisphenol A Modulates Ovarian Cancer Gene Expression Profile and Promotes Epithelial to Mesenchymal Transition Via Canonical Wnt Pathway. *Toxicol. Sci.* **2018**, *164*, 527–538. [CrossRef]
39. Wu, J.; Jiang, Y.; Cao, W.; Li, X.; Xie, C.; Geng, S.; Zhu, M.; Liang, Z.; Zhu, J.; Zhu, W.; et al. miR-19 targeting of PTEN mediates butyl benzyl phthalate-induced proliferation in both ER(+) and ER(−) breast cancer cells. *Toxicol. Lett.* **2018**, *295*, 124–133. [CrossRef] [PubMed]
40. Yin, X.; Ma, T.; Han, R.; Ding, J.; Zhang, H.; Han, X.; Li, D. MiR-301b-3p/3584-5p enhances low-dose mono-n-butyl phthalate (MBP)-induced proliferation by targeting Rasd1 in Sertoli cells. *Toxicol. Vitr.* **2018**, *47*, 79–88. [CrossRef]
41. Scarano, W.R.; Bedrat, A.; Alonso-Costa, L.G.; Aquino, A.M.; Fantinatti, B.E.; Justulin, L.A.; Barbisan, L.F.; Freire, P.P.; Flaws, J.A.; Lemos, B. Exposure to an Environmentally Relevant Phthalate Mixture During Prostate Development Induces MicroRNA Upregulation and Transcriptome Modulation in Rats. *Toxicol. Sci.* **2019**, *171*, 84–97. [CrossRef]
42. Wang, M.; Qiu, Y.; Zhang, R.; Gao, L.; Wang, X.; Bi, L.; Wang, Y. MEHP promotes the proliferation of oral cancer cells via down regulation of miR-27b-5p and miR-372-5p. *Toxicol. Vitr.* **2019**, *58*, 35–41. [CrossRef] [PubMed]
43. Zhu, M.; Wu, J.; Ma, X.; Huang, C.; Wu, R.; Zhu, W.; Li, X.; Liang, Z.; Deng, F.; Zhu, J.; et al. Butyl benzyl phthalate promotes prostate cancer cell proliferation through miR-34a downregulation. *Toxicol. Vitr.* **2019**, *54*, 82–88. [CrossRef]
44. Cui, S.; Wang, L.; Zhao, H.; Lu, F.; Wang, W.; Yuan, Z. Benzyl butyl phthalate (BBP) triggers the migration and invasion of hemangioma cells via upregulation of Zeb1. *Toxicol. Vitr.* **2019**, *60*, 323–329. [CrossRef]
45. Duan, X.-L.; Ma, C.-C.; Hua, J.; Xiao, T.-W.; Luan, J.; Cong-Cong, M. Benzyl butyl phthalate (BBP) triggers the malignancy of acute myeloid leukemia cells via upregulation of PDK4. *Toxicol. Vitr.* **2020**, *62*, 104693. [CrossRef] [PubMed]
46. Chorley, B.N.; Carswell, G.K.; Nelson, G.; Bhat, V.S.; Wood, C.E. Early microRNA indicators of PPARα pathway activation in the liver. *Toxicol. Rep.* **2020**, *7*, 805–815. [CrossRef] [PubMed]
47. Zota, A.R.; Geller, R.J.; Vannoy, B.N.; Marfori, C.Q.; Tabbara, S.; Hu, L.Y.; Baccarelli, A.A.; Moawad, G.N. Phthalate Exposures and MicroRNA Expression in Uterine Fibroids: The FORGE Study. *Epigenetics Insights* **2020**, *13*, 2516865720904057. [CrossRef]
48. Kreike, B.; Hart, G.; Bartelink, H.; Van De Vijver, M.J. Analysis of breast cancer related gene expression using natural splines and the Cox proportional hazard model to identify prognostic associations. *Breast Cancer Res. Treat.* **2009**, *122*, 711–720. [CrossRef] [PubMed]
49. Izzotti, A.; Vargas, G.C.; Pulliero, A.; Coco, S.; Vanni, I.; Colarossi, C.; Blanco, G.; Agodi, A.; Barchitta, M.; Maugeri, A.; et al. Relationship between the miRNA Profiles and Oncogene Mutations in Non-Smoker Lung Cancer. Relevance for Lung Cancer Personalized Screenings and Treatments. *J. Pers. Med.* **2021**, *11*, 182. [CrossRef] [PubMed]
50. Ferrante, M.; Ledda, C.; Conti, G.O.; Fiore, M.; Rapisarda, V.; Copat, C.; Sole, G.; Terzo, N.; Travali, S. Lead exposure and plasma mRNA expression in ERBB2 gene. *Mol. Med. Rep.* **2017**, *15*, 3361–3365. [CrossRef]

Article

MicroRNA Expression Profile Distinguishes Glioblastoma Stem Cells from Differentiated Tumor Cells

Sara Tomei [1,*], Andrea Volontè [2], Shilpa Ravindran [1], Stefania Mazzoleni [3,†], Ena Wang [4,‡], Rossella Galli [3] and Cristina Maccalli [1]

1. Research Department, Sidra Medicine, Doha PO26999, Qatar; ravindranshilpa@gmail.com (S.R.); cmaccalli@sidra.org (C.M.)
2. Unit of Immuno-Biotherapy of Melanoma and Solid Tumors, Division of Molecular Oncology, San Raffaele Foundation Scientific Institute, 20132 Milan, Italy; andrea.volo87@gmail.com
3. Neural Stem Cell Biology Unit, Division of Neuroscience, San Raffaele Scientific Institute, 20132 Milan, Italy; stefania.mazzoleni@genenta.com (S.M.); galli.rossella@hsr.it (R.G.)
4. Infectious Disease and Immunogenetics Section (IDIS), Department of Transfusion Medicine, Clinical Center, and Center for Human Immunology (CHI) National Institutes of Health, Bethesda, MD 20892, USA; Ewang911@gmail.com
* Correspondence: stomei@sidra.org; Tel.: +974-4003-7681
† Current Affiliation: Genenta Science, 20132 Milan, Italy.
‡ Current Affiliation: Translational Oncology, Allogene Therapeutics, San Francisco Bay, CA 94080, USA.

Abstract: Glioblastoma (GBM) represents the most common and aggressive tumor of the brain. Despite the fact that several studies have recently addressed the molecular mechanisms underlying the disease, its etiology and pathogenesis are still poorly understood. GBM displays poor prognosis and its resistance to common therapeutic approaches makes it a highly recurrent tumor. Several studies have identified a subpopulation of tumor cells, known as GBM cancer stem cells (CSCs) characterized by the ability of self-renewal, tumor initiation and propagation. GBM CSCs have been shown to survive GBM chemotherapy and radiotherapy. Thus, targeting CSCs represents a promising approach to treat GBM. Recent evidence has shown that GBM is characterized by a dysregulated expression of microRNA (miRNAs). In this study we have investigated the difference between human GBM CSCs and their paired autologous differentiated tumor cells. Array-based profiling and quantitative Real-Time PCR (qRT-PCR) were performed to identify miRNAs differentially expressed in CSCs. The Cancer Genome Atlas (TCGA) data were also interrogated, and functional interpretation analysis was performed. We have identified 14 miRNAs significantly differentially expressed in GBM CSCs ($p < 0.005$). MiR-21 and miR-95 were among the most significantly deregulated miRNAs, and their expression was also associated to patient survival. We believe that the data provided here carry important implications for future studies aiming at elucidating the molecular mechanisms underlying GBM.

Keywords: glioblastoma; microRNAs; cancer; qPCR; cancer stem cells

1. Introduction

Glioblastoma is the deadliest malignant intracranial tumor in adults. In the United States its annual incidence is 3.2 cases per 100,000 people [1,2], while in Europe the incidence is 3–5 cases per 100,000 people [3]. Its progression is accompanied by a rapid spread, an infiltrative growth and high cellular heterogeneity [4,5]. The current management of Glioblastoma (GBM) patients includes surgical resection, radiotherapy, chemotherapy and tumor treating fields (TTFields) [4,6]. Among the chemotherapeutic agents, temozolomide (TMZ) is the most common alkylating agent employed in the clinical management of GBM patients. However, GBM has been shown to acquire resistance to TMZ, thus explaining GBM recurrence [4,6]. GBM prognosis is generally poor and the median survival is only 14 months, while the 5-year survival rate is unfortunately between 5%–10% [7–10].

Overall, 90% of GBM originate de novo while the remaining 10% arise from lower-grade glioma [11,12]. Although the exact etiology of GBM is still being explored, it has been reported that ionizing radiation at high-dose and rare genetic disorders could facilitate the onset of GBM [13]. Advancements on the molecular understanding of GBM onset and progression are warranted to help the clinical management of GBM.

The most important molecular biomarkers for GBM include the methylation status of O-6-methylguanine-FNA methyltransferase (MGMT) promoter, and the mutational status of the isocitrate dehydrogenase 1 and 2 (IDH1, IDH2). When the MGMT promoter is found methylated, GBM has been reported to have a better outcome [13]. Furthermore, IDH1 and IDH2 mutations have been found correlating with a less aggressive GBM phenotype [1]. Nevertheless, the shortage in molecular biomarkers for GBM underscores the importance to implement new studies for the identification of novel biomarkers, such as microRNAs (miRNAs). MiRNAs are small non-coding RNAs 18–25 nucleotides long. They are transcribed by the RNA polymerase II and processed into their mature form through a series of steps involving Drosha/DGCR8 complex, for the generation of pre-miRNAs, and Dicer, which generates the mature form of miRNAs. Several technologies are now being applied for the study of miRNAs [14]. MiRNAs recognize the complementary sequences in the 3′ untranslated regions (3′UTR) of given transcripts to cause their degradation or translational repression [15,16]. Different types of cancers display miRNA expression dysregulation through different mechanisms, encompassing genomic variations in miRNA encoding genes, deregulation of miRNA transcription, epigenetic mechanisms and disruption of the miRNA synthesis machinery [17,18]. Several miRNAs have been shown to be dysregulated in GBM as compared to normal brain samples [19].

Increasing scientific evidence has pointed to the existence within tumor lesions of a cell subpopulation with stem-like properties, defined "cancer stem cells" (CSCs). GBM CSCs have the ability to self-renew, differentiate multi-potentially in the three lineages of the central nervous system (CNS) and to give rise to tumor when transplanted experimentally [20–23]. Additionally, CSCs have been shown to resist radiotherapy and chemotherapy, thus inducing continued proliferation and possibly mediating tumor recurrence [4,24–27]. Moreover, it has been shown that CSCs display intrinsic ability to protect themselves from both natural and adaptive immune responses [22,28–31]. Targeting GBM CSCs represents an ideal approach to treat GBM and overcome tumor recurrence. Despite the fact that there exists good epidemiological evidence of GBM, the molecular mechanisms underlying its onset and progression are only recently starting to be elucidated.

Currently, studies aimed at evaluating miRNA expression in GBM CSCs are scarce. This study aims at identifying miRNAs potentially explaining GBM CSC properties and their potential immunological resistance. We have employed an array-based quantitative real-time PCR approach and evaluated the differences in the expression of miRNAs in pairs of autologous CSCs and differentiated tumor cells obtained from the same GBM patients. Finally, we have also performed functional pathway analysis and interrogated The Cancer Genome Atlas (TCGA) for validation purposes.

2. Results

2.1. MiRNAs Differentially Expressed between CSCs and Autologous Differentiated Cells

The characterization of the profile of miRNAs in different CSC lines ($n = 11$) vs. differentiated bulk tumor cells ($n = 4$) in GBM was initially performed utilizing custom-made arrays for the detection of 713 human, mammary and viral miRNAs. Class comparison between the two groups identified 20 miRNAs differentially expressed at a significance level of $p < 0.01$ (Supplementary Figure S1A). This analysis was refined by utilizing only the 3 CSCs and their 3 corresponding autologous differentiated cells (from here on denominated "FBS" as they were grown in fetal bovine serum (FBS); Supplementary Figure S1B).

We then validated the differential profile of CSC lines vs. FBS cell lines through quantitative Real-Time PCR (qRT-PCR) of 704 mature miRNAs, annotated by the Sanger miRBase Release 14. To test whether the assignment of the samples to the CSC and

FBS groups would have translated in a different miRNA expression, we have applied principal component analysis (PCA) to the complete miRNA data set. The assignment of the individual samples to the CSC and FBS groups predicted their distribution in a three-dimensional space suggesting that CSCs and FBS samples displayed a differential expression of the miRNAs included in the complete dataset (Figure 1A). Interestingly, samples belonging to the same individual pairs clustered closely to each other compared to the other samples (Figure 1B), suggesting that the intra-individual miRNA expression variability was lower than the inter-individual miRNA expression variability.

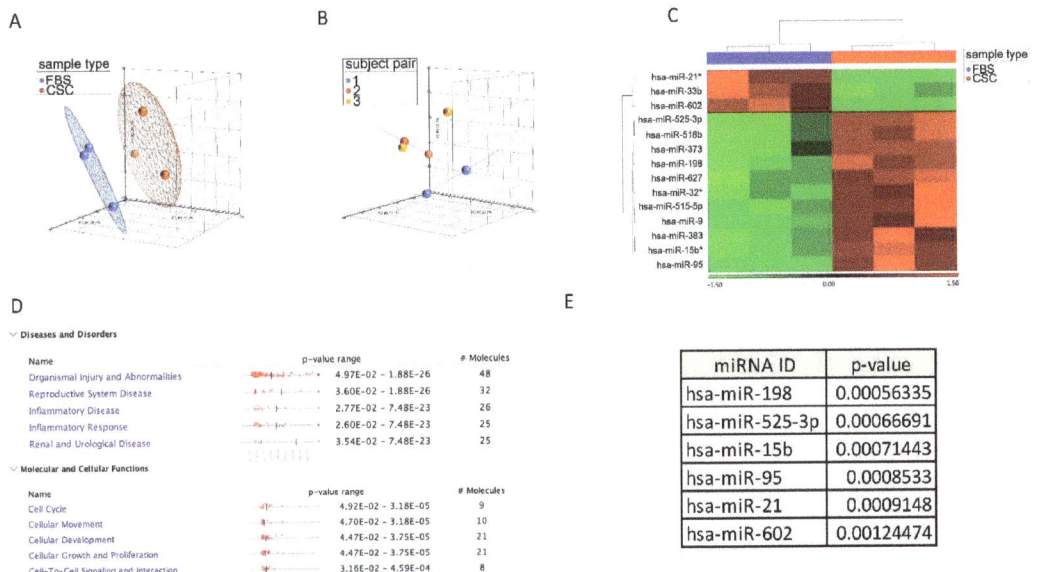

Figure 1. Principal Component Analysis (PCA) of CSC (in red) and FBS (in blue) samples based on the complete miRNA expression data set (**A**). Principal Component Analysis (PCA) of the samples according to their individual pair (**B**). Hierarchical clustering of the 14 significantly differentially expressed miRNAs ($p < 0.005$); miRNAs marked with the asterisk (*) correspond to a less abundant form (**C**). Functional Interpretation analysis of 67 differentially expressed miRNAs at a statistical level of $p < 0.05$ (**D**). List of the 6 most significant differentially expressed miRNAs between CSC and FBS samples (**E**).

The miRNA expression data were next used to identify miRNA discriminating the CSC and FBS samples. At a significance level of $p < 0.05$, 67 miRNAs resulted differentially expressed between CSC and FBS samples. When using a more stringent p-value ($p < 0.005$), 14 miRNAs were differentially expressed, with miR-21, miR-33b and miR-602 being up-regulated in the FBS cells compared to CSCs, while the remaining miRNAs (miR-525, miR-518, miR-373, miR-198, miR-627, miR-32, miR-515, miR-9, miR-383, miR-15 and miR-95) were up-regulated in CSCs compared to their paired FBS cells (Figure 1C).

The functional interpretation by Ingenuity Pathway Analysis (IPA) of the 67 miRNAs differentially expressed at $p < 0.05$ revealed that they were associated with inflammatory disorders as well as functions relating to the cell cycle, cell movement, cell development and cell proliferation (Figure 1D).

2.2. Functional Interpretation Analysis and Interrogation of miRDB and TargetScan

Out of the 14 miRNAs significantly differentially expressed between GBM CSCs and their autologous differentiated cells, we have selected the top ranking 6 miRNAs and queried them for further analyses (Figure 1E). We have used two available online miRNA resources to interrogate miRNA target genes, namely TargetScan and miRDB [32–34]. With the assumption that target genes identified by both platforms for the same miRNA would be more indicative of a real miRNA-target gene interaction, we have generated Venn diagrams for the six most significant miRNAs (Figure 2A). The target genes in the intersection of the six Venn diagrams were combined in a unique list and submitted for functional interpretation analysis to Ingenuity Pathway Analysis (IPA). The analysis revealed an enrichment of genes related to neuronal signaling, cell differentiation and cell cycle regulation as well as pathways associated with the molecular mechanisms of cancer, the regulation of epithelial-mesenchymal transition (EMT) and the Hippo pathway. Several of these pathways were relevant for "stemness" properties. These findings support the role of the 6 top-ranking miRNAs and their target genes in regulating GBM CSC biology (Figure 2B). Nevertheless, the list of the top-ranking canonical pathways included also immune-related signaling pathways, such as the Transforming Growth Factor (TGF)-β signaling and STAT3 signaling pathways, suggesting a potential role of these miRNAs and their target genes in regulating immune-related functions. The functional interpretation analysis was also carried at the individual miRNA level (Supplementary Figure S2). Such analysis highlighted that additional immune-related pathways (e.g., Interleukin (IL)-1, Interferon (IFN), NF-kB, Toll-like receptor and T cell proliferation or exhaustion) could be regulated by the miRNAs differentially expressed in CSCs vs. FBC cell lines.

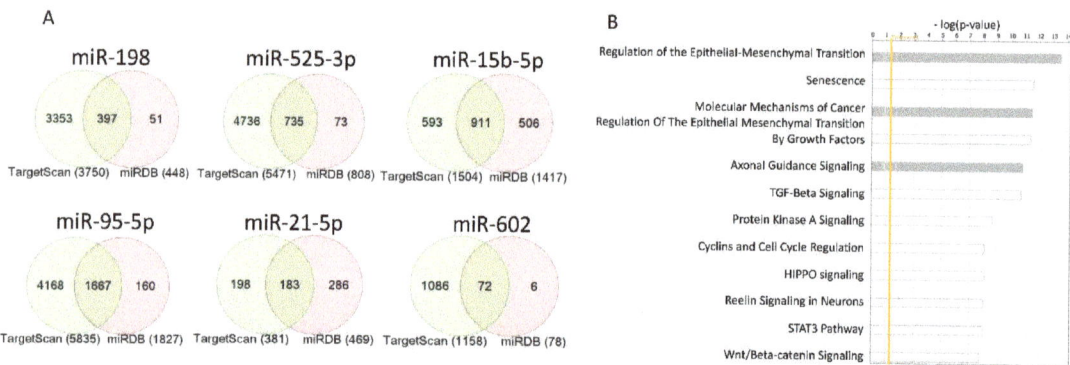

Figure 2. Venn diagrams of the target genes identified by TargetScan and miRDB for the six most significant miRNAs (**A**). Top canonical pathway identified on IPA from the list of the target genes in the intersections of the Venn diagram of the six most significant miRNAs (**B**). The significance values (p-value of overlap) for the canonical pathways are calculated by the right-tailed Fisher's Exact Test. The x-axis displays the -log of the p-value. The orange line indicates the significance threshold. Gray bars indicate pathways for which no prediction of activation or inhibition can be made due to insufficient evidence in the Knowledge Base for confident activity predictions across datasets. White bars indicate pathways with z-scores at or very close to 0.

2.3. Validation on the TCGA Dataset

We interrogated the role of the six most significant differentially expressed miRNAs using the Glioblastoma Bio Discovery Portal (GBM-BioDP) [35]. GBM-BioDP is an online visualization platform that allows the access of miRNAs differentially expressed across GBM samples from the TCGA database [36]. The genomic profiling of GBM from TCGA has led to the definition of four GBM subtypes, namely the classical, the mesenchymal, the neural and the proneural subtypes. Such subtypes might develop through different and independent molecular mechanisms [36]. Among the four subtypes, the mesenchymal one displays a higher necrosis percentage and inflammation features, potentially due to the activation of the NF-kB signaling pathway. The mesenchymal subtype also displays poor prognosis as compared to the other subtypes [37].

To further explore whether the significantly differentially expressed miRNAs between CSCs and differentiated cells found in this study were related to GBM transcriptional subgroups, we have interrogated the six most significantly deregulated miRNAs in GBM against GBM-BioDP. Among them, we found that miR-95 and miR-21 expression was significantly different in the mesenchymal group as compared to the other groups (Figure 3). Specifically, miR-95, which we found upregulated in CSCs, was significantly downregulated in the mesenchymal group compared to the proneural and neural subtypes ($p = 0.017$ and $p = 0.008$, respectively), while miR-21, which was downregulated in CSCs, resulted upregulated in the mesenchymal group as compared to the proneural and neural subtypes ($p = 0.013$ and $p = 0.001$, respectively).

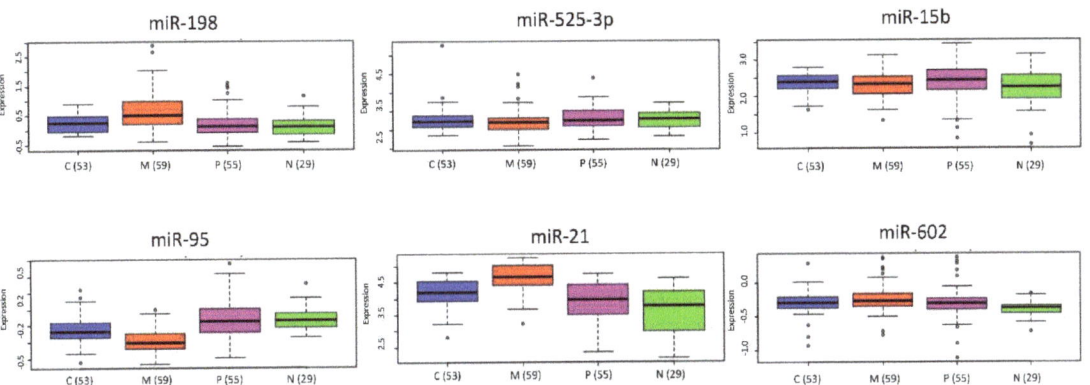

Figure 3. Boxplots of the six most significant miRNAs expression distribution in four subtypes of Glioblastoma (GBM) of The Cancer Genome Atlas (TCGA) patients.

We further questioned whether the expression of miR-95 and miR-21 was associated to survival outcome. The Kaplan–Meier analysis obtained from GBM-BioDP showed an association of a higher expression of miR-21 and a lower expression of miR-95 to a better survival for the neural subtype ($p = 0.012$ and $p = 0.016$, respectively), although no significant association was found for the other subtypes (Figure 4). Genes known to be the targets of miR-95 and miR-21 have also been interrogated against GBM-BioDP. When their expression across the TCGA GBM subtypes was inversed to the one reported for their corresponding miRNA, we assumed this observation to be more indicative of a real miRNA-target gene interaction. The analysis of miR-95 targets revealed an inversed expression of several genes involved in EMT (HGF and MAP2K3), STAT3 signaling (IL10RA) and in the role of macrophages, fibroblast, endothelial cells (TGF-β1 and IL-15) (Supplementary Figure S3). The analysis of miR-21 targets revealed an inversed expression of several genes involved in EMT (PIK3R1 and GAB1), TGF-β signaling (BMPR2) and in IL-1 signaling (GNAZ and MAP2K4) (Supplementary Figure S4).

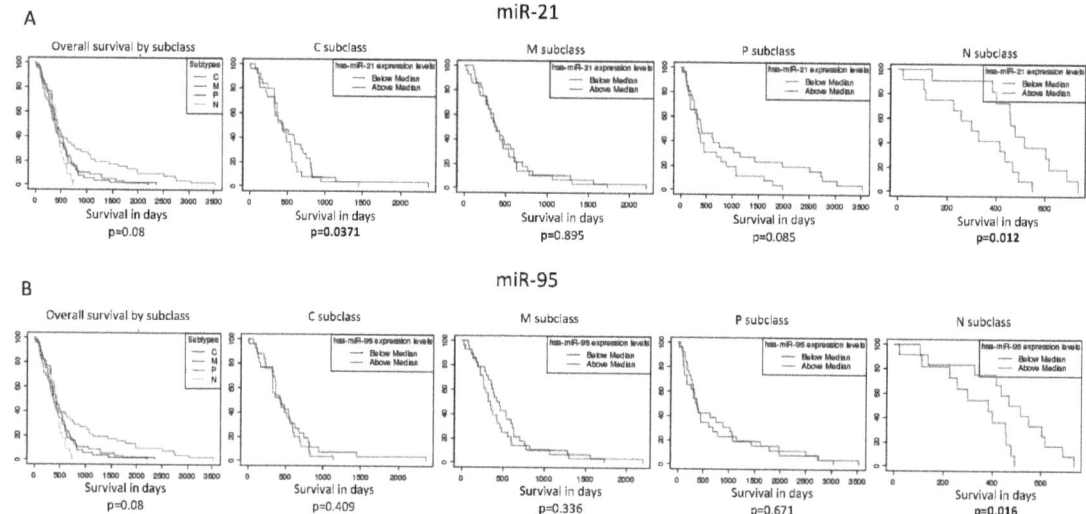

Figure 4. Kaplan–Meier analysis of miR-21 (**A**) and miR-95 (**B**) in the four subtypes of GBM of the TCGA patients.

3. Discussion

GBM remains one of the most lethal solid tumors [38]. Despite the scientific efforts to understand GBM pathogenesis over the last decade, GBM prognosis remains poor, highlighting the challenges in the clinical management of this cancer. GBM displays high level of intratumoral heterogeneity as well as cellular differentiation hierarchy. In fact, increasing scientific evidence supports the existence of a subpopulation of CSCs in GBM with self-renewal capabilities.

MiRNAs are emerging as critical regulators of proliferation and differentiation, and some of them have been shown to carry an important role in CSCs [38]. In this study we questioned the role of miRNA differential expression in CSCs and their corresponding autologous differentiated cells. The PCA analysis on the complete dataset gave a clear separation of the CSCs and the differentiated cells, suggesting that the complete miRNA data set was able to discriminate the two groups, although sample pairs belonging to the same individual clustered more closely compared to the others (Figure 1A,B). The class comparison between CSCs and their autologous differentiated cells identified 67 differentially expressed miRNAs at a significance level of $p < 0.05$. Functional interpretation analysis revealed several cellular functions related to cell growth and proliferation, as expected. When we refined the list to only 14 most significant miRNAs, we found that the majority of miRNAs ($n = 11$) was upregulated in the CSCs as compared to their differentiated counterparts. Among the miRNAs up-regulated in CSCs vs. FBS tumor cells, miR-515, miR-15b and miR-198 resulted as regulators of glioma associated signaling. MiR-95, miR-21 and miR-627 represent key regulators of the EMT signaling that has been shown to be one of the initial mechanisms of CSCs formation [39–41]. Additionally, miR-9, miR-32, miR-383, miR-518, miR-627 and miR-602 are involved in mechanisms regulating the expression/activation of PTEN, p53, Hippo, stem cell pluripotency and Notch signaling that are among the principal pathways involved in stemness-associated features [42–45].

GBM CSCs are endowed with superior self-renewal and tumorigenic ability [20] as compared to the differentiated bulk tumors that might be regulated by the differential miRNA profile. In particular, the aforementioned miRNAs could represent relevant modulators of the expression of target genes involved in signaling pathways associated with stemness properties (e.g., EMT, Notch, Hippo, p53, PTEN etc.).

CSCs also represent the component of tumors responsible of resistance to chemotherapy and radiotherapy [26,27,46]. MiR-383 and miR-525 were also found up-regulated in

CSCs vs. FBS cells, and they were reported to modulate the signaling associated with cell survival and DNA damage that can occur following chemotherapy or radiotherapy [47,48].

To gain further insights on the differential miRNA expression between CSCs and their differentiated paired cells, we looked into the target genes of the six most significant miRNAs. Target genes identified by TargetScan and miRDB of the six most significant miRNAs (Figure 2A) were combined in a unique list and queried for functional interpretation analysis, which identified several GBM-related pathways among the top-ranking canonical pathways (Figure 2B). Additionally, immune-related pathways were also identified, including TGF-β and STAT3 signaling, supporting a potential immune-related role of the six most significant miRNAs and their target genes.

Recurrent genomic alterations in GBM have been largely catalogued by TCGA Network. Based on these alterations, GBM samples have been grouped into four main subtypes, namely the classical, the neural, the proneural and the mesenchymal subtypes, the latter being the subgroup with worst prognosis [36,37]. The mesenchymal subgroup has also been characterized by a higher percentage of necrosis and inflammation features, potentially due to the activation of the NF-kB signaling pathway [37]. When we looked into the expression of the six most significant miRNAs in the TCGA dataset, we found that miR-21 was significantly upregulated, and miR-95 significantly downregulated in the mesenchymal group. Survival analysis also showed that miR-21 upregulation and miR-95 down-regulation were associated with better survival in the neural subtype only. MiR-21 is a well-studied miRNA, which acts as an oncomir and associates with a malignant phenotype [4,49]. It has been very recently reported being significantly downregulated in GBM CSCs compared to astrocytes [11] and has already been shown to associate with a more differentiated phenotype [50,51]. The primary CSCs utilized in the present manuscript have been assessed molecularly and resulted to belong mostly to the proneural transcriptional subgroup [52,53]. However, the mechanisms behind the association of the aforementioned miRNAs need to be further elucidated. MiR-95 has been reported to promote growth in colorectal, pancreas, prostate and breast cancer, but also to have anticancer activity in hepatic, brain and neck cancer [54–56]. In glioma, it was reported that the downregulation of miR-95 decreases the proliferation and invasion while promoting apoptosis of glioma cells [57]. Nevertheless, evidence on the role of miR-95 in GBM is scarce. We believe that our study adds important evidence to the role of miR-95 in GBM.

We acknowledge that to further elucidate the role of miR-95 and miR-21 in particular pathways, it is recommended to establish a knock-down of miRNA and explore the expression of the related downstream targets.

The characterization of the immunological profile of CSCs highlighted a general suboptimal immunogenic potency and susceptibility to cell-mediated immune responses [22,28–31]. Our group has previously reported that GBM-CSCs display a differential immune profile, including HLA molecules, soluble cytokines and growth factors compared to FBS cells, rendering these cells resistant to T cell-mediated responses [22]. Gene and protein expression determination showed a differential profile in the detection of TGF-β1, TGF-β2, IL-6 and IL-8 in GBM CSCs vs FBS cell lines [22]. Of note miR-95 expression inversely correlates with the expression of the target gene TGF-β1, as shown in Supplementary Figure S3. Therefore, the overexpression detected in GBM-CSCs of this miRNA could be responsible of the down-modulation of TGF-β1 observed in CSCs vs FBS cell lines [22]. Moreover, genes associated with IFN and Tumor Necrosis Factor (TNF) signaling were down-modulated in CSCs vs. FBS cells, including targets of miR-383, miR-627 or miR-525, respectively, that are overexpressed in CSCs (Figure 1) [22]. Conversely, the JAK-STAT signaling pathway was up-regulated in cells with stemness properties compared to differentiated cells [22]. Moreover, JAK-STAT signaling can be modulated by miR-9, miR-15, miR-32, miR-95, miR-373 and miR-515 that were differentially expressed in CSCs as compared to their differentiated cells. The molecular make-up of CSCs could be orchestrated by the pattern of miRNAs detected in these cells. STAT3, TGF-β and IFN signaling can be regulated by multiple miRNAs, such as miR-21, miR-32, miR-95, miR-585, miR-373, miR-383 and miR-627. CSCs could efficiently modulate both natural and adaptive immune responses in their relationship with the crosstalk with tumor microenvironment [29,30,58].

Interestingly, the levels of the immune checkpoint Ligand of Programmed Death Ligand 1 (PD-L1) has been reported to be modulated either directly by miR-33 [59] or indirectly through the regulation of the levels of PTEN by miR-21 [60]. PD-L1 has been previously reported to be expressed at high level in GBM-CSCs and, possibly being one of the molecules responsible for the impairment of T-cell mediated immune responses against these cells [22]. Our observations in this study suggest the importance of miR-33 and miR-21 as key regulators of the immunoregulatory properties of GBM-CSCs.

MiR-32 and miR-95, through the modulation of RAC or macrophage-, endothelial- and fibroblast-associated signaling pathways, respectively, could be among the key regulators of this phenomenon. Taken together, the analyses of the miRNA profile in pairs of CSCs vs. the differentiated tumor cells led to the identification of key regulators of signaling involved in stemness and immunological properties of GBM tumor initiating cells. The obtained results corroborate the hypothesis that the profile of miRNAs in CSCs may mediate the resistance of CSCs to immune responses.

We believe that our study provides additional information on the role of GBM CSCs. Previous studies have investigated the role of miRNAs in GBM CSC, nevertheless they employed CSC samples rather than autologous pairs [61–63].

The role of specific miRNAs in GBM CSCs has started being explored [64]. However, further functional investigations are warranted to demonstrate the link between the miRNAs identified in our study and the functions of CSCs. Moreover, additional techniques, such us in situ hybridization and other staining analyses, might help in corroborating our findings. We believe that this evidence paves the way toward the identification of tools that can modulate miRNA expression to optimize the efficacy of targeting GBM CSCs with immunotherapy.

In conclusion, we show here that several miRNAs are associated with GBM CSCs. MiR-21 and miR-95 are among the most significant differentially expressed miRNAs that carry implications on GBM molecular profiling and patient survival. Other miRNAs have been identified as potential regulators of the immunogenicity of CSCs. Additional analyses on larger cohorts are necessary to validate our findings and elucidate the molecular mechanisms behind GBM CSCs in further details.

4. Materials and Methods

4.1. Cell Culture and RNA Isolation

Cancer cells were of human origin. Tumor specimens were collected from $n = 11$ GBM patients admitted at the San Raffaele Hospital Scientific Institute, Milan, Italy. The study was approved by the IRB and patients were enrolled in the study upon signature of the informed consent. GBM cell lines, both CSCs and bulk tumor cells (denominated FBS) were established in vitro from fresh GBM lesions as previously described [22]. Briefly, GBM CSCs were cultured in vitro in the form of neurospheres in the presence of DMEM/F12 medium containing 20 ng/mL of epidermal growth factor (EGF) and fibroblast growth factor (FGF2) (Peprotech, Rocky Hill, NY, USA) plus additives as described in Galli et al. [20]. Primary cells were plated in 25 cm^2 tissue culture flasks at a clonal density of 2500–5000 cells/cm^2. When enough tumor tissue was available, a portion of the cells obtained from the enzymatic digestion was plated in the presence of RPMI 1640 supplemented with 10% FBS (Biowittaker, Lonza, Treviglio, Italy) to generate the aforementioned differentiated tumor cells. Early-in vitro passage ($n = 10$–15) cultures were used for all the experiments.

Total RNA was isolated from 3×10^6 cells using miRNeasy minikit (QIAGEN, Hilden, Germany), according to the manufacturer's protocol. RNA quantity and quality were assessed using Nanodrop Spectrophotometer (Thermo Fisher Scientific, Waltham, MA, USA) and Bioanalyzer (Agilent Technologies, Carlsbad, CA, USA). Samples were evaluated according to their RIN (RNA Integrity Number).

4.2. Array Screening of miRNAs

A miRNA probe set was designed using mature antisense miRNA sequences (Sanger data base, version 9.1) consisting of 827 unique miRNAs from human, mouse, rat and virus plus two control probes. The probes were 5′ amine modified and printed in duplicate on CodeLink activated slides (General Electric, GE Health, Midland Park, NJ, USA) via covalent bonding at the Infectious Disease and Immunogenetics Section of the Department of Transfusion Medicine (DTM) (Clinical Center, NIH, Bethesda, MD, USA). Four µg of total RNA isolated by using Trizol reagent (Invitrogen, Gaithersburg, MD, USA) were directly labelled with miRCURY™ LNA Array Power Labelling Kit (Exiqon, Woburn, MA, USA) according to manufacturer's procedure. The total RNA from the Epstein–Barr virus (EBV)-transformed lymphoblastoid cell line was used as the reference for the miRNA expression array assay. The test sample was labelled with Hy5 and the reference with Hy3. After labelling, the sample and the reference were co-hybridized to the miRNA array at room temperature overnight in the present of blocking reagents as previously described and the slides were washed and scanned by GenePix scanner Pro 4.0 (Axon, Sunnyvale, CA, USA). Resulting data files were analyzed using Partek Genomics Suite. Hierarchical cluster analysis and TreeView [65] software were used for visualization [66].

4.3. Quantitative Real-Time PCR (qRT-PCR) of miRNAs

The quantitative determination of the profile of miRNAs was performed with the RT2 miRNA PCR Array System (QIAGEN). MiRNA Sequence Specific Assays include one universal primer and one gene-specific primer for each miRNA sequence. This kit includes PCR Arrays to determine through a SYBR® Green real-time PCR detection system, the expression of 704 mature miRNAs annotated by the Sanger miRBase Release 14. The panel included SNORD 48, 47, and 44 and U6 as housekeeping assays that were used to normalize the qRT-PCR array data. The kit also included two RNA and PCR quality controls to test the efficiency of the RT2 miRNA first strand kit and efficiency of the polymerase chain reaction, respectively.

Two-hundred ng of small RNA were used for reverse transcription and the first-strand cDNA was synthesized with the RT2 miRNA First Strand Kit according to the manufacturer's instructions (cat. no. 331401). First strand cDNAs were mixed with RT2 SYBR Green qPCR Mastermix and the experimental cocktail was added to each corresponding well of the PCR arrays. PCR conditions were: 10 min at 95 °C and 40 cycles of: 15 s at 95 °C, 30 s at 60 °C and 30 s at 72 °C. The reaction was run on the ABI 7900 HT thermal cycler (Applied Biosystems). A melting curve analysis was performed to check assays' specificity. Samples were run in duplicates. The geometric mean of the housekeeping genes was subtracted from the Ct (Cycle threshold) values of each sample to give a delta Ct value that corrects for different sample amounts. Delta Ct values were then transformed into the negative delta Ct values and used to calculate the $2^{\wedge}$-delta Ct.

4.4. Data Analysis

Principal component analysis (PCA) was applied for visualization when relevant. All the graphical analyses were performed using Partek Genomic Suite tool (Partek, St. Louis, MO, USA). MiRNA expression class comparison between the CSC and FBS cell lines was based on the analysis of variance (ANOVA). All statistical tests were two-sided. p-values lower than 0.05 were considered statistically significant. Functional interpretation analysis was performed using Ingenuity Pathway Analysis (IPA) tools 3.0 (QIAGEN), which transforms large data sets into group of relevant networks including direct and indirect relations among genes based on known interactions established from the literature. Heat-maps are presented based on Partek visualization program.

The TCGA dataset was interrogated for validation purposes. The TCGA data was accessed by using the GBM-BioDP [35]. MiRNA and target genes expression profiles were queried and visualized based on known molecular subtypes [36].

Two-sided *t*-tests comparing the miRNA expression levels between subtypes were performed and their significance values were reported. Kaplan–Meier survival rate analysis was also performed. The dataset included 196 TCGA patients of the following subtypes according to Verhaak et al. [36]: classical ($n = 53$), mesenchymal ($n = 59$), proneural ($n = 55$), and neural ($n = 29$). The mRNA expression of specific miRNA target genes was evaluated using the experiments in the 3-Platform aggregates.

5. Conclusions

Despite the recent scientific efforts to understand GBM etiology and pathogenesis, GBM remains a complex disease and one of the most lethal tumors. Given the low survival rate, it is of primary importance finding biomarkers that could improve the clinical management of GBM patients. This article provides evidence that a group of specific miRNAs can explain the stemness properties and the immunological profile of CSCs in GBM. A further validation of our findings is warranted through studies employing larger cohorts.

Supplementary Materials: The following are available online at https://www.mdpi.com/article/10.3390/jpm11040264/s1, Figure S1: Hierarchical clustering of the 20 significantly differentially expressed miRNAs in $n = 11$ CSCs vs. $n = 4$ FBS cell lines identified through in house made arrays ($p < 0.01$) (A). Hierarchical clustering of the significantly differentially expressed miRNAs in 3 pairs of autologous CSCs and FBS cell lines identified through in house made arrays ($p < 0.01$) (B). Figure S2: Canonical pathways by individual miRNAs. These pathways were identified by querying the target genes (at the intersection of miRDB and TargetScan Venn diagrams) for each individual miRNA of the 14 significant miRNAs ($p < 0.005$). Both the 5p and 3p strands were included. The color legend indicates pathways associated with: 1. Cancer development and stemness features (green); 2. Immune-related functions (orange); 3. Pathways with pro-tumoral and immunological functions (yellow); 4. Cell regulation function that can be aberrantly modulated in cancer (violet); 5. Others (white). Figure S3: Boxplots of the distribution of the expression of miR-95 targets in the four subtypes of GBM of the TCGA patients. We have reported in brackets the molecular pathways associated to the individual target genes. Figure S4: Boxplots of the distribution of the expression of miR-21 targets in the four subtypes of GBM of the TCGA patients. We have reported in brackets the molecular pathways associated to the individual target genes.

Author Contributions: S.R. contributed to data analyses. A.V. performed the experimental part of the study. E.W. participated to the design of the arrays related experiments and data analyses. S.T. participated to the design of the study, data analyses and manuscript preparation. C.M. participated to the design of the study, data analyses and manuscript preparation. S.M. contributed to the establishment in vitro and characterization of cell lines. R.G. supervised the generation and characterization of cell lines, participated to data discussion and revision of the manuscript. All authors have read and agreed to the published version of the manuscript.

Funding: This study has been partially funded by a grant from the Qatar National Research Fund (QNRF) (grant no. NPRP10-0129-170277), Qatar.

Institutional Review Board Statement: The study was conducted according to the guidelines of the Declaration of Helsinki, and approved by the Institutional Review Board of the San Raffaele Scientific Institute, Milan, Italy.

Informed Consent Statement: Informed consent was obtained from all subjects involved in the study.

Data Availability Statement: The data presented in this study are available on request from the corresponding author.

Conflicts of Interest: The authors declare no conflict of interest or relationships relevant to the content of this paper. All authors take responsibility for all aspects of the reliability of the data presented and their discussed interpretation.

Abbreviations

ANOVA	Analysis of Variance
CNS	Central Nervous System
CSC	Cancer Stem Cells
Ct	Cycle threshold
EMT	Epithelial Mesenchymal Transition
EGF	Epidermal Growth Factor
FBS	Fetal Bovine Serum
FGF2	Fibroblast Growth Factor
GBM	Glioblastoma Multiforme
GBM-BioDP	Glioblastoma Bio Discovery Portal
HK	Housekeeping genes
IDH1	isocitrate dehydrogenase 1
IDH2	isocitrate dehydrogenase 2
IL	Interleukin
IFN	Interferon
IPA	Ingenuity Pathway Analysis
MGMT	O-6-methylguanine-FNA methyltransferase
miRNA	micro-RNA
NCI	National Cancer Institute
PCA	Principal Component Analysis
PD-L1	Ligand of Programmed Death Ligand 1
qRT-PCR	quantitative Real Time Polymerase Chain Reaction
RIN	RNA Integrity Number
TCGA	The Cancer Genome Atlas
TGF	Transforming Growth Factor
TNF	Tumor Necrosis Factor
TTFields:	Tumor Treating Fields
TMZ	Temozolomide
UTR	untranslated region

References

1. Alexander, B.M.; Cloughesy, T.F. Adult Glioblastoma. *J. Clin. Oncol.* **2017**, *35*, 2402–2409. [CrossRef] [PubMed]
2. Lin, J.; Zuo, J.; Cui, Y.; Song, C.; Wu, X.; Feng, H.; Li, J.; Li, S.; Xu, Q.; Wei, W.; et al. Characterizing the molecular mechanisms of acquired temozolomide resistance in the U251 glioblastoma cell line by protein microarray. *Oncol. Rep.* **2018**, *39*, 2333–2341. [CrossRef] [PubMed]
3. Crocetti, E.; Trama, A.; Stiller, C.; Caldarella, A.; Soffietti, R.; Jaal, J.; Weber, D.C.; Ricardi, U.; Slowinski, J.; Brandes, A.; et al. Epidemiology of glial and non-glial brain tumours in Europe. *Eur. J. Cancer* **2012**, *48*, 1532–1542. [CrossRef] [PubMed]
4. Guo, X.; Luo, Z.; Xia, T.; Wu, L.; Shi, Y.; Li, Y. Identification of miRNA signature associated with BMP2 and chemosensitivity of TMZ in glioblastoma stem-like cells. *Genes Dis.* **2020**, *7*, 424–439. [CrossRef]
5. Luo, J.W.; Wang, X.; Yang, Y.; Mao, Q. Role of micro-RNA (miRNA) in pathogenesis of glioblastoma. *Eur. Rev. Med. Pharmacol. Sci.* **2015**, *19*, 1630–1639. [PubMed]
6. Wick, W.; Osswald, M.; Wick, A.; Winkler, F. Treatment of glioblastoma in adults. *Ther. Adv. Neurol. Disord.* **2018**, *11*, 1756286418790452. [CrossRef] [PubMed]
7. Delgado-Lopez, P.D.; Corrales-Garcia, E.M. Survival in glioblastoma: A review on the impact of treatment modalities. *Clin. Transl. Oncol.* **2016**, *18*, 1062–1071. [CrossRef] [PubMed]
8. Ohgaki, H.; Kleihues, P. Epidemiology and etiology of gliomas. *Acta Neuropathol.* **2005**, *109*, 93–108. [CrossRef]
9. Jovcevska, I.; Zottel, A.; Samec, N.; Mlakar, J.; Sorokin, M.; Nikitin, D.; Buzdin, A.A.; Komel, R. High FREM2 Gene and Protein Expression Are Associated with Favorable Prognosis of IDH-WT Glioblastomas. *Cancers* **2019**, *11*, 1060. [CrossRef] [PubMed]
10. Noroxe, D.S.; Poulsen, H.S.; Lassen, U. Hallmarks of glioblastoma: A systematic review. *ESMO Open* **2016**, *1*, e000144. [CrossRef]
11. Zottel, A.; Samec, N.; Kump, A.; Raspor Dall'Olio, L.R.; Puzar Dominkus, P.; Romih, R.; Hudoklin, S.; Mlakar, J.; Nikitin, D.; Sorokin, M.; et al. Analysis of miR-9-5p, miR-124-3p, miR-21-5p, miR-138-5p, and miR-1-3p in Glioblastoma Cell Lines and Extracellular Vesicles. *Int. J. Mol. Sci.* **2020**, *21*, 8491. [CrossRef] [PubMed]
12. Miranda, A.; Blanco-Prieto, M.; Sousa, J.; Pais, A.; Vitorino, C. Breaching barriers in glioblastoma. Part I: Molecular pathways and novel treatment approaches. *Int. J. Pharm.* **2017**, *531*, 372–388. [CrossRef] [PubMed]
13. Weller, M.; Wick, W.; Aldape, K.; Brada, M.; Berger, M.; Pfister, S.M.; Nishikawa, R.; Rosenthal, M.; Wen, P.Y.; Stupp, R.; et al. Glioma. *Nat. Rev. Dis. Primers* **2015**, *1*, 15017. [CrossRef] [PubMed]

14. Mathew, R.; Mattei, V.; Al Hashmi, M.; Tomei, S. Updates on the Current Technologies for microRNA Profiling. *Microrna* **2020**, *9*, 17–24. [CrossRef] [PubMed]
15. Leung, A.K.L. The Whereabouts of microRNA Actions: Cytoplasm and Beyond. *Trends Cell Biol.* **2015**, *25*, 601–610. [CrossRef]
16. Yao, Q.; Chen, Y.; Zhou, X. The roles of microRNAs in epigenetic regulation. *Curr. Opin. Chem. Biol.* **2019**, *51*, 11–17. [CrossRef] [PubMed]
17. Peng, Y.; Croce, C.M. The role of MicroRNAs in human cancer. *Signal Transduct. Target Ther.* **2016**, *1*, 15004. [CrossRef] [PubMed]
18. Rezaei, O.; Honarmand, K.; Nateghinia, S.; Taheri, M.; Ghafouri-Fard, S. miRNA signature in glioblastoma: Potential biomarkers and therapeutic targets. *Exp. Mol. Pathol.* **2020**, *117*, 104550. [CrossRef]
19. Moller, H.G.; Rasmussen, A.P.; Andersen, H.H.; Johnsen, K.B.; Henriksen, M.; Duroux, M. A systematic review of microRNA in glioblastoma multiforme: Micro-modulators in the mesenchymal mode of migration and invasion. *Mol. Neurobiol.* **2013**, *47*, 131–144. [CrossRef] [PubMed]
20. Galli, R.; Binda, E.; Orfanelli, U.; Cipelletti, B.; Gritti, A.; De Vitis, S.; Fiocco, R.; Foroni, C.; Dimeco, F.; Vescovi, A. Isolation and characterization of tumorigenic, stem-like neural precursors from human glioblastoma. *Cancer Res.* **2004**, *64*, 7011–7021. [CrossRef] [PubMed]
21. Mazzoleni, S.; Politi, L.S.; Pala, M.; Cominelli, M.; Franzin, A.; Sergi Sergi, L.; Falini, A.; De Palma, M.; Bulfone, A.; Poliani, P.L.; et al. Epidermal growth factor receptor expression identifies functionally and molecularly distinct tumor-initiating cells in human glioblastoma multiforme and is required for gliomagenesis. *Cancer Res.* **2010**, *70*, 7500–7513. [CrossRef] [PubMed]
22. Di Tomaso, T.; Mazzoleni, S.; Wang, E.; Sovena, G.; Clavenna, D.; Franzin, A.; Mortini, P.; Ferrone, S.; Doglioni, C.; Marincola, F.M.; et al. Immunobiological characterization of cancer stem cells isolated from glioblastoma patients. *Clin. Cancer Res.* **2010**, *16*, 800–813. [CrossRef] [PubMed]
23. Lathia, J.D.; Mack, S.C.; Mulkearns-Hubert, E.E.; Valentim, C.L.; Rich, J.N. Cancer stem cells in glioblastoma. *Genes Dev.* **2015**, *29*, 1203–1217. [CrossRef] [PubMed]
24. Sundar, S.J.; Hsieh, J.K.; Manjila, S.; Lathia, J.D.; Sloan, A. The role of cancer stem cells in glioblastoma. *Neurosurg. Focus* **2014**, *37*, E6. [CrossRef]
25. Rycaj, K.; Tang, D.G. Cancer stem cells and radioresistance. *Int. J. Radiat. Biol.* **2014**, *90*, 615–621. [CrossRef]
26. Bao, S.; Wu, Q.; McLendon, R.E.; Hao, Y.; Shi, Q.; Hjelmeland, A.B.; Dewhirst, M.W.; Bigner, D.D.; Rich, J.N. Glioma stem cells promote radioresistance by preferential activation of the DNA damage response. *Nature* **2006**, *444*, 756–760. [CrossRef]
27. Diehn, M.; Clarke, M.F. Cancer stem cells and radiotherapy: New insights into tumor radioresistance. *J. Natl. Cancer Inst.* **2006**, *98*, 1755–1757. [CrossRef]
28. Codony-Servat, J.; Rosell, R. Cancer stem cells and immunoresistance: Clinical implications and solutions. *Transl. Lung Cancer Res.* **2015**, *4*, 689–703. [CrossRef]
29. Maccalli, C.; Rasul, K.I.; Elawad, M.; Ferrone, S. The role of cancer stem cells in the modulation of anti-tumor immune responses. *Semin. Cancer Biol.* **2018**, *53*, 189–200. [CrossRef]
30. Maccalli, C.; Parmiani, G.; Ferrone, S. Immunomodulating and Immunoresistance Properties of Cancer-Initiating Cells: Implications for the Clinical Success of Immunotherapy. *Immunol. Investig.* **2017**, *46*, 221–238. [CrossRef]
31. Maccalli, C.; De Maria, R. Cancer stem cells: Perspectives for therapeutic targeting. *Cancer Immunol. Immunother.* **2015**, *64*, 91–97. [CrossRef] [PubMed]
32. Agarwal, V.; Bell, G.W.; Nam, J.W.; Bartel, D.P. Predicting effective microRNA target sites in mammalian mRNAs. *Elife* **2015**, *4*, e05005. [CrossRef] [PubMed]
33. Liu, W.; Wang, X. Prediction of functional microRNA targets by integrative modeling of microRNA binding and target expression data. *Genome Biol.* **2019**, *20*, 18. [CrossRef]
34. Chen, Y.; Wang, X. miRDB: An online database for prediction of functional microRNA targets. *Nucleic Acids Res.* **2020**, *48*, D127–D131. [CrossRef] [PubMed]
35. Celiku, O.; Johnson, S.; Zhao, S.; Camphausen, K.; Shankavaram, U. Visualizing molecular profiles of glioblastoma with GBM-BioDP. *PLoS ONE* **2014**, *9*, e101239. [CrossRef]
36. Verhaak, R.G.; Hoadley, K.A.; Purdom, E.; Wang, V.; Qi, Y.; Wilkerson, M.D.; Miller, C.R.; Ding, L.; Golub, T.; Mesirov, J.P.; et al. Integrated genomic analysis identifies clinically relevant subtypes of glioblastoma characterized by abnormalities in PDGFRA, IDH1, EGFR, and NF1. *Cancer Cell* **2010**, *17*, 98–110. [CrossRef]
37. Gnanavel, M.; Murugesan, A.; Konda Mani, S.; Yli-Harja, O.; Kandhavelu, M. Identifying the miRNA Signature Association with Aging-Related Senescence in Glioblastoma. *Int. J. Mol. Sci.* **2021**, *22*, 517. [CrossRef] [PubMed]
38. Huang, Z.; Cheng, L.; Guryanova, O.A.; Wu, Q.; Bao, S. Cancer stem cells in glioblastoma—molecular signaling and therapeutic targeting. *Protein Cell* **2010**, *1*, 638–655. [CrossRef]
39. Fantozzi, A.; Gruber, D.C.; Pisarsky, L.; Heck, C.; Kunita, A.; Yilmaz, M.; Meyer-Schaller, N.; Cornille, K.; Hopfer, U.; Bentires-Alj, M.; et al. VEGF-mediated angiogenesis links EMT-induced cancer stemness to tumor initiation. *Cancer Res.* **2014**, *74*, 1566–1575. [CrossRef]
40. Pradella, D.; Naro, C.; Sette, C.; Ghigna, C. EMT and stemness: Flexible processes tuned by alternative splicing in development and cancer progression. *Mol. Cancer* **2017**, *16*, 8. [CrossRef]
41. Singh, A.; Settleman, J. EMT, cancer stem cells and drug resistance: An emerging axis of evil in the war on cancer. *Oncogene* **2010**, *29*, 4741–4751. [CrossRef] [PubMed]

42. Chang, C.J.; Chao, C.H.; Xia, W.; Yang, J.Y.; Xiong, Y.; Li, C.W.; Yu, W.H.; Rehman, S.K.; Hsu, J.L.; Lee, H.H.; et al. p53 regulates epithelial-mesenchymal transition and stem cell properties through modulating miRNAs. *Nat. Cell Biol.* **2011**, *13*, 317–323. [CrossRef]
43. Easwaran, H.; Tsai, H.C.; Baylin, S.B. Cancer epigenetics: Tumor heterogeneity, plasticity of stem-like states, and drug resistance. *Mol. Cell* **2014**, *54*, 716–727. [CrossRef] [PubMed]
44. Eyler, C.E.; Rich, J.N. Survival of the fittest: Cancer stem cells in therapeutic resistance and angiogenesis. *J. Clin. Oncol.* **2008**, *26*, 2839–2845. [CrossRef] [PubMed]
45. Mo, J.S.; Park, H.W.; Guan, K.L. The Hippo signaling pathway in stem cell biology and cancer. *EMBO Rep.* **2014**, *15*, 642–656. [CrossRef] [PubMed]
46. Maugeri-Sacca, M.; Vigneri, P.; De Maria, R. Cancer stem cells and chemosensitivity. *Clin. Cancer Res.* **2011**, *17*, 4942–4947. [CrossRef] [PubMed]
47. Khan, A.Q.; Ahmed, E.I.; Elareer, N.R.; Junejo, K.; Steinhoff, M.; Uddin, S. Role of miRNA-Regulated Cancer Stem Cells in the Pathogenesis of Human Malignancies. *Cells* **2019**, *8*, 840. [CrossRef] [PubMed]
48. Kraemer, A.; Barjaktarovic, Z.; Sarioglu, H.; Winkler, K.; Eckardt-Schupp, F.; Tapio, S.; Atkinson, M.J.; Moertl, S. Cell survival following radiation exposure requires miR-525-3p mediated suppression of ARRB1 and TXN1. *PLoS ONE* **2013**, *8*, e77484. [CrossRef] [PubMed]
49. Masoudi, M.S.; Mehrabian, E.; Mirzaei, H. MiR-21: A key player in glioblastoma pathogenesis. *J. Cell. Biochem.* **2018**, *119*, 1285–1290. [CrossRef] [PubMed]
50. Aldaz, B.; Sagardoy, A.; Nogueira, L.; Guruceaga, E.; Grande, L.; Huse, J.T.; Aznar, M.A.; Diez-Valle, R.; Tejada-Solis, S.; Alonso, M.M.; et al. Involvement of miRNAs in the differentiation of human glioblastoma multiforme stem-like cells. *PLoS ONE* **2013**, *8*, e77098. [CrossRef]
51. Godlewski, J.; Newton, H.B.; Chiocca, E.A.; Lawler, S.E. MicroRNAs and glioblastoma; the stem cell connection. *Cell Death Differ.* **2010**, *17*, 221–228. [CrossRef] [PubMed]
52. Gagliardi, F.; Narayanan, A.; Gallotti, A.L.; Pieri, V.; Mazzoleni, S.; Cominelli, M.; Rezzola, S.; Corsini, M.; Brugnara, G.; Altabella, L.; et al. Enhanced SPARCL1 expression in cancer stem cells improves preclinical modeling of glioblastoma by promoting both tumor infiltration and angiogenesis. *Neurobiol. Dis.* **2020**, *134*, 104705. [CrossRef] [PubMed]
53. Narayanan, A.; Gagliardi, F.; Gallotti, A.L.; Mazzoleni, S.; Cominelli, M.; Fagnocchi, L.; Pala, M.; Piras, I.S.; Zordan, P.; Moretta, N.; et al. The proneural gene ASCL1 governs the transcriptional subgroup affiliation in glioblastoma stem cells by directly repressing the mesenchymal gene NDRG1. *Cell Death Differ.* **2019**, *26*, 1813–1831. [CrossRef] [PubMed]
54. Huang, Z.; Huang, S.; Wang, Q.; Liang, L.; Ni, S.; Wang, L.; Sheng, W.; He, X.; Du, X. MicroRNA-95 promotes cell proliferation and targets sorting Nexin 1 in human colorectal carcinoma. *Cancer Res.* **2011**, *71*, 2582–2589. [CrossRef]
55. Huang, X.; Taeb, S.; Jahangiri, S.; Emmenegger, U.; Tran, E.; Bruce, J.; Mesci, A.; Korpela, E.; Vesprini, D.; Wong, C.S.; et al. miRNA-95 mediates radioresistance in tumors by targeting the sphingolipid phosphatase SGPP1. *Cancer Res.* **2013**, *73*, 6972–6986. [CrossRef]
56. Xiao, Z.; Ching Chow, S.; Han Li, C.; Chun Tang, S.; Tsui, S.K.; Lin, Z.; Chen, Y. Role of microRNA-95 in the anticancer activity of Brucein D in hepatocellular carcinoma. *Eur. J. Pharmacol.* **2014**, *728*, 141–150. [CrossRef]
57. Fan, B.; Jiao, B.H.; Fan, F.S.; Lu, S.K.; Song, J.; Guo, C.Y.; Yang, J.K.; Yang, L. Downregulation of miR-95-3p inhibits proliferation, and invasion promoting apoptosis of glioma cells by targeting CELF2. *Int. J. Oncol.* **2015**, *47*, 1025–1033. [CrossRef]
58. Ravindran, S.; Rasool, S.; Maccalli, C. The Cross Talk between Cancer Stem Cells/Cancer Initiating Cells and Tumor Microenvironment: The Missing Piece of the Puzzle for the Efficient Targeting of these Cells with Immunotherapy. *Cancer Microenviron.* **2019**, *12*, 133–148. [CrossRef] [PubMed]
59. Boldrini, L.; Giordano, M.; Niccoli, C.; Melfi, F.; Lucchi, M.; Mussi, A.; Fontanini, G. Role of microRNA-33a in regulating the expression of PD-1 in lung adenocarcinoma. *Cancer Cell Int.* **2017**, *17*, 105. [CrossRef]
60. Iliopoulos, D.; Jaeger, S.A.; Hirsch, H.A.; Bulyk, M.L.; Struhl, K. STAT3 activation of miR-21 and miR-181b-1 via PTEN and CYLD are part of the epigenetic switch linking inflammation to cancer. *Mol. Cell* **2010**, *39*, 493–506. [CrossRef]
61. Yan, K.; Yang, K.; Rich, J.N. The evolving landscape of glioblastoma stem cells. *Curr. Opin. Neurol.* **2013**, *26*, 701–707. [CrossRef] [PubMed]
62. Po, A.; Abballe, L.; Sabato, C.; Gianno, F.; Chiacchiarini, M.; Catanzaro, G.; De Smaele, E.; Giangaspero, F.; Ferretti, E.; Miele, E.; et al. Sonic Hedgehog Medulloblastoma Cancer Stem Cells Mirnome and Transcriptome Highlight Novel Functional Networks. *Int. J. Mol. Sci.* **2018**, *19*, 2326. [CrossRef] [PubMed]
63. Brower, J.V.; Clark, P.A.; Lyon, W.; Kuo, J.S. MicroRNAs in cancer: Glioblastoma and glioblastoma cancer stem cells. *Neurochem. Int.* **2014**, *77*, 68–77. [CrossRef] [PubMed]
64. Lulli, V.; Buccarelli, M.; Martini, M.; Signore, M.; Biffoni, M.; Giannetti, S.; Morgante, L.; Marziali, G.; Ilari, R.; Pagliuca, A.; et al. miR-135b suppresses tumorigenesis in glioblastoma stem-like cells impairing proliferation, migration and self-renewal. *Oncotarget* **2015**, *6*, 37241–37256. [CrossRef] [PubMed]
65. Eisen, M.B.; Spellman, P.T.; Brown, P.O.; Botstein, D. Cluster analysis and display of genome-wide expression patterns. *Proc. Natl. Acad. Sci. USA* **1998**, *95*, 14863–14868. [CrossRef] [PubMed]
66. Dennis, G., Jr.; Sherman, B.T.; Hosack, D.A.; Yang, J.; Gao, W.; Lane, H.C.; Lempicki, R.A. DAVID: Database for Annotation, Visualization, and Integrated Discovery. *Genome Biol.* **2003**, *4*, 3. [CrossRef]

Article

Relationship between the miRNA Profiles and Oncogene Mutations in Non-Smoker Lung Cancer. Relevance for Lung Cancer Personalized Screenings and Treatments

Alberto Izzotti [1,2,*], Gabriela Coronel Vargas [3], Alessandra Pulliero [3], Simona Coco [4], Irene Vanni [4,5], Cristina Colarossi [6], Giuseppina Blanco [6], Antonella Agodi [7], Martina Barchitta [7], Andrea Maugeri [7], CT-ME-EN Cancer Registry Workers [8,†], Gea Oliveri Conti [7], Margherita Ferrante [6,7] and Salvatore Sciacca [6]

1. Department of Experimental Medicine, University of Genoa, 16132 Genoa, Italy
2. UOC Mutagenesis and Cancer Prevention, IRCCS Ospedale Policlinico San Martino, 16132 Genoa, Italy
3. Department of Health Sciences, University of Genoa, 16132 Genoa, Italy; S3563836@unige.it (G.C.V.); alessandra.pulliero@unige.it (A.P.)
4. Lung Cancer Unit, IRCCS Ospedale Policlinico San Martino, 16132 Genoa, Italy; simona.coco@hsanmartino.it (S.C.); irene.vanni@sanmartino.it (I.V.)
5. Genetics of Rare Cancers, Department of Internal Medicine and Medical Specialties, University of Genoa, 16132 Genoa, Italy
6. Department of Experimental Oncology, Mediterranean Institute of Oncology (IOM), 95029 Catania, Italy; cristina.colarossi@grupposamed.com (C.C.); giusi.blanco@grupposamed.com (G.B.); marfer@unict.it (M.F.); tsciacca42@gmail.com (S.S.)
7. Department of Medical and Surgical Sciences and Advanced Technologies "G.F. Ingrassia", University of Catania, 95123 Catania, Italy; agodia@unict.it (A.A.); martina.barchitta@unict.it (M.B.); andrea.maugeri@unict.it (A.M.); oliericonti@unict.it (G.O.C.)
8. Catania, Messina, Enna Cancer Registry, Via S. Sofia 87, 95123 Catania, Italy; segreteria@registrotumoriintegrato.it
* Correspondence: izzotti@unige.it
† CT-ME-EN Cancer Registry Workers are provided in the Acknowledgments.

Abstract: Oncogene mutations may be drivers of the carcinogenesis process. MicroRNA (miRNA) alterations may be adaptive or pathogenic and can have consequences only when mutation in the controlled oncogenes occurs. The aim of this research was to analyze the interplay between miRNA expression and oncogene mutation. A total of 2549 miRNAs were analyzed in cancer tissue—in surrounding normal lung tissue collected from 64 non-smoking patients and in blood plasma. Mutations in 92 hotspots of 22 oncogenes were tested in the lung cancer tissue. MicroRNA alterations were related to the mutations occurring in cancer patients. Conversely, the frequency of mutation occurrence was variable and spanned from the k-ras and p53 mutation detected in 30% of patients to 20% of patients in which no mutation was detected. The prediction of survival at a 3-year follow up did not occur for mutation analysis but was, conversely, well evident for miRNA analysis highlighting a pattern of miRNA distinguishing between survivors and death in patients 3 years before this clinical onset. A signature of six lung cancer specific miRNAs occurring both in the lungs and blood was identified. The obtained results provide evidence that the analysis of both miRNA and oncogene mutations was more informative than the oncogene mutation analysis currently performed in clinical practice.

Keywords: nonsmokers lung cancer; miRNA; environmental risk factors; oncogenes; mutations

1. Introduction

MicroRNAs (miRNAs) are non-coding RNA molecules that have different regulatory roles in cell differentiation, proliferation, and survival. miRNAs can inhibit complementary mRNA targets, regulating translation through RNA degradation. miRNAs were found to be deregulated in numerous diseases, including cancer, and are frequently altered owing to mutations or transcriptional changes of the enzymes that regulate miRNA biogenesis [1]. miRNAs are also involved in the epithelial–mesenchymal transition, cell growth, proliferation, migration, and invasion [2], as well as processes related to chemotherapy cell resistance. For example, miR-92a expression is increased in *PTEN* deletion cases [3], miR-244 is related to the apoptosis process enhancing the proliferative and migratory effects in non-small cell lung cancer (NSCLC) [4], and miR-200c influences the epithelial–mesenchymal transition in A549 cells [5].

Experimental findings have linked environmental exposure, carcinogenesis, and miRNA profiles. Neither epigenetic nor genetic alteration, when used alone, accurately predict the lung cancer risk in exposed subjects. Indeed, the adverse effects of mutations can be silenced by a functional microRNA machinery and the alteration of the miRNA machinery is devoid of remarkable consequences in absence of genotoxic damage. Early diagnosis of lung cancers using miR-33a-5p and miR-128-3p signatures have been proposed as they are linked to tumor suppression processes [6]. These findings address the identification of a cluster of miRNAs to be used as cancer early predictors considering the high heterogeneity of lung cancer patients.

However, the use of microRNA analysis alone for early lung cancer detection is still questionable. Indeed, despite a variety of miRNA being released extracellularly in the blood from growing cancers [7], the use of blood circulating miRNAs for cancer diagnosis is still a research matter and is not yet applicable to clinical and preventive practices. Several problems still hamper the on-field application of miRNA analysis as a tool for preventive medicine, including (a) the lack of correspondence between cancer and blood miRNAs; (b) the overwhelming effect of miRNA released from large mass organs on cancer miRNAs; (c) the poor reproducibility of miRNA cancer signatures among different studies; (d) the limited predictivity of miRNA analysis when used alone.

MicroRNAs are released not only from growing cancer but also, under physiological conditions, by organs, such as the skeletal muscle, liver, and kidneys (weighting kilos) [8]. The amount of these miRNAs overwhelms those released from the low-size growing cancer mass (weight of a few mg and size of a few mm), a problem increased by the fact that miRNAs are only partly tissue specific, as the same miRNA is expressed, although at different levels, in various body tissues.

The limited predictivity for the cancer occurrence of miRNAs when used alone is because miRNAs are quite unspecific with each one regulating hundreds of genes and, not only one but many, miRNAs play a pathogenic role in cancer progression. The main anti-cancer mechanism exerted by miRNA is the suppression of messenger RNAs produced by mutated oncogenes. This situation occurs in lung cancer for let-7 miRNA suppressing the expression of mutated k-ras oncogene [9] in breast cancer for miR-335 modulating the expression and the biological effects of the mutated BRCA1 oncogene [10].

Accordingly, whenever an oncogene is mutated, but its suppressing miRNA is still functioning, there is no push toward cancer progression, and thus the mutation is devoid of clinical predictivity. Similarly, whenever a microRNA is altered or downregulated, but its controlled genes is not mutated, again, there is no push toward cancer progression, and thus the microRNA alteration mutation is devoid of clinical predictivity. Giving this situation, it appears to be of high relevance to test, in parallel, both microRNA alterations and oncogene mutations to increase the clinical predictivity of these cancer biomarkers.

The study was focused on non or ex-smokers only. Indeed, cigarette smoke exerts a well-documented direct alteration of miRNA expression [11]. Accordingly, we decided to limit the effect of this confounding factor focusing on the relationship between miRNA and oncogenes as related to lung cancer only. This design was more difficult than recruiting current smokers; however, this was the only feasible approach to guarantee that the obtained results reflected cancer-related effects only and were not the results of the direct action of cigarette smoke on the miRNA machinery.

The aim of the herein reported research project is to use integrated mutations and microRNA expression as a new tool to perform lung cancer diagnosis and to identify high risk subjects with reference to lung cancer in non-smokers.

2. Materials and Methods

2.1. Patient Recruitment and Sampling

The enrollment of the patients was performed in the four biggest hospitals of Catania (University Hospital "G. Rodolico—San Marco", "Garibaldi-Nesima" Hospital, "Cannizzaro" Hospital, and "Morgagni" Clinic), and in the "San Vincenzo" Hospital of Taormina of Messina province.

The protocol of this study was approved by the Ethics Committees (n. 11778 released on 17 March 2015. and 346/C.E. released on 28 May 2015) of the involved institutions and performed according to the Declaration of Helsinki.

We used the following inclusion criteria for the patient enrollment: age > 18 years, undergoing lung cancer-surgery, being non-smokers or former smokers for at least 5 years, survival within 3 years, the exclusion of other concurrent diseases, and having signed the written informed consent during the interview. No gender restriction was considered, and no restricted selection was performed regarding the morphology of the reported neoplastic lesions. From the same patient, both neoplastic and healthy tissue samples (lung tissue biopsy) were taken.

The lung tissue samples were sampled directly from the pathological anatomies of the hospitals involved in the project. Instead, the venous blood samples were collected directly from the thoracic surgery units of the hospitals involved. A total of 64 patients were enrolled, including 42 males (66%) and 22 females (34%), aged 69.0 ± 9.5 years, min 43 and max 84 years old.

Through the questionnaire, socio-demographic and lifestyle information, including smoking history, nutrition, home characteristics, and home location, were collected. From the 64 patients enrolled we sampled 64 blood samples, of which, 41 blood samples and 52 lung tissues were dedicated to miRNA profiling and oncogene mutation analysis by Ion-Torrent sequencing. For 35 patients, a 3 years follow up was performed to evaluate their clinical status. These 35 patients were referred to as 'monitored patients'.

2.2. DNA Extraction

Genomic DNA (gDNA) was extracted from 25 mg of fresh frozen lung biopsy DNA using the DNeasy Blood & Tissue kit (Qiagen, Milan, Italy), as described by the manufacturer's protocol. The purification of gDNA was automated on the QIAcube instrument (Qiagen, Milan, Italy). The gDNA quality and quantity were assessed with a NanoDrop 1000 spectrometer and with a Qubit 3.0 Fluorometer using a dsDNA HS Assay Kit (Thermo Fisher Scientific, Carlsbad, CA, USA).

2.3. Somatic Mutation Identification

The mutational status of 22 oncogenes (*KRAS, EGFR, BRAF, PIK3CA, AKT1, ERBB2, PTEN, NRAS, STK11, MAP2K1, ALK, DDR2, CTNNB1, MET, TP53, SMAD4, FBX7, FGFR3, NOTCH1, ERBB4, FGFR1,* and *FGFR2*) associated with lung cancer was analyzed by sequencing using the Colon and Lung Cancer Research Panel v.2 (Thermo Fisher Scientific, Carlsbad, CA, USA), which screens 92 amplicons in hotspots and target regions of these genes. For each sample, 15 ng of gDNA was amplified using the Ion AmpliSeq™ Library Kit 2.0 (Thermo Fisher Scientific, Carlsbad, CA, USA) according to the protocol for gDNA isolated from fresh frozen samples [12].

The quality control of the libraries was assessed by TapeStation 2200 using the High Sensitivity D1000 assay (Agilent Technologies, Santa Clara, CA, USA) and with a Qubit® 2.0 Fluorometer using the dsDNA HS Assay Kit (Thermo Fisher Scientific, Carlsbad, CA, USA). Then, seven multiplexed libraries (100 pM) were amplified and enriched by OneTouch™ and the OneTouch™ ES, respectively using Ion PGM™ Hi-Q™ View OT2

Kit (Thermo Fisher Scientific, Carlsbad, CA, USA). Finally, the template was loaded onto a 316 v.2 chip and sequenced using the Ion PGM™ Hi-Q™ View Sequencing Kit on the Ion PGM™ platform (Thermo Fisher Scientific, Carlsbad, CA, USA). The sequencing data were analyzed using the Ion Torrent Software Suite with the plugin Torrent Variant Caller v.5.10.0.18 (Thermo Fisher Scientific, Carlsbad, CA, USA) applying somatic, high stringency parameters. We considered gene variants with a variant allele frequency up to 1%, if covered at least 1000×. All gene variants were annotated by Ion Reporter™ Software v. 5.10.

2.4. Total RNA Extraction

The total RNA was extracted from lung biopsies and blood plasma using standardized protocols that combined phenol/guanidine-based lysis of samples and silica-membrane-based purification.

Briefly, 3 mL of whole blood were collected in Ethylenediaminetetraacetic acid (EDTA) tubes and layered onto 3 mL Histopaque-1077 (Sigma-Aldrich Chemie Gmbh, Munich, Germany) through centrifugation at $400 \times g$ for 30 min. Plasma and lymphocytes were separately collected and stored at $-20\ °C$ at the Laboratory of Molecular Epidemiology (University of Catania) until analysis. Next, the total RNA from the plasma was extracted using the miRNeasy Serum/Plasma Kit (Qiagen, Milan, Italy), as described by the manufacturer's protocol.

With respect to lung biopsies, 30 mg of fresh starting material was first stabilized in 2.5 mL of RNAlater solution and stored at $-20\ °C$ at the Laboratory of Molecular Epidemiology (University of Catania) until analysis. Next, lung biopsies were disrupted using the TissueRuptor II for 20–40 s and homogenized in 700 µL QIAzol Lysis Reagent (Qiagen, Milan, Italy). The total RNA was purified from the homogenate using the miRNeasy Mini Kit (Qiagen, Milan, Italy), as described by the manufacturer's protocol. The purification of RNA was automated on the QIAcube instrument (Qiagen, Milan, Italy). The quantification of RNA was assessed with a qubit 3.0 Fluorometer using the HS RNA Assay kit (Thermo Fisher Scientific, Carlsbad, CA, USA).

2.5. MiRNA Microarray Analysis

MiRNA profiling was performed by Agilent Platform using Human miRNA 8×60 K Microarray containing 2549 miRNAs (miRBase 21.0) (Agilent Technologies, Santa Clara, CA, USA). For each sample, 50 ng of the total RNA, including the miRNAs, was labeled, and hybridized according to the manufacturer's instructions for miRNA Complete Labeling and the Hyb protocol (v. 3.1.1). The hybridized microarrays were acquired using the G2565CA scanner (Agilent Technologies) and the images were processed by Feature Extraction software v.9.5.3.1 (Agilent Technologies, Santa Clara, CA, USA). All raw data were loaded in the Gene Expression Omnibus (http://www.ncbi.nlm.nih.gov/geo/; GEO number accession requested, 8 March 2021). A tab-delimited text file was analyzed in the R v. 2.7.2 software environment http://www.r-project.org (accessed on 8 March 2021) using the limma package v.2.14.16 of Bioconductor http://www.bioconductor.org accessed on 8 March 2021.

Only spots with a signal minus background that were flagged as positive and significant were used in the following analysis as 'detected' spots. Probes with less than 50% of detected spots across all arrays, and arrays with several detected spots smaller than 50% of all spots on the array were removed. The background-corrected intensities of the replicated spots on each array were averaged. The data were then log2-transformed and normalized for between-array comparison using quintile normalization [13]. MicroRNAs with p-values < 0.05 were selected for further analysis. Given the explorative nature of this study, no correction for multiple testing was applied in the screening procedure aimed at selecting multiple sets of microRNAs for subsequent hierarchical clustering analyses. The agglomerative hierarchical clusters, used to detect similarity relationships in microRNA log2-transformed expressions, were computed using the Euclidean distance between single vectors and the Ward method [14].

2.6. Statistical Analysis

GeneSpring software (GeneSpring Multi-Omic Analysis version 14.9–Build 11939 by Agilent Technologies) was used for the analysis of miRNA expression from lung-tumoral (T = 38), lung-healthy (S = 12), and blood tissues (n = 41).

All lung-tissue-miRNA raw data files from the Agilent Technologies Microarray Scanner System G2505C were imported to GeneSpring using miRNA analysis type, Technology 70156_v21_0, without baseline transformation. The blood miRNA chip raw data were import to GeneSpring with a custom technology as scanner analysis technology was not available. The protocol used was: Analysis type = Expression, Experiment type = Generic Single Color, Normalization algorithm = none, percentile target = 75, and baseline transformation = none.

3. Results

3.1. Mutations in Oncogenes

Despite the presence of lung cancer, no hotspot mutation was observed in 10 out of the 52 examined patients (19.2%). In 42 patients, mutations in oncogenes were observed with the following frequency ranking: *TP53* (36.54%), *KRAS* (30.77%), *EGFR* (25%), *PIK3CA* (13.46%), *ERBB2* (1.92%), *STK11* (5.77%), *BRAF* (3.85%), *PTEN* (9.62%), *MAP2K1* (1.92%), and *FGFR* (1.92%) (Figure 1). Only 14 Patients (26%) carried mutations targetable by available precision medicine therapies (*EGFR* 25 mutations, *BRAF* 2 mutations, and *ALK* 2 mutations), and 25 out of 52 patients presented more than one mutation (Table 1).

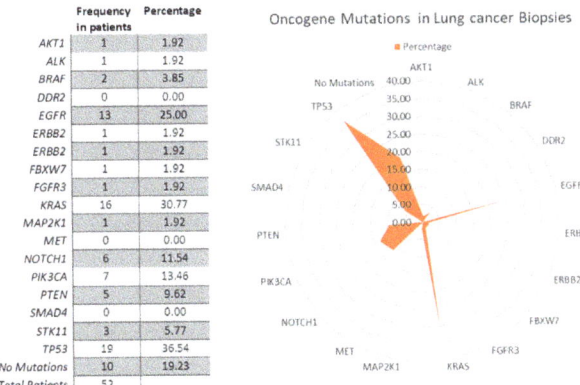

Figure 1. Radar chart showing the frequency of mutations in the lung biopsies of analyzed patients. *TP53* (36.54%), *KRAS* (30.77%), *EGFR* (25%), *PIK3CA* (13.46%), and *NOTCH1* (11.54%) were the most frequent mutations in the analyzed patients.

Table 1. Frequency of single, double, triple, quadruple, and quintuple mutations in lung biopsies from the analyzed patients.

Number of Mutations	Frequency	Percentage
0	10	19.2
1	17	32.7
2	19	36.5
3	2	3.8
4	3	5.8
5	1	1.9
Total	52	100.0

3.2. Relationship between miRNA Profiles and Mutations in Oncogenes

From the 38 patients in which both miRNA and mutations were analyzed, 33 were patients carrying at least one mutation. The mutational status affects the miRNA expression. Indeed, the expression of Cancer Related miRNAs was different between mutation-carrier and mutation-free patients, as shown for each mutation by scatter plot analyses (Figure 2).

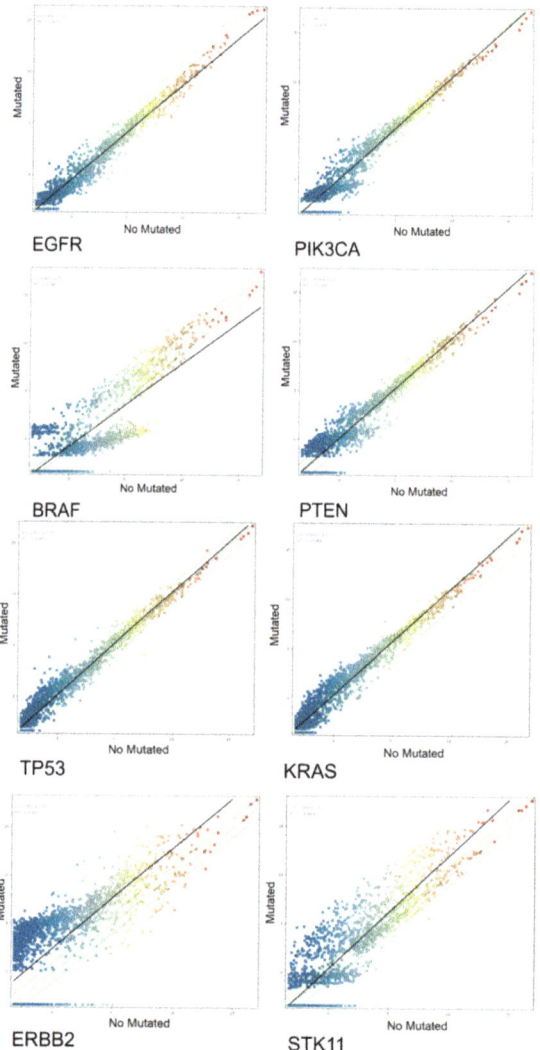

Figure 2. Scatter plot analyses of the miRNA-chip-array results from tumoral lung biopsies of analyzed patients without (horizontal axis) and with (vertical axis) mutations for the oncogenes *TP53*, *KRAS*, *EGFR*, *PIK3CA*, *ERBB2*, *STK11*, *BRAF*, and *PTEN*. The miRNA profile was significantly related with the mutational status of the analyzed oncogenes as demonstrated by the miRNA changing their expression more than two-fold falling outside the two-fold variation interval indicated by the diagonal green lines. The slope of the best fit regression line (black diagonal line) indicates the overall trend toward up or downregulation for the mutational status of each oncogene.

miRNAs altered in tumoral tissue associated with each oncogene mutation were identified by volcano plot analyses (FC > 2.0, $p < 0.05$). Their identity is reported in the supplementary material (Table S1). The number of cancer-related miRNAs altered in tumoral tissue as associated for each oncogene mutation is reported in Table 2.

Table 2. A number of miRNAs significantly changed their expression according to the mutational status of each oncogene. This table lists the number of these miRNAs in patients carrying oncogene mutations.

Gene	Mutated/Total Patients	Number of Entities (Altered miRNAs)	Up	Down	miRNAs Targeting Mutated Oncogene
BRAF	2/33	7	1	6	0
EGFR	9/33	1	0	1	0
ERBB2	1/33	-	-	-	-
ERBB4	1/33	-	-	-	-
FGFR3	1/33	-	-	-	-
KRAS	10/33	13	13	0	2 (hsa-miR-15b-3p, hsa-miR-21-3p)
NOTCH1	3/33	1	1	0	0
PIK3CA	3/33	0	0	0	0
PTEN	2/33	0	0	0	0
STK11	2/33	31	30	1	1 (hsa-miR-548aa)
TP53	10/33	4	4	0	1 (hsa-miR-205-3p)

3.3. Clinical Predictivity of miRNA Profiling

In this study: 9 out of 35 monitored patients died within 3 years of the biopsy. We explored whether the miRNA lung tumor expression profile was predictive of the clinical outcome in the following years after surgery. Indeed, the miRNA expression profile in cancer tissue was different between survivors and non-survivors, as shown by the scatter plot (Figure 3a) and volcano plot analyses (Figure 3b). The list of the 11 miRNAs predictive of patient survival (10 up-regulated (red dots) in survivors as compared to non survivors and 1 down-regulated (blue dot)) is reported in Table S2. A prediction model using the list of these 11 miRNAs related to survival and the GeneSpring Neural Network prediction algorithm was run, obtaining an overall accuracy of 0.92 (+0.11), a higher result than those obtained for all miRNA entities (accuracy 0.81). This high accuracy shows the potential of these 11 cancer-related miRNAs from lung biopsies to be used as survival predictors.

Conversely, the mutation status poorly predicted the survival. Indeed, the rate of survivors (47 out of 60) and non-survivors (13 out of 60) was not different between mutation free (10 out of 52) and mutation carrier (42 out of 52) patients. The patient's detailed information can be found in Table S2. The number of mutations carried by the same patients was not different between survivors and non-survivors as demonstrated by the Chi-squared test ($p = 0.803$) (Figure 4).

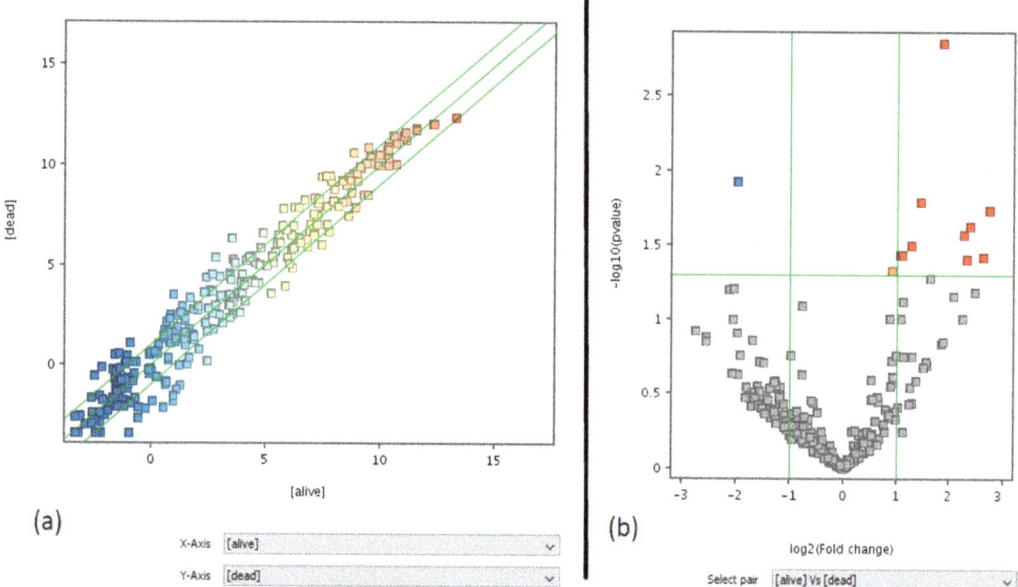

Figure 3. Best-fit line in black, fold change and p-value lines in green. (**a**) Scatter plot analysis = entity list: cancer-related miRNAs (273), interpretation: averaged (alive) vs. (dead), FC $\geq$ 2.0. (**b**) Moderated T-test volcano plot analysis = entity list: cancer-related miRNAs (273), interpretation: averaged (alive) vs. (dead), without multiple testing correction, *p*-value cut-off = 0.05, fold-change cut-off = 2.0.

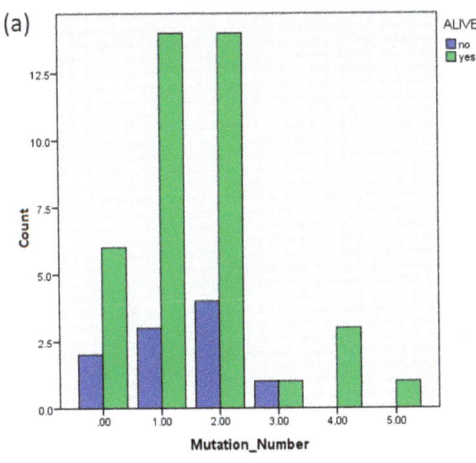

Figure 4. The number of mutations did not predict patient survival. (**a**) Bar plot of the number of patients with zero to five mutations detected separated by survival. (**b**) Same data of (**a**) summarized in a contingency table. (**c**) The Chi-squared test maintained the null hypothesis: the survival and mutation number were independent variables.

3.4. Liquid Biopsy: Lung Versus Blood

The intensity of the expression of circulating blood miRNAs from 41 patients was used to classify miRNAs according to their inter-quartile average intensity expression (0–25% = undetectable, 26–50% = low, 51–75% = intermediate, and 76–100% = high). Out of the 273 Cancer Related miRNAs, 217 entries were also present in miRNA blood arrays. Venn diagram analysis indicated that the majority (n = 121) were undetectable and expressed at a low, 43 were detectable at an intermediate level, and 53 at a high level, i.e., in the upper quartile of the distribution (Table S3).

Accordingly, a signature of 53 cancer related miRNAs present in the blood with a high expression was identified. The panel of these highly detectable miRNAs was compared with their use as possible biomarkers in blood and serum as available in the existing literature (Table 3). Let-7b-5p, miR-150-5p, miR-22-5p, miR-26a-5p, miR-30b-5p, miR-30c-5p, and miR-486-3p were also present in other studies examining circulating miRNAs in the blood as lung cancer biomarkers [15–18].

A similar approach was used to identify the presence in the plasma of lung miRNAs predictive of clinical outcome (survival). Out of the 11 predictive miRNAs identified in the lung cancer tissue (Table S2), Venn diagram analysis indicated that four were expressed at a high level (high inter-quartile intensity) in the plasma. These miRNAs were miR-23a-5p, miR-147b, miR-371b-5p, and miR-2861.

Table 3. Cancer-related miRNAs present in the blood with a high expression falling in the upper quartile of the distribution of intensity expression. The intensity of the miRNA expression was reported in fluorescence units as detected by microarray analysis (middle column). The miRNAs found in our study were compared with the bibliography to evaluate if their dysregulation in the blood could be considered as potential markers for lung cancer (right column).

Tumoral miRNAs in Blood	Average Signal in Blood Plasma Microarray (Fluorescence Units)	Reference in Literature
hsa-let-7b-5p	1556.03	[16,17]
hsa-let-7e-5p	2570.68	[15]
hsa-let-7g-5p	1591.89	ND
hsa-miR-103a-3p	1966.77	ND
hsa-miR-107	2307.96	ND
hsa-miR-1247-5p	1619.35	ND
hsa-miR-143-3p	1517.48	ND
hsa-miR-147b	2867.22	ND
hsa-miR-150-5p	1728.39	[15]
hsa-miR-151a-5p	2375.45	ND
hsa-miR-151b	2375.45	ND
hsa-miR-181a-2-3p	1714.68	ND
hsa-miR-183-3p	4515.51	ND
hsa-miR-184	3097.26	ND
hsa-miR-185-5p	2809.76	ND
hsa-miR-193a-5p	1482.98	ND
hsa-miR-22-5p	1889.39	[15,17]
hsa-miR-224-3p	1805.07	ND
hsa-miR-23a-5p	2880.99	ND
hsa-miR-26a-5p	1497.29	[17]
hsa-miR-2861	3086.05	ND
hsa-miR-29b-2-5p	1481.13	ND
hsa-miR-30b-5p	2117.35	[16]
hsa-miR-30c-2-3p	2919.97	ND
hsa-miR-30c-5p	3299.46	[17,18]
hsa-miR-3149	2367.91	ND
hsa-miR-361-3p	1454.65	ND
hsa-miR-371b-5p	12,583.51	ND
hsa-miR-424-5p	1660.83	ND
hsa-miR-4252	1558.12	ND
hsa-miR-4290	1875.54	ND
hsa-miR-4306	7145.12	ND
hsa-miR-4324	1530.87	ND
hsa-miR-4440	1537.86	ND
hsa-miR-4443	3859.37	ND
hsa-miR-4481	1605.44	ND
hsa-miR-450a-5p	4646.58	ND
hsa-miR-4516	11,603.31	ND
hsa-miR-452-5p	1629.61	ND
hsa-miR-4532	13,231.17	ND
hsa-miR-4634	1884.47	ND
hsa-miR-483-3p	3177.46	ND
hsa-miR-486-3p	2337.52	[14,18]
hsa-miR-490-3p	1882.31	ND
hsa-miR-505-5p	3775.67	ND
hsa-miR-516b-5p	5121.31	ND
hsa-miR-548aa	3480.4	ND
hsa-miR-548q	1453.76	ND
hsa-miR-642b-5p	2070.84	ND
hsa-miR-664b-3p	1539.91	ND
hsa-miR-744-5p	3112.18	ND
hsa-miR-99a-3p	1503.5	ND
hsa-miR-99b-5p	1575.63	ND

ND, Not Detected.

4. Discussion and Conclusions

The identification of novel biomarkers based on miRNA profiles from accessible biological samples, like blood, would help in the near future for a better understanding of a patient's health state. Outcomes, like better malignant tumor tissue early detection, over time therapy effectiveness prediction, and patient survival prediction rates, may become a reality. The identification of useful circulating miRNAs for predictive outcomes may require models based on standardized tissue-specific and blood-based profiles in oncologic patients.

As seen in our results, the presence of different mutations can modify the scatter plot in each case. From the cancer-related miRNAs significantly altered in each mutation, only four were predicted by TargetScan to target the considered genes as follows: hsa-miR-15b-3p and hsa-miR-21-3p for *KRAS*, hsa-miR-548aa for *STK11*, and hsa-miR-205-3p for *TP53*. This suggests that the dysregulation in these miRNAs may worse the mutation condition.

Indeed, functional miRNAs may silence the expression of mutated oncogenes by destroying their encoded mRNA. Accordingly, whenever the miRNA machinery is well functioning, oncogene mutation does not bear relevance for phenotypic changes and progression of the cell in the carcinogenesis process. Conversely, whenever these miRNAs are altered, their efficacy in neutralizing the mRNAs encoded by mutated oncogenes is lost, and oncogene mutation acquires relevance and efficacy for changing cell phenotypes and moving the carcinogenesis process forward.

We found 11 miRNAs as statistically significant predictors of the patients' dead within 3 years: hsa-miR-1227-5p, hsa-miR-147b, hsa-miR-187-5p, hsa-miR-23a-5p, hsa-miR-2861, hsa-miR-3663-5p, hsa-miR-371b-5p, hsa-miR-6068, hsa-miR-6075, hsa-miR-6771-5p, and hsa-miR-7704. At the same time, our analysis confirmed that survival was not correlated to the number of oncogene mutations.

From this list, four miRNAs (miR-187-5p, miR-147b, miR-2861, and miR-6075) appear to be the most promising survival markers. Researchers observed that miR-187-5p suppresses cancer cell progression in non-small cell lung cancer (NSCLC) through the down-regulation of *CYP1B1* [19,20], and that miR-147b promotes lung adenocarcinoma cell aggressiveness through glycoprotein 4 (*MFAP4*) regulation [21]; miR-2861 was proposed as a biomarker of lung cancer stem cells [22]; and miR-6075 was used as a biomarker for lung cancer high-accuracy diagnosis prediction models [23]. As our results demonstrated, from the 59-miRNA signature for blood, the best candidates were let-7b-5p, miR-150-5p, miR-22-5p, miR-26a-5p, miR-30b-5p, miR-30c-5p, and miR-486-3p, as they are also present in other studies regarding circulating miRNA biomarkers in the blood for lung cancer.

The silencing role of microRNA on the expression of mutated oncogenes is well established mainly for lung carcinogenesis. The k-ras let-7 interaction is the best typical example. However, the interaction of miRNAs with the target mRNA may be either specific or unspecific according to the number of complimentary nucleotides recognized on targeted sequences. We cannot exclude that, if the mutations of the oncogenes occurred in their coding regions, this situation could generate escaping mutants not recognized by the miRNA. However, thus far, this situation has not yet been demonstrated, at variance with the presence of experimental data clearly indicating the inhibitory role of miRNA toward oncogene expression.

The main finding of this study was that the evaluation of oncogene mutations alone was poorly predictive of the clinical outcome. The predictive potential was remarkably increased when oncogenes mutation were evaluated in parallel with the analysis of related miRNAs. This approach may be used for the personalized screening of lung cancer to identify high risk subjects to undergo early diagnosis screening by spiral TAC. Indeed, for practical and economic reasons, this approach cannot be applied to the whole population but only to high risk subjects identified by predictive biomarkers.

The obtained results may also be useful for lung cancer treatment, which is currently focused only on the oncogene mutational status. Our results provide evidence that oncogene mutation does not per se directly reflect on clinical outcomes and cancer behavior.

These variables are determined by other important contributing factors, such as miRNA expression. The comparative analysis of oncogene mutations and miRNA alteration may be useful to identify responders to treatments specifically targeting oncogene mutations or those developing resistance to these treatments.

A remarkable results of our study is the correspondence of the results between the liquid biopsy analysis and corresponding data for the target tissue, i.e., the lung. Indeed, we evaluated in parallel in the same patient both blood and lung tissues. The cancer-related signature was evaluated by comparing the miRNA expression between the cancer and healthy surrounding tissue. This signature accounted for 273 miRNAs, 53 of them being well detectable (i.e., in the highest quartile of the distribution) and also by liquid biopsy in the blood plasma. Among these 53 miRNAs, 7 were further confirmed as lung cancer biomarkers in the blood by other independent studies. These results represents a step forward to identify a miRNA blood signature applicable to the early diagnosis of lung cancer.

Overall, the herein reported results provide evidence that the parallel analyses of miRNA and oncogene mutations was more predictive of lung cancer occurrence that the single analysis of only one of these two biomarkers. A tight interconnection between the pattern of miRNA alteration and the mutations occurring was detected, a finding demonstrating the interplay between genetic damage and the postgenomic control exerted by the miRNA machinery. The predictivity of the clinical outcome (survival) was good for the postgenomic miRNA analysis and undetectable for the oncogene mutation analysis. This analysis could be executed by the non-invasive sampling of blood plasma given the fact that both oncogene mutations and specific lung cancer miRNAs can be detected in this body fluid. Such an approach could represent a new tool applicable to cancer preventive and predictive medicine.

These findings support the use of parallel miRNA and oncogene mutation analysis as a new tool to provide clinical and preventive interventions tailored for the individual situation of each subject or patients, thus, realizing a practical approach of personalized medicine applicable to cancer prevention.

Supplementary Materials: The following are available online at https://www.mdpi.com/2075-4426/11/3/182/s1, Table S1: Cancer Related miRNAs altered (FC $\geq$ 2, $p \leq$ 0.05) in Volcano Plot Analysis between average signal in samples with non-small cell lung cancer vs. small cell lung cancer, Table S2: Cancer Related miRNAs run on a Moderated T-Test Volcano Plot analysis (FC $\geq$ 2, $p \leq$ 0.05) for each environmental exposure: (a) passive smoke at home (No vs. Yes), (b) passive smoke at work (No vs. Yes); (c) airborne car traffic pollution (low vs. high); (d) volcano ashes (>60 Km vs. $\leq$60 Km); (e) radon risk (according to house type low vs. high), Table S3: Cancer Related miRNAs altered (FC $\geq$ 2, $p \leq$ 0.05) in Volcano Plot Analysis between average signal in samples of patients alive vs. dead within 3 years since biopsy.

Author Contributions: Conceptualization, A.I. and S.S.; methodology S.C., I.V., A.P., A.A. and M.B.; validation, G.C.V. and A.P.; investigation, G.O.C., M.F.; resources, A.I. and S.S.; data curation, G.C.V.,A.P., S.C.; writing—original draft preparation, G.C.V., A.P. and A.I., all authors; writing—review and editing G.O.C. and A.I.; visualization M.F., supervision A.I.; project administration, A.I.; funding acquisition S.S. and A.I. All authors have read and agreed to the published version of the manuscript.

Funding: This research was supported by Regional CT-ME-EN-Cancer Register fund-2015, and partially by the Italian Association for Cancer Research (AIRC, IG2017-20699 to A.I.).

Institutional Review Board Statement: The study was conducted according to the guidelines of the Declaration of Helsinki, and approved by the Institutional Review Board Ethics Committees (n. 11778 released on 17 March 2015. and 346/C.E. released on 28 May 2015).

Informed Consent Statement: Informed consent was obtained from all subjects involved in the study.

Data Availability Statement: The datasets used and/or analysed during the current study are available from the corresponding author on reasonable request.

Acknowledgments: We would like to thank the members of the staff from CT-ME-EN Cancer Registry Group: Andrea Benedetto, Marine Castaing, Alessia Di Prima, Paolo Fidelbo, Antonella Ippolito, Eleonora Irato, Anna Leone, Fiorella Paderni, Paola Pesce, Alessandra Savasta, Carlo Sciacchitano, Antonietta Torrisi, Antonina Torrisi, Massimo Varvarà and Carmelo Viscosi.

Conflicts of Interest: The authors declare no conflict of interest.

References

1. Rupaimoole, R.; Slack, F.J. MicroRNA therapeutics: Towards a new era for the management of cancer and other diseases. *Nat. Rev. Drug Discov.* **2017**, *16*, 203–222. [CrossRef] [PubMed]
2. Ma, X.; Liang, A.-L.; Liu, Y.-J. Research progress on the relationship between lung cancer drug-resistance and microRNAs. *J. Cancer* **2019**, *10*, 6865–6875. [CrossRef]
3. Ren, P.; Gong, F.; Zhang, Y.; Jiang, J.; Zhang, H. MicroRNA-92a promotes growth, metastasis, and chemoresistance in non-small cell lung cancer cells by targeting PTEN. *Tumor Biol.* **2015**, *37*, 3215–3225. [CrossRef] [PubMed]
4. Cui, R.; Kim, T.; Fassan, M.; Meng, W.; Sun, H.-L.; Jeon, Y.-J. MicroRNA-224 is implicated in lung cancer pathogenesis through targeting caspase-3 and caspase-7. *Oncotarget* **2015**, *6*, 21802. [CrossRef] [PubMed]
5. Zhao, Y.; Han, M.; Xiong, Y.; Wang, L.; Fei, Y.; Shen, X.; Zhu, Y.; Liang, Z.Q. A miRNA-200c/cathepsin L feedback loop determines paclitaxel resistance in human lung cancer A549 cells in vitro through regulating epithelial–mesenchymal transition. *Acta Pharmacol. Sin.* **2018**, *39*, 1034. [CrossRef] [PubMed]
6. Pan, J.; Zhou, C.; Zhao, X.; He, J.; Tian, H.; Shen, W.; Han, Y.; Chen, J.; Fang, S.; Meng, X.; et al. A two-miRNA signature (miR-33a-5p and miR-128-3p) in whole blood as potential biomarker for early diagnosis of lung cancer. *Sci. Rep.* **2018**, *8*, 16699. [CrossRef] [PubMed]
7. Izzotti, A.; Carozzo, S.; Pulliero, A.; Zhabayeva, D.; Ravetti, J.L.; Bersimbaev, R. Extracellular MicroRNA in liquid biopsy: Applicability in cancer diagnosis and prevention. *Am. J. Cancer Res.* **2016**, *6*, 1461–1493. [PubMed]
8. Izzotti, A.; Longobardi, M.G.; La Maestra, S.; Micale, R.T.; Pulliero, A.; Camoirano, A.; Geretto, M.; D'Agostini, F.; Balansky, R.; Miller, M.S.; et al. Release of microRNAs into body fluids form ten organs in mice exposed to cigarette smoke. *Theranostic* **2018**, *8*, 2147–2160. [CrossRef]
9. Izzotti, A.; Pulliero, A. Molecular damage and lung tumors in cigarette smoke exposed mice. *Ann. N. Y. Acad. Sci.* **2015**, *1340*, 75–83. [CrossRef] [PubMed]
10. Heyn, H.; Engelmann, M.; Schreek, S.; Ahrens, P.; Lehmann, U.; Kreipe, H.; Schlegelberger, B.; Beger, C. MicroRNA miR-335 is crucial for the BRCA1 regulatory cascade in breast cancer development. *Int. J. Cancer* **2011**, *129*, 2797–2806. [CrossRef] [PubMed]
11. Izzotti, A.; Calin, G.A.; Arrigo, P.; Steele, V.E.; Croce, C.M.; De Flora, S. Downregulation of microRNA expression in the lungs of rats exposed to cigarette smoke. *FASEB J.* **2009**, *23*, 806–812. [CrossRef]
12. Vanni, I.; Coco, S.; Truini, A.; Rusmini, M.; Dal Bello, M.G.; Alama, A.; Banelli, B.; Mora, M.; Rijavec, E.; Barletta, G.; et al. Next-Generation Sequencing Workflow for NSCLC Critical Samples Using a Targeted Sequencing Approach by Ion Torrent PGM™ Platform. *Int. J. Mol. Sci.* **2015**, *16*, 28765–28782. [CrossRef] [PubMed]
13. Stracquadanio, M.; Dinelli, E.; Trombini, C. Role of volcanic dust in the atmospheric transport and deposition of polycyclic aromatic hydrocarbons and mercury. *J. Environ. Monit.* **2003**, *5*, 984. [CrossRef] [PubMed]
14. Alexandrov, K.; Rojas, M.; Geneste, O.; Castegnaro, M.; Camus, A.M.; Petruzzelli, S.; Giuntini, C.; Bartsch, H. An improved fluorometric assay for dosimetry of benzo(a)pyrene diol-epoxide-DNA adducts in smokers' lung: Comparisons with total bulky adducts and aryl hydrocarbon hydroxylase activity. *Cancer Res.* **1992**, *52*, 6248–6253. [PubMed]
15. Zaporozhchenko, I.A.; Morozkin, E.S.; Ponomaryova, A.A.; Rykova, E.Y.; Cherdyntseva, N.V.; Zheravin, A.A. Profiling of 179 miRNA Expression in Blood Plasma of Lung Cancer Patients and Cancer-Free Individuals. *Sci. Rep.* **2018**, *8*, 1–13. [CrossRef] [PubMed]
16. Kumar, S.; Sharawat, S.K.; Ali, A.; Gaur, V.; Malik, P.S.; Kumar, S.; Mohan, A.; Guleria, R. Identification of differentially expressed circulating serum microRNA for the diagnosis and prognosis of Indian non–small cell lung cancer patients. *Curr. Probl. Cancer* **2020**, 100540. [CrossRef]
17. Bianchi, F.; Nicassio, F.; Marzi, M.; Belloni, E.; Dall'Olio, V.; Bernard, L.; Pelosi, G.; Maisonneuve, P.; Veronesi, G.; Di Fiore, P.P. A serum circulating miRNA diagnostic test to identify asymptomatic high-risk individuals with early stage lung cancer. *Embo Mol. Med.* **2011**, *3*, 495–503. [CrossRef]
18. Boeri, M.; Verri, C.; Conte, D.; Roz, L.; Modena, P.; Facchinetti, F.; Calabrò, E.; Croce, C.M.; Pastorino, U.; Sozzi, G. MicroRNA signatures in tissues and plasma predict development and prognosis of computed tomography detected lung cancer. *Proc. Natl. Acad. Sci. USA* **2011**, *108*, 3713–3718. [CrossRef] [PubMed]
19. Hu, Z.; Chen, X.; Zhao, Y.; Tian, T.; Jin, G.; Shu, Y.; Chen, Y.; Xu, L.; Zen, K.; Zhang, C.; et al. Serum MicroRNA Signatures Identified in a Genome-Wide Serum MicroRNA Expression Profiling Predict Survival of Non–Small-Cell Lung Cancer. *J. Clin. Oncol.* **2010**, *28*, 1721–1726. [CrossRef]
20. Mao, M.; Wu, Z.; Chen, J. MicroRNA-187-5p suppresses cancer cell progression in non-small cell lung cancer (NSCLC) through down-regulation of CYP1B1. *Biochem. Biophys. Res. Commun.* **2016**, *478*, 649–655. [CrossRef] [PubMed]

21. Feng, Y.-Y.; Liu, C.-H.; Xue, Y.; Chen, Y.-Y.; Wang, Y.-L.; Wu, X.-Z. MicroRNA-147b promotes lung adenocarcinoma cell aggressiveness through negatively regulating microfibril-associated glycoprotein 4 (MFAP4) and affects prognosis of lung adenocarcinoma patients. *Gene* **2020**, *730*, 144316. [CrossRef] [PubMed]
22. Zhao, M.; Li, L.; Zhou, J.; Cui, X.; Tian, Q.; Jin, Y.; Zhu, Y. MiR-2861 Behaves as a Biomarker of Lung Cancer Stem Cells and Regulates the HDAC5-ERK System Genes. *Cell. Reprogram.* **2018**, *20*, 99–106. [CrossRef] [PubMed]
23. Asakura, K.; Kadota, T.; Matsuzaki, J.; Yoshida, Y.; Yamamoto, Y.; Nakagawa, K.A. miRNA-based diagnostic model predicts resectable lung cancer in humans with high accuracy. *Commun. Biol.* **2020**, *3*, 1–9. [CrossRef] [PubMed]

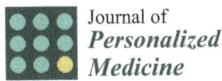

Review

Precision Medicine and Public Health: New Challenges for Effective and Sustainable Health

Deborah Traversi [1,*], Alessandra Pulliero [2], Alberto Izzotti [3,4], Elena Franchitti [1], Licia Iacoviello [5,6], Francesco Gianfagna [5,7], Alessandro Gialluisi [6], Benedetta Izzi [6], Antonella Agodi [8], Martina Barchitta [8], Giovanna Elisa Calabrò [9], Ilda Hoxhaj [9], Michele Sassano [9], Luca Gino Sbrogiò [10], Annamaria Del Sole [11], Francesco Marchiori [12], Erica Pitini [13], Giuseppe Migliara [13], Carolina Marzuillo [13], Corrado De Vito [13], Manuela Tamburro [14], Michela Lucia Sammarco [14], Giancarlo Ripabelli [14], Paolo Villari [13] and Stefania Boccia [9,15]

1. Department of Public Health and Pediatrics, University of Torino, Piazza Polonia 94, 10126 Torino, Italy; elena.franchitti@edu.unito.it
2. Department of Health Sciences School of Medicine, University of Genoa, 16132 Genova, Italy; alessandra.pulliero@unige.it
3. Department of Experimental Medicine, University of Genoa, 16132 Genova, Italy; Alberto.Izzotti@unige.it
4. IRCCS Ospedale Policlinico San Martino, 161632 Genova, Italy
5. Research Center in Epidemiology and Preventive Medicine (EPIMED), Department of Medicine and Surgery, University of Insubria, 21100 Varese, Italy; licia.iacoviello@uninsubria.it (L.I.); francesco.gianfagna@uninsubria.it (F.G.)
6. Department of Epidemiology and Prevention, IRCCS NEUROMED, 86077 Pozzilli, Italy; alessandro.gialluisi@moli-sani.org (A.G.); benedetta.izzi@moli-sani.org (B.I.)
7. Mediterranea Cardiocentro, 80122 Napoli, Italy
8. Department of Medical and Surgical Sciences and Advanced Technologies "GF Ingrassia", University of Catania, 95123 Catania, Italy; agodia@unict.it (A.A.); martina.barchitta@unict.it (M.B.)
9. Section of Hygiene, University Department of Life Sciences and Public Health, Università Cattolica del Sacro Cuore, 00168 Roma, Italy; alisacalabro@icloud.com (G.E.C.); ilda.hoxhaj1@unicatt.it (I.H.); michele.sassano@unicatt.it (M.S.); Stefania.Boccia@unicatt.it (S.B.)
10. Dipartimento di Prevenzione, Az. ULSS3 Serenissima, 30174 Venezia, Italy; LucaGino.Sbrogio@aulss3.veneto.it
11. Dipartimento di Prevenzione, SIAN, Az. ULSS5, 45100 Rovigo, Italy; annamaria.delsole@aulss5.veneto.it
12. Azienda Ospedaliera Universitaria Integrata di Verona, 37126 Verona, Italy; francesco.marchiori@aovr.veneto.it
13. Department of Public Health and Infectious Diseases, Sapienza University of Rome, 00185 Roma, Italy; erica.pitini@uniroma1.it (E.P.); giuseppe.migliara@uniroma1.it (G.M.); carolina.marzuillo@uniroma1.it (C.M.); corrado.devito@uniroma1.it (C.D.V.); paolo.villari@uniroma1.it (P.V.)
14. Department of Medicine and Health Sciences "Vincenzo Tiberio", University of Molise, 86100 Campobasso, Italy; manuela.tamburro@gmail.com (M.T.); sammarco@unimol.it (M.L.S.); ripab@unimol.it (G.R.)
15. Department of Woman and Child Health and Public Health-Public Health Area, Fondazione Policlinico Universitario A. Gemelli IRCCS, 00168 Roma, Italy
* Correspondence: deborah.traversi@unito.it; Tel.: +39-0116705703

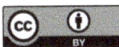

Abstract: The development of high-throughput omics technologies represents an unmissable opportunity for evidence-based prevention of adverse effects on human health. However, the applicability and access to multi-omics tests are limited. In Italy, this is due to the rapid increase of knowledge and the high levels of skill and economic investment initially necessary. The fields of human genetics and public health have highlighted the relevance of an implementation strategy at a national level in Italy, including integration in sanitary regulations and governance instruments. In this review, the emerging field of public health genomics is discussed, including the polygenic scores approach, epigenetic modulation, nutrigenomics, and microbiomes implications. Moreover, the Italian state of implementation is presented. The omics sciences have important implications for the prevention of both communicable and noncommunicable diseases, especially because they can be used to assess the health status during the whole course of life. An effective population health gain is possible if omics tools are implemented for each person after a preliminary assessment of effectiveness in the medium to long term.

Keywords: public health genomics; genetic polymorphisms; epigenetic modulations; miRNA; genetic and microbiome markers; health technology assessment; early disease prevention

1. Introduction

In recent years, statistical genetics and bioinformatics have made progress in the prediction of risk for different complex disorders, i.e., those diseases characterized by several genetic and environmental influences [1]. In particular, genomic markers have shown relatively high predictive power, and promising results are coming from other omics such as epigenomics, transcriptomics, proteomics, and metabolomics. The potentials for interactions among all these biomarkers and environmental data make us hopeful of finding cost-effective and clinically useful novel risk assessment tools for noncommunicable diseases [2].

Genetic susceptibility and environmental exposure alone are not sufficient to explain the pathogenesis of noncommunicable diseases, but should be integrated into a more complex scenario that can manifest pathological phenotypes. Epigenetics is a crucial component of this scenario, as its variations are linked to specific exposures that might be able to highlight the effects of the environment on the genome [3].

Scientific evidence has established that a healthy diet enhances life expectancy and helps prevent diseases. Although in the last few decades there has been huge growth in knowledge of the relationship between dietary components and diseases, the biological mechanisms underlying these effects are not yet well understood [4]. Nutritional epidemiology has contributed significantly to modern public health research and has promoted wellbeing and extended life expectancy. Specifically, researchers have investigated how the main social and behavioral determinants associated with the adherence to a healthy diet, such as the Mediterranean diet, could be useful in understanding and counteracting the global shift toward unhealthy patterns, to promote health and a better quality of life, especially in women of reproductive age [5,6].

Another emerging health determinant is microbiota status. The human microbiota consists of a complex ecosystem of microorganisms that live in the human body. Most of the microbial population is in the gut [7]. The ratio between the number of bacterial and human host genes is about 200:1, and such evidence can have profound effects on host phenotypes, playing critical roles in the host physiology [8]. The gut microbiota influences the evolution of adaptive phenotypic plasticity in mammalian species through the amplification of signals from the external environment, mainly during postnatal development. Therefore, such omics tools have become a crucial element in the risk stratification of the population for high-incidence diseases.

The increasing development of genetic tests has made the evaluation of their risks and benefits crucial to their appropriate translation into clinical practice, especially in the case of the COVID-19 pandemic [9]. The importance of a solid evaluation strategy for this kind of technology has been recognized across Europe and worldwide [10–12].

In this review, an overview of the public health implications is given, focusing on the Italian context. The building of health professionals' and citizens' omics sciences literacy is discussed, as well as the different regional departments' perspectives.

2. Development and Perspectives for Italian Public Health Genomic and Epigenomic Tools

2.1. Promising Perspectives from Clinical Genetics: The Use of Polygenic Scores and Epigenetic Markers

2.1.1. Genetics

In the last few decades, genome-wide association scans (GWAS) have been used to identify the genetic basis of chronic diseases, which revealed the influence of several common genetic variants on their risk. These conditions include but are not limited to cardiovascular disease (CVD) [13,14], cancer [15], and metabolic [16], neurodegenerative [17], and neuropsychiatric disorders [18]. However, despite the high heritability observed for these chronic diseases, the genetic variants identified explained a small proportion of the disease variability. While waiting for novel and larger-scale studies allowing for the analysis of rare variants and numerous gene-gene interactions with machine learning algorithms, many studies analyzed the potential clinical utility of the available variants in disease risk assessment.

Since these variants usually show a small effect size, they are generally condensed into polygenic scores (PGS), also known as polygenic risk scores, when dealing with diseases [19]. These are defined as quantitative factors aggregating the genetic influences of many common genetic variants on a single trait or disease. PGS has usually been computed as the sum of risk alleles that an individual has, weighted by the risk allele effect sizes, as estimated by an independent training GWAS on the phenotype (i.e., Beta or log (Odds Ratio), depending on the phenotype tested). Indeed, PGS represents an estimate of an individual's genetic liability to a trait/disease, calculated according to their genotype profile, using data from independent GWAS as a training model [20]. Thanks to this construction, some PGS have been shown to explain a relatively high amount of the variance in continuous traits [21], like height, with a PGS explaining ~24% of the population phenotypic variance [22]. On the other hand, the variance explained by genetic predisposition to specific disorders is not as high, ranging from <2% for stroke [23] to 7% for schizophrenia [24], although this has revealed interesting genetic overlaps among disorders [25].

As a consequence, the integrated use of PGS with other risk algorithms using environmental factors has been proposed to predict the risk of chronic conditions in common clinical practice [26]. Among the chronic diseases, CVD appears to be the condition with the largest set of data and with potentials for the implementation of a cost-effective PGS [27]. Currently, the clinical guidelines for CVD primary prevention do not recommend the use of genetic data for risk assessment, since all PGS found to have high predictive power failed to modify treatments in a cost-effective manner or to motivate subjects to change their lifestyles [28,29]. Although a significant net risk reclassification improvement of subjects who will develop a particular condition was observed in most large and recent studies [30,31], cost-benefit analyses should be performed to confirm their clinical utility for risk assessment. The number of subjects needed should be considered, along with the cost of biomarker measurements and the treatment of false-positive subjects [32]. The high laboratory costs and the relatively low added predictive power are currently the main barriers.

2.1.2. Epigenetics

Epigenetic biomarkers represent a means by which lifestyle and environment can be taken into account in the study of health and disease [33–35]. DNA methylation, among all epigenetic markers, is very stable and, in principle, can be studied with no special experimental requirements [36] in both fluid and tissue specimens already in use in clinical practice [37–41]. DNA methylation markers are robust, sensitive, and measurable across individuals as well as in population studies. Unfortunately, the progress from preclinical observations to clinical translation of epigenetic biomarkers for noncommunicable diseases is still far from complete [42]. However, there is an interest in finding epigenetic biomarkers, especially in those clinical conditions where a traditional diagnosis fails in the identification of specific cases or where early prediction of the disease leads to a better prognosis or drug response.

The field of oncology is so far the most developed in terms of epigenetic biomarkers. A recognized signature of most cancer types is genome-wide hypomethylation, a hallmark of genome instability, alongside gene-specific hypermethylation (i.e., the silencing of tumor suppressor genes) [43]. The latter clearly defines cancer's specificity and helps with differential diagnosis [44–49]. Among the few FDA-approved epigenetic tests, the screening of early colorectal cancer (CRC) is most frequently used in clinical practice, though it has lower specificity and higher costs than the traditional CRC screening tests [50,51].

Epigenetics is known to play a role in both neurodegenerative and neuropsychiatric diseases, as DNA methylation changes have been described in Alzheimer's disease [52], Parkinson's disease [53], amyotrophic lateral sclerosis [54], schizophrenia [55], major depressive disorder [56], and post-traumatic stress disorder [57]. Multiple studies have also shown the importance of epigenetics in the pathophysiology of type 2 diabetes (T2D) by studying the DNA methylation profiles in several relevant T2D target tissues [58–60], as well as using them for monitoring disease reversion after lifestyle intervention [61,62]. DNA methylation biomarkers in CVD are also far from being implemented into the clinical routine. A large number of epigenome-wide association studies have been performed, but with little reproducibility across cohorts. Despite this evidence, it is worth mentioning a few genes that have been found to have abnormal methylation patterns in association with both CVD and CVD risk factors, such as *GNAS* [63–67], *ZBTB12* [68,69], *BRCA1*, and *CRISP2* [70]. The discovery of these genes could pave the way for future studies along the same lines, possibly serving as good prediction biomarkers of CVD.

One important limitation on the use of epigenetic biomarkers in clinical practice is the tissue-specificity of the methylation patterns, so ideally the target tissue of the disease should be used. Despite this limitation, more and more studies are testing circulating blood as surrogate tissue for epigenetic analysis. Blood is a good source of DNA, obtained from noninvasive liquid biopsy, and is already used for epigenetic biomarker design in clinical practice for many human diseases [33,71]. DNA can be extracted from whole blood, peripheral blood mononuclear cells (PBMCs), single white blood cell (WBC) types, plasma (i.e., exosomes and free circulating-DNA and RNA), or platelets (mitochondrial). Recently, extracellular microRNAs (miRNAs) have been detected in biological fluids and studied as possible cancer markers that can be detected by noninvasive procedures [72].

Very recently, cell-free DNA (cfDNA) epigenetic research has been gaining more attention as a possible means to identify and predict tissue damage or the origin of certain pathological conditions [73]. CancerLOCATOR is a cfDNA-based method that allows for detection and predicts the tissue of origin using CpG methylation profiles [74]. Another study demonstrated that cfDNA methylation profiles were able to identify cardiomyocyte death [75], a possible useful marker of cardiac injury after myocardial infarction. Taken together, these findings suggest a possible use of these markers in clinical practice to predict and/or diagnose a clinical condition, thus better informing further disease prognosis.

Despite their usefulness, the sensitivity and reproducibility of liquid-biopsy-based methods using cfDNA still need to be improved, especially in those applications working with a very low amount of starting sample.

Beyond the lack of evidence of clinical utility for these scores, some issues remain in the field, like transethnic applicability [76] and ethical issues, mainly related to genetic data. However, the integrated use of PGS with other omics data in predicting clinical risk and the analysis of their interactions with environmental factors appears to be the road ahead for personalized medicine.

There is the need for large prospective population-based studies with a large amount of data collected with standardized methods, along with biological samples collected and stored in a biobank. In Italy, recently, the Moli-sani cohort study [77] (24,325 subjects aged 35–99 years, recruited between 2005 and 2010 from the general population) started to measure genomic and epigenomic data on biobank samples.

2.2. Susceptibility to Environmental Pollution, as Inferred from a miRNA Analysis

Environmental pollution is a growing public health burden associated with numerous adverse health effects. It is estimated that around 4.2 million deaths occur each year due to air pollution [78]. Biomarkers reflecting specific air pollution exposures have the potential to measure the internal dose resulting from exposure to complex environmental mixtures [79]. MiRNAs, small noncoding RNAs that regulate gene expression, have been studied as biomarkers in various diseases and have also shown potential as biomarkers of environmental exposure [80,81].

In this context, epigenetics bridges the gap between genetic makeup and environmental exposures to pollution, thus explaining the development of diseases [82].

The epigenome is a plastic entity modifiable by the environment, whose changes may be detected in accessible surrogate tissues (e.g., peripheral blood, urine, buccal cells, etc.). These epigenetic changes show long-term stability; accordingly, the epigenetic pattern may be considered a record of environmental exposures experienced throughout life [83].

The patterns of miRNA alterations are specifically related to the type of environmental pollution to which the organism has been exposed. In studies where smoking-induced changes were investigated, the general observation was a miRNA downregulation of expression, as initially demonstrated in mouse lungs [84] and thereafter confirmed in human bronchial epithelial cells [85]. MiRNA alterations accumulating during carcinogenesis is a prerequisite for full cancer appearance and progression [80,86,87]. MiRNAs are massively dysregulated during lung carcinogenesis, induced by cigarette smoke [84] but also other environmental airborne lung carcinogens and air pollutants [80]. These early alterations are reflected in the extracellular miRNA released from the lungs in the blood during the different stages of carcinogenesis, including the development of microadenoma, adenoma, and adenocarcinoma [88]. However, the transferability of these results to the human situation is quite controversial. Predictive miRNA signatures of lung cancer have been identified in the blood, but they greatly vary between different studies [88]. Many organs contribute to the miRNA burden in the blood, whereas the contribution of the lungs is negligible as compared to that of the muscles and liver. Indeed, miRNA plays a pathogenic role in cancer only when the target oncogene is mutated, and the extracellular release of miRNA corresponds to a cancer-related event and not to an adaptive response to carcinogen exposure. The shift from adaptation to pathogenic alterations of the miRNA machinery depends on the duration of the exposure to environmental pollution. Indeed, long-term exposure leads to irreversible epigenetic alterations [86].

Secondary prevention may be achieved in lung cancer by identifying high-risk individuals using a predictive epigenetic biomarker, such as miRNAs, as analyzed in body fluids. This personalized approach is referred to as "preventive theranostics" and represents an emerging application of personalized medicine to cancer prevention.

Researchers are currently publishing various miRNA signatures that respond to environmental exposure and have shown usefulness as biomarkers. The relative expression of miRNAs can be studied by various techniques, such as microarrays, used as an initial approach to finding the potential candidate miRNAs, or quantitative real-time PCR (qPCR), used to validate highly dysregulated miRNAs. Moreover, miRNAs can be sequenced and quantified using next-generation sequencing (NGS) platforms [89]. Due to their stability, miRNAs have been extensively studied in the peripheral blood and urine.

Future research should focus on (a) identifying the molecular mechanism underlying miRNA expression changes in response to environmental exposures; (b) to determine whether the changes in miRNA expression are an early signal of the pathogenic processes developing in the organism; (c) whether or not this miRNA signature may be used for early detection of cancer identifying high-risk subjects (secondary prevention); and (d) whether miRNA alterations are drivers or passengers in the ongoing carcinogenesis process.

The use of miRNA containing microvesicles is a hot topic in research on the early diagnosis and prognosis of cancer. Given their stability and abundance in blood serum, miRNAs containing micro-vesicles have been proposed as new diagnostic biomarkers for cancer [90]. Extracellular vesicles can transfer information from cell to cell, thus representing a potential mechanism explaining how different environmental exposures interact with the molecular machinery of our organism [91]. Extracellular vesicles play an important role in lung cancer pathogenesis and may have potential as biomarkers [92]. However, the use of extracellular microvesicles as an endpoint in cancer prevention has not yet been fully explored. The association between target-mediated function and miRNA regulation provides a new opportunity for developing novel anticancer preventive strategies, spanning from early diagnosis to the identification of high-risk subjects and prevention of cancer relapses.

2.3. Nutritional and Molecular Epidemiology for Precision Prevention and Health Promotion

The Human Genome Project and the increased use of the omics approach in nutrition science have led researchers to focus on personalized nutrition in order to improve the impact of diet on health status and wellbeing, taking into account individual genetic factors and epigenetic signatures [93]. Precision and personalized medicine are useful tools for preventive strategies and could help with predicting morbidity and mortality and detecting chronic disease much earlier in the disease course, to improve the quality of care and quality of life of the patients and reduced healthcare time, efforts, and costs [94]. It is well established that environmentally related diseases are the result of the "exposome"—the totality of exposure experienced by an individual during life and the health impact of those exposures [95]. Epigenetic phenomena can potentially be modified by environmental and lifestyle factors, including diet, and result in environmental reprogramming of the genome for exposed individuals and future generations of offspring [96]. For example, altered expression of miRNA profiles in maternal blood or placental tissue may reflect not only gestational disorders but also prenatal exposure to environmental pollutants and dietary factors [97]. The protective effect of diet and nutrients can be mediated by reversible epigenetic mechanisms, representing an attractive target for health promotion and the prevention of noncommunicable diseases. For instance, hypomethylation of long interspersed nuclear elements (LINE-1), a surrogate marker of global DNA methylation, has been associated with an increased risk of certain types of cancer, although conflicting findings have also been reported [98]. Blood-based methylation biomarkers, which are easier to obtain and adaptable to population screening for the identification of individuals with cancer or those who are at higher risk, are a new research area of great interest. In particular, LINE-1 methylation, together with other differentially methylated regions, has been proposed for the screening and noninvasive early diagnosis of women at risk of cervical cancer [99]. Interestingly, a dietary pattern characterized by low fruit consumption and folate deficiency has been associated with LINE-1 hypomethylation and thus with higher cancer risk [100]. Therefore, public health interventions to change the unhealthiest dietary patterns in favor of the healthiest options may reduce the risk of hypomethylation and, consequently, of cancer. Moreover, specific foods, nutrients, and healthy dietary habits, such as a Mediterranean-style diet and a diet based on the combined intake of nutrients with antioxidant properties, could help to prevent the progression of persistent high-risk human papillomavirus infection to cervical cancer [101,102]. However, other host factors, including genetic polymorphisms, which may explain some of the individual differences in disease occurrence, should be considered since they could be used to target specific and effective preventive strategies [103].

Although it is reasonable to expect that, in the future, disease prevention and treatment will be formulated at the individual level according to genomics features, at present, the major challenge for public health genomics is represented by the advance of the scientific evidence necessary to demonstrate if and when the use of genomic information in public health can improve health outcomes in a safe, effective, and cost-effective manner, also taking into account the ethical, legal, and social issues [104]. Further studies will examine epigenetic signatures as biomarkers to identify populations that may particularly benefit from incorporating health behavior changes into plans for precision medicine [105].

2.4. The Microbiome of Children: Development and Disease Implications, and Challenges for a Healthy Life

Human-microbiota co-evolution also follows an intergenerational transmission pattern [106]. The origin of the gut microbiota in each human is the placenta microbiome before birth, and its composition is then prominently conditioned by the delivery mode [107]. However, after a few months of life, such differences disappear, and other factors become conditioning. During the postnatal period, the environment changes quickly, so parental care is crucial as food transitions occur. A selection favoring host mechanisms is generated, including innate and adaptive immune mechanisms, to control the gut microbiota for the host's advantage [7].

From such a point of view, the gut microbiota is a selective agent shaping the adaptive evolution of the human diet, phenotypic plasticity, gastrointestinal morphology, and immunity. Therefore, as can be expected, microbiota aberrations (dysbiosis), since childhood, have been associated with a range of communicable [108–110] and noncommunicable diseases, including obesity and metabolic syndrome [111], diabetes [112,113], inflammatory bowel disease, nonalcoholic fatty liver disease [114], asthma, allergies [115], some types of cancer [116], and even certain neuropsychiatric disorders [117] (Table 1).

Table 1. Examples of microbiota modulation involved in disease pathways in children.

Disease	Age	No. of Participants	Study Design	Results	Biological Plausibility	Author, Year
Clostridium difficile infection (CDI)	11 months–23 years old	372 patients (31 were excluded because they had fewer than 60 days of follow-up, six because of refractory CDI)	Cohort study	Fecal Microbiota Transplantation (FMT) had a successful outcome in CDI pediatric patients: 81% had a successful outcome following a single FMT and 86.6% had a successful outcome following a first or repeated FMT; 4.7% had a severe adverse event during the three-month follow-up period, including 10 hospitalizations	There were four independent predictors of FMT success: - fresh donor stool (during a freeze-thaw cycle there may be alterations in the viability of critical taxa for the pediatric population) - delivered by colonoscopy (colonoscopy permits us to identify additional co-morbidities that often confound the diagnosis of CDI) - lack of a feeding tube, which usually is a risk factor - fewer episodes of CDI recurrence	[108]
H. pylori-induced gastritis	4–14 years old	154 (52 *H. pylori*-induced gastritis (HPG), 42 *H. pylori*-negative gastritis (HNG), 62 healthy control (HCG))	Case-control study	Changes in F:B ratio, an increase of *Bacteroidaceae* and *Enterobacteriaceae*, and a decrease of *Lachnospiraceae* and *Bifidobacteriaceae* can be caused by gastritis itself and exacerbated by *H. pylori* infection. These changes may be related to drug resistance and the development of chronic gastrointestinal diseases.	Most of the significant taxa belonged to the Gram-negative bacteria producing LPS. The LPS from the intestinal microbiome induces a chronic subclinical inflammatory process. The upregulation of pro-inflammatory cytokines and downregulation of anti-inflammatory cytokines may be a way to influence gastritis. *Lactobacillus* can change the pH of the intestinal environment to inhibit the growth of pathogenic bacteria and stimulate an immune response.	[109]

Table 1. Cont.

Disease	Age	No. of Participants	Study Design	Results	Biological Plausibility	Author, Year
Tuberculosis	<14 years old	36 (18 diagnosed or probably infected + 18 healthy controls)	Case-control study	Pulmonary TB patients presented an upregulation of *Prevotella*, *Enterococcus*, and a reduction of *Ruminococcaceae*, *Bifidobacteriaceae*, and *F. prausnitzii*.	*Prevotella* is a pro-inflammatory bacterium that may activate inflammatory reactions that aggravate TB. *Enterococcus* is a pathogen associated with intestinal permeability. The translocation of this bacteria into systemic circulation induces an immune-inflammatory reaction. *F. prausnitzii* is an SFCA producer and SCFAs regulate intestinal permeability. Alterations in *Bifidobacteriaceae* may be associated with a reduction in the immune response against the invasion of foreign microbes.	[110]
Recurrent respiratory tract Infections (RRTI)	Under five years old	49 (26 patients and 23 healthy controls)	Case-control study	ROC analysis: *Enterococcus* achieving AUC values of 0.860	Changes in the gut microbiome's constituents, with an increased incidence of opportunistic pathogens like *Enterococcus*, are linked to altered immune responses and homeostasis in the airways.	[118]
Intestinal ischemic injuries	<14 years old	14 patients + 9 healthy controls	Case-control study	Enterobacteriaceae's and *Veillonella dispar*'s increase and a reduction in *Akkermansia muciniphila* might be investigated as a target of intestinal injuries in neonates.	*Enterobacteriaceae* may be related to a pro-inflammatory response by the immature immune system, resulting in homeostasis disruption. *A. muciniphila* stimulates in mice the proliferation of Treg cells and is observed in patients with inflammatory bowel disease, suggesting it may have anti-inflammatory properties. Instead, *V. dispar* has pro-inflammatory effects.	[119]

Table 1. Cont.

Disease	Age	No. of Participants	Study Design	Results	Biological Plausibility	Author, Year
Nonalcoholic Fatty Liver Disease (NAFLD)	8–17 years old	124 (87 biopsy-proven NAFLD, 37 obese controls) N.B. NAFLD patients were more likely to be male	Case-control study	*Prevotella* was more abundant in children with NASH or obesity.	*P. copri* is the dominant *Prevotella* species. Data analysis showed that *P. copri* abundance was the best predictor of fibrosis severity. *P. copri* increases intestinal inflammation to its advantage. Such pro-inflammatory effects may exacerbate liver damage.	[114]
Obesity	111 children aged 6–11; 61 adolescents aged 12–18	172 (76 normal-weight and 96 obese individuals, of whom 46.88% were affected by metabolic syndrome)	Case-control study	Obese children had a higher relative abundance of *Firmicutes* and *Actinobacteria* and decreased *Bacteroidetes*.	*Coriobacteriaceae* family positively correlates with intrahepatic levels of triglycerides and non-HDL plasma concentrations, suggesting an effect on the gut barrier. *Prevotella* is associated with chronic inflammation. *Firmicutes* phylum: *Lactobacillus* is associated with weight gain.	[111]
Type 1 diabetes mellitus (T1D)	Under 18 years old	15 T1DM + 15 nonautoimmune diabetes + 13 healthy controls	Case-control study	Gut microbiota in T1D differs at the taxonomic and functional levels in comparison with healthy subjects and nonautoimmune diabetes patients. T1D was characterized by an increase in *Bacteroidete* and pro-inflammatory bacteria, and a decrease in *Faecalibacterium* and *Roseburia*.	The T1D gut microbiota profile was associated with a loss of epithelial integrity, low-grade inflammation, and autoimmune response, allowing luminal antigens to escape from the gut and promote islet-directed autoimmune responses. The gut microbiota from patients with T1D was significantly enriched with genes for antigen presentation, chemokine production, LPS biosynthesis, and bacterial invasion.	[112]

Table 1. Cont.

Disease	Age	No. of Participants	Study Design	Results	Biological Plausibility	Author, Year
	2 months–6 years old	44 children with a first-degree family history of T1D; 22 were exposed to oral insulin and 22 to a placebo.	Cohort study	There are differences in microbiome composition between children with susceptible and nonsusceptible *INS* genotypes, and after oral insulin treatment in children with the susceptible *INS* AA genotype.	There is an increased abundance of *Bacteroides dorei* in children with the susceptible *INS* AA genotype. There is an increased alpha diversity in children treated with oral insulin, who showed an antibody response compared with those without a response; this observation is consistent with a microbiome-mediated treatment effect.	[120]
	5–10 years old	40 T1D patients and 56 healthy children	Case-control study	Modulation of the T1D risk includes higher Firmicutes levels (OR 7.30; IC 2.26–23.54) and a greater amount of *Bifidobacterium* in the gut (OR 0.13; IC 0.05–0.34)	The origin of the disease process was suspected to be gut microbiota dysbiosis, associated with altered gut permeability and a major vulnerability of the immune system.	[113]
Juvenile idiopathic arthritis (JIA)	1–16 years old	39 JIA diagnosed patients + 42 healthy controls	Case-control study	The relative abundance of four genera, *Anaerostipes, Dialister, Lachnospira,* and *Roseburia,* decreased significantly in the JIA group. 12 genera were identified as potential biomarkers (AUC = 0.7975): *Bifidobacterium, Lachnospira, Dialister, Roseburia, Oscillospira, Akkermansia, Clostridium, Faecalibacterium, Bilophila, Coprococcus, Haemophilus, Anaerostipes.*	*Anaerostipes, Dialister, Lachnospira,* and *Roseburia* in JIA patients decreased, three of which are butyrate-producing microbes; *Dialister* is a propionate-producing microbe. SCFAs have considerable immunomodulatory effects (inducing the differentiation of regulatory T cells, enhancing IL-10 production, and suppressing Th17 cells; butyrate administration suppressed the expression of inflammatory cytokines).	[121]

Table 1. Cont.

Disease	Age	No. of Participants	Study Design	Results	Biological Plausibility	Author, Year
Asthma	2–12 months old	618 children for bacterial 16S rRNA 189 children for fungal ITS region	Case-control study	There is an inverse association of asthma with the measured level of fecal butyrate (OR = 0.28 (0.09–0.91), P = 0.034), bacterial taxa butyrate producers (*Roseburia* and *Coprococcus*, OR = 0.38 (0.17–0.84), P = 0.017) and the relative abundance of the gene encoding butyryl-coenzyme A (CoA): acetate–CoA-transferase, (OR = 0.43 (0.19–0.97), P = 0.042). Children who had grown up on farms had a lower risk of asthma compared to others (OR = 0.56).	Butyrate is the main source of energy for colonic epithelial cells; it contributes to the maintenance of the epithelial gut barrier and has immunomodulatory and anti-inflammatory properties.	[115]
Obstructive sleep apnea syndrome (OSAS)	2–12 years old	16 (divided between patients and healthy controls)	Case-control study	*Faecalibacterium* decrease in children with severe grades of OSAS.	*Faecalibacterium* is involved in the production of butyrate, which improves the gut barrier function, upregulating mucin-associated genes in gut goblet cells and the expression of the tight junction proteins.	[122]
Autism spectrum disease (ASD)	2–6 years old	16 ASD children + 7 controls	Case-control study	Gut microbiota decreased biodiversity: four of the 82 GO terms have a role in the catabolic process of the 3,3phenylpropionate mapped to the *E. coli* group.	3,3phenylpropionate is the conjugate base of 3-phenylpropionic acid deriving from PPA. PPA is an SCFA produced during the bacterial fermentation of carbohydrates. The elevated concentration of propionate metabolites could be due to their reduced degradation because of the *E. coli* drop.	[116]

Table 1. Cont.

Disease	Age	No. of Participants	Study Design	Results	Biological Plausibility	Author, Year
	3–7 years old	78 ASD children + 58 controls	Case-control study	Nine genera and the abundance of seven metallic elements are altered in ASD children. These were used in a diagnostic model in Chinese children with high accuracy (84%).	The diagnostic model is composted by bacterial genera (*Bacteroides*, *Parabacteroides*, *Sutterella*, *Lachnospira*, *Bacillus*, *Bilophila*, *Lactococcus*, *Lachnobacterium*, and *Oscillospira*) and metallic elements (Pb, As, Cu, Zn, Mg, Ca, and Hg). *Parabacteroides* and *Oscillospira* changes could be induced by heavy metal exposure.	[123]
	2–8 years old	43 ASD children (19 with GI symptoms and 24 without) + 31 controls	Case-control study	34 MEs (gut microbiota-associated epitopes) are a potential biomarker of ASD. Those alterations may contribute to abnormalities in gut immunity and/or homeostasis in ASD children.	29 of 34 MEs decreased and were associated with abnormal gut IgA levels and altered gut microbiota composition; 11 of 29 were pathogenic microorganisms' peptides with T or B cell response. ME with homology to a Listeriolysin O peptide from the pathogenic bacterium *Listeria monocytogenes* is increased.	[124]
Acute lymphoblastic leukemia (ALL)	2–25 years old	51 (23 matched patients and a healthy sibling and five unmatched patients)	Case-control study	It was possible to distinguish between the patient and control groups based on their microbiota profiles. *Lachnospiraceae* (which comprises the *Clostridium XIVa*) and *Roseburia* are butyrate-producing bacteria and were greatly reduced in acute leukemia patients compared to a healthy sibling; instead, *Bacteroides* increased.	Bacteria producing butyrate play a major role in the composition of the mucus layer, as butyrate is an important energy source for intestinal epithelial cells and plays a role in the maintenance of colonic homeostasis. Butyrate-producing bacteria may increase the risk of developing chemotherapy-induced mucositis and other GI complications. Antibiotic-induced shifts can increase the susceptibility to *C. difficile* infection.	[125]
Rhabdomyosarcoma	3–7 years old	3 oncologic patients + 2 healthy controls	Case-control study	After radiation exposure, there was an increase in α-diversity related to nonresponsive radiotherapy treatment, and a decrease in *Firmicutes*, associated with a *Proteobacteria* increase. This information could be used for the definition of the therapy.	The decrease of *Firmicutes* could explain the variation in α-diversity and the ability to survive of the *Proteobacteria* phylum and might be related to DNA mutations.	[117]

The developmental origins of health and disease provide a theory by which to understand the pathogenic pathways that explain early-stage environmental factors such as human gut microbiome modulation [126]. Exposure, during the highly plastic period of early life, can determine later disease risk. The first three years of life are fundamental for microbiota development.

The intra-individual (α-diversity) and functional complexity increases with age, while the interindividual variations (β-diversity) become less marked. The ratio among the principal observed microorganisms' families changes with a reduction in the *Enterobacteriaceae* and an increase in the *Bacteriodaceae*. This shift is due to different feeding practices after weaning. The degradation of complex fibers and carbohydrates improves the role of the microbiota in the host metabolism.

The exposure profiles and the gut microbiota change during such a period may then lead to health and disease predisposition in adulthood and can influence aging. Even if a real interconnection and predictive role of the microbiota modulation is not yet clear for most diseases, the clarification of such processes is the key to achieving health improvement for future generations.

From an immunological point of view, various hypothetical models clarify the interconnections of microbiota with the host and the increased prevalence of the disease with an immunological etiology. For example, for type 1 diabetes, five models have been proposed [127], among which there are models with a similar biological plausibility that include the early microbiota development.

From a preventive medicine point of view, knowledge regarding the eubiosis—an equilibrium status that can guarantee the integrity of the gut mucosa—and dysbiosis transitions of the gut microbiota is crucial. The focus could be the identification of validated biomarkers able to describe such a transition. In particular, we need to know about the growth of microorganisms that promote inflammation and the decrease of other groups that can promote host monocytes' collaboration in human homeostasis.

The microbiological methodology seems to privilege a global approach to the complexity of the microbiota, but, on the other hand, a simpler approach based on valid biomarker identification is useful for risk stratification in public health.

The chronic inflammation described in older people is characterized by a reduction in microorganisms such as *Bifidobacterium*, *Akkermansia*, and *Christensenellaceae*.

A recurrent question for diseases associated with dysbiosis status is whether the dysbiosis is a determinant, a risk factor, or a consequence of the disease. Nowadays, the evidence seems to suggest very early modification of the microbiota in disease, so its preventive role as, at least, an early detection opportunity before clinical onset, is fundamental for better clinical management and prognosis.

Dysbiosis not only has an effect on the gut but also on distant organs. Microbial metabolites, such as the induction pathway typical of pathogens and to produce pro-inflammatory cytokines, can reach several organs, also inducing neurodegenerative diseases and cancer. Therefore, even when the identification of the point break between eubiosis and dysbiosis has been identified, how should an intervention proceed?

Different methods have been suggested. The only cost-effective method for the treatment of recurrent vancomycin-resistant *C. difficile* infection is fecal microbiota transplantation. However, such therapeutic intervention—validated from an economical point of view for elderly patients—is not yet common in children because it seems to be associated with a high incidence of adverse effects, including severe adverse effects known in adults (>8%) [128].

Another method consists of the development of a target therapy: for example, using selective antibiotics or phages with the purpose of decreasing the bacteria involved in the pathogenic processes. However, such therapies are uncertain both in terms of the unclear definition of the microbial target and the possible adverse effects [129].

The most common intervention is the intake of a beneficial microorganism probiotic and/or prebiotic, but a wider discussion of the evidence of the beneficial effects is ongoing [8]. The main limitations are a lack of evidence of beneficial effects and a failure to take into account individuals' peculiarities. The microorganisms most commonly used in the probiotics industry belong to the *Lactobacillus* and *Bifidobacterium* genera. In this field, personal beliefs, intuition, and commercial interests, coupled with a lack of sufficient medical regulation, often combine to make objective interpretation difficult [129]. On the other hand, drug-microbiome interactions vary between individuals, demonstrating how the gut microbiome has to be included in drug development and personalized medicine [130].

The most acceptable intervention consists of a variation in nutritional behavior, which can shift the microbiota characteristics and lead to an improvement in the balance of the gut microbiota by increasing health-favoring bacteria. A valuable effect is observable in the medium and long term, but only for as long as the subject maintains the healthy diet [8].

Most of the studies on children today are case-control studies and highlight a significant involvement of the microbiota in the risk modulation for various diseases. In general, a decrease in the level of some microorganisms is a recurrent risk factor—for example, *Bifidobacteriaceae*, *Faecalibacterium* spp., *Ruminococcaceae*, *Dialister*, *Roseburia*, and *Akkermansia*. On the other hand, an increase of *Prevotella* and *Enterococcus* leads to greater risk (Table 1).

The integration of analytic methods, which are not yet standardized for whole-genome sequencing, can provide a more accurate overview of the gut microbiota status.

The corrections possible today mainly include nutritional and behavioral improvement. Gut microbiota research indicates an enormous avoidable burden of disease, considering years of life lost (or healthy years of life for diseases that originate during childhood), but, today, a consolidation of the evidence is needed as a cost-efficacy evaluation. Moreover, a cohort study with long observation during childhood can elucidate the real contribution of microbiota variation.

2.5. A Precision Medicine Approach in COVID-19 Patients: Which Markers Should Be Used for Prognosis?

Precision medicine, also known as personalized or stratified medicine, is an emerging paradigm in disease diagnosis, prevention, and treatment [131,132], aiming at targeted treatments tailored to patient characteristics, which include not only biomarkers, but also individual, social, and economic factors [133]. This represents a novel strategy to rapidly identify, in a noninvasive way, an altered biology and to discern the pathways in individuals suffering from a disease, thereby guiding the most appropriate therapy [134,135]. The approach has as its cornerstone the recent advances in omics sciences, molecular biology, and bioinformatics that support the evaluation and treatment of disorders, focusing on four main principles: prediction—anticipating the disease occurrence based on risk factors, lifestyles, and social determinants; prevention—delaying the disease's evolution before the initial manifestations and once it has settled; personalization—adapting the best therapeutic strategy by analyzing genetic, molecular, and individual factors; and participation—involving biomedical research, academic institutions, health professionals, and the patient [131].

In a multisystemic disease process such as an infection, blood (serum and plasma) analysis provides early detection to characterize the damage, with the use of molecular technologies revealing specific biomarkers associated with certain phenotypes/trait groups, leading to therapeutic changes in patients with diverse clinical presentations [134]. Indeed, personalized medicine encompasses the study of disease pathophysiology and the discovery of mechanisms and gene variants [136,137]. Through big data analysis, personalized medicine is effective at recognizing risk factors and biomarkers, and so is valuable for predicting health outcomes and choosing the best treatment and prevention strategies for a particular patient. Novel therapeutic strategies can be addressed by taking into account genetic information (e.g., underlying genes or variants rather than symptoms) in an integrated system [138]. The study of the pathophysiological mechanisms (endotypes) and clinical disease expression (phenotypes) promotes an approach tailored to the characteristics and needs of a patient, with their active participation in the decision-making [136].

Therefore, models of personalized medicine require large genomic databases, a changed methodology involving clinicians, scientists, patients, and the general population, and collective participation [137]. The principles of personalized medicine have been already applied in the so-called fields of vaccinomics and adversomics to help us understand interindividual variations in vaccine-induced immune responses and vaccine-related adverse side effects [139], providing models for profiling the innate, humoral, and cellular immune responses—integrated at a systems biology level to discover vaccine response biomarkers and obtain a directed approach for vaccine development [140]. This knowledge could significantly improve comprehension for individuals who are at risk of such infections, and help determine the type or dose of vaccine needed [135].

Since the beginning of 2020, the spread of the severe acute respiratory syndrome coronavirus-2 (SARS-CoV-2) has rapidly led to serious challenges for hospital care [141], and coronavirus disease 2019 (COVID-19) has become an emergent epidemiological threat globally, especially for highly vulnerable population groups [142,143]. The SARS-CoV-2 pandemic has severely affected the world population and global healthcare structures, with first aid and intensive care (ICUs) wards under a degree of pressure never experienced before. Consequently, most of the infrastructural and professional resources have been used to counter this unprecedented emergency. At the same time, traditional screening, outpatient, and surgical activities have slowed down and, in some cases, been completely suspended. The combination of these unfavorable conditions has led to a profound crisis in the traditional model of diagnosis and treatment. In Italy, as in other European nations, the number of cases and deaths dramatically increased starting in March 2020 [144]. On 13 December 2020, more than 1,800,000 confirmed cases have been reported in Italy, with over 60,000 deaths, representing one of the highest mortality rates from the initial diffusion [145,146].

Despite the majority of individuals with COVID-19 exhibiting only mild symptoms or even being asymptomatic, there are patients who develop serious complications, underlining the fact that it is crucial to identify who is at higher risk of a worse prognosis and to recognize reliable outcome predictors in a timely manner for improving patient management. As a result, the personalized medicine approach appears to be highly appropriate for the study of COVID-19, considering the wide spectrum of severity and variable phenotypes [147], including asymptomatic, mildly symptomatic, severe symptomatic requiring hospitalization, and respiratory failure due to acute respiratory distress syndrome (ARDS) [148]. Omics-scale studies on SARS-CoV-2 are quickly emerging and have a huge potential to resolve the infection pathophysiology [149], highlighting biologic pathways, modifiable risk factors, and critical information to allow early interventions [150,151]. Hence, comprehension of the underlying mechanisms can be a pivotal step for an individualized therapy [9]. The application of personalized medicine based on the integrated information of the genetic background of COVID-19 patients, individual factors, and clinical data is acquiring great relevance, enabling the detection of predictive biomarkers and paths that are valuable to select specific and effective measures for both prevention and management [132,150,152].

There is growing evidence that COVID-19 occurs more in males [153,154], the elderly, and non-O blood type individuals [155,156]. The inflammatory responses and cytokine storm induced by SARS-CoV-2 are extremely variable [157], and prognosis is conditioned by the host response more than by the infection, since pre-existing comorbidities such as obesity, cardiovascular diseases, arterial hypertension, type 2 diabetes mellitus, and immunosuppression strongly contribute to fatal outcomes [158–162].

To date, research focused on the analysis of single-nucleotide polymorphisms (SNPs) of the angiotensin-converting enzyme 2 (ACE2), a receptor of SARS-CoV-2, revealed that morbidity, clinical course, and mortality depend on ACE D allele frequency [163]. Another study investigated the involvement of genetic factors associated with SARS-CoV-2 infection, particularly ACE-related genes [164], showing a negative correlation with the number of cases and number of deaths due to viral infection, since both decreased with an increasing

ACE1 II genotype frequency; thus, ACE1 polymorphisms could be useful markers for the prediction of high-risk groups and COVID-19 severity. Moreover, investigating 12,343 SARS-CoV-2 genome sequences from patients in six geographic areas, 1234 mutations were found compared with the SARS-CoV-2 reference sequence, and the frequency of several human leukocyte antigen (HLA) alleles was significantly associated with the fatality rate [165]. In particular, through a hierarchical clustering analysis, 28 countries were grouped into three clusters, with Italy in cluster 2, whose average fatality rate was higher than that of countries in clusters 1 and 3. A genome-wide association study on COVID-19 and a severe disease pattern, defined as respiratory failure, which included seven hospitals in Italy and Spain, found an association signal at the ABO blood type locus, and a specific gene cluster as a genetic susceptibility locus in patients with respiratory failure [166]. Indeed, an analysis showed a higher risk in blood type A than in others (Odds Ratio, OR = 1.45), and a protective effect in blood type O as compared with the other groups (OR = 0.65). So far, the relationship between the ABO blood type and SARS-CoV-2 infection has been supported by other studies [167,168] as being valuable for predicting individual risk, with it being reported that the A blood type may be linked to increased infection susceptibility, in contrast to the O blood type's protective effect. The ABO blood types have also been associated with different COVID-19 severity patterns, because patients with blood type A or AB were at increased risk for hospitalization, mechanical ventilation, renal replacement therapy, and prolonged ICU admission compared with those with O or B blood types [169,170]. These findings were previously reported for SARS, and likely explained by the presence of IgG anti-A isoagglutinins in subjects with O blood type, preventing the binding of SARS-CoV-2 to its receptor and the virus's entry into human cells [171]. Consequently, differences in blood type antigen expression could increase or decrease host susceptibility to many infections, modifying the innate immune response and playing a direct role by serving as receptors and/or coreceptors for microorganisms' antigens [172].

In a study, RNA-Seq and high-resolution mass spectrometry on 128 blood samples from COVID-19 positive patients with diverse severity profiles and negative individuals were used to quantify transcripts, proteins, metabolites, and lipids in a relational database, enabling analysis and correlations between molecules and patient prognoses. A total of 219 molecular features were mapped with high significance for severity, mainly involved into complement activation, dysregulated lipid transport, and neutrophil activation [173].

As COVID-19 is characterized by a variable course, with asymptomatic individuals and others experiencing fever, ARDS, or even death, understanding of the antibody response in subjects with severe compared to mild disease is needed. A high-throughput method was used to analyze epitopes of antiviral antibodies in human sera of 232 COVID-19 patients and 190 controls. Results highlighted epitopes ranging from "private", recognized by antibodies in only a small number of subjects, to "public", recognized by antibodies in many individuals, and those with severe COVID-19 exhibited stronger and broader SARS-CoV-2 responses, as well as weaker antibody responses to prior infections [174].

In conclusion, considering the rapid evolution of the current epidemiological situation and the need to ensure adequate continuity of care and contain transmission, precision medicine is the key to fighting the COVID-19 pandemic by creating patient-specific treatment programs tailored to individual needs. This novel approach, implying the integration of clinical, lifestyle, genetic, and biomarker information for patient stratification, could enable us to achieve a better understanding of critical disease pathways and more precise and validated phenotypic recognition. Multi-omics systems could provide critical information to better understand SARS-CoV-2 and COVID-19 features, defining the individual genetic predisposition for both infection and course severity. For example, epigenomic and transcriptomic analyses would allow us to characterize changes in tissues involved in COVID-19, and to understand the interaction between SARS-CoV-2 and patient cells as a reaction to viral infection. Data integration would finally enable the identification of biomarkers and therapeutic targets to stratify patients and allow better interventions and decisions. Hence, an understanding of pathogenic pathways and the classification of phenotypes in SARS-CoV-2-infected patients might significantly contribute to the design of effective prevention strategies, mitigation interventions, and personalized pharmacological options in order to guide public health actions and improve the chances of better outcomes.

2.6. Health Technology Assessment for Public Health Evaluation of Genetic/Genomic Applications on Genetic Tests

The existing evaluation frameworks for genetic tests, and genetic/genomic applications in general, mainly rely on two popular evaluation approaches, i.e., the ACCE model (analytical and clinical validity, clinical utility, ethical, legal, and social implications) and the Health Technology Assessment (HTA) process [175]. The U.S. Centers for Disease Control and Prevention created the ACCE model in the early 2000s, specifically for the evaluation of genetic tests [176]. Its name refers to the evaluation dimensions used, i.e., analytic validity (a test's ability to accurately and reliably measure the genotype of interest), clinical validity (a test's ability to detect or predict the associated disorder), clinical utility (the risks and benefits associated with a test's introduction into practice), and ethical, legal, and social implications (ELSI—regarding the safeguards and impediments surrounding the testing process) [177]. Furthermore, the ACCE model includes under the umbrella of clinical utility some contextual issues related to testing delivery, such as economic benefits and organizational aspects. However, the strength of this model lies in considering specific aspects of genetic tests not adequately addressed by standard methods for a technology assessment, particularly analytic validity and clinical validity. For this reason, the ACCE model has been adopted, often with some adaptations, by various entities both in the United States and worldwide [175].

Unlike the ACCE model, the HTA approach was developed to cover all health technologies. However, since its creation in the USA in the late 1960s, some attempts have been made to adjust it for the evaluation of genetic tests. A notable example is a framework proposed to guide the public coverage of new predictive genetic tests in Ontario, Canada, which proposed the following criteria to assess a genetic test: intended purpose, effectiveness, additional effects, aggregate costs, demand, and cost-effectiveness [175,178]. The main innovation of these HTA-based frameworks is the attempt to adopt a service delivery approach, i.e., extending the scope of the assessment beyond the technical and clinical performance of a test to consider the economic and organizational implications of the whole testing service [179]. This approach is necessary to support decision-makers in securing an efficient and equitable allocation of health care resources and services. Nevertheless, HTA evaluations of genetic tests have not yet reached the comprehensiveness typical of general HTA frameworks in the analysis of delivery models.

Based on these findings, a combination of the ACCE model, with its focus on the unique aspects characterizing the genetic tests, and the HTA process, useful to guide provision and coverage decisions, might represent the best approach to the evaluation of genetic tests. Recently, Sapienza University of Rome tried to realize such an integrated approach and proposed a framework distinguished by a dual focus on both the genetic test and its delivery models [180]. The first section of this new framework addresses the genetic test from a technical and clinical perspective, mostly adopting the ACCE evaluation dimensions (analytic validity, clinical validity, and clinical utility), with the addition of personal utility, a dimension that broadly encompasses the nonclinical outcomes the test may have for patients [181]. The second section addresses the analysis of delivery models, defined as the broad context in which genetic tests are offered to individuals and families with or at risk of genetic disorders [182]. The evaluation dimensions proposed in this section, mostly based on the EUnetHTA HTA core model, are organizational aspects, economic evaluation, ELSI, and, in response to the increasing international interest in patient-centered care, patient perspective [183,184].

Overall, despite the efforts made, several issues still affect the evaluation of genetic/genomic applications. The first one, mainly related to the delivery model approach, is the generalizability of findings, given the context-dependence of economic and organizational issues. Another challenge is the lack of scientific evidence to use for evaluation, especially translation studies [185]. Finally, even if evidence collection represents the core of any technological assessment, a comprehensive process should also include priority setting, as the resources available for evaluation are inadequate to address the increasing development of new genetic tests, and appraisal, as the evidence collected needs to be summarized in final recommendations to inform decisions.

2.7. Fostering the Implementation of Personalized Healthcare by Developing Health Professionals' and Citizens' Omics Science Literacy

Omics sciences can be considered as disruptive innovations that promise a new era of precision health (PH). To fully harness such potential, we envisage some key prerequisites linked to the system' capacity building: (i) health professionals should be enabled to manage the omics knowledge and applications, and (ii) citizens need to gain sufficient health literacy to understand the potential benefits, limits, and risks of omics technologies concerning their health [186].

While several European countries have implemented specific health policies in this field, few countries have integrated public health genomics into the health system offerings [187], e.g., Italy, which since 2010 has included PH as a dedicated pillar in the National Prevention Plans (NPPs) and published in 2013 the first Guidelines on Genomics in Public Health [104]. More recently, the Italian National Innovation Plan of the Healthcare System, based on omics sciences [188], identified educational efforts geared towards professionals, citizens, and decision-makers as a cornerstone for the relevant implementation of omics sciences in healthcare.

Successful personalized healthcare will only be achieved; however, if all stakeholders develop the required awareness of PH, and this can be achieved by improving health professionals' capacity building and citizens' literacy.

The integration of the omics innovation into health system policy and practice requires highly engaged and appropriately trained health professionals [186]. A lack of adequate skills or appropriate attitudes among health professionals might be a barrier to the effective implementation of personalized healthcare. Policymakers and public health experts have emphasized the need for a defined set of core competencies and the inclusion of omics concepts into health professionals' curricula [189]. Several EU countries developed national policies to enhance the preparedness of health professionals and enable the use of omics knowledge for the prevention, diagnosis, and treatment of diseases [190].

In Italy, several initiatives were implemented with the aim of achieving better genomics literacy for both health professionals and the general public. Such educational efforts are in line with the goals of the Italian National Innovation Plan of the Healthcare System, based on omics sciences and published in 2017 [188]. Since 2011, in the context of two different projects funded by the Italian Ministry of Health (MoH), two effective distance training courses on genetics and genomics have been released for physicians [191,192]. Other initiatives in this field are currently underway in Italy, directed at a larger audience of healthcare professionals including biologists, pharmacists, and other professional categories (https://www.eduiss.it/) [193].

With the rapid advances in omics technologies, the demand for well-trained healthcare professionals will grow exponentially, and omics education will need to evolve to keep up with the changing scientific landscape. Therefore, for effective and successful implementation of PH, improving health professionals' literacy will need to be a priority, along with suitable common principles, appropriate policies, and regulatory frameworks.

Among the great challenges that should be addressed to allow for the correct implementation and integration of omics sciences into healthcare practice, citizens' engagement and literacy will play a key role [186]. Citizens are expected to adopt new behaviors in this novel healthcare era, including being involved in shaping and developing personalized healthcare, contributing to research, and being engaged in citizen health projects [194].

A striking example of the potential impact of omics technologies on citizens' health and healthcare systems is direct-to-consumer genetic tests (DTC-GTs). The increasing demand for DTC-GTs among laypeople, together with their peculiar provisional model—i.e., not requiring counseling by health professionals—need not only a careful analysis of the potential benefits and risks by policy-makers [195], but also informed citizens who can be aware of them and, consequently, make appropriate decisions about their health [192]. For these reasons, citizens' literacy in omics sciences, which is poor according to the literature [196], should be increased using appropriate and effective initiatives and strategies. This is what has emerged from a recently published systematic review of the literature [196]. The study summarizes the current knowledge of citizens' literacy, attitudes, and educational needs in omics sciences, underlining the need for strengthening public engagement on this topic. In the Italian context, this has been addressed by authorities through several policy documents [104,188] and different projects funded by the MoH. In fact, as part of one of these projects, a survey conducted in collaboration with a citizens' organization is currently underway, aimed at assessing the real knowledge of Italian citizens about the main issues related to genomics in health.

This further underlines the importance of citizen engagement and literacy in this field, which would allow them to adopt a more active role in the protection of their own health and in shaping more effective strategies for the implementation of personalized healthcare [186].

Several strategic actions will need to be taken to allow for the easy integration of omics knowledge and technologies into healthcare [186].

We could envisage among the main actions:

- developing awareness among stakeholders;
- improving citizens' health literacy to fully empower them;
- fostering health professionals' skills acquisition through extensive educational initiatives in omics sciences;
- shaping sustainable healthcare through the use of evidence-based tools such as a Health Technology Assessment for the omics technologies' evaluation to introduce in healthcare systems.

2.8. The Point of View of the Territorial Department of Prevention and the Community Health District

The Departments of Prevention (DP) are parts of the Local Units of the Italian National Health Service, which oversee public health activities. Their main duties are health promotion, disease prevention, livestock and pet health, and food safety. They promote public well-being by promoting healthy behaviors, preventing infectious and chronic diseases, and improving work safety. They are involved in the strategic planning and evaluation of preventive programs as essential ways to achieve health-related goals. The Direction of the DP guarantees comprehensive governance and integration among the different activity areas and is expected to coordinate and organize public health initiatives [197].

The National Prevention Plan (NPP) it subdivided into regional and local prevention plans, which play a key role in the governance of public health programs. There are some characteristics that public health programs have in common: they

1. are addressed to healthy people in large numbers;
2. represent "proactive" medicine;
3. provide cost-effective and evidence-based technologies;
4. deliver free or co-payment health care services;
5. consider individual as well as community health gain; and
6. are provided in all regions of Italy, as they are mandatory.

These programs are implemented in the following fields:

1. cancer screenings
2. vaccination campaigns
3. risk communication, counseling, health literacy, and empowerment of the target population

4. epidemiological evaluation of the health efficacy in the target population
5. health surveillance activity
6. infectious disease (nowadays, especially COVID-19)

In general, a public health intervention:

- must be efficacy- and value-based;
- needs dedicated resources (personnel, places, technology, software, etc.);
- needs a structured plan from prevention to treatment;
- must avoid inequalities; and
- requires people's advocacy and involvement.

The same fundamental principles can also be applied to the field of "predictive medicine", which, in the public health sector, can be implemented by the DP [198]. Predictive medicine should become an integral part of the duties of the DP, as they have the appropriate methodology, experience, attitudes, and trained personnel. The findings of the basic research should be translated into public health programs. Practical written evidence-based guidelines are essential, as well as an evaluation frame to assess the impact on the population.

The integration of genomics into public health should achieve these results:

- generating more specific and cost-effective public prevention programs;
- enhancing the impact of prevention and risk-reduction campaigns;
- favoring the exchange of information between various branches of the public health sector; and
- maintaining the importance of a central public health author even if the trend is toward personalized medicine.

The NPP 2010–2012 underlined the importance of predictive medicine and its huge potential to identify a population of healthy individuals who are at risk of developing specific diseases [199]. This could provide effective interventions that are specific and personalized. This is in line with the new NPP 2020-2025, which aims to consolidate the focus on the single individual [200]. This can be achieved by targeted interventions to improve health literacy, enhancing the empowerment of individuals to trust and communicate with the public health sector (engagement). The new NPP also claims that, for nontransmissible chronic diseases, it is necessary to combine and integrate a community-based strategy (such as by promoting healthy lifestyles) and personalized strategies (by identifying people at risk or in the early stages of disease).

Therefore, it is necessary to enhance the understanding of predictive medicine and how it can be developed by the DP. Discussion and implementation have just started. To date, predictive medicine has only found a few applications in Italy. Genomic predictive tests are used in public health settings only to investigate monogenic disorders. These include screening for high-penetrance mutations such as breast, ovarian, and colorectal cancer. Genetic screening for complex diseases has been applied to a very limited number of conditions. For example, the NPP 2014-2018, based on the public health genomics approach, aimed to develop organized paths of breast cancer prevention in women with BRCA1/2 mutations [201]. This screening is complementary to the ongoing cancer screening program.

On the other hand, large-scale prevention programs that target large population groups (such as vaccination campaigns, cancer screenings, and cardiovascular disease progression monitoring) are already part of the system and have been used for several years. They can constitute essential background to the introduction of predictive medicine in routine activities of DP [202].

There are many reasons to think that the role of the DP could be central and appropriate:

- consolidated and experienced activity of screening;
- an existing network with clinical disciplines;
- experience of risk communication and counseling;
- experience of follow-up management;
- an appropriate attitude toward the analysis and evaluation of prevention activities;

- appropriate software in use.

In conclusion, predictive medicine in the context of cancer screening is already feasible, but it would require an adaptive process to enhance the knowledge and practical organization. DP healthcare workers will have to increase their specific competences. However, these are often already used in daily activities like screening and health promotion, but should be updated with genomics knowledge. On the other hand, vaccine activities may also profit from genomic screening by taking advantage of the stratification of populations and the identification of nonresponders based on their genetic profile. Additionally, the recent COVID-19 epidemic might open up new uses for predictive medicine to identify individuals at high risk of developing a severe condition.

The "Plan for innovations in the health system based on omics sciences" (published in 2018) defined ways to improve the health system through the application of omics science [203]. This innovation regards prevention, diagnosis, and care based on efficacy and value for the improvement of individual health. The DP has the tendency to lead to changes in the practical organization of all the units of the Italian NHS involved, helping to define policies for the best use of genomics and omics sciences [204].

3. Conclusions

The omics sciences offer a wide range of tools to improve public health: from a single polymorphism detection to the PGS approach, and including whole-genome and exosome sequencing. The interaction between a gene and the environment can be defined by the epigenetic end-point and also by the evaluation of the microbiome shift from eubiosis to dysbiosis, highlighting several prevention opportunities, especially for the early detection of diseases or at-risk conditions. However, the introduction and accessibility of such tools are not yet guaranteed in Italy and they are provided by private bodies, individuals, and sporadic ventures.

In the future, disease prevention and treatment should be formulated at the individual level according to genomic features. However, a current major challenge is a lack or scarcity of scientific evidence, as well as a lack of ethical, legal, and social regulations.

The implementation of omics advancements into clinical practice depends on countries' ability to adopt relevant strategies and innovative approaches. The production, integration, and use of genetic/genomic information in healthcare require significant changes in the way such care is organized and provided to individuals. This is also evident in relation to the COVID-19 pandemic. Therefore, new health policies and specific programs on the omics sciences will be needed to respond to the needs of citizens and all health stakeholders.

Author Contributions: Conceptualization, Section 1, Section 3 and abstract: A.P. and D.T.; Writing of specific sections: Section 2.1—F.G., A.G., B.I. and L.I.; Section 2.2—A.P. and A.I.; Section 2.3—A.A. and M.B.; Section 2.4—E.F. and D.T.; Section 2.5— M.T., M.L.S., and G.R.; Section 2.6—E.P., G.M., C.M., C.D.V., and P.V.; Section 2.7—G.E.C., I.H., M.S., and S.B.; Section 2.8—L.G.S., A.D.S., and F.M.; Writing—review: all authors; Editing: E.F. and D.T.; Coordination assembly and homogenization DT; Supervision: S.B. and P.V. All authors have read and agreed to the published version of the manuscript.

Funding: The APC was funded by SItI Società Italiana di Igiene Medicina Preventiva e Sanità Pubblica. The authors of Section 2.1 have received funding from the European Union's Horizon 2020 research and innovation programme under grant agreement No 798841 and from the Italian Ministry of Health 2018 (Young Investigator grant number: GR-2018-12366528) (BI), moreover they were supported by Fondazione Umberto Veronesi (GA).

Acknowledgments: A special thanks to the SItI Società Italiana di Igiene Medicina Preventiva e Sanità Pubblica and to the numerous specialists who are working daily in Italy for the introduction and accessibility of omics tools for preventive strategies.

Conflicts of Interest: The authors declare no conflict of interest.

References

1. Gwinn, M.; MacCannell, D.R.; Khabbaz, R.F. Integrating Advanced Molecular Technologies into Public Health. *J. Clin. Microbiol.* **2017**, *55*, 703–714. [CrossRef]
2. Williamson, D.A.; Kirk, M.D.; Sintchenko, V.; Howden, B.P. The importance of public health genomics for ensuring health security for Australia. *Med. J. Aust.* **2019**, *210*, 295–297.e1. [CrossRef] [PubMed]
3. Ladd-Acosta, C.; Fallin, M.D. The role of epigenetics in genetic and environmental epidemiology. *Epigenomics* **2016**, *8*, 271–283. [CrossRef]
4. Zhang, Y.; Kutateladze, T.G. Diet and the epigenome. *Nat. Commun.* **2018**, *9*, 9–11. [CrossRef]
5. Maugeri, A.; Barchitta, M.; Fiore, V.; Rosta, G.; Favara, G.; La Mastra, C.; La Rosa, M.C.; San Lio, R.M.; Agodi, A. Determinants of adherence to the mediterranean diet: Findings from a cross-sectional study in women from Southern Italy. *Int. J. Env. Res. Public Health* **2019**, *16*, 2963. [CrossRef] [PubMed]
6. Maugeri, A.; Barchitta, M.; Agrifoglio, O.; Favara, G.; La Mastra, C.; La Rosa, M.C.; Lio, R.M.S.; Panella, M.; Cianci, A.; Agodi, A. The impact of social determinants and lifestyles on dietary patterns during pregnancy: Evidence from the "Mamma & Bambino" study. *Ann. Di Ig.* **2019**, *31*, 81–89.
7. Cani, P.D. Human gut microbiome: Hopes, threats and promises. *Gut* **2018**, *67*, 1716–1725. [CrossRef] [PubMed]
8. Gilbert, J.A.; Blaser, M.J.; Caporaso, J.G.; Jansson, J.K.; Lynch, S.V.; Knight, R. Current understanding of the human microbiome. *Nat. Med.* **2018**, *24*, 392–400. [CrossRef]
9. Shrestha, G.S.; Paneru, H.R.; Vincent, J.L. Precision medicine for COVID-19: A call for better clinical trials. *Crit. Care* **2020**, *24*, 1–3. [CrossRef]
10. Alberg, C.; Burton, H.; Hall, A.; Wright, C.; Zimmern, R. An Independent Response to the House of Lords Science and Technology Committee Report. *PHG Found.* **2010**, *May*, 12–14.
11. Boccia, S.; Federici, A.; Colotto, M.; Villari, P. Implementation of Italian guidelines on public health genomics in Italy: A challenging policy of the NHS TT-Le policy di genomica in sanità pubblica in Italia: Le sfide nella implementazione delle linee guida nel sistema sanitario nazionale. *Epidemiol. Prev.* **2014**, *38*, 29–34.
12. Burke, W.; Atkins, D.; Gwinn, M.; Guttmacher, A.; Haddow, J.; Lau, J.; Palomaki, G.; Press, N.; Richards, C.S.; Wideroff, L.; et al. Genetic test evaluation: Information needs of clinicians, policy makers, and the public. *Am. J. Epidemiol.* **2002**, *156*, 311–318. [CrossRef] [PubMed]
13. Aragam, K.G.; Natarajan, P. Polygenic Scores to Assess Atherosclerotic Cardiovascular Disease Risk: Clinical Perspectives and Basic Implications. *Circ. Res.* **2020**, *126*, 1159–1177. [CrossRef]
14. Hachiya, T.; Hata, J.; Hirakawa, Y.; Yoshida, D.; Furuta, Y.; Kitazono, T.; Shimizu, A.; Ninomiya, T. Genome-wide polygenic score and the risk of ischemic stroke in a prospective cohort: The Hisayama study. *Stroke* **2020**, *51*, 759–765. [CrossRef]
15. Ho, W.K.; Tan, M.M.; Mavaddat, N.; Tai, M.C.; Mariapun, S.; Li, J.; Ho, P.J.; Dennis, J.; Tyrer, J.P.; Bolla, M.K.; et al. European polygenic risk score for prediction of breast cancer shows similar performance in Asian women. *Nat. Commun.* **2020**, *11*, 1–11. [CrossRef]
16. Padilla-Martínez, F.; Collin, F.; Kwasniewski, M.; Kretowski, A. Systematic review of polygenic risk scores for type 1 and type 2 diabetes. *Int. J. Mol. Sci.* **2020**, *21*, 1703. [CrossRef]
17. Ibanez, L.; Farias, F.H.G.; Dube, U.; Mihindukulasuriya, K.A.; Harari, O. Polygenic Risk Scores in Neurodegenerative Diseases: A Review. *Curr. Genet. Med. Rep.* **2019**, *7*, 22–29. [CrossRef]
18. Wendt, F.R.; Pathak, G.A.; Tylee, D.S.; Goswami, A.; Polimanti, R. Heterogeneity and Polygenicity in Psychiatric Disorders: A Genome-Wide Perspective. *Chronic Stress* **2020**, *4*. [CrossRef] [PubMed]
19. Lambert, S.; Gil, L.; Jupp, S.; Ritchie, S.; Xu, Y.; Buniello, A.; Abraham, G.; Chapman, M.; Parkinson, H.; Danesh, J.; et al. The Polygenic Score Catalog: An open database for reproducibility and systematic evaluation. *medRxiv* **2020**. [CrossRef]
20. Choi, S.W.; Mak, T.S.H.; O'Reilly, P.F. Tutorial: A guide to performing polygenic risk score analyses. *Nat. Protoc.* **2020**, *15*, 2759–2772. [CrossRef] [PubMed]
21. Sakaue, S.; Kanai, M.; Karjalainen, J.; Akiyama, M.; Kurki, M.; Matoba, N.; Takahashi, A.; Hirata, M.; Kubo, M.; Matsuda, K.; et al. Trans-biobank analysis with 676,000 individuals elucidates the association of polygenic risk scores of complex traits with human lifespan. *Nat. Med.* **2020**, *26*, 542–548. [CrossRef]
22. Yengo, L.; Sidorenko, J.; Kemper, K.E.; Zheng, Z.; Wood, A.R.; Weedon, M.N.; Frayling, T.M.; Hirschhorn, J.; Yang, J.; Visscher, P.M. Meta-analysis of genome-wide association studies for height and body mass index in ~700 000 individuals of European ancestry. *Hum. Mol. Genet.* **2018**, *27*, 3641–3649. [CrossRef]
23. Malik, R.; Chauhan, G.; Traylor, M.; Sargurupremraj, M.; Okada, Y.; Mishra, A.; Rutten-Jacobs, L.; Giese, A.K.; Van Der Laan, S.W.; Gretarsdottir, S.; et al. Multiancestry genome-wide association study of 520,000 subjects identifies 32 loci associated with stroke and stroke subtypes. *Nat. Genet.* **2018**, *50*, 524–537. [CrossRef]
24. Ripke, S.; Neale, B.M.; Corvin, A.; Walters, J.T.R.; Farh, K.H.; Holmans, P.A.; Lee, P.; Bulik-Sullivan, B.; Collier, D.A.; Huang, H.; et al. Biological insights from 108 schizophrenia-associated genetic loci. *Nature* **2014**, *511*, 421–427.
25. Gialluisi, A.; Andlauer, T.F.M.; Mirza-Schreiber, N.; Moll, K.; Becker, J.; Hoffmann, P.; Ludwig, K.U.; Czamara, D.; Pourcain, B.S.; Honbolygó, F.; et al. Genome-wide association study reveals new insights into the heritability and genetic correlates of developmental dyslexia. *Mol. Psychiatry* **2020**. [CrossRef] [PubMed]

26. Yanes, T.; McInerney-Leo, A.M.; Law, M.H.; Cummings, S. The emerging field of polygenic risk scores and perspective for use in clinical care. *Hum. Mol. Genet.* **2020**, *29*, R165–R176. [CrossRef] [PubMed]
27. Hynninen, Y.; Linna, M.; Vilkkumaa, E. Value of genetic testing in the prevention of cardiovascular events (unpublished). *PLoS ONE* **2019**, *14*, e0210010. [CrossRef]
28. Arnett, D.K.; Blumenthal, R.S.; Albert, M.A.; Buroker, A.B.; Goldberger, Z.D.; Hahn, E.J.; Himmelfarb, C.D.; Khera, A.; Lloyd-Jones, D.; McEvoy, J.W.; et al. 2019 ACC/AHA Guideline on the Primary Prevention of Cardiovascular Disease: A Report of the American College of Cardiology/American Heart Association Task Force on Clinical Practice Guidelines. *J. Am. Coll. Cardiol.* **2019**, *74*, e177–e232. [CrossRef]
29. Piepoli, M.F.; Hoes, A.W.; Agewall, S.; Albus, C.; Brotons, C.; Catapano, A.L.; Cooney, M.T.; Corrà, U.; Cosyns, B.; Deaton, C.; et al. 2016 European Guidelines on cardiovascular disease prevention in clinical practice: The Sixth Joint Task Force of the European Society of Cardiology and Other Societies on Cardiovascular Disease Prevention in Clinical Practice. *Atherosclerosis* **2016**, *252*, 207–274. [CrossRef]
30. Elliott, J.; Bodinier, B.; Bond, T.A.; Chadeau-Hyam, M.; Evangelou, E.; Moons, K.G.M.; Dehghan, A.; Muller, D.C.; Elliott, P.; Tzoulaki, I. Predictive Accuracy of a Polygenic Risk Score-Enhanced Prediction Model vs. a Clinical Risk Score for Coronary Artery Disease. *JAMA J. Am. Med. Assoc.* **2020**, *323*, 636–645. [CrossRef]
31. Läll, K.; Mägi, R.; Morris, A.; Metspalu, A.; Fischer, K. Personalized risk prediction for type 2 diabetes: The potential of genetic risk scores. *Genet. Med.* **2017**, *19*, 322–329. [CrossRef]
32. Pencina, M.J.; D'Agostino, R.B.S.; D'Agostino, R.B.J.; Vasar, R.S. Evaluating the added predictive ability of a new marker: From area under the ROC curve to reclassification and beyond. *Stat. Med.* **2008**, *27*, 157–172. [CrossRef]
33. Garcìa-Gimènez, J.L.; Seco-Cervera, M.; Tollefsbol, T.O.; Romà-Mateo, C.; Peirò-Chova, L.; Lapuzina, P. Epigenetic biomarkers: Current strategies and future challenges for their use in the clinical laboratory. *Crit. Rev. Clin. Lab. Sci.* **2017**, *54*, 529–550. [CrossRef] [PubMed]
34. Relton, C.L.; Hartwig, F.P.; Smith, G.D. From stem cells to the law courts: DNA methylation, the forensic epigenome and the possibility of a biosocial archive. *Int. J. Epidemiol.* **2015**, *44*, 1083–1093. [CrossRef] [PubMed]
35. Andersen, A.M.; Dogan, M.V.; Beach, S.R.H.; Philibert, R.A. Current and future prospects for epigenetic biomarkers of substance use disorders. *Genes* **2015**, *6*, 991–1022. [CrossRef]
36. García-Giménez, J.L.; Mena-Mollá, S.; Beltrán-García, J.; Sanchis-Gomar, F. Challenges in the analysis of epigenetic biomarkers in clinical samples. *Clin. Chem. Lab. Med.* **2017**, *55*, 1474–1477. [CrossRef]
37. Glinge, C.; Clauss, S.; Boddum, K.; Jabbari, R.; Jabbari, J.; Risgaard, B.; Tomsits, P.; Hildebrand, B.; Kaèaèb, S.; Wakili, R.; et al. Stability of circulating blood-based microRNAs-Pre-Analytic methodological considerations. *PLoS ONE* **2017**, *12*, 1–16. [CrossRef]
38. Park, N.J.; Zhou, H.; Elashoff, D.; Henson, B.S.; Kastratovic, D.A.; Abemayor, E.; Wong, D.T. Salivary microRNA: Discovery, characterization, and clinical utility for oral cancer detection. *Clin. Cancer Res.* **2009**, *15*, 5473–5477. [CrossRef]
39. Zubakov, D.; Boersma, A.W.M.; Choi, Y.; Van Kuijk, P.F.; Wiemer, E.A.C.; Kayser, M. MicroRNA markers for forensic body fluid identification obtained from microarray screening and quantitative RT-PCR confirmation. *Int. J. Leg. Med.* **2010**, *124*, 217–226. [CrossRef] [PubMed]
40. Peiró-Chova, L.; Peña-Chilet, M.; López-Guerrero, J.A.; García-Giménez, J.L.; Alonso-Yuste, E.; Burgues, O.; Lluch, A.; Ferrer-Lozano, J.; Ribas, G. High stability of microRNAs in tissue samples of compromised quality. *Virchows Arch.* **2013**, *463*, 765–774. [CrossRef] [PubMed]
41. Patnaik, S.K.; Mallick, R.; Yendamuri, S. Detection of microRNAs in dried serum blots. *Anal. Biochem.* **2010**, *407*, 147–149. [CrossRef] [PubMed]
42. García-Giménez, J.L.; Ushijima, T.; Tollefsbol, T.O. Epigenetic Biomarkers: New Findings, Perspectives, and Future Directions in Diagnostics. In *Epigenetic Biomarkers and Diagnostics*; Elvesier Inc., Ed.; Elvesier: Amsterdam, The Netherlands, 2016; pp. 1–18.
43. Berdasco, M.; Esteller, M. Aberrant Epigenetic Landscape in Cancer: How Cellular Identity Goes Awry. *Dev. Cell* **2010**, *19*, 698–711. [CrossRef]
44. Wang, K.; Yuen, S.T.; Xu, J.; Lee, S.P.; Yan, H.H.N.; Shi, S.T.; Siu, H.C.; Deng, S.; Chu, K.M.; Law, S.; et al. Whole-genome sequencing and comprehensive molecular profiling identify new driver mutations in gastric cancer. *Nat. Genet.* **2014**, *46*, 573–582. [CrossRef] [PubMed]
45. Guinney, J.; Dienstmann, R.; Wang, X.; De Reyniès, A.; Schlicker, A.; Soneson, C.; Marisa, L.; Roepman, P.; Nyamundanda, G.; Angelino, P.; et al. The consensus molecular subtypes of colorectal cancer. *Nat. Med.* **2015**, *21*, 1350–1356. [CrossRef]
46. Bormann, F.; Rodríguez-Paredes, M.; Lasitschka, F.; Edelmann, D.; Musch, T.; Benner, A.; Bergman, Y.; Dieter, S.M.; Ball, C.R.; Glimm, H.; et al. Cell-of-Origin DNA Methylation Signatures Are Maintained during Colorectal Carcinogenesis. *Cell Rep.* **2018**, *23*, 3407–3418. [CrossRef] [PubMed]
47. Pajtler, K.W.; Witt, H.; Sill, M.; Jones, D.T.W.; Hovestadt, V.; Kratochwil, F.; Wani, K.; Tatevossian, R.; Punchihewa, C.; Johann, P.; et al. Molecular Classification of Ependymal Tumors across All CNS Compartments, Histopathological Grades, and Age Groups. *Cancer Cell* **2015**, *27*, 728–743. [CrossRef] [PubMed]
48. Capper, D.; Jones, D.T.W.; Sill, M.; Hovestadt, V.; Schrimpf, D.; Sturm, D.; Koelsche, C.; Sahm, F.; Chavez, L.; Reuss, D.E.; et al. DNA methylation-based classification of central nervous system tumours. *Nature* **2018**, *555*, 469–474. [CrossRef] [PubMed]

49. Rodríguez-Paredes, M.; Bormann, F.; Raddatz, G.; Gutekunst, J.; Lucena-Porcel, C.; Köhler, F.; Wurzer, E.; Schmidt, K.; Gallinat, S.; Wenck, H.; et al. Methylation profiling identifies two subclasses of squamous cell carcinoma related to distinct cells of origin. *Nat. Commun.* **2018**, *9*, 577. [CrossRef]
50. Lamb, Y.N.; Dhillon, S. Epi proColon®2.0 CE: A Blood-Based Screening Test for Colorectal Cancer. *Mol. Diagn.* **2017**, *21*, 225–232. [CrossRef]
51. Ned, R.M.; Melillo, S.; Marrone, M. Fecal DNA testing for Colorectal Cancer Screening: The ColoSure™ test. *PLoS Curr.* **2011**, *22*, RRN1220. [CrossRef]
52. Qazi, T.J.; Quan, Z.; Mir, A.; Qing, H. Epigenetics in Alzheimer's Disease: Perspective of DNA Methylation. *Mol. Neurobiol.* **2018**, *55*, 1026–1044. [CrossRef]
53. Jakubowski, J.L.; Labrie, V. Epigenetic Biomarkers for Parkinson's Disease: From Diagnostics to Therapeutics. *J. Parkinson's Dis.* **2017**, *7*, 1–12. [CrossRef] [PubMed]
54. Paez-Colasante, X.; Figueroa-Romero, C.; Sakowski, S.A.; Goutman, S.A.; Feldman, E.L. Amyotrophic lateral sclerosis: Mechanisms and therapeutics in the epigenomic era. *Nat. Rev. Neurol.* **2015**, *11*, 266–279. [CrossRef]
55. Khavari, B.; Cairns, M.J. Epigenomic Dysregulation in Schizophrenia: In Search of Disease Etiology and Biomarkers. *Cells* **2020**, *9*, 1837. [CrossRef] [PubMed]
56. Penner-Goeke, S.; Binder, E.B. Epigenetics and depression. *Dialogues Clin. Neurosci.* **2019**, *21*, 397–405. [PubMed]
57. Howie, H.; Rijal, C.M.; Ressler, K.J. A review of epigenetic contributions to post-traumatic stress disorder. *Dialogues Clin. Neurosci.* **2019**, *21*, 417–428. [PubMed]
58. Nilsson, E.; Jansson, P.A.; Perfilyev, A.; Volkov, P.; Pedersen, M.; Svensson, M.K.; Poulsen, P.; Ribel-Madsen, R.; Pedersen, N.L.; Almgren, P.; et al. Altered DNA methylation and differential expression of genes influencing metabolism and inflammation in adipose tissue from subjects with type 2 diabetes. *Diabetes* **2014**, *63*, 2962–2976. [CrossRef] [PubMed]
59. Volkmar, M.; Dedeurwaerder, S.; Cunha, D.A.; Ndlovu, M.N.; Defrance, M.; Deplus, R.; Calonne, E.; Volkmar, U.; Igoillo-Esteve, M.; Naamane, N.; et al. DNA methylation profiling identifies epigenetic dysregulation in pancreatic islets from type 2 diabetic patients. *EMBO J.* **2012**, *31*, 1405–1426. [CrossRef] [PubMed]
60. Nitert, M.D.; Dayeh, T.; Volkov, P.; Elgzyri, T.; Hall, E.; Nilsson, E.; Yang, B.T.; Lang, S.; Parikh, H.; Wessman, Y.; et al. Impact of an exercise intervention on DNA methylation in skeletal muscle from first-degree relatives of patients with type 2 diabetes. *Diabetes* **2012**, *61*, 3322–3332. [CrossRef]
61. Impact of Overfeeding and Following Exercise Training in Individuals with and without Increased Risk of Type 2 Diabetes-Full Text View-ClinicalTrials.gov. Available online: https://clinicaltrials.gov/ct2/show/NCT02982408 (accessed on 6 December 2020).
62. Exercise Resistance in Type 2 Diabetes-Full Text View-ClinicalTrials.gov. Available online: https://clinicaltrials.gov/ct2/show/NCT01911104 (accessed on 6 December 2020).
63. Talens, R.P.; Jukema, J.W.; Trompet, S.; Kremer, D.; Westendorp, R.G.J.; Lumey, L.H.; Sattar, N.; Putter, H.; Slagboom, P.E.; Heijmans, B.T. Hypermethylation at loci sensitive to the prenatal environment is associated with increased incidence of myocardial infarction. *Int. J. Epidemiol.* **2012**, *41*, 106–115. [CrossRef]
64. Tarry-Adkins, J.L.; Ozanne, S.E. Nutrition in early life and age-associated diseases. *Ageing Res. Rev.* **2017**, *39*, 96–105. [CrossRef] [PubMed]
65. Freson, K.; Izzi, B.; Labarque, V.; Van Helvoirt, M.; Thys, C.; Wittevrongel, C.; Bex, M.; Bouillon, R.; Godefroid, N.; Proesmans, W.; et al. GNAS defects identified by stimulatory G protein α-subunit signalling studies in platelets. *J. Clin. Endocrinol. Metab.* **2008**, *93*, 4851–4859. [CrossRef]
66. Izzi, B.; Van Geet, C.; Freson, K. Recent Advances in GNAS Epigenetic Research of Pseudohypoparathyroidism. *Curr. Mol. Med.* **2012**, *12*, 566–573. [CrossRef] [PubMed]
67. Freson, K.; Izzi, B.; Van Geet, C. From genetics to epigenetics in platelet research. *Thromb. Res.* **2012**, *129*, 325–329. [CrossRef]
68. Noro, F.; Gianfagna, F.; Gialluisi, A.; De Curtis, A.; Di Castelnuovo, A.; Napoleone, E.; Cerletti, C.; Donati, M.B.; De Gaetano, G.; Hoylaerts, M.F.; et al. ZBTB12 DNA methylation is associated with coagulation- and inflammation-related blood cell parameters: Findings from the Moli-family cohort. *Clin. Epigenetics* **2019**, *11*, 1–10. [CrossRef]
69. Guarrera, S.; Fiorito, G.; Onland-Moret, N.C.; Russo, A.; Agnoli, C.; Allione, A.; Di Gaetano, C.; Mattiello, A.; Ricceri, F.; Chiodini, P.; et al. Gene-specific DNA methylation profiles and LINE-1 hypomethylation are associated with myocardial infarction risk. *Clin. Epigenetics* **2015**, *7*, 1–12. [CrossRef] [PubMed]
70. Istas, G.; Declerck, K.; Pudenz, M.; Szic, K.S.V.; Lendinez-Tortajada, V.; Leon-Latre, M.; Heyninck, K.; Haegeman, G.; Casasnovas, J.A.; Tellez-Plaza, M.; et al. Identification of differentially methylated BRCA1 and CRISP2 DNA regions as blood surrogate markers for cardiovascular disease. *Sci. Rep.* **2017**, *7*, 1–14.
71. Wang, J.; Chen, J.; Sen, S. MicroRNA as Biomarkers and Diagnostics. *J. Cell. Physiol.* **2016**, *231*, 25–30. [CrossRef]
72. Izzotti, A.; Carozzo, S.; Pulliero, A.; Zhabayeva, D.; Ravetti, J.L.; Bersimbaev, R. Extracellular MicroRNA in liquid biopsy: Applicability in cancer diagnosis and prevention. *Am. J. Cancer Res.* **2016**, *6*, 1461–1493.
73. Moss, J.; Magenheim, J.; Neiman, D.; Zemmour, H.; Loyfer, N.; Korach, A.; Samet, Y.; Maoz, M.; Druid, H.; Arner, P.; et al. Comprehensive human cell-type methylation atlas reveals origins of circulating cell-free DNA in health and disease. *Nat. Commun.* **2018**, *9*, 5068. [CrossRef]

74. Kang, S.; Li, Q.; Chen, Q.; Zhou, Y.; Park, S.; Lee, G.; Grimes, B.; Krysan, K.; Yu, M.; Wang, W.; et al. CancerLocator: Non-invasive cancer diagnosis and tissue-of-origin prediction using methylation profiles of cell-free DNA. *Genome Biol.* **2017**, *18*, 1–12. [CrossRef]
75. Zemmour, H.; Planer, D.; Magenheim, J.; Moss, J.; Neiman, D.; Gilon, D.; Korach, A.; Glaser, B.; Shemer, R.; Landesberg, G.; et al. Non-invasive detection of human cardiomyocyte death using methylation patterns of circulating DNA. *Nat. Commun.* **2018**, *9*, 1443. [CrossRef]
76. Duncan, L.; Shen, H.; Gelaye, B.; Meijsen, J.; Ressler, K.; Feldman, M.; Peterson, R.; Domingue, B. Analysis of polygenic risk score usage and performance in diverse human populations. *Nat. Commun.* **2019**, *10*, 3328. [CrossRef] [PubMed]
77. Marotta, A.; Noro, F.; Parisi, R.; Gialluisi, A.; Tirozzi, A.; De Curtis, A.; Costanzo, S.; Di Castelnuovo, A.; Cerletti, C.; Donati, M.B.; et al. NMU DNA methylation in blood is associated with metabolic and inflammatory indices: Results from the Moli-sani study. *Epigenetics* **2021**, *17*, 1–14. [CrossRef]
78. Cohen, A.J.; Brauer, M.; Burnett, R.; Anderson, H.R.; Frostad, J.; Estep, K.; Balakrishnan, K.; Brunekreef, B.; Dandona, L.; Dandona, R.; et al. Estimates and 25-year trends of the global burden of disease attributable to ambient air pollution: An analysis of data from the Global Burden of Diseases Study 2015. *Lancet* **2017**, *389*, 1907–1918. [CrossRef]
79. Kotsyfakis, M.; Patelarou, E. MicroRNAs as biomarkers of harmful environmental and occupational exposures: A systematic review. *Biomarkers* **2019**, *24*, 623–630. [CrossRef]
80. Izzotti, A.; Pulliero, A. The effects of environmental chemical carcinogens on the microRNA machinery. *Int. J. Hyg. Env. Health* **2014**, *217*, 601–627. [CrossRef]
81. Cheng, M.; Wang, B.; Yang, M.; Ma, J.; Ye, Z.; Xie, L.; Zhou, M.; Chen, W. microRNAs expression in relation to particulate matter exposure: A systematic review. *Env. Pollut.* **2020**, *260*, 113961. [CrossRef]
82. Burris, H.H.; Baccarelli, A.A. Environmental epigenetics: From novelty to scientific discipline. *J. Appl. Toxicol.* **2014**, *34*, 113–116. [CrossRef] [PubMed]
83. Duforestel, M.; Briand, J.; Bougras-Carton, G.; Heymann, D.; Frenel, J.-S.; Vallette, F.M.; Carton, P.-F. Cell-free circulating epimarks in cancer monitoring. *Epigenomics* **2020**, *12*, 145–155. [CrossRef] [PubMed]
84. Izzotti, A.; Calin, G.A.; Arrigo, P.; Steele, V.E.; Croce, C.M.; De Flora, S. Downregulation of microRNA expression in the lungs of rats exposed to cigarette smoke. *Faseb J.* **2009**, *23*, 806–812. [CrossRef]
85. Schembri, F.; Sridhar, S.; Perdomo, C.; Gustafson, A.M.; Zhang, X.; Ergun, A.; Lu, J.; Liu, G.; Zhang, X.; Bowers, J.; et al. MicroRNAs as modulators of smoking-induced gene expression changes in human airway epithelium. *Proc. Natl. Acad. Sci. USA* **2009**, *106*, 2319–2324. [CrossRef] [PubMed]
86. Izzotti, A.; Larghero, P.; Longobardi, M.; Cartiglia, C.; Camoirano, A.; Steele, V.E.; De Flora, S. Dose-responsiveness and persistence of microRNA expression alterations induced by cigarette smoke in mouse lung. *Mutat. Res-Fundam. Mol. Mech. Mutagen.* **2011**, *717*, 9–16. [CrossRef]
87. Izzotti, A.; Calin, G.A.; Steele, V.E.; Croce, C.M.; De Flora, S. Relationships of microRNA expression in mouse lung with age and exposure to cigarette smoke and light. *Faseb J.* **2009**, *23*, 3243–3250. [CrossRef] [PubMed]
88. Izzotti, A.; Balansky, R.; Ganchev, G.; Iltcheva, M.; Longobardi, M.; Pulliero, A.; Geretto, M.; Micale, R.T.; La Maestra, S.; Miller, M.S.; et al. Blood and lung microRNAs as biomarkers of pulmonary tumorigenesis in cigarette smoke-exposed mice. *Oncotarget* **2016**, *7*, 84758–84774. [CrossRef]
89. Pulliero, A.; Fazzi, E.; Cartiglia, C.; Orcesi, S.; Balottin, U.; Uggetti, C.; La Piana, R.; Olivieri, I.; Galli, J.; Izzotti, A. The Aicardi-Goutières syndrome. Molecular and clinical features of RNAse deficiency and microRNA overload. *Mutat. Res-Fundam. Mol. Mech. Mutagen.* **2011**, *717*, 99–108. [CrossRef] [PubMed]
90. Ma, P.; Pan, Y.; Li, W.; Sun, C.; Liu, J.; Xu, T.; Shu, Y. Extracellular vesicles-mediated noncoding RNAs transfer in cancer. *J. Hematol. Oncol.* **2017**, *10*, 1–11. [CrossRef]
91. Yáñez-Mó, M.; Siljander, P.R.M.; Andreu, Z.; Zavec, A.B.; Borràs, F.E.; Buzas, E.I.; Buzas, K.; Casal, E.; Cappello, F.; Carvalho, J.; et al. Biological properties of extracellular vesicles and their physiological functions. *J. Extracell. Vesicles* **2015**, *4*, 1–60. [CrossRef]
92. Kadota, T.; Yoshioka, Y.; Fujita, Y.; Kuwano, K.; Ochiya, T. Extracellular vesicles in lung cancer—From bench to bedside. *Semin. Cell Dev. Biol.* **2017**, *67*, 39–47. [CrossRef]
93. Di Renzo, L.; Gualtieri, P.; Romano, L.; Marrone, G.; Noce, A.; Pujia, A.; Perrone, M.A.; Aiello, V.; Colica, C.; De Lorenzo, A. Role of personalized nutrition in chronic-degenerative diseases. *Nutrients* **2019**, *11*, 1707. [CrossRef]
94. Strianese, O.; Rizzo, F.; Ciccarelli, M.; Galasso, G.; D'agostino, Y.; Salvati, A.; Del Giudice, C.; Tesorio, P.; Rusciano, M.R. Precision and personalized medicine: How genomic approach improves the management of cardiovascular and neurodegenerative disease. *Genes* **2020**, *11*, 747. [CrossRef]
95. Wild, C.P. Complementing the genome with an "exposome": The outstanding challenge of environmental exposure measurement in molecular epidemiology. *Cancer Epidemiol. Biomark. Prev.* **2005**, *14*, 1847–1850. [CrossRef]
96. Barchitta, M.; Quattrocchi, A.; Maugeri, A.; Barone, G.; Mazzoleni, P.; Catalfo, A.; De Guidi, G.; Iemmolo, M.; Crimi, N.; Agodi, A. Integrated approach of nutritional and molecular epidemiology, mineralogical and chemical pollutant characterisation: The protocol of a cross-sectional study in women. *BMJ Open* **2017**, *7*, 1–8. [CrossRef] [PubMed]
97. Barchitta, M.; Maugeri, A.; Quattrocchi, A.; Agrifoglio, O.; Agodi, A. The Role of miRNAs as Biomarkers for Pregnancy Outcomes: A Comprehensive Review. *Int. J. Genom.* **2017**, *2017*. [CrossRef] [PubMed]

98. Barchitta, M.; Quattrocchi, A.; Maugeri, A.; Vinciguerra, M.; Agodi, A. LINE-1 hypomethylation in blood and tissue samples as an epigenetic marker for cancer risk: A systematic review and meta-analysis. *PLoS ONE* **2014**, *9*, e109478. [CrossRef]
99. Barchitta, M.; Quattrocchi, A.; Maugeri, A.; Canto, C.; La Rosa, N.; Cantarella, M.A.; Spampinato, G.; Scalisi, A.; Agodi, A. LINE-1 hypermethylation in white blood cell DNA is associated with high-grade cervical intraepithelial neoplasia. *BMC Cancer* **2017**, *17*, 1–10. [CrossRef]
100. Agodi, A.; Barchitta, M.; Quattrocchi, A.; Maugeri, A.; Canto, C.; Marchese, A.E.; Vinciguerra, M. Low fruit consumption and folate deficiency are associated with LINE-1 hypomethylation in women of a cancer-free population. *Genes Nutr.* **2015**, *10*, 1–10. [CrossRef]
101. Barchitta, M.; Maugeri, A.; Quattrocchi, A.; Agrifoglio, O.; Scalisi, A.; Agodi, A. The association of dietary patterns with high-risk human papillomavirus infection and cervical cancer: A cross-sectional study in Italy. *Nutrients* **2018**, *10*, 469. [CrossRef]
102. Barchitta, M.; Maugeri, A.; La Mastra, C.; La Rosa, M.C.; Favara, G.; Lio, R.M.S.; Agodi, A. Dietary antioxidant intake and human papillomavirus infection: Evidence from a cross-sectional study in Italy. *Nutrients* **2020**, *12*, 1384. [CrossRef]
103. Agodi, A.; Barchitta, M.; Cipresso, R.; Marzagalli, R.; La Rosa, N.; Caruso, M.; Castiglione, M.G.; Travali, S. Distribution of p53, GST, and MTHFR polymorphisms and risk of cervical intraepithelial lesions in sicily. *Int. J. Gynecol. Cancer* **2010**, *20*, 141–146. [CrossRef] [PubMed]
104. Simone, B.; Mazzucco, W.; Gualano, M.R.; Agodi, A.; Coviello, D.; Dagna Bricarelli, F.; Dallapiccola, B.; Di Maria, E.; Federici, A.; Genuardi, M.; et al. The policy of public health genomics in Italy. *Health Policy (N.Y.)* **2013**, *110*, 214–219. [CrossRef]
105. Hibler, E.; Huang, L.; Andrade, J.; Spring, B. Impact of a diet and activity health promotion intervention on regional patterns of DNA methylation. *Clin. Epigenetics* **2019**, *11*, 1–12. [CrossRef]
106. Ewald, H.A.S.; Ewald, P.W. Natural selection, microbiomes, and public health. *Yale J. Biol. Med.* **2018**, *91*, 1–34.
107. Derrien, M.; Alvarez, A.S.; de Vos, W.M. The Gut Microbiota in the First Decade of Life. *Trends Microbiol.* **2019**, *27*, 997–1010. [CrossRef] [PubMed]
108. Nicholson, M.R.; Mitchell, P.D.; Alexander, E.; Ballal, S.; Bartlett, M.; Becker, P.; Davidovics, Z.; Docktor, M.; Dole, M.; Felix, G.; et al. Efficacy of Fecal Microbiota Transplantation for Clostridium difficile Infection in Children. *Clin. Gastroenterol. Hepatol.* **2020**, *18*, 612–619.e1. [CrossRef] [PubMed]
109. Yang, L.; Zhang, J.; Xu, J.; Wei, X.; Yang, J.; Liu, Y.; Li, H.; Zhao, C.; Wang, Y.; Zhang, L.; et al. Helicobacter pylori Infection Aggravates Dysbiosis of Gut Microbiome in Children with Gastritis. *Front. Cell. Infect. Microbiol.* **2019**, *9*, 1–14. [CrossRef] [PubMed]
110. Li, W.; Zhu, Y.; Liao, Q.; Wang, Z.; Wan, C. Characterization of gut microbiota in children with pulmonary tuberculosis. *BMC Pediatr.* **2019**, *19*, 1–10. [CrossRef]
111. Nirmalkar, K.; Murugesan, S.; Pizano-Zárate, M.L.; Villalobos-Flores, L.E.; García-González, C.; Morales-Hernández, R.M.; Nuñez-Hernández, J.A.; Hernández-Quiroz, F.; Romero-Figueroa, M.D.S.; Hernández-Guerrero, C.; et al. Gut microbiota and endothelial dysfunction markers in obese Mexican children and adolescents. *Nutrients* **2018**, *10*, 2009. [CrossRef] [PubMed]
112. Leiva-Gea, I.; Sánchez-Alcoholado, L.; Martín-Tejedor, B.; Castellano-Castillo, D.; Moreno-Indias, I.; Urda-Cardona, A.; Tinahones, F.J.; Fernández-García, J.C.; Queipo-Ortuño, M.I. Gut microbiota differs in composition and functionality between children with type 1 diabetes and MODY2 and healthy control subjects: A case-control study. *Diabetes Care* **2018**, *41*, 2385–2395. [CrossRef]
113. Traversi, D.; Rabbone, I.; Scaioli, G.; Vallini, C.; Carletto, G.; Racca, I.; Ala, U.; Durazzo, M.; Collo, A.; Ferro, A.; et al. Risk factors for type 1 diabetes, including environmental, behavioural and gut microbial factors: A case–control study. *Sci. Rep.* **2020**, *10*, 1–13. [CrossRef]
114. Schwimmer, J.B.; Johnson, J.S.; Angeles, J.E.; Behling, C.; Belt, P.H.; Borecki, I.; Bross, C.; Durelle, J.; Goyal, N.P.; Hamilton, G.; et al. Microbiome Signatures Associated with Steatohepatitis and Moderate to Severe Fibrosis in Children with Nonalcoholic Fatty Liver Disease. *Gastroenterology* **2019**, *157*, 1109–1122. [CrossRef] [PubMed]
115. Depner, M.; Taft, D.H.; Kirjavainen, P.V.; Kalanetra, K.M.; Karvonen, A.M.; Peschel, S.; Schmausser-Hechfellner, E.; Roduit, C.; Frei, R.; Lauener, R.; et al. Maturation of the gut microbiome during the first year of life contributes to the protective farm effect on childhood asthma. *Nat. Med.* **2020**, *26*, 1766–1775. [CrossRef]
116. Carissimi, C.; Laudadio, I.; Palone, F.; Fulci, V.; Cesi, V.; Cardona, F.; Alfonsi, C.; Cucchiara, S.; Isoldi, S.; Stronati, L. Functional analysis of gut microbiota and immunoinflammation in children with autism spectrum disorders. *Dig. Liver Dis.* **2019**, *51*, 1366–1374. [CrossRef]
117. Sahly, N.; Moustafa, A.; Zaghloul, M.; Salem, T.Z. Effect of radiotherapy on the gut microbiome in pediatric cancer patients: A pilot study. *PeerJ* **2019**, *7*, 1–17. [CrossRef]
118. Li, L.; Wang, F.; Liu, Y.; Gu, F. Intestinal microbiota dysbiosis in children with recurrent respiratory tract infections. *Microb. Pathog.* **2019**, *136*, 103709. [CrossRef] [PubMed]
119. Romani, L.; Del Chierico, F.; Chiriaco, M.; Foligno, S.; Reddel, S.; Salvatori, G.; Cifaldi, C.; Faraci, S.; Finocchi, A.; Rossi, P.; et al. Gut Mucosal and Fecal Microbiota Profiling Combined to Intestinal Immune System in Neonates Affected by Intestinal Ischemic Injuries. *Front. Cell. Infect. Microbiol.* **2020**, *10*, 1–9. [CrossRef]
120. Assfalg, R.; Knoop, J.; Hoffman, K.L.; Pfirrmann, M.; Zapardiel-Gonzalo, J.M.; Hofelich, A.; Eugster, A.; Weigelt, M.; Matzke, C.; Reinhardt, J.; et al. Oral insulin immunotherapy in children at risk for type 1 diabetes in a randomized trial. *MedRxiv* **2020**. [CrossRef]

121. Qian, X.; Liu, Y.X.; Ye, X.; Zheng, W.; Lv, S.; Mo, M.; Lin, J.; Wang, W.; Wang, W.; Zhang, X.; et al. Gut microbiota in children with juvenile idiopathic arthritis: Characteristics, biomarker identification, and usefulness in clinical prediction. *BMC Genom.* **2020**, *21*, 1–13. [CrossRef]
122. Valentini, F.; Evangelisti, M.; Arpinelli, M.; Di Nardo, G.; Borro, M.; Simmaco, M.; Villa, M.P. Gut microbiota composition in children with Obstructive Sleep Apnoea Syndrome: A pilot study. *Sleep Med.* **2020**, *76*, 140–147. [CrossRef] [PubMed]
123. Zhai, Q.; Cen, S.; Jiang, J.; Zhao, J.; Zhang, H.; Chen, W. Disturbance of trace element and gut microbiota profiles as indicators of autism spectrum disorder: A pilot study of Chinese children. *Env. Res.* **2019**, *171*, 501–509. [CrossRef]
124. Wang, M.; Zhou, J.; He, F.; Cai, C.; Wang, H.; Wang, Y.; Lin, Y.; Rong, H.; Cheng, G.; Xu, R.; et al. Alteration of gut microbiota-associated epitopes in children with autism spectrum disorders. *Brain Behav. Immun.* **2019**, *75*, 192–199. [CrossRef] [PubMed]
125. Rajagopala, S.V.; Yooseph, S.; Harkins, D.M.; Moncera, K.J.; Zabokrtsky, K.B.; Torralba, M.G.; Tovchigrechko, A.; Highlander, S.; Pieper, R.; Sender, L.; et al. Gastrointestinal microbial populations can distinguish pediatric and adolescent Acute Lymphoblastic Leukemia (ALL) at the time of disease diagnosis. *BMC Genom.* **2016**, *17*, 1–10. [CrossRef] [PubMed]
126. Hoffman, D.J.; Reynolds, R.M.; Hardy, D.B. Developmental origins of health and disease: Current knowledge and potential mechanisms. *Nutr. Rev.* **2017**, *75*, 951–970. [CrossRef] [PubMed]
127. Ilonen, J.; Lempainen, J.; Veijola, R. The heterogeneous pathogenesis of type 1 diabetes mellitus. *Nat. Rev. Endocrinol.* **2019**, *15*, 635–650. [CrossRef]
128. Wang, S.; Xu, M.; Wang, W.; Cao, X.; Piao, M.; Khan, S.; Yan, F.; Cao, H.; Wang, B. Systematic review: Adverse events of fecal Microbiota transplantation. *PLoS ONE* **2016**, *11*, 1–24. [CrossRef]
129. Suez, J.; Zmora, N.; Segal, E.; Elinav, E. The pros, cons, and many unknowns of probiotics. *Nat. Med.* **2019**, *25*, 716–729. [CrossRef]
130. Javdan, B.; Lopez, J.G.; Chankhamjon, P.; Lee, Y.C.J.; Hull, R.; Wu, Q.; Wang, X.; Chatterjee, S.; Donia, M.S. Personalized Mapping of Drug Metabolism by the Human Gut Microbiome. *Cell* **2020**, *181*, 1661–1679.e22. [CrossRef] [PubMed]
131. Sagner, M.; McNeil, A.; Puska, P.; Auffray, C.; Price, N.D.; Hood, L.; Lavie, C.J.; Han, Z.G.; Chen, Z.; Brahmachari, S.K.; et al. The P4 Health Spectrum–A Predictive, Preventive, Personalized and Participatory Continuum for Promoting Healthspan. *Prog. Cardiovasc. Dis.* **2017**, *59*, 506–521. [CrossRef]
132. Crisci, C.D.; Ardusso, L.R.F.; Mossuz, A.; Müller, L. A Precision Medicine Approach to SARS-CoV-2 Pandemic Management. *Curr. Treat. Options Allergy* **2020**, *7*, 422–440. [CrossRef]
133. Sigman, M. Introduction: Personalized medicine: What is it and what are the challenges? *Fertil. Steril.* **2018**, *109*, 944–945. [CrossRef]
134. Prokop, J.W.; Shankar, R.; Gupta, R.; Leimanis, M.L.; Nedveck, D.; Uhl, K.; Chen, B.; Hartog, N.L.; Van Veen, J.; Sisco, J.S.; et al. Virus-induced genetics revealed by multidimensional precision medicine transcriptional workflow applicable to COVID-19. *Physiol. Genom.* **2020**, *52*, 255–268. [CrossRef]
135. Poland, G.A.; Ovsyannikova, I.G.; Kennedy, R.B.; Haralambieva, I.H.; Jacobson, R.M. Vaccinomics and a new paradigm for the development of preventive vaccines against viral infections. *Omics.* **2011**, *15*, 625–636. [CrossRef] [PubMed]
136. Hamburg, M.A.; Collins, F.S. The path to personalized medicine. *N. Engl. J. Med.* **2010**, *363*, 301–304. [CrossRef] [PubMed]
137. McGonigle, I.V. The collective nature of personalized medicine. *Genet. Res. (Camb)* **2016**, *98*, e3. [CrossRef] [PubMed]
138. Shomron, N. Prioritizing personalized medicine. *Genet. Res. (Camb)* **2014**, *96*, 19–20. [CrossRef]
139. Poland, G.A. Pharmacology, vaccinomics, and the second golden age of vaccinology. *Clin. Pharm.* **2007**, *82*, 623–626. [CrossRef] [PubMed]
140. Poland, G.A.; Ovsyannikova, I.G.; Kennedy, R.B. Personalized vaccinology: A review. *Vaccine* **2018**, *36*, 5350–5357. [CrossRef]
141. Wollenstein-Betech, S.; Cassandras, C.G.; Paschalidis, I.C. Personalized predictive models for symptomatic COVID-19 patients using basic preconditions: Hospitalizations, mortality, and the need for and ICU or ventilator. *Int. J. Med. Inform.* **2020**, *123*, 11–22. [CrossRef]
142. Baj, J.; Karakuła-Juchnowicz, H.; Teresiński, G.; Buszewicz, G.; Ciesielka, M.; Sitarz, E.; Forma, A.; Karakuła, K.; Flieger, W.; Portincasa, P.; et al. COVID-19: Specific and Non-Specific Clinical Manifestations and Symptoms: The Current State of Knowledge. *J. Clin. Med.* **2020**, *9*, 1753. [CrossRef]
143. Rubino, S.; Kelvin, N.; Bermejo-Martin, J.F.; Kelvin, D.J. As COVID-19 cases, deaths and fatality rates surge in Italy, underlying causes require investigation. *J. Infect. Dev. Ctries.* **2020**, *14*, 265–267. [CrossRef]
144. Cesari, M.; Montero-Odasso, M. COVID-19 and older adults. lessons learned from the Italian epicenter. *Can. Geriatr. J.* **2020**, *23*, 155–159. [CrossRef] [PubMed]
145. Iosa, M.; Paolucci, S.; Morone, G. Covid-19: A Dynamic Analysis of Fatality Risk in Italy. *Front. Med.* **2020**, *7*, 1–5. [CrossRef]
146. Onder, G.; Rezza, G.; Brusaferro, S. Case-Fatality Rate and Characteristics of Patients Dying in Relation to COVID-19 in Italy. *Jama J. Am. Med. Assoc.* **2020**, *323*, 1775–1776. [CrossRef] [PubMed]
147. Parisi, V.; Leosco, D. Precision Medicine in COVID-19: IL-1β a Potential Target. *Jacc Basic Transl. Sci.* **2020**, *5*, 543–544. [CrossRef] [PubMed]
148. Sepulchre, E.; Pittie, G.; Stojkovic, V.; Haesbroek, G.; Crama, Y.; Schyns, M.; Paridaens, H.; de Marchin, J.; Degesves, S.; Biemar, C.; et al. Covid-19: Contribution of clinical characteristics and laboratory features for early detection of patients with high risk of severe evolution. *Acta Clin. Belg. Int. J. Clin. Lab. Med.* **2020**, 1–7. [CrossRef]
149. Ray, S.; Srivastava, S. COVID-19 pandemic: Hopes from proteomics and multiomics research. *Omics.* **2020**, *24*, 457–459. [CrossRef]

150. Ahmed, Z. Practicing precision medicine with intelligently integrative clinical and multi-omics data analysis. *Hum. Genom.* **2020**, *14*, 1–5. [CrossRef]
151. Eckhardt, M.; Hultquist, J.F.; Kaake, R.M.; Hüttenhain, R.; Krogan, N.J. A systems approach to infectious disease. *Nat. Rev. Genet.* **2020**, *21*, 339–354. [CrossRef]
152. Omersel, J.; Karas Kuželički, N. Vaccinomics and Adversomics in the Era of Precision Medicine: A Review Based on HBV, MMR, HPV, and COVID-19 Vaccines. *J. Clin. Med.* **2020**, *9*, 3561. [CrossRef] [PubMed]
153. Bhopal, S.S.; Bhopal, R. Sex differential in COVID-19 mortality varies markedly by age. *Lancet* **2020**, *396*, 532–533. [CrossRef]
154. Michelozzi, P.; De'Donato, F.; Scortichini, M.; De Sario, M.; Noccioli, F.; Rossi, P.; Davoli, M. Mortality impacts of the coronavirus disease (COVID-19) outbreak by sex and age: Rapid mortality surveillance system, Italy, 1 February to 18 April 2020. *Eurosurveillance* **2020**, *25*, 1–5. [CrossRef]
155. Franchini, M.; Glingani, C.; Del Fante, C.; Capuzzo, M.; Di Stasi, V.; Rastrelli, G.; Vignozzi, L.; De Donno, G.; Perotti, C. The protective effect of O blood type against SARS-CoV-2 infection. *Vox Sang.* **2020**, 1–2. [CrossRef]
156. Golinelli, D.; Boetto, E.; Maietti, E.; Fantini, M.P. The association between ABO blood group and SARS-CoV-2 infection: A meta-analysis. *PLoS ONE* **2020**, *15*, 1–14. [CrossRef]
157. Sherwani, S.; Khan, M.W.A. Cytokine response in SARS-CoV-2 infection in the Elderly. *J. Inflamm. Res.* **2020**, *13*, 737–747. [CrossRef]
158. Fadini, G.P.; Morieri, M.L.; Boscari, F.; Fioretto, P.; Maran, A.; Busetto, L.; Bonora, B.M.; Selmin, E.; Arcidiacono, G.; Pinelli, S.; et al. Newly-diagnosed diabetes and admission hyperglycemia predict COVID-19 severity by aggravating respiratory deterioration. *Diabetes Res. Clin. Pr.* **2020**, *168*, 108374. [CrossRef]
159. Figliozzi, S.; Masci, P.G.; Ahmadi, N.; Tondi, L.; Koutli, E.; Aimo, A.; Stamatelopoulos, K.; Dimopoulos, M.A.; Caforio, A.L.P.; Georgiopoulos, G. Predictors of adverse prognosis in COVID-19: A systematic review and meta-analysis. *Eur. J. Clin. Invest.* **2020**, *50*, 1–15. [CrossRef] [PubMed]
160. La Vignera, S.; Cannarella, R.; Condorelli, R.A.; Torre, F.; Aversa, A.; Calogero, A.E. Sex-specific SARS-CoV2 mortality: Among hormone-modulated ACE2 expression, risk of venous thromboembolism and hypovitaminosis D. *Int. J. Mol. Sci.* **2020**, *21*, 2948. [CrossRef]
161. Maddaloni, E.; D'Onofrio, L.; Alessandri, F.; Mignogna, C.; Leto, G.; Pascarella, G.; Mezzaroma, I.; Lichtner, M.; Pozzilli, P.; Agrò, F.E.; et al. Cardiometabolic multimorbidity is associated with a worse Covid-19 prognosis than individual cardiometabolic risk factors: A multicentre retrospective study (CoViDiab II). *Cardiovasc. Diabetol.* **2020**, *19*, 1–11. [CrossRef]
162. Ciceri, F.; Castagna, A.; Rovere-Querini, P.; De Cobelli, F.; Ruggeri, A.; Galli, L.; Conte, C.; De Lorenzo, R.; Poli, A.; Ambrosio, A.; et al. Early predictors of clinical outcomes of COVID-19 outbreak in Milan, Italy. *Clin. Immunol.* **2020**, *217*, 108509. [CrossRef] [PubMed]
163. Sieńko, J.; Kotowski, M.; Bogacz, A.; Lechowicz, K.; Drożdżal, S.; Rosik, J.; Sietnicki, M.; Sieńko, M.; Kotfis, K. COVID-19: The influence of ACE genotype and ACE-I and ARBs on the course of SARS-CoV-2 infection in elderly patients. *Clin. Interv. Aging* **2020**, *15*, 1231–1240. [CrossRef] [PubMed]
164. Yamamoto, N.; Ariumi, Y.; Nishida, N.; Yamamoto, R.; Bauer, G.; Gojobori, T.; Shimotohno, K.; Mizokami, M. SARS-CoV-2 infections and COVID-19 mortalities strongly correlate with ACE1 I/D genotype. *Gene* **2020**, *758*, 144944. [CrossRef] [PubMed]
165. Toyoshima, Y.; Nemoto, K.; Matsumoto, S.; Nakamura, Y.; Kiyotani, K. SARS-CoV-2 genomic variations associated with mortality rate of COVID-19. *J. Hum. Genet.* **2020**, *65*, 1075–1082. [CrossRef]
166. The Sever Covid-19 GWAS Group Genomewide Association Study of Severe Covid-19 with Respiratory Failure. *N. Engl. J. Med.* **2020**, *383*, 1522–1534. [CrossRef]
167. Barnkob, M.B.; Pottegård, A.; Støvring, H.; Haunstrup, T.M.; Homburg, K.; Larsen, R.; Hansen, M.B.; Titlestad, K.; Aagaard, B.; Møller, B.K.; et al. Reduced prevalence of SARS-CoV-2 infection in ABO blood group O. *Blood Adv.* **2020**, *4*, 4990–4993. [CrossRef] [PubMed]
168. Latz, C.A.; DeCarlo, C.; Boitano, L.; Png, C.Y.M.; Patell, R.; Conrad, M.F.; Eagleton, M.; Dua, A. Blood type and outcomes in patients with COVID-19. *Ann. Hematol.* **2020**, *99*, 2113–2118. [CrossRef] [PubMed]
169. Hoiland, R.L.; Fergusson, N.A.; Mitra, A.R.; Griesdale, D.E.G.; Devine, D.V.; Stukas, S.; Cooper, J.; Thiara, S.; Foster, D.; Chen, L.Y.C.; et al. The association of ABO blood group with indices of disease severity and multiorgan dysfunction in COVID-19. *Blood Adv.* **2020**, *4*, 4981–4989. [CrossRef]
170. Zhao, J.; Yang, Y.; Huang, H.; Li, D.; Gu, D.; Lu, X.; Zhang, Z.; Liu, L.; Liu, T. Relationship between the ABO Blood Group and the COVID-19 Susceptibilit. *Clin. Infect. Dis.* **2020**. [CrossRef]
171. Focosi, D. Anti-A isohaemagglutinin titres and SARS-CoV-2 neutralization: Implications for children and convalescent plasma selection. *Br. J. Haematol.* **2020**, *190*, e148–e150. [CrossRef] [PubMed]
172. Cooling, L. Blood groups in infection and host susceptibility. *Clin. Microbiol. Rev.* **2015**, *28*, 801–870. [CrossRef] [PubMed]
173. Overmyer, K.A.; Shishkova, E.; Miller, I.J.; Balnis, J.; Bernstein, M.N.; Peters-Clarke, T.M.; Meyer, J.G.; Quan, Q.; Muehlbauer, L.K.; Trujillo, E.A.; et al. Large-Scale Multi-omic Analysis of COVID-19 Severity. *Cell Syst.* **2020**, *12*, 1–18. [CrossRef]
174. Shrock, E.; Fujimura, E.; Kula, T.; Timms, R.T.; Lee, I.-H.; Leng, Y.; Robinson, M.L.; Sie, B.M.; Li, M.Z.; Chen, Y.; et al. Viral epitope profiling of COVID-19 patients reveals cross-reactivity and correlates of severity. *Science* **2020**, *370*, eabd4250. [CrossRef]
175. Pitini, E.; De Vito, C.; Marzuillo, C.; D'Andrea, E.; Rosso, A.; Federici, A.; Di Maria, E.; Villari, P. How is genetic testing evaluated? A systematic review of the literature. *Eur. J. Hum. Genet.* **2018**, *26*, 605–615. [CrossRef]

176. ACCE Model Process for Evaluating Genetic Tests | CDC. Available online: https://www.cdc.gov/genomics/gtesting/acce/index.htm (accessed on 6 December 2020).
177. Haddow, J.E.; Palomaki, G. *ACCE: A Model Process for Evaluating Data on Emerging Genetic Tests*; Khoury, M., Little, J., Burke, W., Eds.; ACCE (CDC USA.gov): Washington, DC, USA, 2004.
178. Giacomini, M.; Miller, F.; Browman, G. Confronting the "Gray Zones" of Technology Assessment: Evaluating genetic testing services for public insurance coverage in Canada. *Int. J. Technol. Assess. Health Care* **2003**, *19*, 301–316. [CrossRef] [PubMed]
179. Battista, R.N. Expanding the scientific basis of health technology assessment: A research agenda for the next decade. *Int. J. Technol. Assess. Health Care* **2006**, *22*, 275–280. [CrossRef]
180. Pitini, E.; D'Andrea, E.; De Vito, C.; Rosso, A.; Unim, B.; Marzuillo, C.; Federici, A.; Di Maria, E.; Villari, P. A proposal of a new evaluation framework towards implementation of genetic tests. *PLoS ONE* **2019**, *14*, 1–15. [CrossRef] [PubMed]
181. Kohler, J.N.; Turbitt, E.; Biesecker, B.B. Personal utility in genomic testing: A systematic literature review. *Eur. J. Hum. Genet.* **2017**, *25*, 662–668. [CrossRef]
182. Unim, B.; Pitini, E.; Lagerberg, T.; Adamo, G.; De Vito, C.; Marzuillo, C.; Villari, P. Current genetic service delivery models for the provision of genetic testing in Europe: A systematic review of the literature. *Front. Genet.* **2019**, *10*, 1–27. [CrossRef] [PubMed]
183. The EUnetHTA JA 2 HTA Core Model ®Online User guide. *Eunethta JA* **2015**, *2*, 1–27.
184. NEJM Catalyst What Is Patient-Centered Care? Available online: https://catalyst.nejm.org/doi/full/10.1056/CAT.17.0559 (accessed on 6 December 2020).
185. Khoury, M.J. No shortcuts on the long road to evidence-based genomic medicine. *Jama J. Am. Med. Assoc.* **2017**, *318*, 27–28. [CrossRef] [PubMed]
186. Ricciardi, W.; Boccia, S. New challenges of public health: Bringing the future of personalised healthcare into focus. *Eur. J. Public Health* **2017**, *27*, 36–39. [CrossRef]
187. Mazzucco, W.; Pastorino, R.; Lagerberg, T.; Colotto, M.; D'Andrea, E.; Marotta, C.; Marzuillo, C.; Villari, P.; Federici, A.; Ricciardi, W.; et al. Current state of genomic policies in healthcare among EU member states: Results of a survey of chief medical officers. *Eur. J. Public Health* **2017**, *27*, 931–937. [CrossRef]
188. Boccia, S.; Federici, A.; Siliquini, R.; Calabrò, G.E.; Ricciardi, W. Implementation of genomic policies in Italy: The new national plan for innovation of the health system based on omics sciences. *Epidemiol. Biostat. Public Health* **2017**.
189. Boccia, S.; Pastorino, R.; Ricciardi, W.; Ádány, R.; Barnhoorn, F.; Boffetta, P.; Cornel, M.C.; De Vito, C.; Gray, M.; Jani, A.; et al. How to Integrate Personalized Medicine into Prevention? Recommendations from the Personalized Prevention of Chronic Diseases (PRECeDI) Consortium. *Public Health Genom.* **2019**, *22*, 208–214. [CrossRef]
190. Pritchard, D.E.; Moeckel, F.; Villa, M.S.; Housman, L.T.; McCarty, C.A.; McLeod, H.L. Strategies for integrating personalized medicine into healthcare practice. *Pers. Med.* **2017**, *14*, 141–152. [CrossRef] [PubMed]
191. Michelazzo, M.B.; Pastorino, R.; Mazzucco, W.; Boccia, S. Distance learning training in genetics and genomics testing for Italian health professionals: Results of a pre and post-test evaluation. *Epidemiol. Biostat. Public Health* **2015**, *12*, e11516-1–e11516-6.
192. Calabrò, G.E.; Tognetto, A.; Mazzaccara, A.; Barbina, D.; Carbone, P.; Guerrera, D.; Federici, A.; Ricciardi, W.; Boccia, S. Omic sciences and capacity building of health professionals: A distance learning training course for Italian physicians, 2017–2018. *Ig. Sanita Pubblica* **2019**, *75*, 105–124.
193. Eduiss.it. Available online: https://www.eduiss.it/ (accessed on 12 December 2020).
194. Budin-Ljøsne, I.; Harris, J.R. Ask not what personalized medicine can do for you-Ask what you can do for personalized medicine. *Public Health Genom.* **2015**, *18*, 131–138. [CrossRef]
195. Su, P. Direct-to-Consumer Genetic Testing: A Comprehensive View. *Yale J. Biol. Med.* **2013**, *86*, 359–365.
196. Calabrò, G.E.; Sassano, M.; Tognetto, A.; Boccia, S. Citizens' Attitudes, Knowledge, and Educational Needs in the Field of Omics Sciences: A Systematic Literature Review. *Front. Genet.* **2020**, *11*, 570649. [CrossRef]
197. Boccia, S.; Del Sole, A.; Simone, B.; Sbrogiò, L. Genomica di sanità pubblica e medicina predittiva. *Rapp. Prev.* **2011**, *1*, 613–636.
198. Sbrogiò, L.; Banovich, F.; Favaretto, A.; Vigiani, N.; Del Sole, A. *La Medicina Predittiva: Quali Prospettive Operative per i Dipartimenti di Prevenzione*; atti 44° Congresso Nazionale S.It.I.: Venezia, Italy, 2010.
199. Ministero della Salute. *Piano Nazionale di Prevenzione 2010–2012*; Ministero della Salute: Roma, Italy, 2010.
200. Ministero della Salute. *Piano Nazionale della Prevenzione 2020–2025*; Ministero della Salute: Roma, Italy, 2020.
201. Ministero della Salute. *Piano nazionale della prevenzione 2014–2018*; Ministero della Salute: Roma, Italy, 2015.
202. Ministero della Salute. *Intesa Stato Regioni del 13 Marzo 2013 "Linee di Indirizzo Sulla Genomica in Sanità Pubblica"*; Ministero della Salute: Roma, Italy, 2013.
203. Ministero della Salute. *Intesa Stato Regioni del 26 Ottobre 2017 "Piano per L'innovazione del Sistema Sanitario Basata Sulle Scienze Omiche"*; Ministero della Salute: Roma, Italy, 2017.
204. DPCM. *Definizione e Aggiornamento dei Livelli Essenziali di Assistenza, di cui All'articolo 1, Comma 7, del Decreto Legislativo 30 Dicembre 1992, n. 502*; Ministero della Salute: Roma, Italy, 2017.

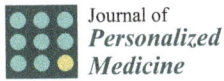

Article

Potential Role of miRNAs in the Acquisition of Chemoresistance in Neuroblastoma

Barbara Marengo [1,*,†], Alessandra Pulliero [2,†], Maria Valeria Corrias [3,†], Riccardo Leardi [4], Emanuele Farinini [4], Gilberto Fronza [5], Paola Menichini [5], Paola Monti [5], Lorenzo Monteleone [1], Giulia Elda Valenti [1], Andrea Speciale [5], Patrizia Perri [3], Francesca Madia [6], Alberto Izzotti [1,5,†] and Cinzia Domenicotti [1,†]

1. Department of Experimental Medicine, University of Genova, 16100 Genova, Italy; lolloleo92@gmail.com (L.M.); giuliaelda.valenti@edu.unige.it (G.E.V.); alberto.izzotti@unige.it (A.I.); cinzia.domenicotti@unige.it (C.D.)
2. Department of Health Sciences, University of Genova, 16100 Genova, Italy; alessandra.pulliero@unige.it
3. Laboratory of Experimental Therapies in Oncology, IRCCS Istituto Giannina Gaslini, 16100 Genova, Italy; mariavaleriacorrias@gaslini.org (M.V.C.); patriziaperri@gaslini.org (P.P.)
4. Department of Pharmacy, University of Genova, 16100 Genova, Italy; riclea@difar.unige.it (R.L.); farinini@difar.unige.it (E.F.)
5. UOC Mutagenesis and Cancer Prevention, IRCCS Ospedale Policlinico San Martino, 16100 Genova, Italy; gilberto.fronza@hsanmartino.it (G.F.); paola.menichini@hsanmartino.it (P.M.); paola.monti@hsanmartino.it (P.M.); andreaspeciale@alice.it (A.S.)
6. Medical Genetics Unit, IRCCS Giannina Gaslini Institute, 16100 Genova, Italy; francescamadia@gaslini.org
* Correspondence: barbara.marengo@unige.it; Tel.: +39-010-3538831
† These authors contributed equally to this work.

Abstract: Neuroblastoma (NB) accounts for about 8–10% of pediatric cancers, and the main causes of death are the presence of metastases and the acquisition of chemoresistance. Metastatic NB is characterized by *MYCN* amplification that correlates with changes in the expression of miRNAs, which are small non-coding RNA sequences, playing a crucial role in NB development and chemoresistance. In the present study, miRNA expression was analyzed in two human *MYCN*-amplified NB cell lines, one sensitive (HTLA-230) and one resistant to Etoposide (ER-HTLA), by microarray and RT-qPCR techniques. These analyses showed that miRNA-15a, -16-1, -19b, -218, and -338 were down-regulated in ER-HTLA cells. In order to validate the presence of this down-regulation in vivo, the expression of these miRNAs was analyzed in primary tumors, metastases, and bone marrow of therapy responder and non-responder pediatric patients. Principal component analysis data showed that the expression of miRNA-19b, -218, and -338 influenced metastases, and that the expression levels of all miRNAs analyzed were higher in therapy responders in respect to non-responders. Collectively, these findings suggest that these miRNAs might be involved in the regulation of the drug response, and could be employed for therapeutic purposes.

Keywords: neuroblastoma; miRNA; *MYCN* amplification; metastases; chemoresistance

1. Introduction

Neuroblastoma (NB) is an extracranial pediatric tumor originating from the aberrant development of neural crest-derived sympathoadrenal lineage [1], and is characterized by a high clinical and biological heterogeneity [2]. In fact, NB can be classified as a low-risk tumor, capable of spontaneously regressing, as well as a high-risk tumor, responsible for a high mortality rate and characterized by the presence of metastases.

The therapy used in high-risk patients is multimodal, and although the response to treatments is initially positive, subsequently, following the onset of chemoresistance, a large number of patients die as a consequence of relapse and metastasis formation [3]. NB metastasizes in vascularized tissue, and bone marrow (BM) is the preferential site of recurrence, being considered as the "fertile soil" for tumor cells and, in particular, for the chemoresistant cells [4,5]. In fact, BM spread is considered a negative prognostic factor [6].

Among the prognostic markers of poor patient outcome, the amplification of the *MYCN* oncogene characterizes the most aggressive high-risk NB subtype [7,8]. More than ten years ago, it was proposed that another approach to classifying the risk group of NB patients could be to evaluate the expression levels of miRNAs [9]. Considering that *MYCN* modulates the expression of several miRNAs [10], the evaluation of these small non-coding RNA sequences has become an accurate predictor of NB outcome [11].

Furthermore, since miRNA expression is related to tumor grade, metastasis, and chemoresistance, they could represent a new class of potential therapeutic targets. In this context, we have recently demonstrated in an NB cell line-based model [12] that Etoposide resistance is associated with miRNA-15a/16-1 down-regulation, highlighting that miRNAs could have a role as both markers of chemoresistance and new possible therapeutic targets [13]. Therefore, in the present study, the expression of these miRNAs, amongst others, was analyzed in primary tumors, metastases, and bone marrow of therapy responder and non-responder NB patients in order to identify the specific miRNAs involved in NB progression and chemoresistance.

2. Materials and Methods

2.1. Cell Cultures

The *MYCN*-amplified human stage-IV NB cell line, HTLA-230, was obtained from Dr. L. Raffaghello (G. Gaslini Institute, Genoa, Italy), while the Etoposide-resistant cell line (ER-HTLA) was selected as previously reported [12,13]. Cells were periodically tested for mycoplasma contamination (Mycoplasma Reagent Set, Aurogene s.p.a, Pavia, Italy). Cells were cultured in RPMI 1640 (Euroclone SpA, Pavia, Italy) and supplemented with 10% fetal bovine serum (FBS; Euroclone SpA, Pavia, Italy), 2 mM of glutamine (Euroclone SpA, Pavia, Italy), 1% penicillin/streptomycin (Euroclone SpA, Pavia, Italy), 1% sodium pyruvate (Sigma-Aldrich, Saint Louis, MO, USA), and 1% amino acid solution (Sigma-Aldrich, Saint Louis, MO, USA).

2.2. Patient Samples

The patients included in the study were diagnosed with NB stage M between January 2002 and December 2015. Written consent for the use of samples and clinical data for research was obtained by their legal guardians. The study was approved by the Gaslini Institute Ethical Committee, and all analyses were performed according to the Helsinki declaration.

The samples used originated from two groups of patients. With regard to the first group, whole bone marrow (BM) samples were collected in PAXgene™ Blood RNA tubes originating from patients who, after diagnosis, were treated according to the high-risk European protocol. The drugs used in the induction therapy were Cisplatin, Etoposide, Vincristine, Cyclophosphamide, and either Carboplatin or Adriamycin. Patients were divided into two subgroups, responders and non-responders: responders being the patients that could proceed with high-dose chemotherapy and stem cell transplants, and non-responders being the patients who could not proceed and were referred to second-line therapy.

With regards to the second group, the samples were represented by tumor specimens containing more than 70% of neoplastic cells and immune-selected metastases from BM samples, as described [14,15] and containing 95% tumor cells. All patient samples were taken at diagnosis before starting with the treatment.

2.3. RNA Extraction

Total RNA was extracted from cultured cells using TRIZOL reagent (LifeTechnologies, Carlsbad, CA, USA) according to the manufacturer's instructions. Total RNA (1 µg) was reverse-transcribed into cDNA by a random hexamer primer and SuperScript™ II Reverse Transcriptase (LifeTechnologies, Carlsbad, CA, USA).

Total RNA and miRNA fractions were extracted from tumor cells and metastases using the miRNeasyMini kit (Qiagen, Hilden, Germany), according to the manufacturer's protocols. Total RNA and miRNA fractions were extracted from whole BM samples using the PAXgene extraction Kit (Qiagen, Hilden, Germany), according to manufacturer's protocol. The quality of the RNA fractions was evaluated in the BioAnalyzer 2100 system (Agilent Technologies, Santa Clara, CA, USA).

2.4. MiRNA Microarray Analysis

MiRNA expression profiling was carried out by the Agilent platform following the miRNA Microarray protocol v.3.1.1 (Agilent Technologies, Santa Clara, CA, USA). Briefly, 50 ng of total RNA, containing miRNAs and spike-in controls, underwent dephosphorylation and a labeling step with Cyanine 3-pCp. The Cy3-labeled RNA was then purified using the Micro Bio-Spin P-6 Gel Column (Bio-Rad Laboratories, Inc., Hercules, CA, USA), and hybridized on human miRNA microarray slides 8 × 60 K (Agilent Technologies; including 2549 miRNAs, miRBase 21.0) at 55 °C for 20 hours. After washing, the slides were scanned by a G2565CA scanner (Agilent Technologies, Santa Clara, CA, USA), and the images were extracted by Feature Extraction software v.10 (Agilent Technologies, Santa Clara, CA, USA). Tab-delimited text files were analyzed in R v.2.7.2 software environment http://www.r-project.org using the limma package v.2.14.16 of Bioconductor http://www.bioconductor.org. Only spots with a signal minus background flagged as positive and significant were used in the following analysis as detected spots. Probes with less than 50% of detected spots across all arrays and arrays with a number of detected spots smaller than 50% of all spots on the array were removed. Background corrected intensities of replicated spots on each array were averaged. Data were then log2-transformed and normalized for between-array comparison using quantile normalization [16]. MicroRNAs with p-values < 0.05 were selected for further analysis. Given the explorative nature of this study, no correction for multiple testing was applied to the screening procedure aimed at selecting multiple sets of microRNAs for subsequent hierarchical clustering analyses. The agglomerative hierarchical clusters, used to detect similarity relationships in microRNA log2-transformed expressions, were computed by the Euclidean distance between single vectors and the Ward method [17].

2.5. Real Time PCR Analysis

Total RNA (10 ng) was reverse transcribed using miR-specific stem-loop RT primers (TaqMan MicroRNA Assays; Applied Biosystems, Thermo-Fisher, Waltam, MA, USA) and components of the High Capacity cDNA Reverse Transcription kit (Life Technologies, Carlsbad, CA, USA), according to the manufacturer's protocols. Expression levels of individual miRNAs were detected by subsequent RQ-PCR using TaqMan MicroRNA assays (Life Technologies, Carlsbad, CA, USA) and a Rotor Gene 3000 PCR System Corbett (Qiagen, Hilden, Germany) with standard thermal cycling conditions, in accordance with manufacturer recommendations. PCR reactions were performed in triplicate in final volumes of 30 µl, including inter-assay controls (IAC) to account for variations between runs. RT-PCR (TaqMan MicroRNA Assays; Applied Biosystems, Thermo-Fisher) was used to quantify the expression of has-miR-16, has-miR-15a, has-miR-19b, has-miR-26b, has-miR-27b, has-miR-29c, has-miR-34c, has-miR-126, has-miR-218, has-miR-338, and has-miR-497, according to the manufacturer's instructions. To normalize the data for quantifying miRNAs, the universal small nuclear RNU38B (RNU38B Assay ID 001004; Applied Biosystems, Thermo-Fisher, Waltam, MA, USA) as an endogenous control was used [18].

The delta–delta Ct method was employed to calculate the fold change. In brief, each 15 µL of the reaction system contained 0.15 µL of 100 mM dNTPs with dTTP, 1 µL of MultiScribe Reverse Transcriptase (50 U/µL), 1.5 µL of RT buffer (×10), 0.1 µL of RNase inhibitor (20 U/µL), 6.25 µL of nuclease-free water, 5 µL of small RNA, and 3 µL of RT primer. Small RNAs were quantified by a Qubit 3 fluorimeter (Life Technologies, Carlsbad,

CA, USA). Thermal cycling conditions were 30 min at 16 °C, 30 min at 42 °C, and 5 min at 85 °C. Each 20 µL of the reaction system for real-time quantitative PCR contained 1 µL of real-time primer, 1.33 µL of product from the RT reaction, 10 µL of TaqMan Universal PCR Master Mix, and 7.67 µL of nuclease-free water. The reactions were performed in triplicate on a Rotor Gene 3000 PCR System Corbett for 10 min at 95 °C, followed by 40 cycles of 15 s at 95 °C and 1 min at 60 °C. Along with the Cq values calculated automatically by the SDS software (threshold value = 0.2, baseline setting: cycles 3–15), raw fluorescence data (Rn values) were exported for further analyses.

2.6. Comparative Genomic Hybridization (CGH) Analysis

Array CGH analyses were performed using the Human Genome array-CGH 8 × 60 K Microarray (Agilent Technologies, Palo Alto, CA), with an average probe spacing of around 55 Kb.

The arrays were performed using Agilent Reference DNAs, analyzed with the Agilent Microarray Scanner Feature Extraction Software version 11.5, and Agilent Genomic Workbench 7.0.4.0 software using the ADM-2 algorithm. Genomic positions of the rearrangements refer to the public UCSC database GRCh37.

2.7. PCA Analysis

Principal components analysis (PCA) is a data display method for multivariate data.

Given a data set in which each sample is described by n variables, the PCA aims to find new directions and linear combinations of the original ones [19,20].

The first component (PC1) corresponds to the direction explaining the maximum variance, while PC2 is the direction, orthogonal to PC1, explaining the maximum variance not explained by PC1, and so on. The result of such a transformation is that a limited number of components is sufficient to explain the relevant part of the information.

The loadings are the coefficients of the linear combinations corresponding to the PCs. By plotting them in a loading plot, it is possible to understand the relationships among the variables in the multivariate space.

On the other side, the score plot (the scores being the coordinates of the samples in the new space defined by the PCs) allows the visualization of the location of samples in the space described by the PCs, making it possible to check similarities and differences among the samples.

The elaborations and the plots were carried out through the software CAT (Chemometric Agile Tool, www.gruppochemiometria.it) [21].

2.8. Statistical Analysis

Results were expressed as mean ± SEM from at least three independent experiments. The statistical significance of the parametric differences among the sets of experimental data was evaluated by one-way ANOVA and Dunnett's test for multiple comparisons. Statistical analysis of the mitotic index and reporter assays data was performed using the Fisher's exact test.

3. Results and Discussion

3.1. miRNA Expression Profiling of HTLA-230 and ER-HTLA Cells.

In order to identify the miRNAs involved in chemoresistance, miRNA microarray analyses were performed on HTLA-230 and ER-HTLA cells.

As shown in Figure 1, miRNAs were differently expressed when comparing these two cell populations. The scatter plot analysis showed that a total of 152 miRNAs changed their expression more than 1.5 fold, 41 being up-regulated and 111 down-regulated (Figure 1).

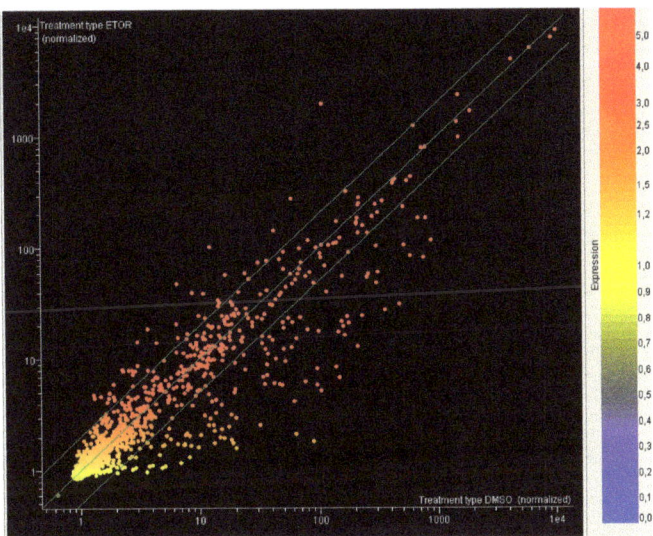

Figure 1. Scatter plot analysis reporting the variation of miRNA expression between HTLA-230 (horizontal axis) and ER-HTLA cells (vertical axis). Each dot represents one miRNA colored according to its level of expression. Green diagonal lines indicate the 1.5-fold variation interval.

Volcano plot analyses, considering threshold values of five-fold for fold variation and $p < 0.01$ for statistical significance, showed that a total of 35 miRNAs significantly changed their expression, three being up-regulated and 32 down-regulated. The list of these 35 miRNAs is available in the Supplementary Material (Table S1).

Given the mechanism of action of miRNAs in regulating gene expression, we focused our attention on the down-regulated ones, and, in order to restrict the number of miRNAs to be studied, from the literature we searched for miRNAs that had been specifically involved in NB biology and/or chemoresistance. Using this criterion, 11 miRNAs were selected (Table 1), and their expression was tested by RT-qPCR analysis.

Table 1. miRNAs differently expressed in HTLA-230 and ER-HTLA cell lines that are involved in NB biology and in general cancer chemoresistance.

miRNA	HTLA-230/ ER-HTLA Ratio	Expression in Neuroblastoma	Expression in Other Chemoresistant Cancers
miR-15a	11.38	Down-regulated in MYCN-amplified chemoresistant NB [13,22–24]	Down-regulated in Burkitt Lymphoma [25], pancreatic ductal adenocarcinoma [26], colorectal [27], and ovarian cancer [28]
miR-16	7.89	Down-regulated in MYCN-amplified NB [22,29] and in chemoresistant NB [13]	Down-regulated in cervical [30], breast [31,32] gastric [32,33], and lung [34] cancer, osteosarcoma [35], and mesothelioma [36]
miR-19b	7.75	Up-regulated in chemoresistant NB [37]	Down-regulated in breast [38] and colon [39] cancer and leukemia [40]
miR-26b	47.87	Not evaluated	Down-regulated in chemoresistant colorectal [41], gastric [42], laryngeal [43], and hepatocellular carcinoma [44,45] cancer and in glioma [46]

Table 1. Cont.

miRNA	HTLA-230/ ER-HTLA Ratio	Expression in Neuroblastoma	Expression in Other Chemoresistant Cancers
miR-27b	8.29	Down-regulated in NB [47]	Down-regulated in lung [48], breast [49], and gastric cancer [50]
miR-29c	9.27	Not evaluated	Down-regulated in ovarian [51], endometrial [52], gastric [53], and small cell lung [54] cancer, glioma [55,56], and leukemia [57,58]
miR-34c	7.49	Not evaluated	Down-regulated in colon [59], gastric [60,61], and ovarian [62,63] cancer, and osteosarcoma [64]
miR-126a	9.66	Not evaluated	Down-regulated in colorectal [65] and breast cancer [66] and in renal cell carcinoma [67]
miR-218	12.30	Up-regulated in MYCN-amplified and in metastatic NB [68–70]	Down-regulated in glioma cells [71], colorectal [72], gallbladder [73], bladder [74], and lung cancer [75,76]
miR-338	15.99	Down-regulated in resistant NB [77,78]	Down-regulated in esophageal squamous carcinoma cells [79]
miR-497	6.92	Down-regulated in chemoresistant NB [24], in MYCN-amplified NB [80]	Down-regulated in lung [81], colorectal [82], ovarian [83], and pancreatic [84] cancer, and lymphoma [85]

As shown in Figure 2, only six miRNAs (i.e., miR-15a, -16-1, -19b, -27b, -126, and -218) among the selected miRNAs were confirmed to be down-regulated in ER-HTLA cells in respect to HTLA-230 parental ones. In detail, miR-27b and miR-16-1 expression levels were found to be reduced by 33.1 and 23.5 fold, respectively, and miR-218 expression was diminished by 9.09 fold, while miR-15a, miR-126, and miR-19b were down-regulated (slightly, but significantly) by 2.8, 2.7, and 1.73 fold, respectively.

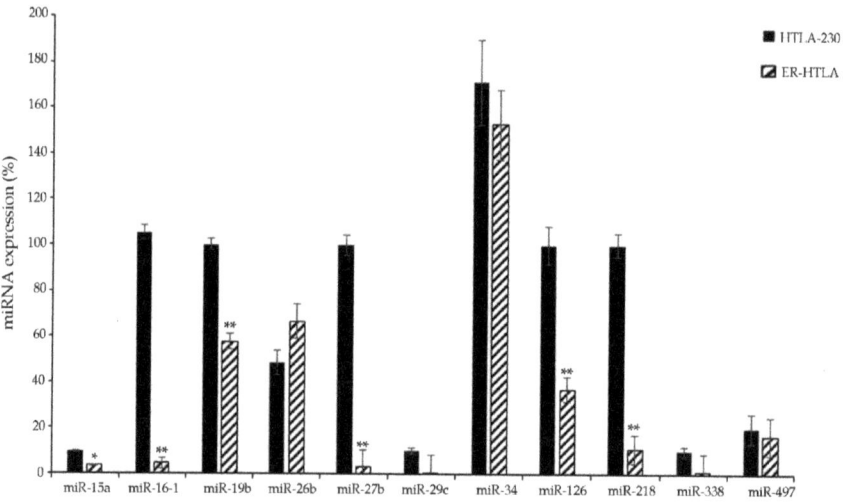

Figure 2. Evaluation of the expression level of the 11 selected miRNAs (Table 1) in HTLA-230 and ER-HTLA cell lines by RT-qPCR analysis. Data is reported as % variation vs. the universal small nuclear RNU38B. * $p < 0.05$ vs. HTLA-230 ** $p < 0.01$ vs. HTLA-230.

For the first time, to our knowledge, this data confers a possible role in NB chemoresistance to miR-27 and miR-218. In fact, despite their expression being found to be downregulated in several chemoresistant cancers (see Table 1) [48–50,71–75], their involvement in chemoresistance of NB has never been reported in the literature. Notably, although miRNA-218 was found to be up-regulated in *MYCN*-amplified and metastatic NB [68–70], this data is not in contradiction with the down-regulation of miRNA-218 that we have observed after chronic Etoposide exposure of *MYCN*-amplified NB cells (ER-HTLA).

In addition, these results confirm the down-regulation of miR-15 and miR-16 in ER-HTLA cells, as found in our previous study [13]. Moreover, for the first time, miR-19b expression was found to be reduced in chemoresistant NB in conformity with other malignancies (Table 1) [38–40]. In fact, only one study has reported an up-regulation of miR-19b in chemoresistant NB cells [37]. This discrepancy could be due to the fact that, in this same study, NB cells were exposed to the drug for only 24 hours while, in our present study, the ER-HTLA cells were selected by chronically treating parental cells (HTLA-230) with Etoposide for six months (i.e., a condition that better mimics in vivo treatment).

3.2. Comparative Genomic Hybridization (CGH) on HTLA-230 and ER-HTLA Cells

Since both genetic and epigenetic mechanisms have been demonstrated to influence NB biology [86], in order to better characterize the chemoresistant phenotype, CGH analysis was performed. DNAs from HTLA-230 and ER-HTLA cells were hybridized to obtain a comparison of gains and losses that could be connected to the acquisition of chemoresistance. As reported in Table 2, an intriguing finding was the presence of several alterations in chromosome 13, where miR-15a, miR-16-1, and miR-19b were mapped, and, in chromosome 17, where miR-338 was localized.

Table 2. CGH analysis on HTLA-ER cells in comparison to HTLA-230 cells.

CHR	START	STOP	CYTO	SIZE KB	VALUE	Control (HTLA-230)
1	152,079,488	155,154,990	q21.3–q22	3.075	1.5	Absent
3	73,792,065	75,028,724	p13–p12.3	1.236	−0.7	Absent
5	20,160,410	44,924,503	p14.3–p12	24.764	−0.7	Absent
8	112,697,432	146,280,020	q23.3–q24.3	33.582	−1/−0.4	Duplicated
9	204,193	38,815,475	p24.3–p13.1	38.611	−0.7/−3	Absent
10	43,020,732	60,914,512	q11.21–q21.1	17.893	−0.7/−1.2	Duplicated
12	38,805,636	48,103,580	q12–q13.11	9.297	0.7/0.4/1.4	Absent
13	20,412,619	39,841,779	q12.11–q13.3	19.429	0.3/0.6	Absent
13	39,900,189	86,110,407	q13.3–q31.1	46.210	−0.5	Absent
13	86,151,801	111,106,213	q31.1–q34	24.954	0.5	Absent
13	111,181,035	113,538,619	q34	2.357	−0.8	Absent
13	113,610,612	115,092,648	q34	1.482	0.4	Absent
17	44,684	625,475	p13.3	580	−0.7	Absent
17	25,654,874	40,109,636	q11.1–q21.2	14.454	−0.7/−1.2	Duplicated
19	32,783,771	36,293,337	q13.11–q13.12	3.509	−0.6	Duplicated
20	60,747	19,483,849	p13–p11.23	19.423	0.5	Deleted or mosaic
21	15,538,980	32,776,404	q11.2–q22.11	17.237	−0.6	Absent

Moreover, our data, identifying some chromosomal regions that are more frequently altered in ER-HTLA cells, is in line with the results obtained in a previous paper reporting a gain of 13q14.1-32 and a loss of 17q in other NB chemoresistant cell lines [87]. Since these chromosome traits (e.g., chromosome 13) contain the locus in which miRNAs, involved in the acquisition of Etoposide resistance, are mapped, it is possible to hypothesize that the evaluation of these miRNAs in patient samples might be used as prognostic markers that are able to early identify chemoresistant signatures.

3.3. miRNA Expression Profiling of Therapy-Sensitive (Responder) and Therapy-Resistant (Non-Responder) NB Patients

In order to evaluate in vivo the expression of miRNAs and their potential role in NB chemoresistance, ten whole BM samples, taken at diagnosis from NB patients either sensitive (responder) or resistant (non-responder) to induction therapy, were randomly selected from our biobank, and six miRNAs from Table 1 (i.e., miR-15a, -16-1, 19b, -27b, -126, and -218) were analyzed. NB patient characteristics are reported in Table 3.

Table 3. NB characteristics and patient clinical outcomes.

N	MYCN Status	Age (Months)	EFS (Months)	OS (Months)	INRG Stage	Induction Response	Relapse	Follow-Up
2	Amplified	55	71.25	71.25	M	Yes	No	Alive
3	Not evaluated	41	81.06	81.06	M	Yes	No	Alive
4	Single copy	12	60.53	60.53	M	Yes	No	Alive
6	Amplified	62	50.83	50.83	M	Yes	No	Alive
9	Amplified	21	55.38	55.38	M	Yes	No	Alive
1	Amplified	17	6.86	7.10	M	No	Yes	Dead
5	Single copy	47	22.94	26.17	M	No	Yes	Dead
7	Amplified	20	9.54	19.27	M	No	Yes	Dead
8	Amplified	21	5.54	7.00	M	No	Yes	Dead
10	Amplified	16	4.69	8.98	M	No	Yes	Dead

EFS, event-free survival; OS, overall survival; INRG, International Neuroblastoma Risk Group.

By comparing the expression of miRNAs in therapy-sensitive and therapy-resistant NB patients, only miR-16 was significantly down-regulated in the bone marrow of non-responder patients (Figure 3), while the other miRNAs analyzed were not significantly modified, even though a slight trend of reduction in non-responder patients was observed.

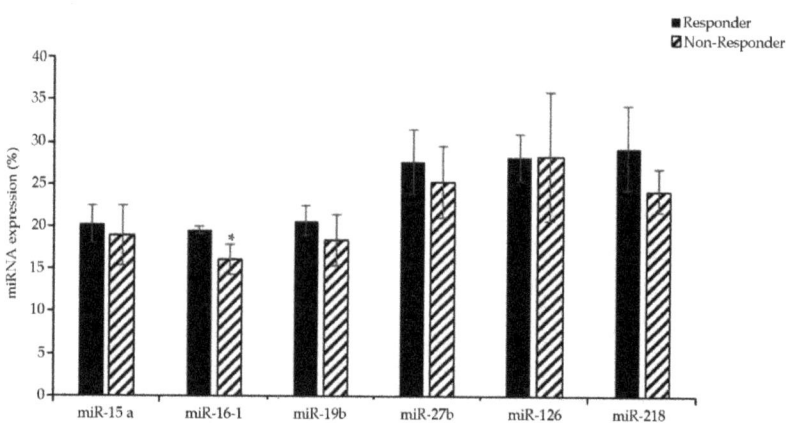

Figure 3. Evaluation of the expression levels of selected miRNAs in the bone marrow of patients sensitive (responder) or resistant (non-responder) to therapy by RT-qPCR analysis. Data is reported as % variation vs. the universal small nuclear RNU38B. * $p < 0.05$ vs. responder.

These findings, while confirming a potential role of miR-16 in delivering intrinsic chemoresistance of NB, do not confirm the other results obtained from ER-HTLA cells. However, this is not unusual when comparing in vitro with in vivo data, most likely due to the variability found in individual patients. Nevertheless, it should be noted that the content of NB cells in the BM samples ranged from 5% to 35%, making the normal hematopoietic cells prevalent, and thus potentially masking miRNA down-regulation occurring in neoplastic cells.

3.4. miRNA Expression Profiling of NB Primary Tumors and Metastases

Therefore, in order to better understand the role that these miRNAs could possibly have in NB biology, their expression was tested in ten primary tumors and ten immune-magnetically-enriched NB metastases from stage M NB patients, randomly selected from our biobank. The NB patients' features of this new set of samples are reported in Table 4. Since it has been recently reported [13] and herein confirmed that ER-HTLA cells have a monoallelic deletion of the 13q14.3 locus, which maps for miR-15/16, particular attention was given to those miRNAs whose locus was found mutated. The analysis was also extended to miR-338 and miR-218, even though the corresponding locus had not been altered, because their expression has been demonstrated to be strictly related to NB chemoresistance [77,78] and to Etoposide refractoriness [76].

Table 4. Features of NB primary tumors and metastases and patients' clinical outcomes.

	N	MYCN Status	Age (Years)	EFS (Months)	OS (Months)
Tumors	1	Amplified	1.99	46.2	84.8
	2	Not amplified	3.18	5.3	9.3
	3	Not amplified	1.27	187.2	187.2
	4	Amplified	1.13	4.3	7.4
	5	Amplified	3.88	70.0	114.5
	6	Amplified	6.30	36.2	47.7
	7	Amplified	2.07	3.2	10.3
	8	Amplified	4.76	114,9	114,9
	9	Amplified	4.57	21.7	22.4
	10	Amplified	1.44	26.8	33.0
Metastases	11	Not amplified	1.68	58.88	58.88
	12	Not amplified	3	24.52	35.98
	13	Amplified	6.8	8.68	42.41
	14	Amplified	0.9	11.06	11.06
	15	Not amplified	2.55	70.73	70.73
	16	Not amplified	3.34	13,3	21.22
	17	Amplified	8.2	8.61	8.61
	18	Amplified	1.67	9.6	14.98
	19	Amplified	6.89	29.04	29.04
	20	Amplified	1.7	13.3	23

EFS, event-free survival; OS, overall survival.

As reported in Figure 4, miRNA-19b, -218, and -338 were down-regulated in *MYCN*-amplified metastases by about 30% as compared to *MYCN*-amplified tumors, while no significant changes were observed in the expression of the other miRNAs. It is interesting to note that the *MYCN* status did not influence the expression of these latter miRNAs, neither in tumors nor in metastases (Figure 4).

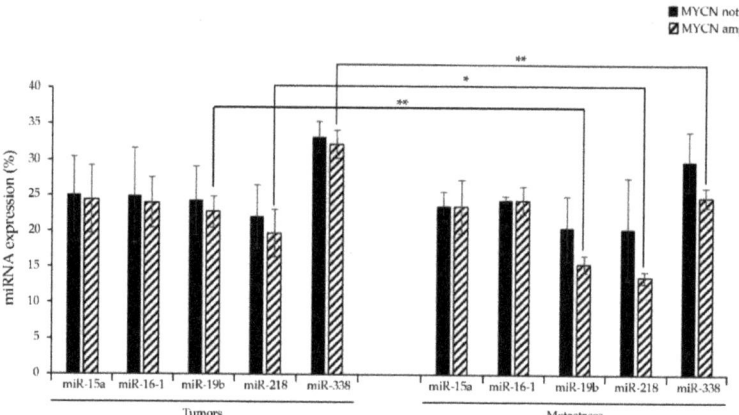

Figure 4. RT-qPCR analysis of the selected miRNA expression levels in tumors and metastases samples of NB patients. Data is reported as % variation vs. the universal small nuclear RNU38B. * $p < 0.05$ vs. MYCN-amplified tumors; ** $p < 0.01$ vs. MYCN-amplified tumors.

miR-338 down-regulation in NB metastases has been previously reported by Chen et al., who demonstrated that this miRNA could exert an inhibitory role on the migration, proliferation, and invasion of NB cells through the modulation of the PTEN/Akt pathway [77]. However, while miR-19b expression has been found to be reduced in metastatic clear renal cell carcinoma [88] and miR-218 expression down-regulated in metastatic prostate [89], breast [90], gastric [91], cervical [92], and lung [93] cancer, to our knowledge, this is the first time that a down-regulation of miR-19b has been detected in metastatic NB in vivo. In addition, miRNA-218 has also been found to be down-regulated in NB metastases. This result obtained from analyses of patients' tissues is in contrast with previous studies reporting an up-regulation of this miRNA [70] in patients' serum, but this discrepancy could be due to the different nature of the analyzed samples. In fact, it is conceivable that the increased levels of miRNA-218 in the serum might be due to a response of peritumoral tissue, and not originating from the tumor.

3.5. Principal Component Analysis (PCA) of the Results Obtained in Patients' Samples

In order to better extract the information from the dataset about NB biology and chemoresistance, principal component analysis (PCA) was carried out by collecting miRNA expression profiles analyzed in bone marrows infiltrates, tumors, and metastases. The first PCA has been performed on responder (four) and non-responder (four) patients' samples. The loading plot showed that all of the variables had similar positive loadings on PC1, meaning that the score on PC1 can be considered as a global quantitative index. On the other hand, PC2 mainly explains the contrast between miR-15, miR-218, and -16 variables (Figure 5, left panel). By analyzing the score plot, although only a few subjects were available, it was possible to observe that all of the responder patients' samples (red) were well-separated from the non-responders (black) and located in a specific region in the PC space: compared to the non-responders, all of the responders were mainly characterized by higher values of the variables miR-218 and miR-16 (Figure 5, right panel).

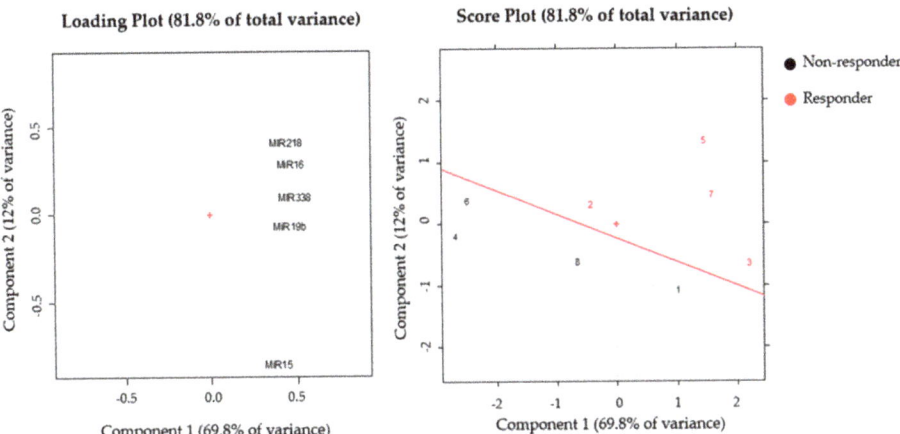

Figure 5. PCA performed on responder and non-responder patients' samples. The loading (left panel) and the score plot (right panel) were reported. In the score plot, the samples were indicated by the number reported in Table 3. + represents the point with coordinates 0 and 0 for x and y axes, respectively. This points is the reference to define the multivariate space.

Furthermore, a second PCA was carried out on tumor and metastasized patients' samples. The loading plot showed correlations between the variables miR-19b, -218, and -338, all characterized by negative loadings on PC1 (group 1), and between miR-15 and -16, which had positive loadings on PC2 (group 2). The two groups of correlated variables were uncorrelated, since their directions from the origin were orthogonal (Figure 6, left panel). The score plot showed that the metastasized patients' samples were characterized by intermediate values of the variables miR-15 and -16. On the other hand, the majority of the non-metastasized patients' samples had extreme values of both variables miR-15 and -16 (Figure 6, right panel).

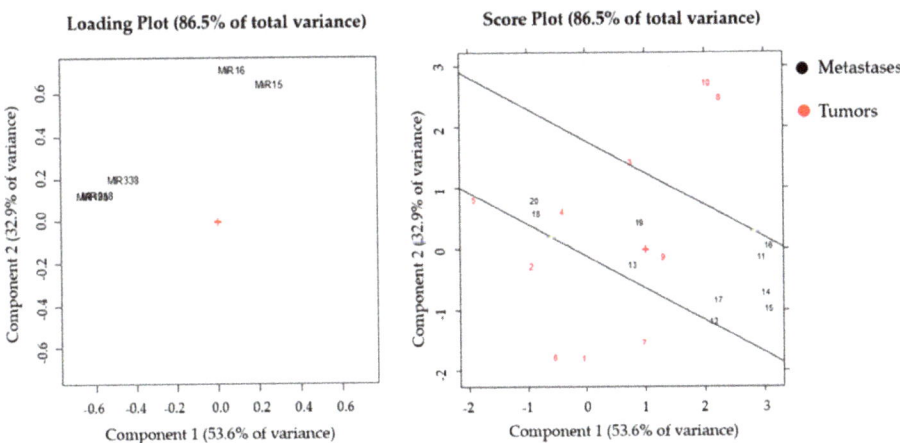

Figure 6. PCA performed on tumors and metastases samples. The loading (left panel) and the score plot (right panel) were reported. In the score plot, the samples were indicated by the number reported in Table 4. + represents the point with coordinates 0 and 0 for x and y axes, respectively. This points is the reference to define the multivariate space.

4. Conclusions

The presence of chemoresistant cells in the primary tumor and within bone marrow is the most powerful negative prognostic factor for patients with NB. The acquisition of chemoresistance and the ability to metastasize are the results of genetic and epigenetic mechanisms and, among them, miRNAs can play a crucial role [94]. In fact, their expression is frequently de-regulated in several chemoresistant malignancies and, as supported by the results herein, in NB. Indeed, the evaluation of miRNA expression could have a double value. In fact, on the one hand, the modulation of a specific miRNA or of a cluster of miRNAs could be used as a prognostic and predictive factor advantageous for monitoring the acquisition of chemoresistance. On the other hand, miRNAs might also have therapeutic potential, since many current studies are focused on discovering the best mechanism that is able to restore the expression of miRNAs in oncologic patients [95]. In the present study, our findings demonstrate, for the first time, that the down-regulation of miR-16-1 is strictly related to the acquisition of NB chemoresistance. In fact, among the six miRNAs whose expression is found down-regulated in our in vitro model of Etoposide resistance, only miR-16-1 is significantly down-regulated in non-responder NB patients treated with the induction therapy comprised of Etoposide (Figure 7). This data suggests that the restoration of miR-16 could be a valid strategy to counteract chemoresistance (Figure 7).

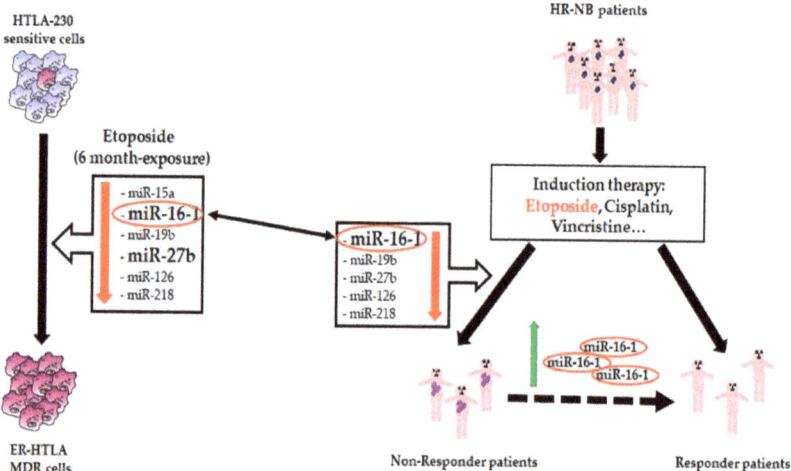

Figure 7. Role of miR-16-1 in NB chemoresistance. The acquisition of chemoresistance in multidrug resistant (MDR) cells and in high-risk (HR) patients is characterized by miR-16-1 down-regulation, suggesting a potential role of miR-16-1 as a chemosensitizer.

In addition, miR-19b, miR-338, and partially miR-218, whose down-regulation correlates with the metastatic process, could have prognostic value as biomarkers of NB progression.

Supplementary Materials: The following are available online at https://www.mdpi.com/2075-4426/11/2/107/s1, Table S1: miRNAs differently expressed in HTLA-230 and ER-HTLA cells.

Author Contributions: Conceptualization, B.M., A.P., M.V.C., A.I., and C.D.; methodology, B.M., A.P., and M.V.C.; validation, G.F., P.M., P.M., and A.S.; formal analysis, B.M., A.P., R.L., and E.F.; investigation, B.M., A.P., M.V.C., L.M., G.E.V., P.P., and F.M.; resources, B.M., A.P., A.I., and C.D.; data curation, B.M., A.P., A.I., and C.D.; writing—original draft preparation, B.M., A.P., M.V.C., G.F., P.M. (Paola Menichini), and P.M. (Paola Monti); writing—review and editing, B.M., A.I., and C.D.; visualization, B.M., A.P., M.V.C., and F.M.; supervision, B.M. and C.D.; project administration, B.M., A.I., and C.D.; funding acquisition, B.M. and C.D. All authors have read and agreed to the published version of the manuscript.

Funding: This research was supported by the University of Genoa and by the Italian Association for Cancer research (AIRC) IG-2017 Id.20699.

Institutional Review Board Statement: The study was approved by the Gaslini Institute Ethical Committee and all analyses were performed according to the Declaration of Helsinki.

Informed Consent Statement: Informed consent was obtained from all subjects involved in the study.

Data Availability Statement: Data are available upon request from the corresponding author. Data are not publicly available due to patients' privacy.

Acknowledgments: We would like to thank Giuseppe Catalano (DIMES-University of Genoa) for his technical assistance and Suzanne Patten for her language editing.

Conflicts of Interest: The authors declare no conflict of interest.

References

1. Maris, J.M. Recent advances in neuroblastoma. *N. Engl. J. Med.* **2010**, *362*, 2202–2211. [CrossRef] [PubMed]
2. Brodeur, G.M. Neuroblastoma: Biological insights into a clinical enigma. *Nat. Rev. Cancer* **2003**, *3*, 203–216. [CrossRef] [PubMed]
3. Pinto, N.R.; Applebaum, M.A.; Volchenboum, S.L.; Matthay, K.K.; London, W.B.; Ambros, P.F.; Nakagawara, A.; Berthold, F.; Schleiermacher, G.; Park, J.R.; et al. Advances in Risk Classification and Treatment Strategies for Neuroblastoma. *J. Clin. Oncol.* **2015**, *33*, 3008–3017. [CrossRef]
4. Hochheuser, C.; van Zogchel, L.M.J.; Kleijer, M.; Kuijk, C.; Tol, S.; van der Schoot, C.E.; Voermans, C.; Tytgat, G.A.M.; Timmerman, I. The Metastatic Bone Marrow Niche in Neuroblastoma: Altered Phenotype and Function of Mesenchymal Stromal Cells. *Cancers* **2020**, *12*, 3231. [CrossRef]
5. Seeger, R.C.; Reynolds, C.P.; Gallego, R.; Stram, D.O.; Gerbing, R.B.; Matthay, K.K. Quantitative tumor cell content of bone marrow and blood as a predictor of outcome in stage IV neuroblastoma: A Children's Cancer Group Study. *J. Clin. Oncol.* **2000**, *18*, 4067–4076. [CrossRef] [PubMed]
6. Cai, J.Y.; Pan, C.; Tang, Y.J.; Chen, J.; Ye, Q.D.; Zhou, M.; Xue, H.; Tang, J.Y. Minimal residual disease is a prognostic marker for neuroblastoma with bone marrow infiltration. *Am. J. Clin. Oncol.* **2012**, *35*, 275–278. [CrossRef]
7. Stallings, R.L. Are chromosomal imbalances important in cancer? *Trends Genet.* **2007**, *23*, 278–283. [CrossRef]
8. Brodeur, G.M.; Seeger, R.C.; Schwab, M.; Varmus, H.E.; Bishop, J.M. Amplification of N-myc in untreated human neuroblastomas correlates with advanced disease stage. *Science* **1984**, *224*, 1121–1124. [CrossRef]
9. Lin, R.J.; Lin, Y.C.; Chen, J.; Kuo, H.H.; Chen, Y.Y.; Diccianni, M.B.; London, W.B.; Chang, C.H.; Yu, A.L. microRNA signature and expression of Dicer and Drosha can predict prognosis and delineate risk groups in neuroblastoma. *Cancer Res.* **2010**, *70*, 7841–7850. [CrossRef] [PubMed]
10. Schulte, J.H.; Schowe, B.; Mestdagh, P.; Kaderali, L.; Kalaghatgi, P.; Schlierf, S.; Vermeulen, J.; Brockmeyer, B.; Pajtler, K.; Thor, T.; et al. Accurate prediction of neuroblastoma outcome based on miRNA expression profiles. *Int. J. Cancer* **2010**, *127*, 2374–2385. [CrossRef]
11. Mohammadi, M.; Goodarzi, M.; Jaafari, M.R.; Mirzaei, H.R.; Mirzaei, H. Circulating microRNA: A new candidate for diagnostic biomarker in neuroblastoma. *Cancer Gene Ther.* **2016**, *23*, 371–372. [CrossRef]
12. Colla, R.; Izzotti, A.; De Ciucis, C.; Fenoglio, D.; Ravera, S.; Speciale, A.; Ricciarelli, R.; Furfaro, A.L.; Pulliero, A.; Passalacqua, M.; et al. Glutathione-mediated antioxidant response and aerobic metabolism: Two crucial factors involved in determining the multi-drug resistance of high-risk neuroblastoma. *Oncotarget* **2016**, *7*, 70715–70737. [CrossRef] [PubMed]
13. Marengo, B.; Monti, P.; Miele, M.; Menichini, P.; Ottaggio, L.; Foggetti, G.; Pulliero, A.; Izzotti, A.; Speciale, A.; Garbarino, O.; et al. Etoposide-resistance in a neuroblastoma model cell line is associated with 13q14.3 mono-allelic deletion and miRNA-15a/16-1 down-regulation. *Sci. Rep.* **2018**, *8*, 13762. [CrossRef] [PubMed]
14. Scaruffi, P.; Morandi, F.; Gallo, F.; Stigliani, S.; Parodi, S.; Moretti, S.; Bonassi, S.; Fardin, P.; Garaventa, A.; Zanazzo, G.; et al. Bone marrow of neuroblastoma patients shows downregulation of CXCL12 expression and presence of IFN signature. *Pediatr. Blood Cancer* **2012**, *59*, 44–51. [CrossRef]
15. Morandi, F.; Scaruffi, P.; Gallo, F.; Stigliani, S.; Moretti, S.; Bonassi, S.; Gambini, C.; Mazzocco, K.; Fardin, P.; Haupt, R.; et al. Bone marrow-infiltrating human neuroblastoma cells express high levels of calprotectin and HLA-G proteins. *PLoS ONE* **2012**, *7*, e29922. [CrossRef] [PubMed]
16. Stracquadanio, M.; Dinelli, E.; Trombini, C. Role of volcanic dust in the atmospheric transport and deposition of polycyclic aromatic hydrocarbons and mercury. *J. Environ. Monit.* **2003**, *5*, 984–988. [CrossRef]
17. Alexandrov, K.; Rojas, M.; Geneste, O.; Castegnaro, M.; Camus, A.M.; Petruzzelli, S.; Giuntini, C.; Bartsch, H. An improved fluorometric assay for dosimetry of benzo(a)pyrene diol-epoxide-DNA adducts in smokers' lung: Comparisons with total bulky adducts and aryl hydrocarbon hydroxylase activity. *Cancer Res.* **1992**, *52*, 6248–6253.

18. Torres, A.; Torres, K.; Wdowiak, P.; Paszkowski, T.; Maciejewski, R. Selection and validation of endogenous controls for microRNA expression studies in endometrioid endometrial cancer tissues. *Gynecol. Oncol.* **2013**, *130*, 588–594. [CrossRef]
19. Davies, T.; Fearn, T. *Back to Basics: The Principles of Principal Component Analysis*; Spectroscopy Europe: Charlston, Chichester, UK, 2004; p. 20.
20. Leardi, R. Chemometric methods in food authentication. In *Modern Techniques for Food Authentication*, 2nd ed.; Elsevier: Amsterdam, The Netherlands, 2018; pp. 687–729.
21. Leardi, R.; Melzi, C.; Polotti, G. CAT (Chemometric Agile Software). Available online: http://gruppochemiometria.it/index.php/software (accessed on 18 December 2020).
22. Chava, S.; Reynolds, C.P.; Pathania, A.S.; Gorantla, S.; Poluektova, L.Y.; Coulter, D.W.; Gupta, S.C.; Pandey, M.K.; Challagundla, K.B. miR-15a-5p, miR-15b-5p, and miR-16-5p inhibit tumor progression by directly targeting MYCN in neuroblastoma. *Mol. Oncol.* **2020**, *14*, 180–196. [CrossRef]
23. Pouliot, L.M.; Chen, Y.C.; Bai, J.; Guha, R.; Martin, S.E.; Gottesman, M.M.; Hall, M.D. Cisplatin sensitivity mediated by WEE1 and CHK1 is mediated by miR-155 and the miR-15 family. *Cancer Res.* **2012**, *72*, 5945–5955. [CrossRef] [PubMed]
24. Soriano, A.; París-Coderch, L.; Jubierre, L.; Martínez, A.; Zhou, X.; Piskareva, O.; Bray, I.; Vidal, I.; Almazán-Moga, A.; Molist, C.; et al. MicroRNA-497 impairs the growth of chemoresistant neuroblastoma cells by targeting cell cycle, survival and vascular permeability genes. *Oncotarget* **2016**, *7*, 9271–9287. [CrossRef] [PubMed]
25. Guo, C.; Gong, M.; Li, Z. Knockdown of lncRNA MCM3AP-AS1 Attenuates Chemoresistance of Burkitt Lymphoma to Doxorubicin Treatment via Targeting the miR-15a/EIF4E Axis. *Cancer Manag. Res.* **2020**, *12*, 5845–5855. [CrossRef] [PubMed]
26. Guo, S.; Fesler, A.; Huang, W.; Wang, Y.; Yang, J.; Wang, X.; Zheng, Y.; Hwang, G.R.; Wang, H.; Ju, J. Functional Significance and Therapeutic Potential of miR-15a Mimic in Pancreatic Ductal Adenocarcinoma. *Mol. Ther. Nucleic Acids* **2020**, *19*, 228–239. [CrossRef] [PubMed]
27. Fesler, A.; Liu, H.; Ju, J. Modified miR-15a has therapeutic potential for improving treatment of advanced stage colorectal cancer through inhibition of BCL2, BMI1, YAP1 and DCLK1. *Oncotarget* **2017**, *9*, 2367–2383. [CrossRef]
28. Dwivedi, S.K.; Mustafi, S.B.; Mangala, L.S.; Jiang, D.; Pradeep, S.; Rodriguez-Aguayo, C.; Ling, H.; Ivan, C.; Mukherjee, P.; Calin, G.A.; et al. Therapeutic evaluation of microRNA-15a and microRNA-16 in ovarian cancer. *Oncotarget* **2016**, *7*, 15093–15104. [CrossRef]
29. Zhang, X.; Zhang, J.; Liu, Q.; Zhao, Y.; Zhang, W.; Yang, H. Circ-CUX1 Accelerates the Progression of Neuroblastoma via miR-16-5p/DMRT2 Axis. *Neurochem. Res.* **2020**, *45*, 2840–2855. [CrossRef]
30. Zhao, Z.; Ji, M.; Wang, Q.; He, N.; Li, Y. miR-16-5p/PDK4-Mediated Metabolic Reprogramming Is Involved in Chemoresistance of Cervical Cancer. *Mol. Ther. Oncolytics* **2020**, *17*, 509–517. [CrossRef]
31. Patel, N.; Garikapati, K.R.; Pandita, R.K.; Singh, D.K.; Pandita, T.K.; Bhadra, U.; Bhadra, M.P. miR-15a/miR-16 down-regulates BMI1, impacting Ub-H2A mediated DNA repair and breast cancer cell sensitivity to doxorubicin. *Sci. Rep.* **2017**, *7*, 4263. [CrossRef] [PubMed]
32. Venturutti, L.; Russo, R.I.C.; Rivas, M.A.; Mercogliano, M.F.; Izzo, F.; Oakley, R.H.; Pereyra, M.G.; De Martino, M.; Proietti, C.J.; Yankilevich, P.; et al. MiR-16 mediates trastuzumab and lapatinib response in ErbB-2-positive breast and gastric cancer via its novel targets CCNJ and FUBP1. *Oncogene* **2016**, *35*, 6189–6202. [CrossRef]
33. Xia, L.; Zhang, D.; Du, R.; Pan, Y.; Zhao, L.; Sun, S.; Hong, L.; Liu, J.; Fan, D. miR-15b and miR-16 modulate multidrug resistance by targeting BCL2 in human gastric cancer cells. *Int. J. Cancer* **2008**, *123*, 372–379. [CrossRef]
34. Chatterjee, A.; Chattopadhyay, D.; Chakrabarti, G. MiR-16 targets Bcl-2 in paclitaxel-resistant lung cancer cells and overexpression of miR-16 along with miR-17 causes unprecedented sensitivity by simultaneously modulating autophagy and apoptosis. *Cell. Signal.* **2015**, *27*, 189–203. [CrossRef]
35. Liu, Y.; Gu, S.; Li, H.; Wang, J.; Wei, C.; Liu, Q. SNHG16 promotes osteosarcoma progression and enhances cisplatin resistance by sponging miR-16 to upregulate ATG4B expression. *Biochem. Biophys. Res. Commun.* **2019**, *518*, 127–133. [CrossRef]
36. Fennell, D. miR-16: Expanding the range of molecular targets in mesothelioma. *Lancet Oncol.* **2017**, *18*, 1296–1297. [CrossRef]
37. Chen, Y.; Tsai, Y.H.; Tseng, B.J.; Pan, H.Y.; Tseng, S.H. Suppression of miR-19b enhanced the cytotoxic effects of mTOR inhibitors in human neuroblastoma cells. *J. Pediatr. Surg.* **2016**, *51*, 1818–1825. [CrossRef]
38. Thorne, J.L.; Battaglia, S.; Baxter, D.E.; Hayes, J.L.; Hutchinson, S.A.; Jana, S.; Millican-Slater, R.A.; Smith, L.; Teske, M.C.; Wastall, L.M.; et al. MiR-19b non-canonical binding is directed by HuR and confers chemosensitivity through regulation of P-glycoprotein in breast cancer. *Biochim. Biophys. Acta Gene Regul. Mech.* **2018**, *1861*, 996–1006. [CrossRef]
39. Jiang, T.; Ye, L.; Han, Z.; Liu, Y.; Yang, Y.; Peng, Z.; Fan, J. miR-19b-3p promotes colon cancer proliferation and oxaliplatin-based chemoresistance by targeting SMAD4: Validation by bioinformatics and experimental analyses. *J. Exp. Clin. Cancer Res.* **2017**, *36*, 131. [CrossRef] [PubMed]
40. Bouvy, C.; Wannez, A.; Laloy, J.; Chatelain, C.; Dogné, J.M. Transfer of multidrug resistance among acute myeloid leukemia cells via extracellular vesicles and their microRNA cargo. *Leuk. Res.* **2017**, *62*, 70–76. [CrossRef] [PubMed]
41. Wang, B.; Lu, F.Y.; Shi, R.H.; Feng, Y.D.; Zhao, X.D.; Lu, Z.P.; Xiao, L.; Zhou, G.Q.; Qiu, J.M.; Cheng, C.E. MiR-26b regulates 5-FU-resistance in human colorectal cancer via down-regulation of Pgp. *Am. J. Cancer Res.* **2018**, *8*, 2518–2527.
42. Zhao, B.; Zhang, J.; Chen, X.; Xu, H.; Huang, B. Mir-26b inhibits growth and resistance to paclitaxel chemotherapy by silencing the CDC6 gene in gastric cancer. *Arch. Med. Sci.* **2019**, *15*, 498–503. [CrossRef]

43. Tian, L.; Zhang, J.; Ren, X.; Liu, X.; Gao, W.; Zhang, C.; Sun, Y.; Liu, M. Overexpression of miR-26b decreases the cisplatin-esistance in laryngeal cancer by targeting ATF2. *Oncotarget* **2017**, *8*, 79023–79033. [CrossRef]
44. Jin, F.; Wang, Y.; Li, M.; Zhu, Y.; Liang, H.; Wang, C.; Wang, F.; Zhang, C.Y.; Zen, K.; Li, L. MiR-26 enhances chemosensitivity and promotes apoptosis of hepatocellular carcinoma cells through inhibiting autophagy. *Cell Death Dis.* **2017**, *8*, e2540. [CrossRef]
45. Zhao, N.; Wang, R.; Zhou, L.; Zhu, Y.; Gong, J.; Zhuang, S.M. MicroRNA-26b suppresses the NF-κB signaling and enhances the chemosensitivity of hepatocellular carcinoma cells by targeting TAK1 and TAB3. *Mol. Cancer* **2014**, *13*, 35. [CrossRef]
46. Wang, L.; Su, J.; Zhao, Z.; Hou, Y.; Yin, X.; Zheng, N.; Zhou, X.; Yan, J.; Xia, J.; Wang, Z. MiR-26b reverses temozolomide resistance via targeting Wee1 in glioma cells. *Cell Cycle* **2017**, *16*, 1954–1964. [CrossRef] [PubMed]
47. Lee, J.J.; Drakaki, A.; Iliopoulos, D.; Struhl, K. MiR-27b targets PPARγ to inhibit growth, tumor progression and the inflammatory response in neuroblastoma cells. *Oncogene* **2012**, *31*, 3818–3825. [CrossRef]
48. Zhang, J.; Hua, X.; Qi, N.; Han, G.; Yu, J.; Yu, Y.; Wei, X.; Li, H.; Chen, X.; Leng, C.; et al. MiR-27b suppresses epithelial-mesenchymal transition and chemoresistance in lung cancer by targeting Snail1. *Life Sci.* **2020**, *254*, 117238. [CrossRef]
49. Chen, D.; Si, W.; Shen, J.; Du, C.; Lou, W.; Bao, C.; Zheng, H.; Pan, J.; Zhong, G.; Xu, L.; et al. miR-27b-3p inhibits proliferation and potentially reverses multi-chemoresistance by targeting CBLB/GRB2 in breast cancer cells. *Cell Death Dis.* **2018**, *9*, 188. [CrossRef]
50. Shang, Y.; Feng, B.; Zhou, L.; Ren, G.; Zhang, Z.; Fan, X.; Sun, Y.; Luo, G.; Liang, J.; Wu, K.; et al. The miR27b-CCNG1-P53-miR-508-5p axis regulates multidrug resistance of gastric cancer. *Oncotarget* **2016**, *7*, 538–549. [CrossRef]
51. Hu, Z.; Cai, M.; Zhang, Y.; Tao, L.; Guo, R. miR-29c-3p inhibits autophagy and cisplatin resistance in ovarian cancer by regulating FOXP1/ATG14 pathway. *Cell Cycle* **2020**, *19*, 193–206. [CrossRef] [PubMed]
52. Li, L.; Shou, H.; Wang, Q.; Liu, S. Investigation of the potential theranostic role of KDM5B/miR-29c signaling axis in paclitaxel resistant endometrial carcinoma. *Gene* **2019**, *694*, 76–82. [CrossRef] [PubMed]
53. Wang, L.; Yu, T.; Li, W.; Li, M.; Zuo, Q.; Zou, Q.; Xiao, B. The miR-29c-KIAA1199 axis regulates gastric cancer migration by binding with WBP11 and PTP4A3. *Oncogene* **2019**, *38*, 3134–3150. [CrossRef] [PubMed]
54. Sun, D.M.; Tang, B.F.; Li, Z.X.; Guo, H.B.; Cheng, J.L.; Song, P.P.; Zhao, X. MiR-29c reduces the cisplatin resistance of non-small cell lung cancer cells by negatively regulating the PI3K/Akt pathway. *Sci. Rep.* **2018**, *8*, 8007. [CrossRef] [PubMed]
55. Xiao, S.; Yang, Z.; Qiu, X.; Lv, R.; Liu, J.; Wu, M.; Liao, Y.; Liu, Q. miR-29c contribute to glioma cells temozolomide sensitivity by targeting O6-methylguanine-DNA methyltransferases indirectly. *Oncotarget* **2016**, *7*, 50229–50238. [CrossRef] [PubMed]
56. Wang, Y.; Li, Y.; Sun, J.; Wang, Q.; Sun, C.; Yan, Y.; Yu, L.; Cheng, D.; An, T.; Shi, C.; et al. Tumor-suppressive effects of miR-29c on gliomas. *Neuroreport* **2013**, *24*, 637–645. [CrossRef] [PubMed]
57. Tang, L.J.; Sun, G.K.; Zhang, T.J.; Wu, D.H.; Zhou, J.D.; Ma, B.B.; Xu, Z.J.; Wen, X.M.; Chen, Q.; Yao, D.M.; et al. Down-regulation of miR-29c is a prognostic biomarker in acute myeloid leukemia and can reduce the sensitivity of leukemic cells to decitabine. *Cancer Cell Int.* **2019**, *19*, 177. [CrossRef]
58. Mraz, M.; Malinova, K.; Kotaskova, J.; Pavlova, S.; Tichy, B.; Malcikova, J.; Stano Kozubik, K.; Smardova, J.; Brychtova, Y.; Doubek, M.; et al. miR-34a, miR-29c and miR-17-5p are downregulated in CLL patients with TP53 abnormalities. *Leukemia* **2009**, *23*, 1159–1163. [CrossRef]
59. Ye, S.; Sun, B.; Wu, W.; Yu, C.; Tian, T.; Lian, Z.; Liang, Q.; Zhou, Y. LINC01123 facilitates proliferation, invasion and chemoresistance of colon cancer cells. *Biosci. Rep.* **2020**, *40*, BSR20194062. [CrossRef] [PubMed]
60. Zheng, H.; Wang, J.J.; Yang, X.R.; Yu, Y.L. Upregulation of miR-34c after silencing E2F transcription factor 1 inhibits paclitaxel combined with cisplatin resistance in gastric cancer cells. *World J. Gastroenterol.* **2020**, *26*, 499–513. [CrossRef]
61. Wu, H.; Huang, M.; Lu, M.; Zhu, W.; Shu, Y.; Cao, P.; Liu, P. Regulation of microtubule-associated protein tau (MAPT) by miR-34c-5p determines the chemosensitivity of gastric cancer to paclitaxel. *Cancer Chemother. Pharmacol.* **2013**, *71*, 1159–1171. [CrossRef]
62. Xiao, S.; Li, Y.; Pan, Q.; Ye, M.; He, S.; Tian, Q.; Xue, M. MiR-34c/SOX9 axis regulates the chemoresistance of ovarian cancer cell to cisplatin-based chemotherapy. *J. Cell Biochem.* **2019**, *120*, 2940–2953. [CrossRef]
63. Tung, S.L.; Huang, W.C.; Hsu, F.C.; Yang, Z.P.; Jang, T.H.; Chang, J.W.; Chuang, C.M.; Lai, C.R.; Wang, L.H. miRNA-34c-5p inhibits amphiregulin-induced ovarian cancer stemness and drug resistance via downregulation of the AREG-EGFR-ERK pathway. *Oncogenesis* **2017**, *6*, e326. [CrossRef]
64. Xu, M.; Jin, H.; Xu, C.X.; Bi, W.Z.; Wang, Y. MiR-34c inhibits osteosarcoma metastasis and chemoresistance. *Med. Oncol.* **2014**, *31*, 972. [CrossRef]
65. Liu, C.; Hou, J.; Shan, F.; Wang, L.; Lu, H.; Ren, T. Long Non-Coding RNA CRNDE Promotes Colorectal Carcinoma Cell Progression and Paclitaxel Resistance by Regulating miR-126-5p/ATAD2 Axis. *Onco Targets Ther.* **2020**, *13*, 4931–4942. [CrossRef]
66. Fu, R.; Tong, J.S. miR-126 reduces trastuzumab resistance by targeting PIK3R2 and regulating AKT/mTOR pathway in breast cancer cells. *J. Cell. Mol. Med.* **2020**, *24*, 7600–7608. [CrossRef] [PubMed]
67. Liu, W.; Chen, H.; Wong, N.; Haynes, W.; Baker, C.M.; Wang, X. Pseudohypoxia induced by miR-126 deactivation promotes migration and therapeutic resistance in renal cell carcinoma. *Cancer Lett.* **2017**, *394*, 65–75. [CrossRef] [PubMed]
68. Murray, M.J.; Raby, K.L.; Saini, H.K.; Bailey, S.; Wool, S.V.; Tunnacliffe, J.M.; Enright, A.J.; Nicholson, J.C.; Coleman, N. Solid tumors of childhood display specific serum microRNA profiles. *Cancer Epidemiol. Biomark. Prev.* **2015**, *24*, 350–360. [CrossRef]
69. Wei, J.S.; Johansson, P.; Chen, Q.R.; Song, Y.K.; Durinck, S.; Wen, X.; Cheuk, A.T.; Smith, M.A.; Houghton, P.; Morton, C.; et al. microRNA profiling identifies cancer-specific and prognostic signatures in pediatric malignancies. *Clin. Cancer Res.* **2009**, *15*, 5560–5568. [CrossRef]

70. Zeka, F.; Decock, A.; Van Goethem, A.; Vanderheyden, K.; Demuynck, F.; Lammens, T.; Helsmoortel, H.H.; Vermeulen, J.; Noguera, R.; Berbegall, A.P.; et al. Circulating microRNA biomarkers for metastatic disease in neuroblastoma patients. *JCI Insight* **2018**, *3*, e97021. [CrossRef]
71. Su, Y.K.; Lin, J.W.; Shih, J.W.; Chuang, H.Y.; Fong, I.H.; Yeh, C.T.; Lin, C.M. Targeting BC200/miR218-5p Signaling Axis for Overcoming Temozolomide Resistance and Suppressing Glioma Stemness. *Cells* **2020**, *9*, 1859. [CrossRef] [PubMed]
72. Liu, T.; Zhang, X.; Du, L.; Wang, Y.; Liu, X.; Tian, H.; Wang, L.; Li, P.; Zhao, Y.; Duan, W.; et al. Exosome-transmitted miR-128-3p increase chemosensitivity of oxaliplatin-resistant colorectal cancer. *Mol. Cancer* **2019**, *18*, 43. [CrossRef]
73. Wang, H.; Zhan, M.; Xu, S.W.; Chen, W.; Long, M.M.; Shi, Y.H.; Liu, Q.; Mohan, M.; Wang, J. miR-218-5p restores sensitivity to gemcitabine through PRKCE/MDR1 axis in gallbladder cancer. *Cell Death Dis.* **2017**, *8*, e2770. [CrossRef]
74. Li, P.; Yang, X.; Cheng, Y.; Zhang, X.; Yang, C.; Deng, X.; Li, P.; Tao, J.; Yang, H.; Wei, J.; et al. MicroRNA-218 Increases the Sensitivity of Bladder Cancer to Cisplatin by Targeting Glut1. *Cell Physiol. Biochem.* **2017**, *41*, 921–932. [CrossRef]
75. Zarogoulidis, P.; Petanidis, S.; Kioseoglou, E.; Domvri, K.; Anestakis, D.; Zarogoulidis, K. MiR-205 and miR-218 expression is associated with carboplatin chemoresistance and regulation of apoptosis via Mcl-1 and Survivin in lung cancer cells. *Cell. Signal.* **2015**, *27*, 1576–1588. [CrossRef]
76. Zeng, F.; Wang, Q.; Wang, S.; Liang, S.; Huang, W.; Guo, Y.; Peng, J.; Li, M.; Zhu, W.; Guo, L. Linc00173 promotes chemoresistance and progression of small cell lung cancer by sponging miR-218 to regulate Etk expression. *Oncogene* **2020**, *39*, 293–307. [CrossRef]
77. Chen, X.; Pan, M.; Han, L.; Lu, H.; Hao, X.; Dong, Q. miR-338-3p suppresses neuroblastoma proliferation, invasion and migration through targeting PREX2a. *FEBS Lett.* **2013**, *587*, 3729–3737. [CrossRef] [PubMed]
78. Xu, Z.; Sun, Y.; Wang, D.; Sun, H.; Liu, X. SNHG16 promotes tumorigenesis and cisplatin resistance by regulating miR-338-3p/PLK4 pathway in neuroblastoma cells. *Cancer Cell Int.* **2020**, *20*, 236. [CrossRef] [PubMed]
79. Han, L.; Cui, D.; Li, B.; Xu, W.W.; Lam, A.K.Y.; Chan, K.T.; Zhu, Y.; Lee, N.P.Y.; Law, S.Y.K.; Guan, X.Y.; et al. MicroRNA-338-5p reverses chemoresistance and inhibits invasion of esophageal squamous cell carcinoma cells by targeting Id-1. *Cancer Sci.* **2019**, *110*, 3677–3688. [CrossRef] [PubMed]
80. Creevey, L.; Ryan, J.; Harvey, H.; Bray, I.M.; Meehan, M.; Khan, A.R.; Stallings, R.L. MicroRNA-497 increases apoptosis in MYCN amplified neuroblastoma cells by targeting the key cell cycle regulator WEE1. *Mol. Cancer* **2013**, *12*, 23. [CrossRef]
81. Wang, J.; Ji, X.B.; Wang, L.H.; Qiu, J.G.; Zhou, F.M.; Liu, W.J.; Wan, D.D.; Lin, M.C.; Liu, L.Z.; Zhang, J.Y.; et al. Regulation of MicroRNA-497-Targeting AKT2 Influences Tumor Growth and Chemoresistance to Cisplatin in Lung Cancer. *Front. Cell Dev. Biol.* **2020**, *8*, 840. [CrossRef]
82. Wang, L.; Jiang, C.F.; Li, D.M.; Ge, X.; Shi, Z.M.; Li, C.Y.; Liu, X.; Yin, Y.; Zhen, L.; Liu, L.Z.; et al. MicroRNA-497 inhibits tumor growth and increases chemosensitivity to 5-fluorouracil treatment by targeting KSR1. *Oncotarget* **2016**, *7*, 2660–2671. [CrossRef]
83. Xu, S.; Fu, G.B.; Tao, Z.; Yang, J.O.; Kong, F.; Jiang, B.H.; Wan, X.; Chen, K. MiR-497 decreases cisplatin resistance in ovarian cancer cells by targeting mTOR/P70S6K1. *Oncotarget* **2015**, *6*, 26457–26471. [CrossRef]
84. Xu, J.; Wang, T.; Cao, Z.; Huang, H.; Li, J.; Liu, W.; Liu, S.; You, L.; Zhou, L.; Zhang, T.; et al. MiR-497 downregulation contributes to the malignancy of pancreatic cancer and associates with a poor prognosis. *Oncotarget* **2014**, *5*, 6983–6993. [CrossRef] [PubMed]
85. Hoareau-Aveilla, C.; Quelen, C.; Congras, A.; Caillet, N.; Labourdette, D.; Dozier, C.; Brousset, P.; Lamant, L.; Meggetto, F. miR-497 suppresses cycle progression through an axis involving CDK6 in ALK-positive cells. *Haematologica* **2019**, *104*, 347–359. [CrossRef] [PubMed]
86. Domingo-Fernandez, R.; Watters, K.; Piskareva, O.; Stallings, R.L.; Bray, I. The role of genetic and epigenetic alterations in neuroblastoma disease pathogenesis. *Pediatr. Surg. Int.* **2013**, *29*, 101–119. [CrossRef]
87. Bedrnicek, J.; Vicha, A.; Jarosova, M.; Holzerova, M.; Cinatl, J., Jr.; Michaelis, M.; Cinatl, J.; Eckschlager, T. Characterization of drug-resistant neuroblastoma cell lines by comparative genomic hybridization. *Neoplasma* **2005**, *52*, 415–419. [PubMed]
88. Wang, L.; Yang, G.; Zhao, D.; Wang, J.; Bai, Y.; Peng, Q.; Wang, H.; Fang, R.; Chen, G.; Wang, Z.; et al. CD103-positive CSC exosome promotes EMT of clear cell renal cell carcinoma: Role of remote MiR-19b-3p. *Mol. Cancer* **2019**, *18*, 86. [CrossRef] [PubMed]
89. Peng, P.; Chen, T.; Wang, Q.; Zhang, Y.; Zheng, F.; Huang, S.; Tang, Y.; Yang, C.; Ding, W.; Ren, D.; et al. Decreased miR-218-5p Levels as a Serum Biomarker in Bone Metastasis of Prostate Cancer. *Oncol. Res. Treat.* **2019**, *42*, 165–185. [CrossRef]
90. Ahmadinejad, F.; Mowla, S.J.; Honardoost, M.A.; Arjenaki, M.G.; Moazeni-Bistgani, M.; Kheiri, S.; Teimori, H. Lower expression of miR-218 in human breast cancer is associated with lymph node metastases, higher grades, and poorer prognosis. *Tumour Biol.* **2017**, *39*. [CrossRef]
91. Deng, M.; Zeng, C.; Lu, X.; He, X.; Zhang, R.; Qiu, Q.; Zheng, G.; Jia, X.; Liu, H.; He, Z. miR-218 suppresses gastric cancer cell cycle progression through the CDK6/Cyclin D1/E2F1 axis in a feedback loop. *Cancer Lett.* **2017**, *403*, 175–185. [CrossRef]
92. Jiang, Z.; Song, Q.; Zeng, R.; Li, J.; Li, J.; Lin, X.; Chen, X.; Zhang, J.; Zheng, Y. MicroRNA-218 inhibits EMT, migration and invasion by targeting SFMBT1 and DCUN1D1 in cervical cancer. *Oncotarget* **2016**, *7*, 45622–45636. [CrossRef]
93. Chiu, K.L.; Kuo, T.T.; Kuok, Q.Y.; Lin, Y.S.; Hua, C.H.; Lin, C.Y.; Su, P.Y.; Lai, L.C.; Sher, Y.P. ADAM9 enhances CDCP1 protein expression by suppressing miR-218 for lung tumor metastasis. *Sci. Rep.* **2015**, *5*, 16426. [CrossRef]

94. Marengo, B.; Pulliero, A.; Izzotti, A.; Domenicotti, C. miRNA Regulation of Glutathione Homeostasis in Cancer Initiation, Progression and Therapy Resistance. *Microrna* **2020**, *9*, 187–197. [CrossRef] [PubMed]
95. Stigliani, S.; Scaruffi, P.; Lagazio, C.; Persico, L.; Carlini, B.; Varesio, L.; Morandi, F.; Morini, M.; Gigliotti, A.R.; Esposito, M.R.; et al. Deregulation of focal adhesion pathway mediated by miR-659-3p is implicated in bone marrow infiltration of stage M neuroblastoma patients. *Oncotarget* **2015**, *6*, 13295–13308. [CrossRef] [PubMed]

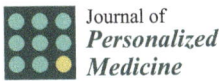

Review

Salivary Micro-RNA and Oral Squamous Cell Carcinoma: A Systematic Review

Maria Menini [1,*], Emanuele De Giovanni [1], Francesco Bagnasco [1], Francesca Delucchi [1], Francesco Pera [2], Domenico Baldi [1] and Paolo Pesce [1]

1. Division of Prosthodontics and Implant Prosthodontics, Department of Surgical Sciences (DISC), University of Genova, 16126 Genova, Italy; lele9-90@hotmail.it (E.D.G.); fcbagna5@hotmail.it (F.B.); dafne.1995@libero.it (F.D.); domenico.baldi@unige.it (D.B.); paolo.pesce@unige.it (P.P.)
2. Department of Surgical Sciences, CIR-Dental School, University of Turin, 10126 Turin, Italy; francesco.pera@unito.it
* Correspondence: maria.menini@unige.it; Tel.: +39-010-3537421

Abstract: Oral squamous cell carcinoma (OSCC) is a widespread malignancy with high mortality. In particular, a delay in its diagnosis dramatically decreases the survival rate. The aim of this systematic review was to investigate and summarize clinical results in the literature, regarding the potential use of salivary microRNAs (miRNAs) as diagnostic and prognostic biomarkers for OSCC patients. Twelve papers were selected, including both case–control and cohort studies, and all of them detected significantly dysregulated miRNAs in OSCC patients compared to healthy controls. Based on our results, salivary miRNAs might provide a non-invasive and cost-effective method in the diagnosis of OSCC, and also to monitor more easily its evolution and therapeutic response and therefore aid in the establishment of specific therapeutic strategies.

Keywords: oral squamous cell carcinoma; miRNAs; diagnosis; prognosis; saliva; biomarker

1. Introduction

Oral cavity cancer is the most frequent malignancy of the head and neck. It represents the 16th most common malignancy and the 15th leading cause of death worldwide, with an incidence of oral cancer (age adjusted) in the world of four cases per 100,000 people, with a wide variation across the globe which depends on gender, age groups, countries, races and ethnic groups and socio-economic conditions [1].

Roughly 90% of oral cancers histologically originate from squamous cells and are classified as oral squamous cell carcinoma (OSCC). OSCC develops in the oral cavity and oropharynx and can occur due to many etiological factors; smoking and alcohol remain the most common risk factors especially in the western world. Other risk factors include diet, immunodeficiency and high-risk HPV 16/18 [2]. There are also several genetic alterations involved in oral carcinogenesis. Among these, alterations in oncosuppressors (APC, p53), proto-oncogenes (Myc), oncogenes (Ras), and genes that control normal cellular processes (EIF3E, GSTM1) play a fundamental role in cancer development [3].

Despite advances in therapies, the overall 5-year survival rate has remained unchanged during the past decades. While at early stages the survival rate is approximately 89%, at late stages it decreases to 39%. Unfortunately, oral cancer patients are still frequently diagnosed in advanced stages despite educational interventions for prevention and early diagnosis, that is the most important prognostic factor for predicting survival [4].

To date, the gold standard for OSCC diagnosis is represented by a clinical oral examination integrated by a histological investigation on tissue biopsies of suspicious lesions [5]. However, cancer research is currently focusing on finding less invasive and cost-effective methods to provide a more comprehensive view of the cancer profile, also to more easily monitor its evolution and therapeutic response and therefore aid in the establishment of specific therapeutic strategies [6]. MicroRNAs (miRNAs) might provide a useful tool in this regard.

MiRNAs are small noncoding RNAs (ncRNAs) of approximately 22 nucleotides responsible for specific regulation of gene expression in a post-transcriptional manner. They are the main regulator of gene transcription and bear relevance in predicting clinical outcomes. Indeed, only less than 5% of expressed genes producing messenger RNA is really translated into proteins while miRNAs are fully functionally active in cell cytoplasm; they are responsible for various cellular and metabolic pathways, including cell proliferation, differentiation, and survival [7,8]. Deregulation of miRNAs has been reported in a number of diseases. In Implant Dentistry miRNAs have been found to be predictors of dental implants clinical outcomes and may be used as biomarkers for diagnostic and prognostic purposes [9,10].

In recent years, researchers have found that miRNA expression is dysregulated in human malignant tumor cells [11]. Due to their stability in human peripheral blood and body fluids and disease specific expression, an increasing number of studies indicate that miRNAs may represent an ideal set of biomarkers applied in early diagnosis and prognosis of cancers [12]. Related to OSCC, a growing number of studies has demonstrated that certain miRNAs are differentially expressed in oral cancer and analyses have indicated that the differentially expressed miRNAs may help distinguishing patients with oral cancer from healthy subjects [13]. In addition, dysregulation due to distinct polymorphisms in mature miRNAs, particularly miR-196a2 rs11614913 C>T, miR-146a rs2910164 G>C, miR-149 rs2292832 C>T, and miR-499 rs3746444 A>G, are associated with the risk of OSCC [14,15]. Several recent systematic reviews focused on the role of miRNAs in oral cancer. These papers show that miRNAs may assist in the prognosis of head and neck cancer and they can also predict resistance to chemotherapeutic agents, recurrence and metastasis [16–18]. Most of the reviews focused on oral cancer in general [19,20] or the evaluation of circulating miRNAs from serum or plasma [17,18]. Repetitive blood sampling can often be time consuming and physically intrusive, adding excessive stress and pain to patients, thereby leading to poor patient compliance. In the last years, salivary diagnostics has attracted significant attention among clinicians and scientists since the method of sample collection for disease is cost-effective, accurate and noninvasive. Moreover, oral cancer cells are immersed in the salivary milieu. Unlike other kinds of body fluid, oral tissues are continually immersed in saliva. Therefore, saliva may provide direct information regarding the disease status of oral mucosa. Saliva has been used as a diagnostic medium for OSCC, and saliva analytes such as proteins and DNA have been used to detect OSCC [21]. Thousands of miRNAs are present in saliva, and a panel of salivary miRNAs can be used for oral cancer detection [22]. Salivary miRNAs appear to enter the oral cavity through various sources, including the three major saliva glands, gingival crevice fluid, and desquamated oral epithelial cells. The majority of salivary miRNAs appear to be present as partially degraded forms. These partially degraded miRNAs maintain their stability in saliva through their association with unidentified macromolecules [23].

The aim of the present systematic review was to investigate and summarize results in the literature, regarding the potential use of salivary miRNAs as diagnostic and prognostic biomarkers for OSCC patients. In particular, the salivary miRNAs differently expressed in the saliva of patients with OSCC compared to healthy subjects were investigated.

2. Materials and Methods

The present systematic review was conducted according to guidelines reported in the indications of the Preferred Reporting Items for Systematic Review and Meta-Analysis (PRISMA) [24].

The focused question was: "What are the miRNAs differently expressed in the saliva of patients with oral squamous cell carcinoma (OSCC) compared to patients without OSCC?"

2.1. Search Strategy

The following Internet sources were used to search for papers that satisfied the study purpose: the National Library of Medicine (MEDLINE—PubMed), Scopus and Cochrane Library. In addition, a partial research of the gray literature was carried out through Google Scholar. The last search was done on 8 December 2020. We used the following search terms to search all databases: microRNA, microRNAs, miRNA, miRNAs, miR, mi-RNA combined with "oral squamous cell carcinoma" or OSCC.

All the clinical studies investigating miRNAs in patients with OSCC were included if they met the following inclusion criteria:

- Patients diagnosed with OSCC;
- Minimum of 10 patients included;
- Study subjects included cancer patients and healthy controls;
- Possibility to extrapolate data for patients with OSCC (data regarding oral cancer in general or head and neck cancer were excluded).

Eligible articles included: cross-sectional, case–control and cohort studies. Publications that did not report salivary miRNAs and their role as diagnostic/prognostic biomarkers in OSCC and did not meet the above inclusion criteria were excluded. Papers that were not dealing with original clinical cases (e.g., reviews, conference abstracts, personal opinions, editorials, etc.) and multiple publications from the same pool of patients (redundant publications) were also excluded. No restrictions in terms of year or language of publication were applied. No publication status restrictions were imposed. In addition, full-text articles of narrative and systematic reviews published between 2018 and 2020 and dealing with miRNAs and oral cancer were obtained. A hand search was performed by screening these reviews and the reference list of all included publications.

2.2. Screening and Selection

Titles and abstracts of the searches were screened by two independent reviewers (EDG and MM) for possible inclusion. Disagreements between reviewers were resolved by discussion between the two review authors; if no agreement could be reached, a third author decided (PP). The full texts of all studies of possible relevance were then obtained for independent assessment by the reviewers. If title and abstract did not provide sufficient information to determine eligibility of the study, the full report was obtained as well.

2.3. Data Extraction

Data from the studies included in the final selection were extracted by one of the authors using Microsoft Excel spreadsheet software (Excel 16.4, Microsoft CO, Redmond, WA, USA) (EDG). The accuracy of data was verified independently by another coauthor (FD). The following data were extracted: author(s), publication year, title, study design, nation where the study was conducted, sample size of both cases and controls (individuals with OSCC and healthy subjects respectively), diagnostic stage of disease, follow-up period, miRNAs detection method, name of the miRNA(s) identified as dysregulated, type of dysregulation recorded and main outcomes.

2.4. Quality Assessment

The risk of bias of included studies was assessed using the Newcastle Ottawa scale (NOS). Two reviewers (EDG, FB) independently evaluated the quality of studies based on the following parameters: Selection, Comparability, and Outcome/Exposure. A maximum of 4 stars in selection domain, 2 stars in comparability domain and 4 stars in outcome/exposure domain were given. The included studies were qualified as "Good", "Fair" and "Poor" quality based on the total NOS score they achieved. Studies with a NOS score ≥ 7 were considered good-quality studies.

3. Results

3.1. Bibliographic Search and Study Selection

The initial database search yielded a total of 1880 entries; of which 977 were found in PubMed®/MEDLINE, 898 in Scopus, and five in Cochrane library. In addition, a partial research of the gray literature was carried out through Google Scholar. A flow chart that depicts the screening process is displayed in Figure 1. After excluding all duplicates, the total number of entries was reduced to 1021. A total of 974 articles were excluded after review of title and abstract. Hence, full-text examination was conducted for 47 articles. A total of 35 additional articles were excluded after full-text review and application of the eligibility criteria. The final selection consisted of 12 articles. Detailed data for the 12 included studies are listed in Table 1.

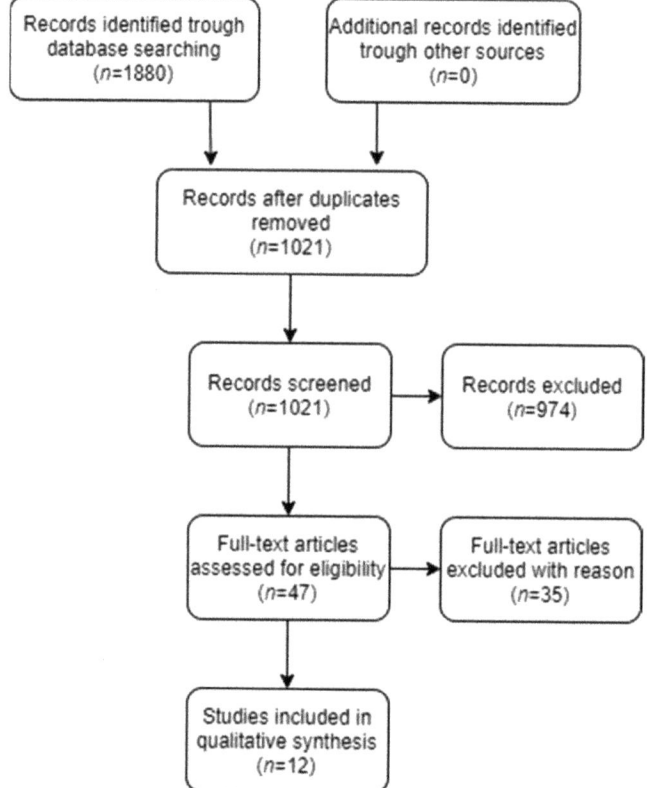

Figure 1. Preferred reporting of systematic reviews and meta-analyses (PRISMA) flow diagram related to bibliographic searching and study selection.

Table 1. Main characteristics of the included studies.

Authors (Year)	Cases (OSCC Patients)	Controls (Healthy Subjects)	Tumor Histological Stage or Grade	miRNAs Detection Method	Salivary miRNAs—Disregulation in OSCC Patients	Application	Follow-Up	Main Outcomes
Park et al. 2009 [25].	50 OSCC	50	10 patients were at tumor stage I, 14 were at stage II, 16 were at stage III, 10 were at stage IV	RT-PCR preampqPCR Saliva miRNA stability assay	miR142-3p miR200a miR125a miR-93 Downregulation	Diagnosis	ND	miRNAs are present in both whole saliva and supernatant saliva. miR-125a and miR-200a, are downregulated in the saliva of OSCC patients compared to healthy controls
Wiklund et al. 2011 [26].	15 OSCC	7	ND	TaqManH low density array qRT-PCR	miR-34b miR-137 miR-155 miR-200c-141 miR-203 mir-205 miR-375 mir-410 Aberrant expression and DNA hypermethylation	Diagnosis	ND	Compared to healthy subjects, OSCC patients had deregulated miRNAs with associated DNA methylation patterns. Particularly, repression of miR-375 and methylation on miR-137, miR-200c-141, and miR-200 s/miR-205 loci were found in OSCC patients vs. healthy patients, being promising candidates to develop OSCC-specific miRNA signatures.
Liu et al. 2012 [27].	45 OSCC	24	21 stage I-II 24 stage III-IV	qRT-PCR	miR-31 Upregulation	Diagnosis and follow-up	4–6 weeks after surgery	Salivary miR-31 was significantly increased in patients with OSCC at all clinical stages, including very early stages. In addition, it was shown to be more abundant in saliva than in plasma, and after tumor surgical removal its expression was reduced.

Table 1. *Cont.*

Authors (Year)	Cases (OSCC Patients)	Controls (Healthy Subjects)	Tumor Histological Stage or Grade	miRNAs Detection Method	Salivary miRNAs—Disregulation in OSCC Patients	Application	Follow-Up	Main Outcomes
Momen-Heravi et al. 2014 [28].	9 OSCC (before treatment), 8 OSCC-r (in remission)	9	ND	RT-qPCR	miR136 miR147 miR1250 miR148a miR632 miR646 miR668 miR877 miR503 miR220a miR323-5p underexpressed miR-24 miR27b overexpressed	Diagnosis	ND	miRNA profiles derived from OSCC, OSCC-r, and healthy controls were distinctively different. In particular, overexpression of miRNA-27b was found in OSCC saliva samples and not in the saliva of the other two groups
Zarhan et al. 2015 [29].	100 Oral cancer (20 OSCC)	20	Grade III (high grade) LN involvement: 7 Grade II, LN involvement (2 LN): 1 Grade II, no LN involvement: 7 No record available: 3	qRT-PCR	miR-21 upregulation miR184 upregulation miR145 downregulation	Diagnosis	ND	Salivary miRNA-21, miRNA-145, and miRNA-184 were differentially expressed in OSCC and healthy saliva samples, with miRNA-184 having the best diagnostic value
Duz et al. 2016 [30].	25 OSCC	25	2 grade 1 16 grade 2 4 grade 3 3 ND	qRT-PCR Microarray-based miRNA	miR139-5p downregulation	Diagnosis and follow-up	4–6 weeks after surgery	Salivary miR-139-5p was significantly reduced in TSCC patients compared to controls, and its level turned back to normal after surgery.
Seung-Ki Min et al. 2017 [31].	18 OSCC	ND	ND	RT-qPCR miRNA Microarray	miR-146a-5p upregulated	Diagnosis	ND	miR-146a-5p expression was highly upregulated in OSCC patients.

Table 1. *Cont.*

Authors (Year)	Cases (OSCC Patients)	Controls (Healthy Subjects)	Tumor Histological Stage or Grade	miRNAs Detection Method	Salivary miRNAs—Disregulation in OSCC Patients	Application	Follow-Up	Main Outcomes
Yap T et al. 2018 [32].	30 OSCC	30	14 stage 1 3 stage 2 3 stage 3 10 stage 4	RT-qPCR	miR-24 miR-21 miR-31 upregulation miR-99a let-7c miR-100 downregulation	Diagnosis	ND	Upregulation of miR-31 and miR-21 and downregulation of miR-99a, let-7c, miR-125b, and miR-100 were found in OSCC and controls in both FFPE and fresh-frozen samples. These miRNAs were studied in oral swirls to develop a dysregulation score with the classification tree identifying 100% (15/15) of OSCC and 67% (10/15) of controls.
Mehdipour et al. 2018 [33].	30 OLP 15 OSCC	15	ND	qRT-PCR	miR-21 upregulation miR-125a downregulation miR-31 upregulation miR-200a downregulation	Diagnosis	ND	miR-21 levels were significantly increased in saliva samples derived from patients with OLP, dysplastic OLP and OSCC, compared to those from healthy controls. Conversely, significant decreases in miR-125a levels were found in the OLP, dysplastic OLP and OSCC samples, compared to those from healthy controls. Significant increases in miR-31 levels were found in samples derived from dysplastic OLP and OSCC patients, but not in nondysplastic OLP, compared to healthy controls. miR-200a levels were significantly decreased only in samples derived from OSCC patients

Table 1. Cont.

Authors (Year)	Cases (OSCC Patients)	Controls (Healthy Subjects)	Tumor Histological Stage or Grade	miRNAs Detection Method	Salivary miRNAs—Disregulation in OSCC Patients	Application	Follow-Up	Main Outcomes
Gai C et al. 2018 [34].	21 OSCC	11	T1 (n = 7), T2 (n = 8), T3 (n = 3), T4 (n = 3)	qRT-PCR array qRT-PCR	miR-412- 3p, miR-489-3p, miR-512-3p, miR-597-5p, and miR-603 upregulated miR-193b-3p, miR-30e3p, miR-376c-3p, miR-484, miR-720, and miR-93-3p downregulated	Diagnosis	ND	miR-302b-3p and miR-517b-3p were expressed only in EVs from OSCC patients and miR-512-3p and miR-412-3p were up-regulated in salivary EVs from OSCC patients compared to controls with the ROC curve showing a good discrimination power for OSCC diagnosis
Yap T et al. 2019 [35].	53 OSCC	54	24 T1 10 T2 3 T3 15 T4a 1 not specified	RT-qPCR	miR-24-3p, miR-21-5p, let-7c-5p, miR-99a-5p, miR-100-5p	Diagnosis	ND	MicroRNAs can be predictably isolated from oral swirls. A high-risk dysregulation signature was found to be accurate in indicating the presence of OSCC with 86.8% sensitivity and 81.5% specificity
He L et al. 2020 [36].	49 OSCC	14	ND	Microarray analysis qRT-PCR	miR-7975, miR-1246 and miR-24-3p upregulated	Diagnosis	ND	The authors identified a significant increase of miR-24-3p in the salivary exosomes from 45 preoperative OSCC patients compared to healthy individuals

OSCC—Oral squamous cell carcinoma; ND—Undeclared; OLP—Oral lichen planus; qRT-PCR—Quantitative reverse transcription polymerase chain reaction; RT-qPCR—Real-time quantitative polymerase chain reaction; qPCR—Quantitative polymerase chain reaction; RT-preamp-qPCR—reverse transcriptase preamplification-quantitative; FFPE—formalin-fixed paraffin-embedded; EV—extracellular vesicle.

3.2. Description of Included Studies

Detailed data for the 12 included studies are listed in Table 1. All studies included in the present review are studies performed on humans.

Two studies were conducted in USA [25,28]; two in Australia [32,35]; one in Denmark [26]; one in Taiwan [27]; one in Turkey [30]; one in Iran [33]; one in Korea [31], one in Italy [34] one in Egypt [29], and one in China [36].

All the studies utilized real time quantitative polymerase chain reaction (RTq-PCR) to quantify salivary miRNAs. Three studies (Duz et al. 2016; Seung-Ki Min et al. 2017; He L et al. 2020) also utilized microarray-based miRNA analysis.

All the papers included identified a set of significantly dysregulated miRNAs in OSCC patients compared to healthy controls. Different types of miRNAs were found to be upregulated and other downregulated in OSCC patients. In particular, mir21 was identified as upregulated in OSCC patients compared to healthy controls in three studies (Zahran et al. 2015; Yap T et al. 2018; Mehdipour et al. 2018); and mir31 was identified as upregulated in OSCC patients compared to healthy controls in other three papers (Liu et al. 2012; Yap T et al. 2018; Mehdipour et al. 2018).

Two studies (Park et al. 2009; Mehdipour et al. 2018) identified mir200a and mir125a as downregulated in OSCC patients compared to healthy controls.

The other studies did not report superimposable outcomes.

3.3. Excluded Studies

Out of 47 papers for which the full-text was analyzed, 35 articles [37–71]. were excluded from the systematic review. (Table A1). The main reasons for exclusion were the following: study type; miRNAs detected in samples different from saliva and data regarding not OSCC but oral cancer in general or premalignant conditions.

3.4. Quality Assessment of Included Studies

The risk of bias of included studies was assessed using the Newcastle Ottawa scale (NOS). Outcomes are reported in Table 2.

Table 2. Risk of bias of included studies.

Study	Selection	Comparability	Outcome/Exposure	NOS Score
Park et al. 2009	●●○●	○●	○○●●	6
Wiklund et al. 2011	●●○●	●○	○○●●	6
Liu et al. 2012	●●○●	●●	○○●●	7
Momen-Heravi et al. 2014	●●○●	●○	○○●●	6
Zarhan et al. 2015	●●○●	●○	○○●●	6
Duz et al. 2016	●●○●	●●	○○●●	7
Yap T et al. 2018	●●○●	○●	○○●●	6
Mehdipour et al. 2018	●●○●	●○	○○●●	6
Gai C et al. 2018	●●○●	●●	○○●●	7
Yap T et al. 2019	●●○●	●○	○○●●	6
He L et al. 2020	●●○●	●●	○○●●	7
Seung-Ki Min et al. 2017	●○○●	●○	○○●●	5

NOS-Newcastle Ottawa Scale.

4. Discussion

The 5-year survival rates in OSCC depends on the stage at diagnosis. Patients have better survival and favorable outcomes if detected early, as compared to those diagnosed in advanced stages. There are several screening and awareness programs implemented, but they have not been able to lower the incidence of OSCC.

Traditional diagnostics for malignant tumors such as tissue biopsy and mucosal scraping examination can often be time-consuming and physically intrusive, adding excessive stress and pain to patients, thereby leading to poor patient compliance. In this context, the addition of a non-invasive diagnostic test based on a liquid biopsy would be beneficial in the early diagnosis and prognosis of such diseases as an alternative to solid biopsies. Liquid biopsy is a novel approach that relies on the study of circulating cells, circulating DNA, micro-RNA, microvesicles and exosomes in body fluids supporting the concept of personalized medicine [72,73]. In recent decades, saliva has been widely investigated as a promising source of OSCC biomarkers for liquid biopsy [74].

There are many advantages to employing saliva as a substrate for diagnostic analysis. Its sampling is inexpensive and non-invasive. Aberrant expression profiles of salivary miRNAs have been detected in different types of cancer, showing their power as a discriminatory clinical method [75]. A recent systematic review and meta-analysis demonstrated a high diagnostic accuracy of salivary and blood miRNAs to differentiate OSCC patients from healthy individuals, with sensitivity, specificity, and AUC (area under the SROC curve) values of 0.78, 0.82, and 0.91, respectively [43]. However, considerable heterogeneity was detected among the included studies and the authors suggested the need for further research on the topic.

A total of 12 papers were included in the present systematic review. Four of them were considered of good quality (NOS score equal to 7), and the remaining eight studies were considered at high risk of bias (NOS score 6 or 5), demonstrating the need for further studies with a more rigorous design on the topic.

The studies included applied heterogeneous methodologies to investigate the role of miRNAs in OSCC patients. In particular, the time of sampling (i.e., before and/or after surgery/radiotherapy) was not reported in all the studies. The research protocols included stimulated or unstimulated saliva for analysis of either whole saliva or salivary supernatant. In addition, salivary samples were taken at different clinical stages of OSCC and the studies differed regarding patients' demographic characteristics (i.e., smoke, alcohol consumption, positivity to HPV, patients' age and sex, etc.) and possible comorbidities possibly affecting the outcomes. Some of the studies included did not account for such patients' characteristics nor for the site of OSCC (buccal mucosa, gingiva, tongue, etc.). For this reason, the realization of a metanalysis was contraindicated and it is difficult to draw comprehensive conclusions on the topic. These heterogeneities might also explain why the type of miRNAs identified and the dysregulations detected in the various studies were mostly not superimposable.

Differently from the other investigations included, the study by He et al. analyzed miRNAs in salivary exosomes. The lipid bilayer of exosomes can protect miRNAs from degradation by RNase in body fluids. However, the use of salivary exosomal miRNAs as biomarkers for human disease remains controversial. A critical limitation of using salivary exosomes for cancer screening is that differences in isolation techniques may alter the composition of purified subpopulations and the purity of the exosome pellets. Gai et al. analyzed miRNAs in salivary extracellular vesicles (EVs, including exosomes, microvesicles or ectosomes, and apoptotic bodies). A previous study [76]. showed that most of the salivary RNA was associated with EVs. However, miRNAs can be differentially represented in whole saliva and salivary EVs, as it has been previously described for total plasma or plasma-derived EVs [77,78].

Despite the limitations listed above, our data overall demonstrate that there is strong evidence for a role of miRNAs in OSCC behavior. In fact, all the 12 papers included detected significantly dysregulated miRNAs in OSCC patients compared to healthy controls. In particular, some miRNAs were identified as differently expressed in OSCC patients in different papers: mir21, mir31, mir200a and mir125a. This panel of four miRNAs appears to have a significant predictive value in OSCC. Further longitudinal studies are needed in order to confirm which specific salivary miRNAs are the most effective biomarkers for the diagnosis and management of OSCC patients.

In conclusion, the present systematic review suggests that salivary miRNAs might provide a non-invasive and cost-effective method in the diagnosis of OSCC, and also to monitor more easily its evolution and therapeutic response and therefore aid in the establishment of specific therapeutic strategies.

Author Contributions: Conceptualization, M.M. and P.P.; methodology, M.M., P.P. and E.D.G.; investigation, E.D.G., F.B, F.D., F.P.; resources, M.M. and P.P.; writing—original draft preparation, M.M., E.D.G. and F.B.; writing—review and editing, M.M., D.B., F.P. and P.P.; supervision, M.M. and P.P.; project administration, M.M. and D.B. All authors have read and agreed to the published version of the manuscript.

Funding: This research received no external funding.

Conflicts of Interest: The authors declare no conflict of interest.

Appendix A

Table A1. Table reporting the 35 excluded studies and reasons for exclusion.

Article Excluded	Reason for Exclusion
Dumache R et al. 2017	Review article
Cristaldi M et al. 2019	Review article
Gaba et al. 2018	Review article
Salazar-Ruales et al. 2018	Oral cancer in general
Lay YH et al. 2018	In vitro study
Arantes et al. 2018	Review article
Rapado-Gonzalez et al. 2019	Review article
Wan Y et al. 2017	Oral cancer in general
Greither T et al. 2017	No control group
Fadhil et al. 2020	Oral cancer in general
Yeh LY et al. 2015	Oral cancer in general
Pentenero et al. 2019	Review article
Coon J et al. 2020	In vitro study
Brinkmann O et al. 2011	Review article
Langevin S et al. 2017	In vitro study
Shaidi M et al. 2017	Oral lichen planus
Dharmawardana N et al. 2019	Review article
Dumache R et al. 2015	Review article
Peacock B et al. 2018	Tissue sample
Patil S et al. 2019	Review article
Li et al. 2018	Tissue sample
Sun C et al. 2018	Tissue sample
Salazar C et al. 2014	Oral cancer in general
Gallo A et al. 2013	Descriptive article
Chen M et al. 2020	In vitro study
Yang et al. 2013	Oral premalignant lesion
Al Makey et al. 2015	Oral cancer in general
Hung et al. 2016	Oral premalignant lesion
Maheswari et al. 2020	Oral premalignant lesion
Petronacci et al. 2019	Tissue sample
Wang Y et al. 2018	Tissue sample
Pedersen et al. 2018	Tissue sample and plasma
Gissi et al. 2018	Tissue sample
Yang et al. 2017	Tissue sample
Moratin et al. 2016	Tissue sample

References

1. Ferlay, J.; Colombet, M.; Soerjomataram, I.; Mathers, C.; Parkin, D.M.; Pineros, M.; Znaor, A.; Bray, F. Estimating the global cancer incidence and mortality in 2018: GLOBOCAN sources and methods. *Int. J. Cancer* **2019**, *144*, 1941–1953. [CrossRef] [PubMed]
2. Bugshan, A.; Farooq, I. Oral squamous cell carcinoma: Metastasis, potentially associated malignant disorders, etiology and recent advancements in diagnosis. *F1000Research* **2020**, *9*, 229. [CrossRef] [PubMed]
3. Ali, J.; Sabiha, B.; Jan, H.U.; Haider, S.A.; Khan, A.A.; Ali, S.S. Genetic etiology of oral cancer. *Oral Oncol.* **2017**, *70*, 23–28. [CrossRef]
4. Gigliotti, J.; Madathil, S.; Makhoul, N. Delays in oral cavity cancer. *Int. J. Oral Maxillofac. Surg.* **2019**, *48*, 1131–1137. [CrossRef]
5. Fuller, C.; Camilon, R.; Nguyen, S.; Jennings, J.; Day, T.; Gillespie, M.B. Adjunctive diagnostic techniques for oral lesions of unknown malignant potential: Systematic review with meta-analysis. *Head Neck* **2015**, *37*, 755–762. [CrossRef]
6. Wang, J.; Chang, S.; Li, G.; Sun, Y. Application of liquid biopsy in precision medicine: Opportunities and challenges. *Front. Med.* **2017**, *11*, 522–527. [CrossRef]
7. Izzotti, A. Molecular medicine and development of cancer chemopreventive agents. *Ann. N. Y. Acad. Sci.* **2012**, *1259*, 26–32. [CrossRef]
8. Hwang, H.-W.; Mendell, J.T. MicroRNAs in cell proliferation, cell death, and tumorigenesis. *Br. J. Cancer* **2006**, *94*, 776–778. [CrossRef] [PubMed]
9. Menini, M.; Dellepiane, E.; Baldi, D.; Longobardi, M.G.; Pera, P.; Izzotti, A. Microarray expression in peri-implant tissue next to different titanium implant surfaces predicts clinical outcomes: A split-mouth study. *Clin. Oral. Implant. Res.* **2017**, *28*, e121–e134. [CrossRef]
10. Menini, M.; Pesce, P.; Baldi, D.; Coronel Vargas, G.; Pera, P.; Izzotti, A. Prediction of Titanium Implant Success by Analysis of microRNA Expression in Peri-Implant Tissue. A 5-Year Follow-Up Study. *J. Clin. Med.* **2019**, *8*, 888. [CrossRef]
11. Di Leva, G.; Garofalo, M.; Croce, C.M. MicroRNAs in cancer. *Annu. Rev. Pathol.* **2014**, *9*, 287–314. [CrossRef]
12. Chen, X.; Ba, Y.; Ma, L.; Cai, X.; Yin, Y.; Wang, K.; Guo, J.; Zhang, Y.; Chen, J.; Guo, X.; et al. Characterization of microRNAs in serum: A novel class of biomarkers for diagnosis of cancer and other diseases. *Cell Res.* **2008**, *18*, 997–1006. [CrossRef]
13. Wang, J.; Lv, N.; Lu, X.; Yuan, R.; Chen, Z.; Yu, J. Diagnostic and therapeutic role of microRNAs in oral cancer. *Oncol. Rep.* **2020**, *45*, 58–64. [CrossRef]
14. Hou, Y.Y.; Lee, J.H.; Chen, H.C.; Yang, C.M.; Huang, S.J.; Liou, H.H.; Chi, C.-C.; Tsai, K.-W.; Ger, L.-P. The association between miR-499a polymorphism and oral squamous cell carcinoma progression. *Oral Dis.* **2015**, *21*, 195–206. [CrossRef] [PubMed]
15. Liu, C.J.; Tsai, M.M.; Tu, H.F.; Lui, M.T.; Cheng, H.W.; Lin, S.C. miR196a overexpression and miR-196a2 gene polymorphism are prognostic predictors of oral carcinomas. *Ann. Surg. Oncol.* **2013**, *20*, S406–S414. [CrossRef] [PubMed]
16. Sahu, S.; Routray, S. Assessing the analytical efficacy of TEX in diagnosing oral cancer using a systematic review approach. *J. Oral Pathol. Med.* **2020**. Online ahead of print. [CrossRef]
17. Patil, S.; Warnakulasuriya, S. Blood-based circulating microRNAs as potential biomarkers for predicting the prognosis of head and neck cancer-a systematic review. *Clin. Oral Investig.* **2020**, *24*, 3833–3841. [CrossRef]
18. Dioguardi, M.; Caloro, G.A.; Laino, L.; Alovisi, M.; Sovereto, D.; Crincoli, V.; Aiuto, R.; Coccia, E.; Troiano, G.; Lo Muzio, L.; et al. Circulating miR-21 as a potential biomarker for the diagnosis of oral cancer: A systematic review with meta-analysis. *Cancers* **2020**, *12*, 936. [CrossRef]
19. Lamichhane, S.R.; Thachil, T.; Gee, H.; Milic, N. Circulating MicroRNAs as prognostic molecular biomarkers in human head and neck cancer: A systematic review and meta-analysis. dis markers. *Dis. Markers* **2019**, *18*. [CrossRef] [PubMed]
20. Kumarasamy, C.; Devi, A.; Jayaraj, R. Prognostic value of microRNAs in head and neck cancers: A systematic review and meta-analysis protocol. *Syst. Rev.* **2018**, *7*, 150. [CrossRef] [PubMed]
21. Hu, S.; Arellano, M.; Boontheung, P.; Wang, J.; Zhou, H.; Jiang, J.; Elashoff, D.; Wei, R.; Loo, J.A.; Wong, D.T. Salivary proteomics for oral cancer biomarker discovery. *Clin. Cancer Res.* **2008**, *14*, 6246–6252. [CrossRef] [PubMed]
22. Li, Y.; St John, M.A.; Zhou, X.; Kim, Y.; Sinha, U.; Jordan, R.C.; Eisele, D.; Abemayor, E.; Elashoff, D.; Park, N.H.; et al. Salivary transcriptome diagnostics for oral cancer detection. *Clin. Cancer Res.* **2004**, *10*, 8442–8450. [CrossRef] [PubMed]
23. Park, N.J.; Zhou, X.; Yu, T.; Brinkman, B.M.; Zimmermann, B.G.; Palanisamy, V.; Wong, D.T. Characterization of salivary RNA by cDNA library analysis. *Arch. Oral Biol.* **2007**, *52*, 30–35. [CrossRef] [PubMed]
24. Moher, D.; Liberati, A.; Tetzlaff, J.; Altman, D.G. Preferred reporting items for systematic reviews and meta-analyses: The PRISMA statement. *Int. J. Surg.* **2009**, *339*, b2535.
25. Park, N.J.; Zhou, H.; Elashoff, D.; Henson, B.S.; Kastratovic, D.A.; Abemayor, E.; Wong, D.T. Salivary microRNA: Discovery, characterization, and clinical utility for oral cancer detection. *Clin. Cancer Res.* **2009**, *15*, 5473–5477. [CrossRef]
26. Wiklund, E.D.; Gao, S.; Hulf, T.; Sibbritt, T.; Nair, S.; Costea, D.E.; Villadsen, S.B.; Bakholdt, V.; Bramsen, J.B.; Sørensen, J.A.; et al. MicroRNA alterations and associated aberrant DNA methylation patterns across multiple sample types in oral squamous cell carcinoma. *PLoS ONE* **2011**, *6*, e27840. [CrossRef]
27. Liu, C.J.; Lin, S.C.; Yang, C.C.; Cheng, H.W.; Chang, K.W. Exploiting salivary miR-31 as a clinical biomarker of oral squamous cell carcinoma. *Head Neck* **2012**, *34*, 219–224. [CrossRef]
28. Momen-Heravi, F.; Trachtenberg, A.J.; Kuo, W.P.; Cheng, Y.S. Genomewide study of salivary MicroRNAs for detection of oral cancer. *J. Dent. Res.* **2014**, *93*, 86S–93S. [CrossRef]

29. Zahran, F.; Ghalwash, D.; Shaker, O.; Al-Johani, K.; Scully, C. Salivary microRNAs in oral cancer. *Oral Dis.* **2015**, *21*, 739–747. [CrossRef]
30. Duz, M.B.; Karatas, O.F.; Guzel, E.; Turgut, N.F.; Yilmaz, M.; Creighton, C.J.; Ozen, M. Identification of miR-139–5p as a saliva biomarker for tongue squamous cell carcinoma: A pilot study. *Cell Oncol.* **2016**, *39*, 187–193. [CrossRef]
31. Min, S.K.; Jung, S.Y.; Kang, H.K.; Park, S.A.; Lee, J.H.; Kim, M.J.; Min, B.M. Functional diversity of miR-146a-5p and TRAF6 in normal and oral cancer cells. *Int. J. Oncol.* **2017**, *51*, 1541–1552. [CrossRef]
32. Yap, T.; Koo, K.; Cheng, L.; Vella, L.J.; Hill, A.F.; Reynolds, E.; Nastri, A.; Cirillo, N.; Seers, C.; McCullough, M. Predicting the presence of oral squamous cell carcinoma using commonly dysregulated MicroRNA in oral swirls. *Cancer Prev. Res.* **2018**, *11*, 491–502. [CrossRef]
33. Mehdipour, M.; Shahidi, M.; Manifar, S.; Jafari, S.; Mashhadi Abbas, F.; Barati, M.; Mortazavi, H.; Shirkhoda, M.; Farzanegan, A.; Elmi Rankohi, Z.; et al. Diagnostic and prognostic relevance of salivary microRNA-21, -125a, -31 and -200a levels in patients with oral lichen planus-a short report. *Cell. Oncol.* **2018**, *41*, 329–334. [CrossRef]
34. Gai, C.; Camussi, F.; Broccoletti, R.; Gambino, A.; Cabras, M.; Molinaro, L.; Carossa, S.; Camussi, G.; Arduino, P.G. Salivary extracellular vesicle-associated miRNAs as potential biomarkers in oral squamous cell carcinoma. *BMC Cancer* **2018**, *18*, 439. [CrossRef] [PubMed]
35. Yap, T.; Seers, C.; Koo, K.; Cheng, L.; Vella, L.J.; Hill, A.F.; Reynolds, E.; Nastri, A.; Cirillo, N.; McCullough, M.; et al. Non-invasive screening of a microRNA-based dysregulation signature in oral cancer and oral potentially malignant disorders. *Oral Oncol.* **2019**, *96*, 113–120. [CrossRef] [PubMed]
36. He, L.; Ping, F.; Fan, Z.; Zhang, C.; Deng, M.; Cheng, B.; Xia, J. Salivary exosomal miR-24–3p serves as a potential detective biomarker for oral squamous cell carcinoma screening. *Biomed Pharmacother.* **2020**, *121*, 109553. [CrossRef]
37. Dumache, R. Early diagnosis of oral squamous cell carcinoma by salivary microRNAs. *Clin. Lab.* **2017**, *63*, 1771–1776. [CrossRef]
38. Cristaldi, M.; Mauceri, R.; Di Fede, O.; Giuliana, G.; Campisi, G.; Panzarella, V. Salivary biomarkers for oral squamous cell carcinoma diagnosis and follow-up: Current status and perspectives. *Front. Physiol.* **2019**, *10*, 1476. [CrossRef]
39. Gaba, F.I.; Sheth, C.C.; Veses, V. Salivary biomarkers and their efficacies as diagnostic tools for oral squamous cell carcinoma: Systematic review and meta-analysis. *J. Oral Pathol. Med.* **2018**. [CrossRef]
40. Salazar-Ruales, C.; Arguello, J.V.; López-Cortés, A.; Cabrera-Andrade, A.; García-Cárdenas, J.M.; Guevara-Ramírez, P.; Peralta, P.; Leone, P.E.; Paz-y-Miño, C. Salivary MicroRNAs for early detection of head and neck squamous cell carcinoma: A case-control study in the high altitude mestizo ecuadorian population. *Biomed Res. Int.* **2018**, *2018*. [CrossRef]
41. Lai, Y.H.; Liu, H.; Chiang, W.F.; Chen, T.W.; Chu, L.J.; Yu, J.S.; Chen, S.J.; Chen, H.C.; Tan, B.C. MiR-31–5p-ACOX1 axis enhances tumorigenic fitness in oral squamous cell carcinoma via the promigratory prostaglandin E2. *Theranostics* **2018**, *8*, 486–504. [CrossRef]
42. Arantes, L.M.R.B.; De Carvalho, A.C.; Melendez, M.E.; Lopes Carvalho, A. Serum, plasma and saliva biomarkers for head and neck cancer. *Expert Rev. Mol. Diagn.* **2018**, *18*, 85–112. [CrossRef]
43. Rapado-González, Ó.; Martínez-Reglero, C.; Salgado-Barreira, Á.; López-López, R.; Suárez-Cunqueiro, M.M.; Muinelo-Romay, L. miRNAs in liquid biopsy for oral squamous cell carcinoma diagnosis: Systematic review and meta-analysis. *Oral Oncol.* **2019**, *99*, 104465. [CrossRef]
44. Wan, Y.; Vagenas, D.; Salazar, C.; Kenny, L.; Perry, C.; Calvopiña, D.; Punyadeera, C. Salivary miRNA panel to detect HPV-positive and HPV-negative head and neck cancer patients. *Oncotarget* **2017**, *8*, 99990–100001. [CrossRef]
45. Greither, T.; Vorwerk, F.; Kappler, M.; Bache, M.; Taubert, H.; Kuhnt, T.; Hey, J.; Eckert, A.W. Salivary miR-93 and miR-200a as post-radiotherapy biomarkers in head and neck squamous cell carcinoma. *Oncol. Rep.* **2017**, *38*, 1268–1275. [CrossRef]
46. Fadhil, R.S.; Wei, M.Q.; Nikolarakos, D.; Good, D.; Nair, R.G. Salivary microRNA miR-let-7a-5p and miR-3928 could be used as potential diagnostic bio-markers for head and neck squamous cell carcinoma. *PLoS ONE* **2020**, *15*, e0221779. [CrossRef]
47. Yeh, L.Y.; Liu, C.J.; Wong, Y.K.; Chang, C.; Lin, S.C.; Chang, K.W. miR-372 inhibits p62 in head and neck squamous cell carcinoma In Vitro and In Vivo. *Oncotarget* **2015**, *6*, 6062–6075. [CrossRef]
48. Pentenero, M.; Bowers, L.; Jayasinghe, R.; Cheong, S.C.; Farah, C.S.; Kerr, A.R.; Alevizos, I. World workshop on oral medicine VII: Functional pathways involving differentially expressed lncRNAs in oral squamous cell carcinoma. *Oral Dis.* **2019**, *25*, 79–87. [CrossRef]
49. Coon, J.; Kingsley, K.; Howard, K.M. miR-365 (microRNA): Potential biomarker in oral squamous cell carcinoma exosomes and extracellular vesicles. *Int. J. Mol. Sci.* **2020**, *21*, 5317. [CrossRef]
50. Brinkmann, O.; Wong, D.T. Salivary transcriptome biomarkers in oral squamous cell cancer detection. *Adv. Clin. Chem.* **2011**, *55*, 21–34. [PubMed]
51. Langevin, S.; Kuhnell, D.; Parry, T.; Biesiada, J.; Huang, S.; Wise-Draper, T.; Casper, K.; Zhang, X.; Medvedovic, M.; Kasper, S.; et al. Comprehensive microRNA-sequencing of exosomes derived from head and neck carcinoma cells in vitro reveals common secretion profiles and potential utility as salivary biomarkers. *Oncotarget* **2017**, *8*, 82459–82474. [CrossRef] [PubMed]
52. Shahidi, M.; Jafari, S.; Barati, M.; Mahdipour, M.; Gholami, M.S. Predictive value of salivary microRNA-320a, vascular endothelial growth factor receptor 2, CRP and IL-6 in Oral lichen planus progression. *Inflammopharmacology* **2017**, *25*, 577–583. [CrossRef]
53. Dharmawardana, N.; Ooi, E.H.; Woods, C.; Hussey, D. Circulating microRNAs in head and neck cancer: A scoping review of methods. *Clin. Exp. Metastasis* **2019**, *36*, 291–302. [CrossRef]

54. Dumache, R.; Rogobete, A.F.; Andreescu, N.; Puiu, M. Genetic and epigenetic biomarkers of molecular alterations in oral carcinogenesis. *Clin. Lab.* **2015**, *61*, 1373–1381. [CrossRef] [PubMed]
55. Peacock, B.; Rigby, A.; Bradford, J.; Pink, R.; Hunter, K.; Lambert, D.; Hunt, S. Extracellular vesicle microRNA cargo is correlated with HPV status in oropharyngeal carcinoma. *J. Oral. Pathol. Med.* **2018**, *47*, 954–963. [CrossRef]
56. Patil, S.; Arakeri, G.; Alamir, A.W.H.; Awan, K.H.; Baeshen, H.; Ferrari, M.; Patil, S.; Fonseca, F.P.; Brennan, P.A. Role of salivary transcriptomics as potential biomarkers in oral cancer: A systematic review. *J. Oral. Pathol. Med.* **2019**, *48*, 871–879. [CrossRef]
57. Li, Y.Y.; Tao, Y.W.; Gao, S.; Li, P.; Zheng, J.M.; Zhang, S.E.; Liang, J.; Zhang, Y. Cancer-associated fibroblasts contribute to oral cancer cells proliferation and metastasis via exosome-mediated paracrine miR-34a-5p. *EBioMedicine* **2018**, *36*, 209–220. [CrossRef]
58. Sun, C.; Li, J. Expression of MiRNA-137 in oral squamous cell carcinoma and its clinical significance. *J. Buon.* **2018**, *23*, 167–172.
59. Salazar, C.; Nagadia, R.; Pandit, P.; Cooper-White, J.; Banerjee, N.; Dimitrova, N.; Coman, W.B.; Punyadeera, C. A novel saliva-based microRNA biomarker panel to detect head and neck cancers. *Cell Oncol.* **2014**, *37*, 331–338. [CrossRef]
60. Gallo, A.; Alevizos, I. Isolation of circulating microRNA in saliva. *Methods Mol. Biol.* **2013**, *1024*, 183–190. [PubMed]
61. Chen, M.; Luo, R.; Li, S.; Li, H.; Qin, Y.; Zhou, D.; Liu, H.; Gong, X.; Chang, J. Paper-based strip for ultrasensitive detection of OSCC-associated salivary MicroRNA via CRISPR/Cas12a coupling with is-primer amplification reaction. *Anal. Chem.* **2020**, *92*, 13336–13342. [CrossRef]
62. Yang, Y.; Li, Y.X.; Yang, X.; Jiang, L.; Zhou, Z.J.; Zhu, Y.Q. Progress risk assessment of oral premalignant lesions with saliva miRNA analysis. *BMC Cancer* **2013**, *13*, 129. [CrossRef]
63. Al-Malkey, M.K.; Abbas, A.A.H. Original research article expression analysis of salivary microrna-31 in oral cancer patients. *Int. J. Curr. Microbiol. Appl. Sci.* **2015**, *4*, 375–382.
64. Hung, K.F.; Liu, C.J.; Chiu, P.C.; Lin, J.S.; Chang, K.W.; Shih, W.Y.; Kao, S.Y.; Tu, H.F. MicroRNA-31 upregulation predicts increased risk of progression of oral potentially malignant disorder. *Oral Oncol.* **2016**, *53*, 42–47. [CrossRef] [PubMed]
65. Uma Maheswari, T.N.; Nivedhitha, M.S.; Ramani, P. Expression profile of salivary microRNA-21 and 31 in oral potentially malignant disorders. *Braz. Oral. Res.* **2020**, *34*, e002. [CrossRef]
66. Chamorro Petronacci, C.M.; Pérez-Sayáns, M.; Padín Iruegas, M.E.; Suárez Peñaranda, J.M.; Lorenzo Pouso, A.I.; Blanco Carrión, A.; García García, A. miRNAs expression of oral squamous cell carcinoma patients: Validation of two putative biomarkers. *Medicine* **2019**, *98*, e14922. [CrossRef]
67. Wang, Y.F.; Li, B.W.; Sun, S.; Li, X.; Su, W.; Wang, Z.H.; Wang, F.; Zhang, W.; Yang, H.Y. Circular RNA expression in oral squamous cell carcinoma. *Front. Oncol.* **2018**, *8*, 398. [CrossRef]
68. Pedersen, N.J.; Jensen, D.H.; Lelkaitis, G.; Kiss, K.; Charabi, B.W.; Ullum, H.; Specht, L.; Schmidt, A.Y.; Nielsen, F.C.; von Buchwald, C. MicroRNA-based classifiers for diagnosis of oral cavity squamous cell carcinoma in tissue and plasma. *Oral Oncol.* **2018**, *83*, 46–52. [CrossRef]
69. Gissi, D.B.; Morandi, L.; Gabusi, A.; Tarsitano, A.; Marchetti, C.; Cura, F.; Palmieri, A.; Montebugnoli, L.; Asioli, S.; Foschini, M.P.; et al. A noninvasive test for MicroRNA expression in oral squamous cell carcinoma. *Int. J. Mol. Sci.* **2018**, *19*, 1789. [CrossRef]
70. Yang, X.; Ruan, H.; Hu, X.; Cao, A.; Song, L. miR-381-3p suppresses the proliferation of oral squamous cell carcinoma cells by directly targeting FGFR. *Am. J. Cancer Res.* **2017**, *7*, 913–922.
71. Moratin, J.; Hartmann, S.; Brands, R.; Brisam, M.; Mutzbauer, G.; Scholz, C.; Seher, A.; Müller-Richter, U.; Kübler, A.C.; Linz, C.; et al. Evaluation of miRNA-expression and clinical tumour parameters in oral squamous cell carcinoma (OSCC). *J. Craniomaxillofac Surg.* **2016**, *44*, 876–881. [CrossRef] [PubMed]
72. Izzotti, A.; Carozzo, S.; Pulliero, A.; Zhabayeva, D.; Ravetti, J.L.; Bersimbaev, R. Extracellular MicroRNA in liquid biopsy: Applicability in cancer diagnosis and prevention. *Am. J. Cancer Res.* **2016**, *6*, 1461–1493. [PubMed]
73. Lousada-Fernandez, F.; Rapado-Gonzalez, O.; Lopez-Cedrun, J.L.; Lopez-Lopez, R.; Muinelo-Romay, L.; Suarez-Cunqueiro, M.M. Liquid biopsy in oral cancer. *Int. J. Mol. Sci.* **2018**, *8*, 1704. [CrossRef] [PubMed]
74. Kaczor-Urbanowicz, K.E.; Martin Carreras-Presas, C.; Aro, K.; Tu, M.; GarciaGodoy, F.; Wong, D.T.W. Saliva diagnostics-current views and directions. *Exp. Biol. Med.* **2017**, *242*, 459–472. [CrossRef]
75. Rapado-González, Ó.; Majem, B.; Muinelo-Romay, L.; Álvarez-Castro, A.; Santamaría, A.; Gil-Moreno, A.; López-López, R.; Suárez-Cunqueiro, M.M. Human salivary microRNAs in cancer. *J. Cancer* **2018**, *9*, 638–649. [CrossRef]
76. Deregibus, M.C.; Figliolini, F.; D'Antico, S.; Manzini, P.M.; Pasquino, C.; De Lena, M.; Tetta, C.; Brizzi, M.F.; Camussi, G. Charge-based precipitation of extracellular vesicles. *Int. J. Mol. Med.* **2016**, *38*, 1359–1366. [CrossRef]
77. Cheng, L.; Sharples, R.A.; Scicluna, B.J.; Hill, A.F. Exosomes provide a protective and enriched source of miRNA for biomarker profiling compared to intracellular and cell-free blood. *J. Extracell. Vesicles* **2014**, *3*. [CrossRef]
78. Endzeliņš, E.; Berger, A.; Melne, V.; Bajo-Santos, C.; Soboļevska, K.; Ābols, A.; Rodriguez, M.; Šantare, D.; Rudņickiha, A.; Lietuvietis, V.; et al. Detection of circulating miRNAs: Comparative analysis of extracellular vesicle-incorporated miRNAs and cell-free miRNAs in whole plasma of prostate cancer patients. *BMC Cancer* **2017**, *17*, 730. [CrossRef]

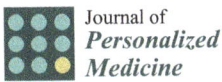

Review

Role of microRNAs in Lung Carcinogenesis Induced by Asbestos

Rakhmetkazhy Bersimbaev *, Olga Bulgakova *, Akmaral Aripova, Assiya Kussainova and Oralbek Ilderbayev

Department of General Biology and Genomics, Institute of Cell Biology and Biotechnology, L.N. Gumilyov Eurasian National University, Nur-Sultan 010008, Kazakhstan; aripova001@gmail.com (A.A.); assya.kussainova@gmail.com (A.K.); oiz5@yandex.ru (O.I.)
* Correspondence: ribers@mail.ru (R.B.); ya.summer13@yandex.kz (O.B.); Tel.: +7-7172-33-53-77 (R.B.); +7-707-432-97-27 (O.B.)

Abstract: MicroRNAs are a class of small noncoding endogenous RNAs 19–25 nucleotides long, which play an important role in the post-transcriptional regulation of gene expression by targeting mRNA targets with subsequent repression of translation. MicroRNAs are involved in the pathogenesis of numerous diseases, including cancer. Lung cancer is the leading cause of cancer death in the world. Lung cancer is usually associated with tobacco smoking. However, about 25% of lung cancer cases occur in people who have never smoked. According to the International Agency for Research on Cancer, asbestos has been classified as one of the cancerogenic factors for lung cancer. The mechanism of malignant transformation under the influence of asbestos is associated with the genotoxic effect of reactive oxygen species, which initiate the processes of DNA damage in the cell. However, epigenetic mechanisms such as changes in the microRNA expression profile may also be implicated in the pathogenesis of asbestos-induced lung cancer. Numerous studies have shown that microRNAs can serve as a biomarker of the effects of various adverse environmental factors on the human body. This review examines the role of microRNAs, the expression profile of which changes upon exposure to asbestos, in key processes of carcinogenesis, such as proliferation, cell survival, metastasis, neo-angiogenesis, and immune response avoidance.

Keywords: carcinogenesis; lung cancer; microRNA; asbestos exposure

1. Introduction

Lung cancer is one of the most frequent forms of cancer and is one of the leading causes of death from malignant neoplasms worldwide [1,2]. Approximately 1.8 million new cases of lung cancer are diagnosed annually in the world, and more than 1.5 million people die from this disease every year. According to experts, the number of deaths from lung cancer will increase to 3 million in 2035 [3]. The five-year survival rate for lung cancer ranges from 5% to 17% (average 15%), depending on the stage of the disease at the time of its diagnosis. The American Cancer Society estimated that there were about 234,000 new cases and about 154,000 deaths for lung cancer in the United States in 2018 [4].

Lung cancer is commonly associated with smoking and exposure to the carcinogenic components of tobacco smoke. About 90% of lung cancers in men and 80% in women are caused by tobacco smoking. Smoking causes about 25% of deaths among women and men [5]. Research estimated that for men and women between the ages of 25 and 70, the mortality rate among smokers was about three times higher than among those who had never smoked [6]. The increased mortality of smokers is mainly associated with neoplasms and respiratory diseases [7]. The life expectancy of smokers is more than 10 years shorter than those who have never smoked [2].

Carcinogenic environmental factors, such as air pollution and air emissions from fuel combustion as well as environmental exposure to radon, asbestos, certain metals (such as chromium, cadmium, and arsenic), and some organic chemicals, also contribute to the development of lung cancer [8]. Environmental carcinogens can cause specific genetic and epigenetic changes in lung tissue, leading to aberrant functions of lung cancer oncogenes and tumor suppressor genes [9]. Research also found that about 25% of lung cancer cases occur in people who have never smoked [7]. Thus, we can say that lung cancer today is an important medical problem, and progress in the treatment of this group of cancers can be achieved by improving our understanding of the molecular basis and biology of the tumor, especially at the level of the cells that trigger the tumor process [9].

2. Asbestos as a Carcinogenic Factor of the Environment

One of the important environmental carcinogen associated with lung cancer is asbestos [10,11]. Asbestos fibers are naturally occurring silicate mineral fibers that have long been used in industry due to their exceptional properties, such as tensile strength, low thermal conductivity, and relative resistance to chemical attack. For these reasons, asbestos has been used for insulation in buildings and as an ingredient in a variety of products, such as roofing shingles, water pipes, and fire-retardant coatings, as well as clutch and brake pads, density rings, and vehicle supports. Asbestos is used as an additive for asphalt concrete to increase the stability of the road surface.

There are six types of asbestos mineral fibers: chrysotile (white asbestos), crocidolite (blue asbestos), amosite (brown or gray asbestos), anthophyllite, tremolite, and actinolite [10]. The main types of asbestos are chrysotile (white asbestos), the spiral-shaped, most common form of asbestos, and crocidolite (blue asbestos). Amphiboles (crocidolite, amosite, anthophyllite, tremolite, and actinolite) are straight rod-shaped fibers that have a needle-like appearance, while serpentines (for example, chrysotile) are curved fibers.

Numerous industrial workers are exposed to asbestos dust, as is a significant proportion of the urban population associated with the extraction, processing, and industrial use of asbestos. Exposure to asbestos fibers is strongly associated with the development of malignant mesothelioma and lung cancer [12,13]. Asbestos-related lung disease is a major health problem worldwide [13,14].

All identified forms of asbestos have been classified as human carcinogens by the International Agency for Research on Cancer. According to World Health Organization (WHO) estimates, 125 million people worldwide are exposed to asbestos, and the use of this substance can cause the development of not only lung cancer but also ovarian and laryngeal cancer as well as mesothelioma [15,16]. Exposure to asbestos also causes diseases such as asbestosis (pulmonary fibrosis) and pleural plaques thickening and effusion. It is estimated that around 110,000 people die annually from lung cancer, mesothelioma, and asbestosis as a result of exposure to asbestos.

Between 5% and 7% of all lung cancer cases in the world have high levels of asbestos as the cause of the disease, mainly due to occupational exposure [17]. Roughly half of the deaths from occupational cancer in workers in the asbestos industry are due to asbestos [18].

There are many industries where workers deal with asbestos. Possible ways of contact with this material are as follows: "Primary", extraction, sorting, grinding; "Industrial", the production of asbestos itself and products from it; "Construction", all kinds of construction and installation work, for example, the installation of boiler equipment, laying pipelines; and "Ecological", the industrial emissions of asbestos industries, which are dangerous for people living in the neighborhood; the destruction of buildings constructed with the use of asbestos and asbestos-containing materials, without observing the relevant standards; and uncontrolled removal, the release of asbestos waste and dust into the natural environment [10,19].

In addition, it is estimated that several thousand deaths annually may be caused by the use of asbestos and asbestos-containing materials in the home; for example, asbestos was widely used at one time in the manufacture of ironing boards. It has also been shown that simultaneous exposure to tobacco smoke and asbestos fibers significantly increases the risk of lung cancer—the more a person smokes, the higher the risk [20,21].

Respirable fibers are the main source of exposure to asbestos [17,21]. With prolonged inhalation of asbestos dust, pneumoconiosis (silicatoses) and chronic dust bronchitis develop, the clinical picture of which has features due to the physicochemical properties of the corresponding types of dust. In industrial environments, exposure to mixed dust containing silicates and free silica is possible. Due to the fibrous structure of asbestos, dust, in addition to its fibrosing effect, causes more pronounced mechanical damage to the mucous membrane of the respiratory tract and lung tissue than other types of industrial dust [17].

The accumulation of asbestos fibers in the lungs leads to fibrosis, inflammation, and carcinogenesis, although the specific effects depend on the dose and type of fiber inhaled [20].

The mechanism of destruction that occurs in the lungs as a result of exposure to asbestos is determined by the efficiency of removing fibers from the cells of the respiratory tract. Longer fibers can penetrate deeper into the respiratory tract and are cleared more slowly than short ones and are associated with a higher carcinogenic potential [11,13,21]. Other elements, such as iron (which can account for up to 30% of the weight of asbestos fibers), embedded in the surface of the fibers can also enhance the pathogenic effects associated with asbestos.

2.1. Asbestos and Lung Diseases

Asbestos causes asbestosis and malignant neoplasms through molecular mechanisms that are not fully understood. The side effects of asbestos generally fall into three categories: pleural disease, lung parenchymal disease, and neoplastic disease. Effects on the pleura include pleural effusions, plaques, and diffuse pleural thickening. In the parenchyma, rounded atelectasis, fibrous cords, and asbestosis are observed. Exposure to asbestos can lead to neoplastic diseases, such as lung cancer pleural mesothelioma, peritoneal mesothelioma, and bronchogenic carcinoma [20]. The mechanisms of action underlying asbestosis, lung cancer, and mesothelioma appear to differ depending on the fiber type, lung clearance, and genetics. The picture of asbestos-induced carcinogenesis is complex with many types and results of molecular aberrations that can arise from exposure [22].

When asbestos dust interacts with human cells, asbestos silicates attract and bind to cations; in the lungs, asbestos fibers hold ions on their surface, thereby contributing to the leaching of the cellular environment [23]. These processes can generate reactive oxygen species (ROS), which initiate the processes of cell and DNA damage and explain the genotoxic effect of asbestos [24,25]. There are at least three sources of ROS production when exposed to asbestos, including (a) fiber surface reactivity, (b) release from immune cells, especially alveolar macrophages, and (c) mitochondrial ROS released from immune and other target cells, such as lung epithelial cells and mesothelial cells [26].

The high iron content in some asbestos fibers and the tendency of asbestos to adsorb iron in vivo have led to the assumption that iron-induced Fenton reactions also contribute to an increase in ROS, inflammation, and carcinogenesis [20]. Likely, it is ROS and the oxidative stress developing as a result of their action that underlie the damage to the lung tissue [13]. Oxidative stress can promote apoptosis, gene mutations, chromosomal aberrations, and, ultimately, cell transformation [17,20]. Inflammation, as mentioned above, is another important source of ROS production, given that all forms of asbestos activate the generation of ROS by neutrophils and alveolar macrophages of rodents and humans during the so-called frustrated phagocytosis, a process that is accompanied by the release of cytokines, chemokines, proteases, and growth factors contributing to the development of an inflammatory response [14,21].

In addition, research demonstrated that oxidative stress caused by exposure to asbestos dust can activate signaling pathways, including mitogen-activated protein kinases, nuclear factor kB (NF-kB), and activator protein 1, which control cell proliferation, apoptosis, and the inflammatory response [14]. The accumulated data strongly suggest that ROS generated from the mitochondria of key target cells mediate pulmonary asbestos toxicity.

Thus, Carter and colleagues demonstrated an important role in the production of H_2O_2 by the mitochondria of alveolar macrophages using an animal model of asbestosis [27,28].

A high level of apoptosis, in turn, can trigger the development of inflammatory processes in lung tissue due to another type of free-circulating nucleic acids—free-circulating mitochondrial DNA (fc mtDNA). The fc mtDNA copy number changes in different types of malignant neoplasias, including lung cancer [29]. Fc mtDNA, through TLR-9 receptors, can also mediate the activation of the NF-kB signaling pathway and, as a consequence, develop aseptic inflammation [28,29]. However, the role of fc mtDNA in the pathogenesis of lung cancer induced by exposure to asbestos dust remains unexplored, despite the fact that, as mentioned above, the mitochondria themselves are directly involved in the development of the cellular and molecular effects of asbestos.

2.2. The Role of microRNAs in Lung Cancer Carcinogenesis

Another type of free-circulating nucleic acids involved in the process of carcinogenesis is microRNA [30,31]. MicroRNAs are small noncoding RNAs that are involved in the regulation of target genes at the posttranscriptional level. MicroRNAs can covalently bind to complementary sequences in the 3' UTR region of the mRNA and thereby inhibit translation. It is known that microRNAs control many cellular processes such as proliferation, differentiation, and cell death (Figure 1).

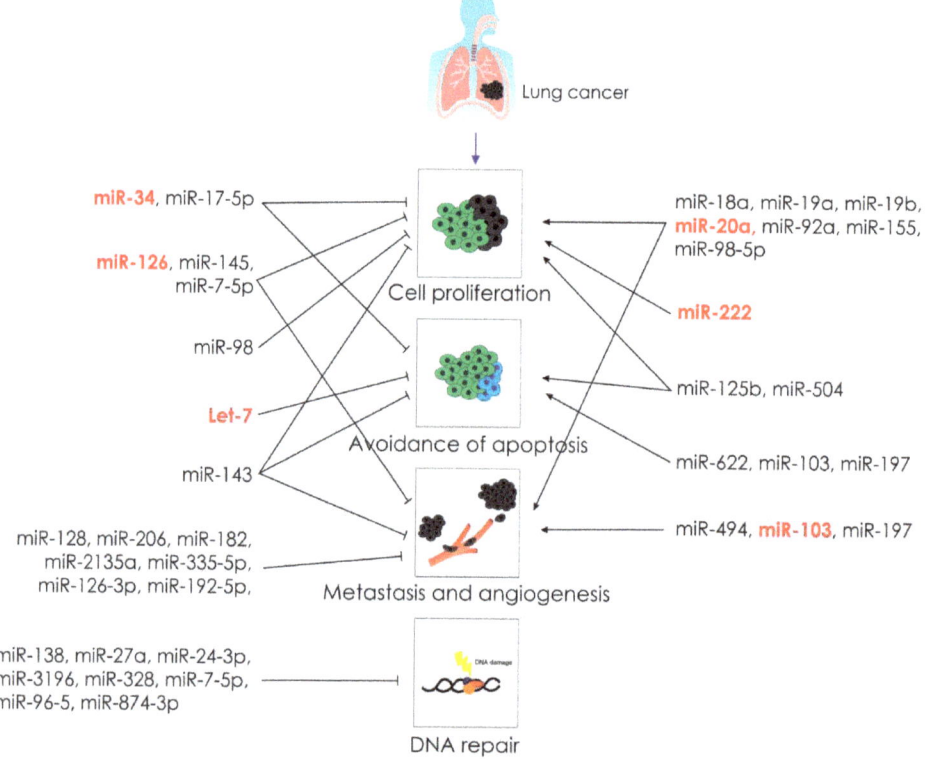

Figure 1. Cellular aspects of lung carcinogenesis with microRNA regulations (microRNAs whose expression profile changed under the influence of asbestos, are highlighted in red).

According to various estimates, microRNAs can control the expression of up to 50% of human genes [32]. MicroRNAs are found in tissue cells, but they are also found in extracellular areas, in blood plasma, and in other body fluids. MicroRNAs have also been found in platelets, erythrocytes, and nucleated blood cells. In the extracellular fluids of the body, they are carried in small membrane vesicles (exosomes), forming complexes with high density lipoproteins or carrier proteins.

At present, microRNAs are isolated into a separate class, most widely represented today, of short noncoding RNAs. According to the latest revision (January 2019), the mirbase.org database contains information on 38,589 hairpin precursors and 48,860 mature microRNAs from 271 species [32].

To date, a large body of evidence has been accumulated on the involvement of microRNAs in the carcinogenesis of various malignant neoplasias: malignant pleura, mesothelioma, prostate cancer, hematological malignant neoplasms, glioblastoma, and others. Subsequently, many studies have shown that the expression of certain microRNAs closely correlates with the development and progression of lung cancer. Research found that microRNAs are directly involved in many types of cancer, including lung cancer. MicroRNAs can not only be regulators of oncogenes but can themselves be regulated by oncogenes or suppressors of oncogenes [33,34].

Although microRNA is not tissue-specific, tumor cells develop a unique genetic profile during oncogenesis. The profiles of circulating microRNAs are different for each microenvironment and stage of cancer progression. Analysis of these microRNA profiles provides a better understanding of tumor pathogenesis and cancer origins. As tumors alter the normal concentration of circulating microRNAs, research suggested that these nucleotides can be used for early diagnosis, staging, follow-up, and the assessment of therapeutic responses and therapy outcomes in certain types of human cancer, including lung cancer [30,33]. MicroRNAs playing the role of oncogenes (OncomiR) and oncosuppressors in the development of lung cancer are shown in Tables 1 and 2.

2.2.1. MicroRNA and Cell Proliferation in Lung Cancer

MicroRNAs play an important role in the control of cell proliferation [35] (Figure 1). An example is the human mir-17 cluster, consisting of six microRNAs: hsa-miRs-17-5p, -18, -19a, -19b, -20, and -92. This cluster is located at 13q31, which is often amplified in several types of lymphomas and solid tumors. Research demonstrated that the oncogenic protein c-MYC binds directly to the genomic locus encoding these microRNAs to activate their transcription. In addition, two microRNAs of this cluster, hsa-miR-17-5p and hsa-miR-20, target the transcription factor E2F1, which regulates the expression of proapoptotic proteins in the cell, thereby avoiding apoptosis and increasing cell proliferation [36].

An example of microRNA oncosuppressors is the let-7 family, whose members target *ras* oncogenes (*H-ras*, *K-ras*, and *N-ras*) [37]. As *ras* overexpression is a key oncogenic event in lung cancer, the involvement of let-7 in the pathogenesis of this disease is beyond doubt. Indeed, let-7 expression in lung cancer cells is significantly reduced as compared to normal tissue. In addition, the RAS protein levels in bronchial epithelial cells are inversely proportional to the let-7 levels, which is consistent with microRNA-mediated translational repression of the *ras* gene [37]. The expression of let-7 in the lung carcinoma cell line A549 directly suppresses the growth of cancer cells in vitro [37], illustrating the effectiveness of targeted antitumor therapy using this microRNA.

Another oncosuppressive microRNA is miR-126. Studies have shown that miR-126 can inhibit the proliferation of NSCLC through the suppression of EGFL7 and PTEN/PI3K/AKT signaling pathways [38,39]. In addition, decreased expression of miR-126 was associated with adhesion, migration, and invasion of NSCLC cells due to an increase in the Crk protein [40]. Hence, miR-126 may function as an important regulatory gene in the development of NSCLC. Research found that miR-145 is involved in the regulation of tumor cell proliferation by disabling the signaling pathways RAS/ERK, PI3K/AKT, ERK5/c-MYC, and p68/p72/β-catenin [41,42].

Recent meta-analysis demonstrated that miR-155 may be a potential biomarker for lung cancer detection. Experiments on an animal model showed that mice that were artificially injected with miR-155 exhibited proliferation of lung tumors [43]. In addition, it was found that overexpression of miR-155-5p significantly extended the malignant phenotype of lung cancer cells, including cell growth, colony formation, migration, invasion, and antiapoptotic effects [44,45].

A recent study indicated that miR-222 overexpression was related to NSCLC risk [46]. It was shown that miR-222 promotes the growth of non-small cell cancer cell lines by targeting oncosuppressor p27, which controls the cell cycle progression at G1 [47].

2.2.2. MicroRNA and Apoptosis in Lung Cancer

MicroRNAs can also have antiproliferative and proapoptotic activities (Figure 1). These molecules function in the cell as tumor suppressors. The main regulator of apoptosis in the cell is the p53 protein. Recent studies indicated the relationship between the profile of certain microRNAs and the expression level of the *TP53* gene. It was shown that the change in the microRNA profile after p53 induction occurs in the direction of an increase in the content of microRNA-34a, 34b, and 34c [48]. The level of these microRNAs increased in response to genotoxic stress with the involvement of p53 both in vitro and in vivo.

The transcription of microRNA-34a, -34b, and -34c at both loci is directly activated by p53. Studies have shown that members of the hsa-miR-34 family inhibit the expression of several targets involved in cell cycle regulation, such as cyclin E2 and cyclin-dependent kinases 4 and 6 (CDK4 and CDK6), and BCL2 [48]. Interestingly, some *TP53* mutations, which were previously associated with oncogenic progression, suppress the expression of some microRNAs [48]. p53 can also serve as a target for some types of microRNAs. Research showed that miR-504 can target the mRNA of p53. Ectopic expression of miR-504 decreases the p53 protein level, which inhibits p53-dependent apoptosis and arrest of the cell cycle in the G1 phase [49]. hsa-miR-125b targets p53 and proapoptotic proteins Bak1 and Puma, which leads to the inhibition of apoptosis [50].

Studies demonstrated the radioprotective role of some types of microRNA. In vitro studies using the WI-38 human fibroblast line showed that the mature form of hsa-miR-155 inhibited radiation-induced premature "cellular senescence" [51]. In this regard, scientists assumed that some microRNAs can determine the resistance of tumor cells to radiation therapy and be used as a predictive biomarker to monitor the effectiveness of cancer treatment.

The suppression of apoptosis may underlie this effect. Thus, the overexpression of hsa-miR-622 in colon cancer cells inhibits the Rb protein, thus inactivating the Rb-E2F1-P/CAF complex, whose participation is a key moment in the activation of proapoptotic genes [52].

In the development and homeostasis process, apoptosis plays a significant role. There are two ways of separating the apoptotic process: external and internal. A series of cascading proteases are triggered by each pathway, and cell death occurs eventually. Tumor cells have the capacity to inhibit apoptosis and thus support the survival of cells. In response to a broad range of endogenous and exogenous signals, including DNA damage, hypoxia, ribosome biogenesis inhibition, food starvation, ribonucleotide triphosphate depletion, and oncogene activation (C-Mus, RAS, and E2F-1), p53 is activated. p53 causes cell cycle arrest, apoptosis, or aging, depending on the cell type, environmental background, and degree of stress, to avoid the spread of damaged cells that may potentially become cancerous [53].

In tumorigenesis, microRNAs are important apoptosis regulators, and cancer cells can control microRNAs in oncogenesis to regulate cell survival. miR-103 expression in the carcinoma tissues of NSCLC patients was found to be increased. After knockdown of miR-103, the number of apoptotic cells increased, the expression level of the proapoptotic protein Bax increased, and the level of the antiapoptotic protein Bcl-2 decreased in A549 and H23 cell lines. In addition, the level of FBW7 protein was increased after the miR-103 knockdown. F-box and WD repeat domain-containing 7 (FBW7) is a tumor inhibiting protein that can inhibit the emergence and development of numerous types of tumors by regulating the cycle, differentiation, apoptosis, proliferation, invasion, and migration of tumor cells [54].

The induction of apoptosis in wild-type p53 cells is the responsibility of two BH3-only NOXA and BMF proteins as new miR-197 targets, identifying miR-197 as a main survival factor in NSCLC. The inhibition of miR-197 is, therefore, proposed as a new therapeutic approach toward lung cancer [55]. The miR-197-3p profile was elevated in the tissues of patients with lung adenocarcinoma. The inhibition of miR-197-3p expression led to increased apoptosis through the activation of caspase-3/7 in lung adenocarcinoma cells. The overexpression of miR-197-3p stimulated proliferation and did not block apoptosis of human bronchial epithelial cells, thus suggesting that miR-197-3p expression has an important role in malignant neoplasms [56].

The content of miR-17 was decreased in T2–T4 pathologic stage NSCLC tissues and SK-MAS-1, A549, SPCA-1, H460, H1229, and HCC827 cell lines. Li et al. demonstrated that miR-17-5p inhibited proliferation and caused apoptosis of H460 NSCLC cells, inhibiting TGFßR2, which was significantly increased in NSCLC tissues and cell lines [57]. An experiment was also conducted in paclitaxel-resistant lung cancer cells. Paclitaxel exerts a cytotoxic effect, inducing apoptosis [58]. However, in drug-resistant cancer, tumor cells overcome this cytotoxic effect of paclitaxel and become resistant to apoptosis. Increased miR-17-5p expression and paclitaxel treatment induced apoptotic cell death in lung cancer cells [59].

An increased expression profile of miR-486 protected against PM2.5-induced cell apoptosis in cell lines A549 [60]. Studies have shown that PM2.5 treatment can cause cell apoptosis, cell necrosis, autophagy, DNA damage, mitochondrial damage, and gene mutations in respiratory tract tissues [61]. Recently, the effect of propofol in the H1299 and H1792 lung cancer cell lines and the role of miR-486 have been studied. When treated with propofol in cell lines, the expression level of miR-486 increased, and cell viability, when combined with propofol with an inhibitor of miR-486, was increased compared to the control and propofol group. The authors indicated that increased expression of miR-486 may contribute to the antitumor activity of propofol [62]. Increased expression of the miR-486-5p profile blocked cell proliferation and invasion by repressing GAB2 in non-small cell lung cancer [63].

The level of expression of miR-98 was reduced simultaneously in both tissues and cell lines A549 and H12999 [63]. Tumor size, TNM level, lymph node metastasis, and survival in pancreatic adenocarcinoma were associated with decreased miR-98 expression [64]. High miR-98 expression patients showed longer average survival than low miR-98 expression patients [65]. Inhibited miR-98 activated PAK1 (P21-activated protein kinase 1), a biomarker of pulmonary cancer, which promotes NSCLC cell proliferation, migration, and invasion [66].

2.2.3. MicroRNA and Angiogenesis in Lung Cancer

Different pro- or antiangiogenic factors manipulate angiogenesis, a key step in tumor growth and metastasis. By modulating the expression of essential angiogenic factors, microRNAs have recently been shown to modulate the angiogenic processes (Figure 1). The function of microRNAs derived from tumors in controlling tumor vascularization remains to be explained [67].

The targeting of PTEN and subsequent activation of the Akt/eNOS pathway mediates the angiogenic effect of miR-494. Importantly, coculture experiments showed that, through a microvesicle-mediated pathway, a lung cancer cell line, A549, secreted and delivered miR-494 into endothelial cells. In addition, in response to hypoxia, the expression of miR-494 was induced in tumor cells, possibly through the HIF-1 alpha-mediated mechanism [68].

A mimic miR-128 significantly suppressed the expression of vascular endothelial growth factor (VEGF)-C. The overexpression of miR-128 in NSCLC cells and human endothelial vein umbilical cells caused a reduction expression of VEGF-A, vascular endothelial growth factor receptor 2, and VEGFR-3, essential factors critical for cancer angiogenesis and lymphangiogenesis, and slightly declined the phosphorylation of extracellular signal-regulated kinase, phosphatidylinositol 3-kinase, and p38 signaling pathways [69]. miR-206 decreased the angiogenic efficiency of NSCLC by inhibiting the 14-3-3ζ/STAT3/HIF-1α/VEGF pathway [70]. miR-135a decreased angiogenesis-related factors VEGF, bFGF, and IL-8 in A549 cells by inhibiting IGF-1 [71].

2.2.4. MicroRNA and Metastasis in Lung Cancer

A large percentage of cancer deaths are associated with the metastasis of primary tumors [72]. The invasion of cancer cells and the formation of metastases is a clinically significant process. The molecular genetics and epigenetic mechanisms of this process are the least studied at the moment.

The spread of tumor metastasis is a complex multistage process that includes the invasion of cancer cells into the lumen of a blood or lymphatic vessel, migration, localization in a new place, the growth of metastases, and the formation of additional blood vessels to feed the metastatic foci.

Lung cancer is often diagnosed at an advanced stage with the formation of metastases [73]. Tumors of the lung have preferred organs for metastasis—the brain, bones, liver, and adrenal glands. Other organs may be affected in the terminal stage of the disease. It has been observed that various histological types of lung cancer typically metastasize to specific organs. In SCLC, metastasis is found mainly in the liver and brain, and adenocarcinoma in the brain and bones, [74,75], while NSCLC affects mainly the bones, brain, adrenal glands, liver, and lymphatic vessels [76].

Molecular genetics and epigenetic changes during metastasis are associated with the epithelial–mesenchymal transition, which is activated by the activity of internal factors—KRAS, Her2, MET, and EGFR, [77–81] as well as external factors TGF-β, EGF, HGF, PDGF, TNF-α, and IL-6 [81]. The role of microRNAs in metastasis was first reported by Ma et al., who found that the overexpression of miR-10b promotes the formation of lung metastases in breast cancer [82]. miR-10b also exhibits oncogenic activity and is involved in the metastasis of NSCLC (Figure 1). The expression of miR-10b in lymphatic vessel metastases was significantly higher compared to the primary tumor in the lungs [83].

The role of miR-646 in the development of metastases in renal cancer [84] and gastric cancer [85] is ambiguous. MiR-646 exhibits tumor suppressive properties in pancreatic cancer [86]. TRIM44 activates the AKT/mTOR signal pathway to induce melanoma progression by stabilizing TLR4. Zhang et al. showed that miR-646 can inhibit proliferation and invasion and can suppress the EMT of NSCLC cells in mice. The FGF2 and CCND2 genes are targets for miR-646. Overexpression of miR-646 significantly suppressed the expression of mRNA and protein FGF2 and CCND2 in NSCLC cell lines [87].

Li et al. showed that overexpression of miR-182 promoted the expression of E-cadherin, which led to the inhibition of EMT. MiR-182 also suppresses AKT phosphorylation and accumulation of the Snail transcription factor, which initiates EMT in lung cancer cells. As mentioned above, the hepatocyte growth factor HGF activates EMT by activating the Met signaling pathway, which, as a result, increases the invasive and metastatic potential of cells. It has been shown that miR-182 can directly bind to Met, thereby negatively regulating Met expression and reducing lung tumor metastasis [88].

miR-7-5p inhibits the proliferation, migration, and invasion of tumor cells by regulating the expression of genes associated with EMT both in vitro and in vivo. miR-7-5p also suppresses NSCLC metastasis by acting on NOVA2 [89], which presumably disrupts the angiogenesis of the resulting metastases and inhibits their further growth [90].

Liao et al. found a decrease in the miR-206 levels in NSCLC. The oncosuppressive mechanism of miR-206 is that this microRNA inhibits the development of NSCLC metastases through the negative regulation of the actin-binding protein coronin 1C (CORO1C) [91]. CORO1C knockdown significantly reduced the ability of cells to grow and metastasize in gastric [92] and breast cancer [93].

Decreased expression of miR-335-5p and increased expression of the ROCK1 oncogene was observed in NSCLC metastases to lymphatic vessels. The overexpression of miR-335-

5p led to inhibition of TGF-β1-mediated EMT in NSCLC as a result of downregulation of ROCK1 [94]. ROCK1 is also known to reduce PTEN activation/phosphorylation and then phosphorylate PI3K/AKT, which leads to the phosphorylation of FAK tyrosine kinase, which plays a key role in cell adhesion and in stimulating cell migration and invasion [95].

2.2.5. MicroRNAs Participating in Epithelial–Mesenchymal Transition (EMT)

A significant decrease in the miR-126-3p expression in NSCLC cell lines and tissues and an increase in the miR-126-3p levels suppressed the migration and invasion of cancer cells (Figure 1). Studies demonstrated that miR-126-3p inhibited NSCLC cell growth and metastasis by acting on chemokine receptor 1 (CCR1) [96]. miR-192-5p was significantly reduced in patients with metastatic lung cancer [97]. This microRNA reduces the migration and invasion of lung cancer by inhibiting TRIM44, which induces EMT by activating the AKT/mTOR signaling pathway [98]. This mechanism of metastasis was also observed in melanoma [99] and esophageal cancer [100].

miR-625 is a suppressor in NSCLC. There was a decrease in miR-625 expression found in NSCLC tissues, which likely contributes to tumor progression and metastasis due to EMT activation via the PI3K/AKT/Snail signaling pathway [101]. Overexpression of miR-652-3p was found in tumor tissues of patients with NSCLC and was significantly higher in patients with lymph node metastases. The probable mechanism of metastasis is the binding of miR-652-3p mRNA of the Lgl1 protein, which promotes cell adhesion and inhibits cell migration by suppressing the expression of MMP2 and MMP14 and re-expression of E-cadherin [102].

Xia et al. noted that miR-143 suppressed NSCLC cell proliferation, induced apoptosis, and suppressed migration and invasion in vitro. Limk1 has been identified as a direct target for miR-143 [103]. Decreases in the Limk1 levels were also noted in prostate [104] and breast [105] cancers. miR-98-5p inhibits translation of the messenger RNA encoding TGFBR1, which is involved in the regulation of cellular processes, including motility, differentiation, adhesion, division, and apoptosis. Decreased TGFBR1 levels led to proliferation, migration, and invasion in A549 and H1299 cell lines [106].

2.2.6. MicroRNAs and DNA Repair in Lung Cancer

Asbestos-related lung cancer has been made of a result of various mutations, lesions caused by DNA-damaging ROS [107]. Typically, DNA damage is recognized and repaired by the DNA repair machinery. When DNA repair fails, the genomic integrity of the cell is disrupted and this can lead to cancer. Recent studies have suggested that microRNAs take a one of the important part in the regulation of the DNA repair network (Figure 1) [108–110].

An example miR-138 knockdown facilitates DNA damage repair, while miR-138 overexpression inhibits DNA damage repair in small-cell lung cancer (SCLC) cells due to a decrease in the level of H2AX expression, and as a result of miR-138 overexpression, reduction of cell growth and a significant inhibition on cell-cycle progression was detected [111].

hsa-miR-526b also suppressed double-stranded breaks (DSB) repair by inhibition of the Ku80, thus significantly suppressing the NSCLC growth both in vitro and in vivo [112]. Another study demonstrated that inhibition of ATM transcript by miR-27a lead to cell survival and cell cycle progression of A549 cell line [113].

It was shown miR-24-3p plays a role as regulator of the cellular response to DNA damage in pathogenesis of Chronic Obstructive Pulmonary Disease (COPD) which is considered one of the risk factors for lung cancer. Nouws et al. have shown that miR-24-3p suppressed homology-directed DNA repair by inhibition of BRCA1 expression in the cells of parenchymal lung tissue [109].

miR-346 suppressed nucleotide excision repair (NER) by inhibition of the XPC, thus caused promotion tumor growth of A549 cells in xenografts mice [110].

Oncomir miR-34a negatively regulates the process of recombinant repair in NSCLC cells by binding to the 3′-untranslated region of RAD51 [114]. RAD51 expression was also significantly reduced in cells overexpressing hsa-miR-96-5p [115].

Mairinger et all. have shown that miR-125b-5p, miR-21-5p and miR-222-3p expression inversely correlates to PARP1 mRNA expression [108]. Lai et al. showed that miR-7-5p expression levels were significantly reduced in Dox-resistant SCLC cells. miR-7-5p inhibited Dox-induced homologous DSB repair by suppressing the expression of Rad51 and BRCA1 by inhibiting PARP1 [116]. It is interesting, that asbestos activates PARP1 which caused accumulation of single-stranded breaks (SSB) lesions in human mesothelial cells [117].

Table 1. OncomiRs in lung cancer.

	MicroRNA	MicroRNA Targets and Mechanism	Role in Carcinogenesis	Ref.
1	2	3	4	5
1	cluster of microRNA miR-17-92 (miR-18a, miR-19a, miR-19b, miR-20a and miR-92a)	miR-19a, miR-19b-1 hsa-miR-20a, and miR-92a inhibit translation of the messenger RNA encoding the tumor suppressor PTEN, enhancing cell proliferation and survival. miR-20a targets RNA encoding the E2F2/E2F3 transcription factors, which play a leading role in the regulation of the cell cycle. Repression of the TGF-β antiproliferative signaling pathway: miR-17 and miR-20a target TGF-β-receptor II (TGFBRII), miR-18a targets the participants of this signaling pathway Smad2 and Smad4; miR-18a and miR-19 directly inhibit the antiangiogenic factor thrombospondin-1 (TSP-1).	Proliferation, cell survival, angiogenesis	[35]
2	miR-155	Inhibits translation of the messenger RNA encoding SHIP1 (negative regulator of proliferation) to promote cell growth; C/EBPβ (transcriptional activator for mir-143, which targets one of the main glycolysis enzymes—hk2); TP53INP1 (tumor suppressor regulating autophagy and apoptosis) leads to the inhibition of cell death; MSH2 and MSH6 (key misfit repair proteins) lead to decreased repair; FOXO3 (a transcription factor that regulates genes whose products are involved in apoptosis—for example, Bim and PUMA) leads to avoidance of apoptosis, SOCS1 (negative regulator of cytokine signal transduction) leads to increased proliferation; increases TNF-α levels by binding to the 3′ UTR region of mRNA and increasing transcript stability; with the participation of histone deacetylase HDAC2, represses BRCA1 transcription, which leads to a decrease in repair	Inhibition of apoptosis, proliferation metastases, Warburg effect	[42–44]
3	miR-125b	Inhibits translation of the messenger RNAs encoding p53 and proapoptotic proteins Bak1 and Puma; inhibits translation of the messenger RNA encoding the oncosuppressor p14ARF	Avoidance of apoptosis, proliferation	[50]
4	miR-504	Inhibits translation of the messenger RNA encoding p53	Avoidance of apoptosis, proliferation	[49]
5	miR-622	Inhibits translation of the messenger RNA encoding Rb protein	Avoidance of apoptosis	[52]
6	miR -103	Inhibits translation of the messenger RNA encoding proapoptotic protein Bax	Avoidance of apoptosis	[54]
7	miR-197	Inhibits translation of the messenger RNA encoding NOXA and BMF	Avoidance of apoptosis	[55,56]

Table 1. Cont.

	MicroRNA	MicroRNA Targets and Mechanism	Role in Carcinogenesis	Ref.
1	2	3	4	5
8	miR-494	Inhibits translation of the messenger RNA encoding PTEN and subsequent activation of the Akt/eNOS pathway	Angiogenic effect	[68]
9	miR-222	Inhibits translation of the messenger RNA encoding cyclin-dependent kinase inhibitor p27Kip1	Proliferation	[46,47]
10	miR-10b	Inhibits translation of the messenger RNA encoding the homeobox D10, which increases expression prometastatic gene RHOC	Lung metastases	[83]
11	miR-652-3p	Inhibits translation of the messenger RNA encoding the Lgl1 protein, which promotes cell adhesion and inhibits cell migration by suppressing the expression of MMP2 and MMP14 and the re-expression of E-cadherin	Metastases	[102]
12	miR-98-5p	Inhibits translation of the messenger RNA encoding TGFBR1	Proliferation, migration and invasion of A549 and H1299 cell lines	[64]
13	miR-27a	Inhibits translation of the messenger RNA encoding ATM	Cell survival and cell cycle progression	[113]
14	miR-346	Inhibits translation of the messenger RNA encoding XPC	Promotion tumor growth	[110]

Table 2. Oncosuppressive microRNAs in lung cancer.

	MicroRNA	MicroRNA Targets and Mechanism	Role in Carcinogenesis	Ref.
1	2	3	4	5
1	Let-7	Inhibits translation of the messenger RNAs encoding oncogenes, such as KRAS, NRAS, MYC, HMGA2, and MCT	Inhibits proliferation, inhibits PI3K-mTOR signaling pathway	[37]
2	miR-34	Inhibits translation of the messenger RNA encoding the N-MUS oncogene; cyclin-dependent kinases CDK4 and CDK6; transmembrane receptor protein NOTCH1, involved in the signaling pathway of cancer stem cells; ubiquitin ligase MDMX, involved in p53 degradation; antiapoptotic protein BCL2; sirtuin 1 (SIRT1 gene) involved in p53 degradation; transcription factor E2F3; transcription factors involved in self-renewal of undifferentiated embryonic stem cells: NANOG and SOX2; an integral cellular glycoprotein that plays an important role in cell–cell interactions, cell adhesion, and CD44 migration	Inhibits proliferation, promotes cell cycle arrest and apoptosis	[48]

Table 2. *Cont.*

1	MicroRNA	MicroRNA Targets and Mechanism	Role in Carcinogenesis	Ref.
1	2	3	4	5
3	miR-126	Inhibits translation of the messenger RNA encoding S1PR2, thereby inhibiting the PI3K/Akt signaling pathway; inhibits tumor angiogenesis by targeting VEGF-A	Inhibits proliferation and angiogenesis	[38,39]
4	miR-17-5p	Inhibits translation of the messenger RNA encoding TGFßR2, which is significantly increased in NSCLC tissues and cell lines	Inhibits proliferation, causes apoptosis of H460 NSCLC cells	[59]
5	miR-98	Inhibits translation of the messenger RNA encoding PAK1, which promotes NSCLC cell proliferation, migration, and invasion	Inhibits proliferation	[66]
6	miR-128	Inhibits translation of the messenger RNA encoding VEGF-A, vascular endothelial growth factor receptor 2, and VEGFR-3	Inhibits angiogenesis	[69]
7	miR-206	Inhibits the 14-3-3ζ/STAT3/HIF-1α/VEGF pathway	Inhibits angiogenesis	[70]
8	miR-135a	Decreased angiogenesis-related factors VEGF, bFGF, and IL-8	Inhibits angiogenesis	[71]
9	miR-145	Inhibits translation of the messenger RNA encoding mTOR/p70S6K1	Inhibits proliferation	[41,42]
10	miR-646	Inhibits translation of the messenger RNA encoding FGF2 and CCND2	Inhibits proliferation, invasion, and suppress EMT of NSCLC cells in mice	[87]
11	miR-182	Suppresses AKT phosphorylation and accumulation of the Snail transcription factor, which initiates EMT in lung cancer cells. Inhibits translation of the messenger RNA encoding the Met	Promotes the expression of E-cadherin, which leads to inhibition of EMT	[88]
12	miR-7-5p	Inhibits translation of the messenger RNA encoding NOVA2, which disrupts the angiogenesis	Inhibits proliferation, migration, and invasion of tumor	[89]
13	miR-206	Inhibits translation of the messenger RNA encoding the actin-binding protein coronin 1C (CORO1C)	Reduces the ability of cells to grow and metastasize	[91]
14	miR-335-5p	Inhibits translation of the messenger RNA encoding ROCK1	Leads to inhibition of TGF-β1-mediated EMT	[94]

Table 2. Cont.

	MicroRNA	MicroRNA Targets and Mechanism	Role in Carcinogenesis	Ref.
1	2	3	4	5
15	miR-126-3p	Inhibits translation of the messenger RNA encoding chemokine receptor 1 (CCR1)	Inhibits NSCLC cell growth and metastasis	[96]
16	miR-192-5p	Inhibits translation of the messenger RNA encoding TRIM44	Reduces migration and invasion	[97]
17	miR-143	Inhibits translation of the messenger RNA encoding Limk1	Suppresses NSCLC cell proliferation, induced apoptosis, and suppresses migration and invasion in vitro	[103]
18	miR-138	Inhibits translation of the messenger RNA encoding H2AX	Inhibition on cell-cycle progression and cell grow	[111]
19	hsa-miR-526b	Inhibits translation of the messenger RNA encoding Ku80	Suppresses NSCLC growth	[112]

3. MicroRNAs as Biomarkers of Environmental Factors

As shown in several studies, the microRNA profile can change due to exposure to both chemicals [118,119] and physical environmental factors [120–123]. Ionizing radiation can cause changes in the microRNA expression profile in human fibroblasts [124] and immortalized cell lines [125]. Changes in the expression of microRNAs under the influence of radiation have a dose-dependent effect [126], which indicates the possibility of using microRNAs as biomarkers of radiation exposure [127]. Cui and colleagues showed that the expression profile of several microRNAs in BEAS2B cells changed upon exposure to radon [128].

We examined 136 subjects, including 49 patients with lung cancer exposed to radon, 37 patients with lung cancer without radon exposure, and 50 volunteers as a control group. The level of free-circulating microRNA hsa-miR-19b-3p was significantly higher in groups of patients with lung cancer compared with healthy individuals. However, no differences were found in the expression level of hsa-miR-19b-3p between patients with radon-induced lung cancer and those who were not exposed to radon. These results indicate that the detection of hsa-miR-19b-3p levels in blood plasma can potentially be used as a noninvasive method for diagnosing lung cancer. However, this microRNA is not suitable as a biomarker for radon exposure [129].

Considering that asbestos is one of the causes of lung cancer and that microRNAs are involved in carcinogenesis, the study of the role of microRNAs in asbestos-induced lung damage is relevant.

4. Asbestos and MicroRNA

Extensive research over the past several decades has identified many important pathogenic mechanisms of asbestos fibers for lung cancer; however, the exact molecular mechanisms involved and the cross-linkages between the pathways involved are not fully understood. The significant presence of asbestos in buildings, combined with a long latency period of 30–40 years between exposure and pulmonary toxicity, suggests that asbestos-related lung disease will continue to spread in all countries.

Many studies have examined microRNAs associated with asbestos-induced genetic and epigenetic changes in mesothelioma (highly specific cancer induced by exposure to asbestos) [17,20,130–132]. Thus, it was shown that asbestos causes the overexpression of seven microRNAs (miR-374a, miR-24-1, let-7d, Let-7e, miR-199b-5p, miR-331-3p, and miR-96) in lung tumors (Figure 1), and five microRNAs (miR-939, miR-671-5p, miR-605, miR-1224-5p, and miR-202) demonstrate reduced expression under the influence of asbestos [17,21,131,132]. MicroRNAs whose expression profile changes under the influence of asbestos are shown in Table 3.

Santarelli et al. [132] recently established that four microRNAs, namely, miR-126, miR-205, miR-222, and miR-520g, are involved in asbestos-related malignant diseases. Notably, increased expression of miR-126 and miR-222 has been found in asbestos-exposed subjects, and both microRNAs are involved in major pathways associated with cancer development. Epigenetic changes and cross-linking between cancer and stroma can induce miR-126 repression to facilitate tumor formation, angiogenesis, and invasion.

The study included four patient groups, including patients with asbestos and non-asbestos-related non-small cell lung cancer or malignant pleural mesothelioma, as well as healthy subjects. Selected microRNAs were evaluated in the asbestos-exposed population. This study indicated that microRNAs are potentially involved in asbestos-related malignancies, and their expression describes the mechanisms by which microRNAs may be involved in the asbestos-induced pathogenesis of bronchopulmonary diseases [132].

Nymark and coauthors [130] investigated 26 tumors from highly asbestos-exposed and untreated patients and from normal lung tissue control samples that were analyzed for microRNA expression data. They found thirteen microRNAs associated with asbestos, and, among them, eight microRNAs were overexpressed: miR-148b, miR-374a, miR-24-1, Let-7d, Let-7e, miR-199b-5p, miR-331-3p, and miR-96 and five were downregulated: miR-939, miR-671-5p, miR-605, miR-1224-5p, and miR-202. New microRNAs associated with asbestos and histology were identified.

In addition, an inverse correlation of specific target genes was found using an integrative analysis of microRNA and mRNA data from the same patient samples.

A link between the hypermethylation of promotor DNA and inflammation has been shown in many forms of cancer, including asbestos-related lung cancer [133,134]. Molecular genetic analysis have shown changes in the number of DNA copies, changes in the profiles of many microRNAs, and dysregulation of the expression of certain genes in asbestos-associated lung cancer [130,133,134]. However, how asbestos fibers directly or indirectly affect cells in lung cancer and how they interact with cells at the molecular level is currently not known [17].

Asbestos causes pulmonary toxicity, and thus there are several molecular changes: the generation of ROS, which causes tissue and cell damage, apoptosis of alveolar macrophages, and the release of various cytokines and chemokines.

Transcription factors and the tumor suppressor protein p53 are involved in destroying cellular response DNA, causing mitochondrial dysfunction and apoptosis. Activated p53 affects various genes that inhibit cell growth and partially promote apoptosis due to the mitochondrial-regulated pathway of death [135]. The *TP53* oncosuppressor gene, localized on chromosome 17p13, is expressed in all cell types and encodes the p53 protein, which serves as a transcription factor [136]. Several studies have been performed on the genotoxicity and function of *TP53* in the pathogenesis of lung cancer and pleural mesothelioma [136–138].

Mitochondrial dysfunction and apoptosis in p53-dependent transcription in an asbestos-induced A549 cell line was determined. When the human papillomavirus E6 protein was transfected to A549 cells, the E6 protein inhibited the function of the p53 gene and lost checkpoint in G1 control. A549-empty vector cells exposed to asbestos revealed dose-dependent mitochondrial dysfunction and apoptosis. Panduri et al. demonstrated that asbestos promoted p53 activity, mRNA levels, protein expression, and translocation of Bax and p53 mitochondria. Inhibitors of p53-dependent transcriptional activation blocked asbestos-induced A549 cell activation of caspase 9 and apoptosis [138].

miR-30d expression levels were decreased in plasma subjects exposed to asbestos, the mesothelial cell line NCI-H2452, and the normal mesothelial cell line MeT-5A treated with chrysotile. After transfection of miR-30d to the NCI-H2452 cell line, a percentage difference in G1/S/G2 stages was not found; however, the overall rate of apoptosis increased [139]. The expression of miR-30d was reduced in NSCLC tissue, and the NSCLC stage I/II was upregulated compared with the NSCLC stage III. Hosseini et al. proposed that this expression level could distinguish between different stages of malignancies [140].

In vitro experiments indicated that miR-30d could attenuate the proliferation and viability of NSCLC cells [141]. The aberrant expression of miR-30a in lung cancer stimulated the expression of myocyte enhancer factor 2D (MEF2D) protein [142]. The myocyte enhancer factor 2 (MEF2) family of human transcription factors, consisting of four subtypes, MEF2-A, -B, -C, and -D, has a diversity of functions in different tissues and has been implicated in numerous diseases. MEF2s play an important role in the activation of the genetic processes that control the cell differentiation, proliferation, and apoptosis in lung cancer. miR-30a prevented the growth and formation of lung cancer cells in a colony by inducing apoptosis [143,144].

Research demonstrated that c-Met, which triggers cell growth in tumor formation, was activated through the suppression of p53-regulated miR-34a in mouse malignant mesothelioma cells [145]. miR-34 also regulated the SNAIL1 gene in EMT in A549 cell lines and targeted an essential p53 tumor suppressor [146].

Researchers found that aberrant methylation and silence of miR-34b and miR-34c were observed in asbestos-induced pleural mesothelioma [147]. In lung cancer, the AXL tyrosine kinase receptor is often overexpressed. Via the JNK pathway, the AXL tyrosine kinase receptor activated the ELK1 transcription factor. ELK1, in turn, controlled miR-34a expression by direct activation of the promoter, and miR-34a returned to suppress AXL mRNA. JNK1 overexpression significantly decreased the expression of AXL and caused G1 arrest and apoptosis in lung cancer cells [148]. This allows us to conclude that miR-34 may be involved in the pathogenesis of asbestos-induced lung cancer.

Weber et al. showed that, in the blood of malignant mesothelioma patients exposed to asbestos, miR-20a and miR-103 were downregulated [149]. As we noted above, both of these microRNAs play the role of oncomiRs in the development of lung cancer [35,53], which suggests the presence of different mechanisms of carcinogenesis during the development of asbestos-induced mesothelioma and asbestos-induced lung cancer with the participation of microRNAs.

It is known that asbestos promotes the generation of ROS, which caused the formation of DSB [150,151]. As a result of DSB, changes occur in the chromatin structure, which leads to phosphorylation of the nucleosomal protein H2A and further damage repair. Msiska et al. showed an increase in the amount of γ-H2AX in human lung cell lines (SAE) and lung adenocarcinoma cells (A549) as a result of asbestos-induced DSB formation [152]. Accumulation of γ-H2AX in both cell lines suggests either impaired DSB repair or long-term production of ROS due to asbestos exposure. It should be noted that the level of γ-H2AX in normal cells was higher than in A549. Histone H2AX plays an important role in apoptosis. Xu et al. showed that knockdown of H2AX in A549 cells affects miR-3196 expression. miR-3196 inhibits apoptosis in A549 cells by acting on the PUMA protein. γH2AX binds to the miR-3196 promoter, inhibits the binding of RNA polymerase II to the miR-3196 promoter, leading to inhibition of miR-3196 transcription [153]. Histone H2AX has been identified as a target for miR-138 [111]. However, there is no information on the change in the expression level of this microRNA due to asbestos exposure. Further research is needed to determine the role of microRNAs involved in DNA repair network in the pathogenesis of asbestos-related lung cancer.

In total, we identified 20 microRNAs, whose expression changed upon exposure to asbestos (Table 3).

Table 3. MicroRNAs whose expression profile changed under the influence of asbestos.

	MicroRNA	Expression Level	Type of Cancer	Sample	Ref.
1	miR-374a	Overexpression	Lung cancer	Lung tissue	[130]
2	miR-24-1	Overexpression	Lung cancer	Lung tissue	[130]
3	let-7d	Overexpression	Lung cancer	Lung tissue	[130]
4	let-7e	Overexpression	Lung cancer	Lung tissue	[130]
5	miR-199b-5p	Overexpression	Lung cancer	Lung tissue	[130]
6	miR-331-3p	Overexpression	Lung cancer	Lung tissue	[130]
7	miR-96	Overexpression	Lung cancer	Lung tissue	[130]
8	miR-148b	Overexpression	Lung cancer	Lung tissue	[130]
9	miR-126	Overexpression	Lung cancer	serum	[132]
10	miR-222	Overexpression	Lung cancer	serum	[132]
11	miR-939	down regulation	Lung cancer	Lung tissue	[130]
12	miR-671-5p	down regulation	Lung cancer	Lung tissue	[130]
13	miR-605	down regulation	Lung cancer	Lung tissue	[130]
14	miR-1224-5p	down regulation	Lung cancer	Lung tissue	[130]
15	miR-202	down regulation	Lung cancer	Lung tissue	[130]
16	miR-30d	down regulation	Lung cancer	Lung tissue	[140]
17	miR-34b	down regulation	mesothelioma	serum	[147]
18	miR-34c	down regulation	mesothelioma	serum	[147]
19	miR-20a	down regulation	mesothelioma	blood	[149]
20	miR-103	down regulation	mesothelioma	blood	[149]

Comparative analysis of the microRNAs involved in the development of lung cancer and microRNAs whose expression profile changed upon exposure to asbestos made it possible to identify three microRNAs as possible biomarkers of asbestos-induced lung cancer: miR-222, miR-34b, and miR-34c (Figure 2).

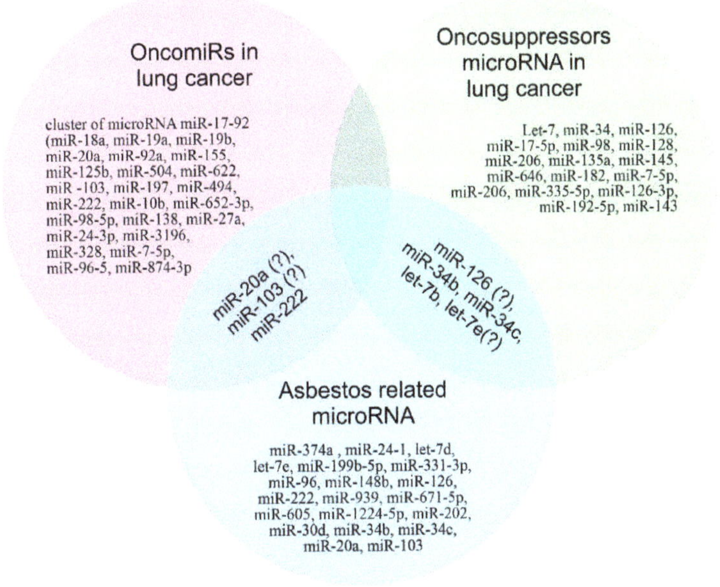

Figure 2. Asbestos-related lung cancer microRNAs.

Three microRNAs (let-7d, let-7e, and miR-126), which act as tumor suppressors and reduce the risk of developing lung cancer, had an increased level of expression in individuals exposed to asbestos. This indicates the need to study the role of microRNAs in asbestos-induced lung cancer and possibly a different mechanism of carcinogenesis in a malignant different mechanism of carcinogenesis in malignant mesothelioma and lung cancer.

Most of the reviews, including systematic reviews [154], devoted to the issue of the relationship of asbestos and microRNAs precisely highlight the changes in the microRNA profile in mesothelioma; however, as we can see, this does not always correspond to lung cancer induced by asbestos.

As this review has shown, further studies are needed to answer the question of whether it is possible to use microRNAs as biomarkers of lung damage caused by asbestos for the diagnosis of lung cancer.

Author Contributions: These authors contributed equally to this work. All authors have read and agreed to the published version of the manuscript.

Funding: This study was partially supported by Ministry of Science and Education of the Republic of Kazakhstan (Grant №– AP09259700).

Institutional Review Board Statement: Not applicable.

Informed Consent Statement: Not applicable.

Conflicts of Interest: The authors declare no conflict of interest.

References

1. Barta, J.A.; Powell, C.A.; Wisnivesky, J.P. Global epidemiology of lung cancer. *Ann. Glob. Health* **2019**, *85*, 1–16. [CrossRef]
2. Siegel, R.L.; Miller, K.D.; Jemal, A. Cancer statistics, 2019. *CA Cancer J. Clin.* **2019**, *69*, 7–34. [CrossRef] [PubMed]
3. Didkowska, J.; Wojciechowska, U.; Manczuk, M.; Lobaszewski, J. Lung cancer epidemiology: Contemporary and future challenges worldwide. *Ann. Transl. Med.* **2016**, *4*, 150. [CrossRef] [PubMed]
4. Miller, K.D.; Nogueira, L.; Mariotto, A.B.; Rowland, J.H.; Yabroff, K.R.; Alfano, C.M.; Jemal, A.; Kramer, J.L.; Siegel, R.L. Cancer treatment and survivorship statistics, 2019. *CA Cancer J. Clin.* **2019**, *69*, 363–385. [CrossRef] [PubMed]

5. Rahal, Z.E.; Nemr, S.; Sinjab, A.; Chami, H.; Tfayli, A.; Kadara, H. Smoking and lung cancer: A Geo-Regional Perspective. *Front. Oncol* **2017**, *7*, 194. [CrossRef]
6. Dicker, D.; Nguyen, G.; Abate, D. GBD 2017 Mortality Collaborators. Global, regional, and national age-sex-specific mortality and life expectancy, 1950-2017: A systematic analysis for the Global Burden of Disease Study 2017. *Lancet* **2018**, *392*, 1684–1735. [CrossRef]
7. Pallis, A.G.; Syrigos, K.N. Lung cancer in never smokers: Disease characteristics and risk factors. *Crit. Rev. Oncol. Hematol.* **2013**, *88*, 494–503. [CrossRef]
8. Martinez, V.D.; Sage, A.P.; Marshall, E.A.; Suzuki, M.; Goodarzi, A.A.; Dellaire, G.; Lam, W.L. Oncogenetics of Lung Cancer induced by environmental carcinogens. *Oncog. Carcinog.* **2019**. [CrossRef]
9. Testa, U.; Castelli, G.; Pelosi, E. Lung Cancers: Molecular Characterization, Clonal Heterogeneity and Evolution, and Cancer Stem Cells. *Cancers* **2018**, *10*, 248. [CrossRef]
10. IARC. Asbestos (chrystolyte, amosite, crocidolite, trmolite, actioolite and antropolite). *IARC Monogr. Eval. Carcinog. Risks Hum.* **2012**, *100c*, 219–309. Available online: monographs.iarc.fr?ENG/Monographs/vol100c/index.php (accessed on 30 January 2021).
11. Asbestos Safety and Eradication Agency. About Asbestos. 2019. Available online: https://www.asbestossafety.gov.au/about-asbestos (accessed on 11 November 2019).
12. Takahashi, K.; Landrigan, P.J. The Global health dimensions of asbestos and asbestos-related diseases. *Ann. Glob. Health* **2016**, *82*, 209–213. [CrossRef] [PubMed]
13. Norbet, C.; Joseph, A.; Rossi, S.S. Asbestos-related lung disease: A pictorial review. *Curr. Probl. Diagn. Radiol.* **2015**, *44*, 371–382. [CrossRef] [PubMed]
14. Huang, S.X.; Jaurand, M.C.; Kamp, D.W.; Whysner, J.; Hei, T.K. Role of mutagenicity in asbestos fiber induced carcinogenicity and other diseases. *J. Toxicol. Environ. Health Part B Crit. Rev.* **2011**, *14*, 179–245. [CrossRef] [PubMed]
15. The Mesothelioma Center. Asbestos-Related Lung Cancer. 2019. Available online: https://www.asbestos.com/cancer/lung-cancer/ (accessed on 11 November 2019).
16. Kameda, T.; Takahashi, K.; Kim, R.; Jiang, Y.; Movahed, M.; Park, E.-K.; Rantanen, J. Asbestos: Use, bans and disease burden in Europe. *Bull. World Health Organ.* **2014**, *92*, 790–797. [CrossRef]
17. Ospina, D.; Villegas, V.E.; Rodriguez-Leguizamon, G.; Rondon-Lagos, M. Analyzing biological and molecular charachteristics and genomic damage induced by exposure to asbestos. *Cancer Manag. Res.* **2019**, *11*, 4997–5012. [CrossRef]
18. Wolff, H.; Vehmas, T.; Oksa, P.; Rantanen, J.; Vainio, H. Asbestos, asbestosis, and cancer, the Helsinki criteria for diagnosis and attribution 2014: Recommendations. *Scand. J. Work Environ. Health* **2015**, *41*, 5–15. [CrossRef]
19. The International Ban Asbestos Secretariat. Current Asbestos Bans. 2018. Available online: http://www.ibasecretariat.org/alpha_ban_list.php (accessed on 1 April 2018).
20. Liu, G.; Cheresh, P.; Kamp, D.W. Molecular basis of asbestos-induced lung disease. *Annu. Rev. Pathol.* **2013**, *24*, 161–187. [CrossRef]
21. Mossman, B.T.; Lippmann, M.; Hesterberg, T.W.; Kelsey, K.T.; Barchowsky, A.; Bonner, J.C. Pulmonary endpoints (lung carcinomas and asbestosis) following inhalation exposure to asbestos. *J. Toxicol. Environ. Health B Crit. Rev.* **2011**, *14*, 76–121. [CrossRef]
22. Markowitz, S. Asbestos-related lung cancer and malignant mesothelioma of the pleura: Selected current issues. *Semin. Respir. Crit. Care Med.* **2015**, *36*, 334–346. [CrossRef]
23. Baldys, A.; Aust, A.E. Role of iron in inactivation of epidermal growth factor receptor after asbestos treatment of human lung and pleural target cells. *Am. J. Respir. Cell Mol. Biol.* **2005**, *32*, 436–442. [CrossRef]
24. Aljandali, A.; Pollack, H.; Yeldandi, A. Asbestos causes apoptosis in alveolar epithelial cells: Role of iron-induced free radicals. *J. Lab. Clin. Med.* **2001**, *137*, 330–339. [CrossRef] [PubMed]
25. Upadhyay, D.; Kamp, D.W. Asbestos-induced pulmonary toxicity: Role of DNA damage and apoptosis. *Exp. Biol. Med.* **2003**, *228*, 650–659. [CrossRef] [PubMed]
26. Arsenic, M. *Fibers and Dust International Agency for Research on Cancer (IARC) Monographs*; International Agency for Research on Cancer: Lyon, France, 2012.
27. Murthy, S.; Ryan, A.; He, C.; Mallampalli, R.K. Carter AB. Rac1-mediated mitochondrial H2O2 generation regulates MMP-9 gene expression in macrophages via inhibition of SP-1 and AP-1. *J. Biol. Chem.* **2010**, *285*, 25062–25073. [CrossRef] [PubMed]
28. He, C.; Murthy, S.; McCormick, M.L.; Spitz, D.R.; Ryan, A.J.; Carter, A.B. Mitochondrial Cu, Zn-superoxide dismutase mediates pulmonary fibrosis by augmenting H2O2 generation. *J. Biol. Chem.* **2011**, *286*, 15597–15607. [CrossRef]
29. Bulgakova, O.; Kussainova, A.; Kausbekova, A.; Bersimbaev, R. The free-circulating mtDNA copies number in plasma of patients with NSCLC. *Ann. Oncol.* **2019**, *30*, 467. [CrossRef]
30. Wu, K.L.; Tsai, Y.M.; Lien, C.T.; Kuo, P.L.; Hung, J.Y. The Roles of MicroRNA in Lung Cancer. *Int. J. Mol. Sci.* **2019**, *20*, 1611. [CrossRef]
31. Wang, Y.; Wang, L.; Chen, C.; Chu, X. New insights into the regulatory role of microRNA in tumor angiogenesis and clinical implications. *Mol. Cancer* **2018**, *17*, 22. [CrossRef]
32. Kozomara, A.; Birgaoanu, M.; Griffiths-Jones, S. miRBase: From microRNA sequences to function. *Nucleic Acids Res.* **2019**, *47*, D155–D162. [CrossRef]
33. Izzotti, A.; Carozzo, S.; Pulliero, A.; Zhabayeva, D.; Ravetti, J.L.; Bersimbaev, R. Extracellular MicroRNA in liquid biopsy: Applicability in cancer diagnosis and prevention. *Am. J. Cancer Res.* **2016**, *6*, 1461–1493.

34. Bersimbaev, R.; Pulliero, A.; Bulgakova, O.; Kussainova, A.A.; Aripova, A.; Izzotti, A. Radon Biomonitoring and microRNA in Lung Cancer. *Int. J. Mol. Sci.* **2020**, *21*, 2154. [CrossRef]
35. Hwang, H.W.; Mendell, J.T. MicroRNAs in cell proliferation, cell death, and tumorigenesis. *Br. J. Cancer* **2006**, *94*, 776–780. [CrossRef] [PubMed]
36. García-Martínez, A.; López-Muñoz, B.; Fajardo, C.; Cámara, R.; Lamas, C.; Silva-Ortega, S.; Aranda, I.; Picó, A. Increased E2F1 mRNA and miR-17-5p Expression Is Correlated to Invasiveness and Proliferation of Pituitary Neuroendocrine Tumours. *Diagnostics* **2020**, *10*, 227. [CrossRef] [PubMed]
37. Chen, Z.; Wang, D.; Gu, C.; Liu, X.; Pei, W.; Li, J.; Cao, Y.; Jiao, Y.; Tong, J.; Nie, J. Down-regulation of let-7 microRNA increased K-ras expression in lung damage induced by radon. *Environ. Toxicol. Pharmacol.* **2015**, *40*, 541–548. [CrossRef] [PubMed]
38. Song, L.; Li, D.; Gu, Y.; Wen, Z.M.; Jie, J.; Zhao, D.; Peng, L.P. MicroRNA-126 Targeting PIK3R2 Inhibits NSCLC A549 Cell Proliferation, Migration, and Invasion by Regulation of PTEN/PI3K/AKT Pathway. *Clin. Lung Cancer* **2016**, *17*, e65–e75. [CrossRef] [PubMed]
39. Chen, Q.; Chen, S.; Zhao, J.; Zhou, Y.; Xu, L. MicroRNA-126: A new and promising player in lung cancer (Review). *Oncol. Lett.* **2020**, *21*, 1. [CrossRef]
40. Tsay, J.J.; Tchou-Wong, K.M.; Yie, T.; Leibert, E.; Segal, L.N.; Greenberg, A.; Pass, H.; Rom, W.N. Bronchial brushings' microRNA and field cancerization in lung adenocarcinoma. *Am. J. Respir. Crit. Care Med.* **2013**, *187*, A4753.
41. Ye, D.; Shen, Z.; Zhou, S. Function of microRNA-145 and mechanisms underlying its role in malignant tumor diagnosis and treatment. *Cancer Manag. Res.* **2019**, *11*, 969–979. [CrossRef]
42. Xu, Q.; Liu, L.Z.; Qian, X.; Chen, Q.; Jiang, Y.; Li, D.; Lai, L.; Jiang, B.H. MiR-145 directly targets p70S6K1 in cancer cells to inhibit tumor growth and angiogenesis. *Nucleic Acids Res.* **2012**, *40*, 761–774. [CrossRef]
43. Shao, C.; Yang, F.; Qin, Z.; Jing, X.; Shu, Y.; Shen, H. The value of miR-155 as a biomarker for the diagnosis and prognosis of lung cancer: A systematic review with meta-analysis. *BMC Cancer* **2019**, *19*, 1103. [CrossRef]
44. Xiang, X.; Zhuang, X.; Ju, S.; Zhang, S.; Jiang, H.; Mu, J.; Zhang, L.; Miller, D.; Grizzle, W.; Zhang, H.G. miR-155 promotes macroscopic tumor formation yet inhibits tumor dissemination from mammary fat pads to the lung by preventing EMT. *Oncogene* **2011**, *30*, 3440–3453. [CrossRef]
45. Kaipeng, X.H.; Cheng, L.; Cheng, W.; Na, Q.; Wei, S.; Yayun, G.; Caiwang, Y.; Kai, Z.; Ningbin, D.; Meng, Z.; et al. A functional variant in miR-155 regulation region contributes to lung cancer risk and survival. *Oncotarget* **2015**, *6*, 42781–42792.
46. Zaporozhchenko, I.A.; Morozkin, E.S.; Ponomaryova, A.A.; Rykova, E.Y.; Cherdyntseva, N.V.; Zheravin, A.A.; Pashkovskaya, O.A.; Pokushalov, E.A.; Vlassov, V.V.; Laktionov, P.P. Profiling of 179 microRNA Expression in Blood Plasma of Lung Cancer Patients and Cancer-Free Individuals. *Sci. Rep.* **2018**, *8*, 6348. [CrossRef] [PubMed]
47. Zhong, C.; Ding, S.; Xu, Y.; Huang, H. MicroRNA-222 promotes human non-small cell lung cancer H460 growth by targeting p27. *Int. J. Clin. Exp. Med.* **2015**, *8*, 5534–5540. [PubMed]
48. Navarro, F.; Lieberman, J. miR-34 and p53: New Insights into a Complex Functional Relationship. *PLoS ONE* **2015**, *10*, e0132767. [CrossRef] [PubMed]
49. Bublik, D.R.; Bursać, S.; Sheffer, M.; Oršolić, I.; Shalit, T.; Tarcic, O.; Kotler, E.; Mouhadeb, O.; Hoffman, Y.; Fuchs, G.; et al. Regulatory module involving FGF13, miR-504, and p53 regulates ribosomal biogenesis and supports cancer cell survival. *Proc. Natl. Acad. Sci. USA* **2017**, *114*, E496–E505. [CrossRef] [PubMed]
50. Banzhaf-Strathmann, J.; Edbauer, D. Good guy or bad guy: The opposing roles of microRNA 125b in cancer. *CCS* **2014**, *12*, 30. [CrossRef]
51. Wang, Y.; Scheiber, M.N.; Neumann, C.; Calin, G.A.; Zhou, D. MicroRNA regulation of ionizing radiation-induced premature senescence. *Int. J. Radiat. Oncol. Biol. Phys.* **2011**, *81*, 839–848. [CrossRef] [PubMed]
52. Ma, W.; Yu, J.; Qi, X.; Liang, L.; Zhang, Y.; Ding, Y.; Lin, X.; Li, G.; Ding, Y. Radiation-induced microRNA-622 causes radioresistance in colorectal cancer cells by down-regulating Rb. *Oncotarget* **2015**, *6*, 15984–15994. [CrossRef]
53. Zevine, A.J.; Hu, W.; Feng, Z. The P53 pathway: What questions remain to be explored? *Cell Death Differ.* **2006**, *13*, 1027–1036.
54. Zhou, J.; Zhang, H.; Chen, L.; Song, Q. Effect of miR 103 on proliferation and apoptosis of non small cell lung cancer by inhibition of FBW7 expression. *Oncol. Lett.* **2020**. [CrossRef]
55. Fiori, M.; Barbini, C.; Haas, T.L.; Marroncelli, N.; Patrizii, M.; Biffoni, M.; De Maria, R. Antitumor effect of miR-197 targeting in p53 wild-type lung cancer. *Cell Death Differ.* **2014**, *21*, 774–782. [CrossRef] [PubMed]
56. Chen, Y.; Yang, C. miR-197-3p induced downregulation of lysine 63 deubiquitinase promotes cell proliferation and inhibits cell apoptosis in lung adenocarcinoma cell lines. *Mol. Med. Rep.* **2018**, *17*, 3921–3927. [CrossRef] [PubMed]
57. Li, H.; Zhou, H.; Luo, J.; Huang, J. MicroRNA-17-5p inhibits proliferation and triggers apoptosis in non-small cell lung cancer by targeting transforming growth factor β receptor 2. *Exp. Med.* **2017**, *13*, 2715–2722. [CrossRef]
58. Chi, E.Y.; Viriyapak, B.; Kwack, H.S.; Lee, Y.K.; Kim, S.I.; Lee, K.H.; Park, T.C. Regulation of paclitaxel-induced programmed cell death by autophagic induction: A model for cervical cancer. *Obstet. Gynecol. Sci.* **2013**, *56*, 84. [CrossRef] [PubMed]
59. Chatterjee, A.; Chattopadhyay, D.; Chakrabarti, G. miR-17-5p Downregulation Contributes to Paclitaxel Resistance of Lung Cancer Cells through Altering Beclin1 Expression. *PLoS ONE* **2014**, *9*, e95716. [CrossRef]
60. Li, J.; Zhou, Q.; Liang, Y.; Pan, W.; Bei, Y.; Zhang, Y.; Wang, J.; Jiao, Z. miR-486 inhibits PM2.5-induced apoptosis and oxidative stress in human lung alveolar epithelial A549 cells. *Ann. Transl. Med.* **2018**, *6*, 209. [CrossRef]

61. Ahn, M.J.; Kang, K.A.; Ryu, Y.S.; Hyun, Y.J.; Shilnikova, K.; Zhen, A.X.; Jeong, J.W.; Choi, Y.H.; Kang, H.K.; Koh, Y.S.; et al. Particulate matter 2.5 damages skin cells by inducing oxidative stress, subcellular organelle dysfunction, and apoptosis. *Arch. Toxicol.* **2018**, *92*, 2077–2091.
62. Yang, N.; Liang, Y.; Yang, P.; Yang, T.; Jiang, L. Propofol inhibits lung cancer cell viability and induces cell apoptosis by upregulating microRNA-486 expression. *Braz. J. Med. Biol. Res.* **2017**, *50*. [CrossRef]
63. Yu, S.; Geng, S.; Hu, Y. miR-486-5p inhibits cell proliferation and invasion through repressing GAB2 in non-small cell lung cancer. *Oncol. Lett.* **2018**, *16*, 3525–3530. [CrossRef]
64. Zhou, H.; Huang, Z.; Chen, X.; Chen, S. miR-98 inhibits expression of TWIST to prevent progression of non-small cell lung cancers. *Biomed. Pharmacother.* **2017**, *89*, 1453–1461. [CrossRef] [PubMed]
65. Fu, Y.; Liu, X.; Chen, Q.; Liu, T.; Lu, C.; Yu, J.; Miao, Y.; Wei, J. Downregulated miR-98-5p promotes PDAC proliferation and metastasis by reversely regulating MAP4K4. *J. Exp. Clin. Cancer Res.* **2018**, *37*, 130. [CrossRef] [PubMed]
66. Yang, G.; Zhang, X.; Shi, J. MiR-98 inhibits cell proliferation and invasion of non-small cell carcinoma lung cancer by targeting PAK1. *Int. J. Clin. Exp. Med.* **2015**, *8*, 20135–20145. [PubMed]
67. Lou, W.; Liu, J.; Gao, Y.; Zhong, G.; Chen, D.; Shen, J.; Bao, C.; Xu, L.; Pan, J.; Cheng, J.; et al. MicroRNAs in cancer metastasis and angiogenesis. *Oncotarget* **2017**, *8*, 115787–115802. [CrossRef] [PubMed]
68. Mao, G.; Liu, Y.; Fang, X.; Liu, Y.; Fang, L.; Lin, L.; Liu, X.; Wang, N. Tumor-derived microRNA-494 promotes angiogenesis in non-small cell lung cancer. *Angiogenesis* **2015**, *18*, 373–382. [CrossRef]
69. Hu, J.; Cheng, Y.; Li, Y.; Jin, Z.; Pan, Y.; Liu, G.; Fu, S.; Zhang, Y.; Feng, K.; Feng, Y. microRNA-128 plays a critical role in human non-small cell lung cancer tumourigenesis, angiogenesis and lymphangiogenesis by directly targeting vascular endothelial growth factor-C. *Eur. J. Cancer* **2014**, *50*, 2336–2350. [CrossRef]
70. Xue, D.; Yang, Y.; Liu, Y.; Wang, P.; Dai, Y.; Liu, Q.; Chen, L.; Shen, J.; Ju, H.; Li, Y.; et al. MicroRNA-206 attenuates the growth and angiogenesis in non-small cell lung cancer cells by blocking the 14-3-3ζ/STAT3/HIF-1α/VEGF signaling. *Oncotarget* **2016**, *7*, 79805–79813. [CrossRef]
71. Zhou, Y.; Li, S.; Li, J.; Wang, D.; Li, Q. Effect of microRNA-135a on Cell Proliferation, Migration, Invasion, Apoptosis and Tumor Angiogenesis Through the IGF-1/PI3K/Akt Signaling Pathway in Non-Small Cell Lung Cancer. *Cell Physiol. Biochem.* **2017**, *42*, 1431–1446. [CrossRef]
72. Chaffer, C.L.; Weinberg, R.A. A perspective on cancer cell metastasis. *Science* **2011**, *331*, 1559–1564. [CrossRef]
73. Wu, S.G.; Chang, T.H.; Liu, Y.N.; Shih, J.Y. MicroRNA in Lung Cancer Metastasis. *Cancers* **2019**, *11*, 265. [CrossRef]
74. Shin, D.Y.; Na, I.I.; Kim, C.H.; Park, S.; Baek, H.; Yang, S.H. EGFR mutation and brain metastasis in pulmonary adenocarcinomas. *J. Thorac. Oncol.* **2014**, *9*, 195–199. [CrossRef]
75. Cho, Y.J.; Cho, Y.M.; Kim, S.H.; Shin, K.H.; Jung, S.T.; Kim, H.S. Clinical analysis of patients with skeletal metastasis of lung cancer. *BMC Cancer* **2019**, *19*, 303. [CrossRef] [PubMed]
76. Tamura, T.; Kurishima, K.; Nakazawa, K.; Kagohashi, K.; Ishikawa, H.; Satoh, H.; Hizawa, N. Specific organ metastases and survival in metastatic non-small-cell lung cancer. *Mol. Clin. Oncol.* **2015**, *3*, 217–221. [CrossRef] [PubMed]
77. Edme, N.; Downward, J.; Thiery, J.P.; Boyer, B. Ras induces NBT-II epithelial cell scattering through the coordinate activities of Ras and MAPK pathways. *J. Cell Sci.* **2002**, *115*, 2591–2601. [PubMed]
78. Jenndahl, L.E.; Isakson, P.; Baeckstrom, D. c-erbB2-induced epithelial-mesenchymal transition in mammary epithelial cells is suppressed by cell-cell contact and initiated prior to E-cadherin downregulation. *Int. J. Oncol.* **2005**, *27*, 439–448. [CrossRef]
79. Wise, R.; Zolkiewska, A. Metalloprotease-dependent activation of EGFR modulates CD44(+)/CD24(-) populations in triple negative breast cancer cells through the MEK/ERK pathway. *Breast Cancer Res. Treat.* **2017**, *166*, 421–433. [CrossRef]
80. Claperon, A.; Mergey, M.; Ho-Bouldoires, T.H.N.; Vignjevic, D.; Wendum, D.; Chretien, Y.; Merabtene, F.; Frazao, A.; Paradis, V.; Housset, C.; et al. EGF/EGFR axis contributes to the progression of cholangiocarcinoma through the induction of an epithelial-mesenchymal transition. *J. Hepatol.* **2014**, *61*, 325–332. [CrossRef]
81. Thiery, J.P.; Acloque, H.; Huang, R.Y.; Nieto, M.A. Epithelial-mesenchymal transitions in development and disease. *Cell* **2009**, *139*, 871–890. [CrossRef]
82. Ma, L.; Teruya-Feldstein, J.; Weinberg, R.A. Tumour invasion and metastasis initiated by microRNA-10b in breast cancer. *Nature* **2007**, *449*, 682–688. [CrossRef]
83. Li, Y.; Li, Y.; Liu, J.; Fan, Y.; Li, X.; Dong, M.; Liu, H.; Chen, J. Expression levels of microRNA-145 and microRNA-10b are associated with metastasis in non-small cell lung cancer. *Cancer Biol.* **2016**, *17*, 272–279. [CrossRef]
84. Li, W.; Liu, M.; Feng, Y.; Xu, Y.-F.; Huang, Y.-F.; Che, J.-P.; Wang, G.-C.; Yao, X.-D.; Zheng, J.-H. Downregulated miR-646 in clear cell renal carcinoma correlated with tumour metastasis by targeting the nin one binding protein (NOB1). *Br. J. Cancer* **2014**, *111*, 1188–1200. [CrossRef]
85. Zhang, P.; Tang, W.M.; Zhang, H.; Li, Y.Q.; Peng, Y.; Wang, J.D.; Liu, G.N.; Huang, X.T.; Zhao, J.J.; Li, G.X.; et al. MiR-646 inhibited cell proliferation and EMT-induced metastasis by targeting FOXK1 in gastric cancer. *Br. J. Cancer* **2017**, *117*, 525–534. [CrossRef] [PubMed]
86. Niu, Y.; Jin, Y.; Deng, S.-C.; Deng, S.-J.; Zhu, S.; Liu, Y.; Li, X.; He, C.; Liu, M.-L.; Zeng, Z.; et al. MicroRNA-646-mediated reciprocal repression between HIF-1alpha and MIIP contributes to tumorigenesis of pancreatic cancer. *Oncogene* **2018**, *37*, 1743–1758. [CrossRef] [PubMed]

87. Zhang, L.; Wu, J.; Li, Y.; Jiang, Y.; Wang, L.; Chen, Y.; Lv, Y.; Zou, Y.; Ding, X. Circ_0000527 promotes the progression of retinoblastoma by regulating miR-646/LRP6 axis. *Cancer Cell Int.* **2020**, *20*, 1. [CrossRef] [PubMed]
88. Li, Y.; Zhang, H.; Li, Y.; Zhao, C.; Fan, Y.; Liu, J.; Li, X.; Liu, H.; Chen, J. MiR-182 inhibits the epithelial to mesenchymal transition and metastasis of lung cancer cells by targeting the Met gene. *Mol. Carcinog.* **2018**, *57*, 125–136. [CrossRef] [PubMed]
89. Xiao, H. MiR-7-5p suppresses tumor metastasis of non-small cell lung cancer by targeting NOVA2. *Cell. Mol. Biol. Lett.* **2019**, *24*, 60. [CrossRef] [PubMed]
90. Giampietro, C.; Deflorian, G.; Gallo, S.; Di Matteo, A.; Pradella, D.; Bonomi, S.; Belloni, E.; Nyqvist, D.; Quaranta, V.; Confalonieri, S.; et al. The alternative splicing factor Nova2 regulates vascular development and lumen formation. *Nat. Commun.* **2015**, *6*, 8479. [CrossRef] [PubMed]
91. Liao, M.; Peng, L. MiR-206 may suppress non-small lung cancer metastasis by targeting CORO1C. *Cell. Mol. Biol. Lett.* **2020**, *25*, 22. [CrossRef]
92. Cheng, X.; Wang, X.; Wu, Z.; Tan, S.; Zhu, T.; Ding, K. CORO1C expression is associated with poor survival rates in gastric cancer and promotes metastasis in vitro. *FEBS Open Bio* **2019**, *9*, 1097–1108. [CrossRef]
93. Lim, J.P.; Shyamasundar, S.; Gunaratne, J.; Scully, O.J.; Matsumoto, K.; Bay, B.H. YBX1 gene silencing inhibits migratory and invasive potential via CORO1C in breast cancer in vitro. *BMC Cancer* **2017**, *17*, 201. [CrossRef]
94. Du, W.; Tang, H.; Lei, Z.; Zhu, J.; Zeng, Y.; Liu, Z.; Huang, J.-A. miR-335-5p inhibits TGF-β1-induced epithelial–mesenchymal transition in non-small cell lung cancer via ROCK1. *Respir. Res.* **2019**, *20*, 225. [CrossRef]
95. Hu, C.; Zhou, H.; Liu, Y.; Huang, J.; Liu, W.; Zhang, Q.; Tang, Q.; Sheng, F.; Li, G.; Zhang, R. ROCK1 promotes migration and invasion of non-small-cell lung cancer cells through the PTEN/PI3K/FAK pathway. *Int. J. Oncol.* **2019**, *55*, 833–844. [CrossRef] [PubMed]
96. Liu, R.; Zhang, Y.-S.; Zhang, S.; Cheng, Z.-M.; Yu, J.-L.; Zhou, S.; Song, J. MiR-126-3p suppresses the growth, migration and invasion of NSCLC via targeting CCR1. *Eur. Rev. Med. Pharm. Sci.* **2019**, *23*, 679–689.
97. Zou, P.; Zhu, M.; Lian, C.; Wang, J.; Chen, Z.; Zhang, X.; Yang, Y.; Chen, X.; Cui, X.; Liu, J.; et al. miR-192-5p suppresses the progression of lung cancer bone metastasis by targeting TRIM44. *Sci. Rep.* **2019**, *9*, 19619. [CrossRef] [PubMed]
98. Xing, Y.; Meng, Q.; Chen, X.; Zhao, Y.; Liu, W.; Hu, J.; Xue, F.; Wang, X.; Cai, L. TRIM44 promotes proliferation and metastasis in non-small cell lung cancer via mTOR signaling pathway. *Oncotarget* **2016**, *7*, 30479–30491. [CrossRef] [PubMed]
99. Wei, C.Y.; Wang, L.; Zhu, M.X.; Deng, X.Y.; Wang, D.H.; Zhang, S.M.; Ying, J.H.; Yuan, X.; Wang, Q.; Xuan, T.F.; et al. TRIM44 activates the AKT/mTOR signal pathway to induce melanoma progression by stabilizing TLR4. *J. Exp. Clin. Cancer Res.* **2019**, *38*, 137. [CrossRef]
100. Xiong, D.; Jin, C.; Ye, X.; Qiu, B.; Jianjun, X.; Zhu, S.; Xiang, L.; Wu, H.; Yongbing, W. TRIM44 promotes human esophageal cancer progression via the AKT/mTOR pathway. *Cancer Sci.* **2018**, *109*, 3080–3092. [CrossRef]
101. Zhao, Y.; Zheng, R.; Ning, D.; Xie, F. MiR-625 Inhibits Tumor Cell Invasion, Migration and EMT by Negatively Regulating the Expression of Resistin in Non-Small Cell Lung. *Cancer Manag. Res.* **2020**, *12*, 4171–4180. [CrossRef]
102. Yang, W.; Zhou, C.; Luo, M.; Shi, X.; Li, Y.; Sun, Z.; Zhou, F.; Chen, Z.; He, J. MiR-652-3p is upregulated in non-small cell lung cancer and promotes proliferation and metastasis by directly targeting Lgl1. *Oncotarget* **2016**, *7*, 16703–16715. [CrossRef]
103. Xia, H.; Sun, S.; Wang, B.; Wang, T.; Liang, C.; Li, G.; Huang, C.; Qi, D.; Chu, X. miR-143 Inhibits NSCLC Cell Growth and Metastasis by Targeting Limk1. *Int. J. Mol. Sci* **2014**, *15*, 11973–11983. [CrossRef]
104. Tapia, T.; Ottman, R.; Chakrabarti, R. LIM kinase1 modulates function of membrane type matrix metalloproteinase 1: Implication in invasion of prostate cancer cells. *Mol. Cancer* **2011**, *10*, 6. [CrossRef]
105. Bagheri-Yarmand, R.; Mazumdar, A.; Sahin, A.A.; Kumar, R. LIM kinase 1 increases tumor metastasis of human breast cancer cells via regulation of the urokinase-type plasminogen activator system. *Int. J. Cancer* **2006**, *118*, 2703–2710. [CrossRef] [PubMed]
106. Jiang, F.; Yu, Q.; Chu, Y.; Zhu, X.; Lu, W.; Liu, Q.; Wang, Q. MicroRNA-98-5p inhibits proliferation and metastasis in non-small cell lung cancer by targeting TGFBR1. *Int. J. Oncol.* **2019**, *54*, 128–138. [CrossRef] [PubMed]
107. Cui, Y.; Zha, Y.; Li, T.; Bai, J.; Tang, L.; Deng, J.; He, R.; Dong, F.; Zhang, Q. Oxidative effects of lungs in Wistar rats caused by long-term exposure to four kinds of China representative chrysotile. *Environ. Sci. Pollut. Res. Int.* **2019**, *26*, 18708–18718. [CrossRef] [PubMed]
108. Mairinger, F.D.; Werner, R.; Flom, E.; Schmeller, J.; Borchert, S.; Wessolly, M.; Wohlschlaeger, J.; Hager, T.; Mairinger, T.; Kollmeier, J.; et al. miRNA regulation is important for DNA damage repair and recognition in malignant pleural mesothelioma. *Virchows Arch.* **2017**, *470*, 627–637. [CrossRef] [PubMed]
109. Nouws, J.; Wan, F.; Finnemore, E.; Roque, W.; Kim, S.J.; Bazan, I.S.; Li, C.X.; Sköld, C.M.; Dai, Q.; Yan, X.; et al. MicroRNA miR-24-3p reduces DNA damage responses, apoptosis, and susceptibility to chronic obstructive pulmonary disease. *JCI Insight* **2020**, *8*, 134218. [CrossRef]
110. Szatkowska, M.; Krupa, R. Regulation of DNA Damage Response and Homologous Recombination Repair by microRNA in Human Cells Exposed to Ionizing Radiation. *Cancers* **2020**, *12*, 1838. [CrossRef]
111. Yang, H.; Luo, J.; Liu, Z.; Zhou, R.; Luo, H. MicroRNA-138 Regulates DNA Damage Response in Small Cell Lung Cancer Cells by Directly Targeting H2AX. *Cancer Investig.* **2015**, *33*, 126–136. [CrossRef]
112. Zhang, Z.Y.; Fu, S.L.; Xu, S.Q.; Zhou, X.; Liu, X.S.; Xu, Y.J.; Zhao, J.P.; Wei, S. By downregulating Ku80, HSA-miR-526b suppresses non-small cell lung cancer. *Oncotarget* **2015**, *6*, 1462–1477. [CrossRef]

113. Di Francesco, A.; De Pittà, C.; Moret, F.; Barbieri, V.; Celotti, L.; Mognato, M. The DNA-damage response to γ-radiation is affected by miR-27a in A549 cells. *Int. J. Mol. Sci.* **2013**, *14*, 17881–17896. [CrossRef]
114. Cortez, M.A.; Valdecanas, D.; Niknam, S.; Peltier, H.J.; Diao, L.; Giri, U.; Komaki, R.; Calin, G.A.; Gomez, D.R.; Chang, J.Y.; et al. In Vivo Delivery of miR-34a Sensitizes Lung Tumors to Radiation Through RAD51 Regulation. *Mol. Ther. Nucleic Acids* **2015**, *4*, e270. [CrossRef]
115. Piotto, C.; Biscontin, A.; Millino, C.; Mognato, M. Functional validation of miRNAs targeting genes of DNA double-strand break repair to radiosensitize non-small lung cancer cells. *Biochim. Biophys. Acta Gene Regul. Mech.* **2018**, *1861*, 1102–1118. [CrossRef] [PubMed]
116. Lai, J.; Yang, H.; Zhu, Y.; Ruan, M.; Huang, Y.; Zhang, Q. MiR-7-5p-mediated downregulation of PARP1 impacts DNA homologous recombination repair and resistance to doxorubicin in small cell lung cancer. *BMC Cancer* **2019**, *19*, 602. [CrossRef]
117. Yang, H.; Rivera, Z.; Jube, S.; Nasu, M.; Bertino, P.; Goparaju, C.; Franzoso, G.; Lotze, M.; Krausz, T.; Pass, H.I.; et al. Programmed necrosis induced by asbestos in human mesothelial cells causes high-mobility group box 1 protein release and resultant inflammation. *Proc. Natl. Acad. Sci. USA* **2010**, *107*, 12611–12616. [CrossRef] [PubMed]
118. Valencia-Quintana, R.; Sánchez-Alarcón, J.; Tenorio-Arvide, M.G.; Deng, Y.; Montiel-González, J.M.; Gómez-Arroyo, S.; Villalobos-Pietrini, R.; Cortés-Eslava, J.; Flores-Márquez, A.R.; Arenas-Huertero, F. The microRNAs as potential biomarkers for predicting the onset of aflatoxin exposure in human beings: A review. *Front. Microbiol.* **2014**, *5*, 1–14. [CrossRef] [PubMed]
119. Izzotti, A.; Pulliero, A. The effects of environmental chemical carcinogens on the microRNA machinery. *Int. J. Hyg. Environ. Health* **2014**, *217*, 601–627. [CrossRef]
120. Jayanthy, A.; Setaluri, V. Light-regulated MicroRNAs. *Photochem. Photobiol.* **2015**, *91*, 163–172. [CrossRef]
121. Metheetrairut, C.; Slack, F.J. MicroRNAs in the ionizing radiation response and in radiotherapy. *Curr. Opin. Genet. Dev.* **2013**, *23*, 12–19. [CrossRef]
122. Czochor, J.R.; Glazer, P.M. microRNAs in cancer cell response to ionizing radiation. *Antioxid. Redox Signal.* **2014**, *21*, 293–312. [CrossRef]
123. Halimi, M.; Asghari, S.M.; Sariri, R.; Moslemi, D.; Parsian, H. Cellular response to ionizing radiation: A microRNA story. *Int. J. Mol. Cell. Med.* **2012**, *1*, 178–184.
124. Simone, N.L.; Soule, B.P.; Ly, D.; Saleh, A.D.; Savage, J.E.; Degraff, W.; Cook, J.; Harris, C.C.; Gius, D.; Mitchell, J.B. Ionizing radiation-induced oxidative stress alters microRNA expression. *PLoS ONE* **2009**, *4*, e6377. [CrossRef]
125. Shin, S.; Cha, H.J.; Lee, E.M.; Lee, S.J.; Seo, S.K.; Jin, H.O.; Park, I.C.; Jin, Y.W.; An, S. Alteration of microRNA profiles by ionizing radiation in A549 human non-small cell lung cancer cells. *Int. J. Oncol.* **2009**, *35*, 81–86.
126. Templin, T.; Young, E.F.; Smilenov, L.B. Whole mouse blood microRNA as biomarkers for exposure to -rays and (56) Fe ion. *Int. J. Radiat. Biol.* **2011**, *87*, 653–662. [CrossRef] [PubMed]
127. Templin, T.; Young, E.F.; Smilenov, L.B. Proton radiation-induced microRNA signatures in mouse blood: Characterization and comparison with 56Fe-ion and gamma radiation. *Int. J. Radiat. Biol.* **2012**, *88*, 531–539. [CrossRef] [PubMed]
128. Cui, F.M.; Li, J.X.; Chen, Q.; Du, H.B.; Zhang, S.Y.; Nie, J.H.; Cao, J.P.; Zhou, P.K.; Hei, T.K.; Tong, J. Radon-induced alterations in micro-RNA expression profiles in transformed BEAS2B cells. *J. Toxicol. Environ. Health* **2013**, *76*, 107–119. [CrossRef] [PubMed]
129. Bulgakova, O.; Zhabayeva, D.; Kussainova, A.; Pulliero, A.; Izzotti, A.; Bersimbaev, R. miR-19 in blood plasma reflects lung cancer occurrence but is not specifically associated with radon exposure. *Oncol. Lett.* **2018**, *15*, 8816–8824. [CrossRef] [PubMed]
130. Nymark, P.; Guled, M.; Borze, I.; Faisal, A.; Lahti, L.; Salmenkivi, K.; Kettunen, E.; Anttila, S.; Knuutila, S. Integrative analysis of microRNA, mRNA and aCGH data reveals asbestos- and histology-related changes in lung cancer. *Genes Chromosom. Cancer* **2011**, *50*, 585–597. [CrossRef] [PubMed]
131. Kettunen, E.; Aavikko, M.; Nymark, P.; Ruosaari, S.; Wikman, H.; Vanhala, E.; Salmenkivi, K.; Pirinen, R.; Karjalainen, A.; Kuosma, E.; et al. DNA copy number loss and allelic imbalance at 2p16 in lung cancer associated with asbestos exposure. *Br. J. Cancer* **2009**, *100*, 1336–1342. [CrossRef]
132. Santarelli, L.; Gaetani, S.; Monaco, F.; Bracci, M.; Valentino, M.; Amati, M.; Rubini, C.; Sabbatini, A.; Pasquini, E.; Zanotta, N.; et al. Four-miRNA Signature to identify asbestos related lung malignancies. *Cancer Epidemiol. Biomark. Prev.* **2019**, *28*. [CrossRef]
133. Kettunen, E.; Hernandez-Vargas, H.; Cros, M.-P.; Durand, G.; Le Calvez-Kelm, F.; Stuopelyte, K.; Jarmalaite, S.; Salmenkivi, K.; Anttila, S.; Wolff, H.; et al. Asbestos-associated genome-wide DNA methylation changes in lung cancer. *Int. J. Cancer* **2017**, *141*, 2014–2029. [CrossRef]
134. Cheng, Y.Y.; Rath, E.M.; Linton, A.; Yuen, M.L.; Takahashi, K.; Lee, K. The current understanding of asbestos-induced epigenetic changes associated with lung cancer. *Lung Cancer* **2020**, *11*, 1–11. [CrossRef]
135. Oren, M. Decision making by p53: Life, death and cancer. *Cell Death Differ.* **2003**, *10*, 431–442. [CrossRef] [PubMed]
136. Andujar, P.; Pairon, J.C.; Renier, A.; Descatha, A.; Hysi, I. Differential mutation profiles and similar intronic TP53 polymorphisms in asbestos-related lung cancer and pleural mesothelioma. *Mutagenesis* **2013**, *28*, 323–331. [CrossRef] [PubMed]
137. Inamura, K.; Ninomiya, H.; Nomura, K.; Tsuchiya, E.; Satoh, Y.; Okumura, S.; Nakagawa, K.; Takata, A.; Kohyama, N.; Ishikawa, Y. Combined effects of asbestos and cigarette smoke on the development of lung adenocarcinoma: Different carcinogens may cause different genomic changes. *Oncol. Rep.* **2014**, *32*, 475–482. [CrossRef] [PubMed]
138. Panduri, V.; Surapureddi, S.; Soberanes, S.; Weitzman, S.A.; Chandel, N.; Kamp, D.W. P53 Mediates Amosite Asbestos–Induced Alveolar Epithelial Cell Mitochondria-Regulated Apoptosis. *Am. J. Respir. Cell Mol. Biol.* **2006**, *34*, 443–452. [CrossRef]

139. Ju, L.; Wu, W.; Yin, X.; Xiao, Y.; Jia, Z.; Lou, J.; Zhu, L. miR-30d is related to asbestos exposure and inhibits migration and invasion in NCI-H2452 cells. *FEBS Open Bio* **2017**, *7*, 1469–1479. [CrossRef] [PubMed]
140. Hosseini, S.M.; Soltani, B.M.; Tavallaei, M.; Mowla, S.J.; Tafsiri, E.; Bagheri, A.; Khorshid, H.R.K. Clinically Significant Dysregulation of hsa-miR-30d-5p and hsa-let-7b Expression in Patients with Surgically Resected Non-Small Cell Lung Cancer. *Avicenna J. Med. Biotechnol.* **2018**, *10*, 98–104.
141. Gao, L.; He, R.; Wu, H.-Y.; Zhang, T.-T.; Liang, H.; Ye, Z.-H.; Li, Z.-Y.; Xie, T.-T.; Shi, Q.; Ma, J.; et al. Expression Signature and Role of miR-30d-5p in Non-Small Cell Lung Cancer: A Comprehensive Study Based on in Silico Analysis of Public Databases and *In Vitro* Experiments. *Cell Physiol. Biochem.* **2018**, *50*, 1964–1987. [CrossRef]
142. Luan, N.; Wang, Y.; Liu, X. Absent expression of miR-30a promotes the growth of lung cancer cells by targeting MEF2D. *Oncol. Lett.* **2018**, *16*, 1173–1179. [CrossRef] [PubMed]
143. Zhu, H.-X.; Shi, L.; Zhang, Y.; Zhu, Y.; Bai, C.; Wang, X.; Zhou, J.-B. Myocyte enhancer factor 2D provides a cross-talk between chronic inflammation and lung cancer. *J. Transl. Med.* **2015**, *15*, 65. [CrossRef]
144. Hylebos, M.; Guy, V.C. The Genetic Landscape of Malignant Pleural Mesothelioma: Results from Massively Parallel Sequencing. *J. Thorac. Oncol.* **2016**, *11*, 1615–1626. [CrossRef]
145. Menges, C.W.; Kadariya, Y.; Altomare, D.; Kadariya, Y.; Altomare, D. Tumor suppressor alterations cooperate to drive aggressive mesotheliomas with enriched cancer stem cells via a p53-miR-34a-c-Met axis. *Cancer Res.* **2014**, *74*, 1261–1271. [CrossRef] [PubMed]
146. Kim, N.H.; Kim, H.S.; Li, X.Y.; Lee, I.; Choi, H.S.; Kang, S.E.; Cha, S.Y.; Ryu, J.K.; Yoon, D.; Fearon, E.R.; et al. A p53/microRNA-34 axis regulates Snail1-dependent cancer cell epithelial-mesenchymal transition. *J. Cell Biol.* **2011**, *195*, 417–433. [CrossRef] [PubMed]
147. Muraoka, T.; Soh, J.; Toyooka, S.; Aoe, K.; Fujimoto, N.; Hashida, S.; Maki, Y.; Tanaka, N.; Shien, K.; Furukawa, M.; et al. The degree of microRNA-34b/c methylation in serum-circulating DNA is associated with malignant pleural mesothelioma. *Lung Cancer* **2013**, *82*, 485–490. [CrossRef] [PubMed]
148. Cho, C.Y.; Huang, J.S.; Shiah, S.; Chung, S.Y.; Lay, J.D.; Yang, Y.Y.; Lai, G.M.; Cheng, A.L.; Chen, L.T.; Chuang, S.E. Negative feedback regulation of AXL by miR-34a modulates apoptosis in lung cancer cells. *RNA* **2016**, *22*, 303–315. [CrossRef]
149. Weber, D.G.; Johnen, G.; Bryk, O.; Jöckel, K.H.; Brüning, T. Identification of miRNA-103 in the cellular fraction of human peripheral blood as a potential biomarker for malignant mesothelioma—A pilot study. *PLoS ONE* **2012**, *7*, e30221. [CrossRef]
150. Okayasu, R.; Takahashi, S.; Yamada, S.; Hei, T.K.; Ullrich, R.L. Asbestos and DNA double strand breaks. *Cancer Res.* **1999**, *59*, 298–300.
151. Castranova, V. Signaling pathways controlling the production of inflammatory mediators in response to crystalline silica exposure: Role of reactive oxygen/nitrogen species. *Free Radic Biol. Med.* **2004**, *37*, 916–925. [CrossRef]
152. Msiska, Z.; Pacurari, M.; Mishra, A.; Leonard, S.S.; Castranova, V.; Vallyathan, V. DNA double-strand breaks by asbestos, silica, and titanium dioxide: Possible biomarker of carcinogenic potential? *Am. J. Respir. Cell Mol. Biol.* **2010**, *43*, 210–219. [CrossRef]
153. Xu, C.; Zhang, L.; Duan, L.; Lu, C. MicroRNA-3196 is inhibited by H2AX phosphorylation and attenuates lung cancer cell apoptosis by downregulating PUMA. *Oncotarget* **2016**, *7*, 77764–77776. [CrossRef]
154. Micolucci, L.; Akhtar, M.M.; Olivieri, F.; Rippo, M.R.; Procopio, A.D. Diagnostic value of microRNAs in asbestos exposure and malignant mesothelioma: Systematic review and qualitative meta-analysis. *Oncotarget* **2016**, *7*, 58606–58637. [CrossRef]

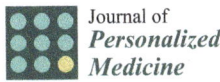

Review

The Impact of Air Pollution Exposure on the MicroRNA Machinery and Lung Cancer Development

Michal Sima [1], Andrea Rossnerova [2], Zuzana Simova [1] and Pavel Rossner Jr. [1,*]

1 Department of Nanotoxicology and Molecular Epidemiology, Institute of Experimental Medicine CAS, Videnska 1083, 142 20 Prague, Czech Republic; michal.sima@iem.cas.cz (M.S.); zuzana.simova@iem.cas.cz (Z.S.)
2 Department of Genetic Toxicology and Epigenetics, Institute of Experimental Medicine CAS, Videnska 1083, 142 20 Prague, Czech Republic; andrea.rossnerova@iem.cas.cz
* Correspondence: pavel.rossner@iem.cas.cz; Tel.: +420-241-062-763

Abstract: Small non-coding RNA molecules (miRNAs) play an important role in the epigenetic regulation of gene expression. As these molecules have been repeatedly implicated in human cancers, they have been suggested as biomarkers of the disease. Additionally, miRNA levels have been shown to be affected by environmental pollutants, including airborne contaminants. In this review, we searched the current literature for miRNAs involved in lung cancer, as well as miRNAs deregulated as a result of exposure to air pollutants. We then performed a synthesis of the data and identified those molecules commonly deregulated under both conditions. We detected a total of 25 miRNAs meeting the criteria, among them, miR-222, miR-21, miR-126-3p, miR-155 and miR-425 being the most prominent. We propose these miRNAs as biomarkers of choice for the identification of human populations exposed to air pollution with a significant risk of developing lung cancer.

Keywords: air pollution; biomarker; exposure; human; lung cancer; miRNA

Citation: Sima, M.; Rossnerova, A.; Simova, Z.; Rossner, P., Jr. The Impact of Air Pollution Exposure on the MicroRNA Machinery and Lung Cancer Development. *J. Pers. Med.* **2021**, *11*, 60. https://doi.org/10.3390/jpm11010060

Academic Editor: Alessandra Pulliero
Received: 23 December 2020
Accepted: 15 January 2021
Published: 19 January 2021

Publisher's Note: MDPI stays neutral with regard to jurisdictional claims in published maps and institutional affiliations.

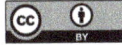

Copyright: © 2021 by the authors. Licensee MDPI, Basel, Switzerland. This article is an open access article distributed under the terms and conditions of the Creative Commons Attribution (CC BY) license (https://creativecommons.org/licenses/by/4.0/).

1. Introduction to miRNA

1.1. Basic Information on miRNA

Small non-coding microRNA molecules (miRNAs) were the **most studied RNA** throughout the last decade. The history of their research started in 1993 in Victor R. Ambros' laboratory, during an investigation of the developmental pathways of the soil nematode *Caenorhabditis elegans*, when lin-4 miRNA, the first miRNA, was described [1]. These single-strand, approximately 22 nucleotide long RNA molecules, which play a crucial role in the epigenetic regulation of gene expression, represent a broad group of nucleic acids described in various species including humans. Regarding miRNAs role in the process of effectivity of translation, these molecules attract the interest of numerous researchers from various fields of biomonitoring research. At the end of 2020, more than 27 years after miRNA discovery, almost 112,000 research articles focused on miRNA molecules can be identified in the PubMed database. This intensive research contributes to revealing new miRNAs every year. Their database, including miRNA sequences, is updated in the miRbase biological catalogue [2]. The latest version released in March 2018 (v22) contains sequences from 48,860 mature miRNAs of various species including 2656 molecules relevant to humans [3,4].

Besides mature miRNAs, many immature miRNA molecules are present in cells during their development, as their maturation is a relatively complex process [5,6]. Their **biogenesis** starts in the nucleus by transcription of the primary miRNA (pri-miRNA), which is an approximately 500-3000 bases long molecule created by transcription of the miRNA gene or intron by RNA polymerase II or III. This process is followed by cleavage of pri-miRNA to an approximately 70 base long precursor miRNA (pre-miRNA) by the Drosha-Pasha (DGCR8) complex. The steps that follow in cytoplasm are started by the export of pre-miRNA from the nucleus by the protein Exportin 5. The next step of maturation; the cleavage of pre-miRNA hairpin to miRNA duplex form, is assisted by RNase III enzyme Dicer, bound to the dsRNA-binding TRBP protein. Finally, this double stranded RNA duplex is transformed into a functional, mature single stranded form of miRNA together with Argonaute proteins. Formation of the RNA-induced silencing complex (RISC) with mature miRNA follows. It has a crucial role in miRNA function related to mRNA degradation in the case of perfect complementarity, or inhibition of translation in the case of non-complementarity of thereof.

miRNA nomenclature has evolved to distinguish mature sequences (denoted miR-XX) from precursors (mir-XX), as well as mature identical sequences originating from different genes (miR-XX-1; miR-XX-2). Adding a lower case letter (a, b . . .) at the end of the molecule name indicates a close relation among miRNAs with the same number differing only by one or two nucleotides (miR-XXa/b). The -3p or -5p suffix at the miRNA name indicates that miRNAs are excised on the $3'$ or $5'$ end of the same precursor, respectively (miR-XX-3p; miR-XX-5p) [7].

1.2. Methodological Approaches for miRNA Investigation

Along with knowledge of the processes of miRNA maturation and expression, two important aspects should be considered during the planning of human biomonitoring studies. First, the selection of biological material used in the particular study is crucial, as the expression machinery substantially differs between tissue and biological fluids, as plasma or urine. Second, a selected methodological approach can impact the overall interpretation of the results. To date, three major **methodological strategies** of miRNA analysis have been used. They are based on amplification, hybridization, or sequencing protocols [8–10]. Their choice for individual studies strongly depends on the aim of the experiment, the quality and quantity of samples as well as on the budget of the researcher.

Among **amplification-based** approaches, quantitative real-time polymerase chain reaction (qRT-PCR) is the most available method, which is still considered the gold standard due to its specificity, accuracy, sensitivity, and relatively low price. This approach can be used for individual miRNA detection, as well as for predefined sets of a few hundred molecules in an array format. Two variants of qRT-PCR differing in cost, nucleotide labeling and specificity are commonly used: CYBR Green or TaqMan. The CYBR Green approach is cheaper but there is a possibility of non-specific dsDNA-fluorescent dye binding which may negatively affect the results. In contrast, the TaqMan assays work based on a dual labeled oligonucleotide and exonuclease activity of Taq polymerase enzyme which increase the specificity [11]. However, to assure accuracy, for both qRT-PCR variants normalization of the data to the expression of an internal reference gene is mandatory. The reference gene, usually a housekeeping or another constitutively expressed gene, should be stably expressed in different cell types and under various experimental and treatment conditions [12].

The **hybridization method** represents a more advanced approach that is based on binding of miRNAs in a sample to specific complementary probes immobilized on surface of glass slides (microarrays). The current microarrays available on the market allow for the detection of a relatively high number of human miRNAs included in the previous version of miRNA release (v21 = 2549 miRNAs). However, this approach is limited to the already described miRNAs only. Additionally, due to the risk of false-positive results, verification of the data by qRT-PCR is required. The **sequencing strategy** by next generation sequencing (NGS) allows for the analysis of a full set of small RNA including miRNAs presented in a sample with the possibility to discover novel miRNAs, or other non-coding RNAs. The relatively high cost and demanding data processing could be a limitation for application in some studies.

1.3. miRNA as a Biomarker

Specific miRNA pattern has been repeatedly used as a biomarker of various diseases, including cardiovascular, neurodegenerative, or retinal disorders, as well as cancer [13–15]. The presence of specific miRNAs serves as an important diagnostic, prognostic, and therapeutic marker especially in relation to various **cancers**. Even though this record only started in 2002 when the deregulation of miR-15 and miR-16 was described in patients with chronic lymphocytic leukemia (CLL) [16], more than 53,000 studies have already been published according to a PubMed database search for keywords: "miRNA" and "cancer".

Various environmental and chemical **exposures** affect humans on a daily basis. These stressors are considered important risk factors for disease development. According to the World Health Organization (WHO), air pollution exposure is considered the greatest environmental risk factor of ill health [17]. The most recent data (related to year 2016) estimates that 4.2 million premature deaths occur each year due to outdoor air pollution and 3.8 million deaths are related to household air pollution. Among them, the majority were associated with ischemic heart disease and stroke, pneumonia, chronic obstructive pulmonary disease, and lung cancer which are estimated to account for more than half a million cases per year. These facts along with new methodology development, resulted in investigation of the epigenetic markers, including DNA methylation, miRNA expression or histone modification.

Similar to the research on diseases, many exposure studies linked to various environmental stressors revealed a specific miRNA expression pattern. The number of these studies has also increased during recent years. More than 3000 reports can be found using PubMed database search for keywords "miRNA" and "exposure".

Nowadays, links between **environmental exposure and risk of cancer related to deregulation of specific miRNAs** have also been described. Even though a huge number of publications related to miRNA, environmental exposure and cancer have been published and reviewed [18–23], we attempted to go deeper into these topics and concentrated in detail on the narrower part of this research. The main **aim of this review** was to find an intersection of specific miRNAs expressed in relation to (i) lung cancer, as the most common cancer related to air pollution exposure (see Section 2), (ii) air pollution exposure which is relevant to human populations living in polluted areas (see Section 3) and identify the specific miRNA expression changes related to air pollution and potentially leading to lung cancer. To fulfil the aim, we focused on particular exposure conditions in studied populations (chronic, acute, or seasonally changed) including the concentrations of environmental stressors (e.g., particulate matter (PM) of various aerodynamic diameter), the age of the studied human population, as well as the methodological approach used for miRNA pattern investigation due to their different complexity.

2. Lung Cancer and miRNA

Since the discovery of the relationship between miRNA deregulation and CLL [16], many research groups have focused their attention to investigation of the connection between miRNA and various cancers (reviewed by [24]).

The mechanisms of miRNA deregulation in cancer are frequently linked with alterations in genomic miRNA copy number and gene locations. There are also other processes, which could influence miRNA expression, such as dysregulation of key transcription factors, epigenetic modulation, or mutation or aberrant expression of any component of the miRNA biogenesis pathway (reviewed by [25]). In cancer, miRNAs can serve as oncogenes or tumor suppressors. The miRNA-suppressors inhibit oncogenes and/or apoptosis- or cell differentiation-controlling genes which results in tumor suppression. On the contrary, the miRNA-oncogenes support tumor development usually by inhibiting tumor suppressor genes and/or genes involved in cell differentiation or apoptosis (reviewed by [26]). The role of miRNAs (e.g., miR-126, miR-221, miR-222) in angiogenesis, an important process associated with progression of several diseases, including cancer has also been reported.

During angiogenesis, endothelial cells are activated and proliferate resulting in formation of tubular structures and supporting tumor growth [27].

In 2004, the role of miRNA in human lung cancer was highlighted and connected to shortened postoperative survival [28]. WHO classified lung cancer into two clinicopathological categories–contentious and intermittently metastatic small cell lung cancer (SCLC) and the more prevalent but less destructive non-small cell lung cancer (NSCLC) [29]. Even if new detection and therapeutic methods are in progress, lung cancer is often diagnosed in the later stage with survival rate around 20% [30].

In 2015, Feng et al. reviewed the role and importance of miRNA deregulation for lung cancer diagnostics and possible treatment. From previously published papers, they concluded, that several miRNAs are highly expressed in NSCLC patients when compared to healthy individuals but, on the other hand, other miRNAs are specifically under-expressed in lung cancer cases [31]. Based on that, miRNAs could serve as biomarkers for early detection of NSCLC which in effect could decrease the high risks of lung cancer deaths.

The searching of PubMed database for keywords "miRNA AND lung cancer AND human cases" produced 284 hits. In order not to repeat the previously summarized data, from the review mentioned above [31] until the present time, the number of publications was reduced to 158. From this amount, we further excluded review articles, meta-analyses, non-human or cell-based-only studies or studies where only cancer patients (without controls) were involved. After this specification, 54 papers met the conditions: miRNA expression was compared between lung cancer patients and healthy subjects (or other than tumor tissue from NSCLC patients).

Overall, four various input materials were used for miRNA detection: blood (4 studies), plasma (6 studies), serum (10 studies), and, the most common, tumor tissue (34 studies). Patniak et al. (2017) suggested, that whole blood is probably not suitable for the later miRNA quantification due to a lack of differences in expression levels based on microarray and qRT-PCR [32]. In disagreement with this finding, two studies observed deregulated miRNA in LC patients [33,34]. In the majority of reports (47) researchers utilized qRT-PCR for the quantification of miRNA levels, in the remaining studies, microarrays [35–37] or the novel method of PCR-droplet digital PCR [38–40] were used. For one study, only the abstract, without this information, was available [41].

In addition to being a biomarker, which could reveal the early stage of LC, in more than twenty publications the role of miRNAs in lung cancer development has been proposed. Some miRNAs have been described as **oncogenes**: miR-675 was associated with NSCLC progression through activation of nuclear factor-κB signaling pathway [42], miR-198-5p was downregulated in the early stage of lung squamous cell carcinoma and could play an important role via its target genes [43]. The metastasis suppressor 1 was repressed by miR-29a which resulted in tumor proliferation [44], leucine zipper putative tumor suppressor 3 was deregulated due to its connection to miR-1275 [45] and the level of miR-99a-5p was connected to poor survival in surgically resected lung adenocarcinoma specimen [46]. In the pulmonary adenocarcinoma, miR-210 and miR-183 were upregulated and served as oncogenes [47].

Alternatively, the **onco-suppressor** role has been described for miR-218-5p, miR-497, miR-34c due to their inhibition of cancer cell proliferation and migration [47–49], as well as for miR-451 and its link with macrophage migration inhibitory factor [50]. The onco-suppression was further linked with miR-219 that targets the high mobility group AT-hook 2 [51], and with miR-504 that is upregulated and inhibits cell invasion and proliferation [52]. The signal transducer and activator of transcription-3 is the direct target of miR-454 [53] and the transforming growth factor β receptor 2 is downregulated by miR-107 [54], other onco-suppressors.

Twelve miRNAs have been specifically proposed as **possible therapeutic targets**: miR-34b-3p that targets cyclin-dependent kinase 4 [37]; miR-588 whose silencing causes the increased expression of prostaglandin [55]; miR-103 that deregulates the programmed cell death 10 [56]; miR-491-5p that might reduce the expression of matrix metallopeptidase 9 [57];

miR-140-5p whose restoration may support the current LC therapies [58]; miR-12528 that controls the insulin-like growth factor 1 receptor, which is overexpressed in most of the cancer types [59]; miR-1260b that acts as onco-miRNA when inhibiting protein tyrosine phosphatase receptor type kappa and therefore might serve as a novel target for treatment [60]. The connection of p53 tumor-suppressor and miR-101 is important for tumor suppression due to the link with nucleolar stress [61]. miR-196b-5p is involved in Quaking-GATA binding protein 6-tetraspanin 12 pathway [62]. SRY-Box transcription factor 18 and its mRNA levels are influenced by the deregulation of miR-7a and miR-24-3p [38,39] and the expression of RUNX family transcription factor 2 is connected to miR23-b [63]. Therefore, their deregulation is suggested as a potential therapeutic strategy.

Altogether, in the 28 remaining studies, 97 various miRNAs were suggested as being biomarkers, which could help to reveal lung cancer in the early stages leading to a possible survival rate increase. In the following paragraph, several studies with the most commonly detected differentially expressed miRNAs are described. The total overview is summarized in Table 1.

Table 1. An overview of studies focused on relationships between lung cancer and miRNA expression.

miRNA	Tissue	Patients	Main Output	Method	Reference
let-7a-5p, miR-214-3p, miR-1291, miR-1-3p, miR-375	Serum	744	DB	qRT-PCR	[64]
miR-29a-5p, miR-4491, miR-542-3p, miR-135a-5p	Blood	145	DB	Microarray + qRT-PCR	[33]
miR-2114, miR-2115, miR-449c	Blood	NS	DB	qRT-PCR	[34]
miR-210-3p, miR-126-3p, miR-145, miR-205-5p	Plasma	471	DB	qRT-PCR	[65]
miR-25	Plasma	114	DB	qRT-PCR	[66]
miR-26a-5p, miR-126-5p, miR-139-5p, miR-152-3p, miR-200c-3p, miR-3135b, miR-151a-3p, miR-151a-5p, miR-151b, miR-550a-3p	Plasma	437	DB	qRT-PCR	[67]
miR-339-5p, miR-21	Plasma	28	DB	Microarray + qRT-PCR	[68]
miR-532, miR-628-3p, miR-425	Plasma	201	DB	qRT-PCR	[69]
let-7c, miR-122, miR-182, miR-193a-5p, miR-200c, miR-203, miR-218, miR-155, let-7b, miR-411, miR-450b-5p, miR-485-3p, miR-519a, miR-642, miR-517b, miR-520f, miR-206, miR-566, miR-661, miR-340, miR-1243, miR-720, miR-543, miR-1267	Plasma	100	DB	Microarray	[35]
miR-107	Serum	NS	OS	qRT-PCR	[54]
miR-223	Serum	75	DB	ddPCR	[40]
miR-21-5p, miR-140-5p, miR-126-3p	Serum	23	DB	qRT-PCR	[70]
miR-661	Serum	150	DB	qRT-PCR	[71]
miR-23b, miR-423-3p, miR-148b, miR-221	Serum	50	DB	qRT-PCR	[72]
miR-21	Serum	50	DB	NS	[41]
miR-22, miR-126	Serum	127	DB	qRT-PCR	[73]
miR-451, miR-1290, miR-636, miR-30c, miR-22-3p, miR-19b, miR-486-5p, miR-20b, miR-93, miR-34b, miR-185, miR-126-5p, miR-93-3p, miR-1274a, miR-142-5p, miR-628-5p, miR-486-3p, miR-425, miR-645, miR-24	Serum	253	DB	Microarray	[36]
miR-21	Serum	50	DB	qRT-PCR	[74]
miR-483-5p, miR-193a-3p, miR-25, miR-214, miR-7	Serum	221	DB	Microarray + RT-PCR	[75]

235

Table 1. Cont.

miRNA	Tissue	Patients	Main Output	Method	Reference
miR-196b-5p	Tissue	713	PTT	qRT-PCR	[62]
miR-497	Tissue	15	OS	qRT-PCR	[49]
miR-661-3p	Tissue	12	DB	qRT-PCR	[76]
miR-99a-5p	Tissue	50	OG	qRT-PCR	[46]
miR-29a	Tissue	55	OG	qRT-PCR	[44]
miR-101	Tissue	200	PTT	qRT-PCR	[61]
miR-21	Tissue	89	DB	qRT-PCR	[77]
miR-1275	Tissue	70	OG	qRT-PCR	[45]
miR-12528	Tissue	20	PTT	qRT-PCR	[59]
miR-182-5p	Tissue	23	DB	qRT-PCR	[78]
miR-491-5p	Tissue	100	PTT	qRT-PCR	[57]
miR-1260b	Tissue	26	PTT	qRT-PCR	[60]
miR-198-5p	Tissue	23	OG	Microarray + qRT-PCR	[43]
miR-454	Tissue	67	OS	qRT-PCR	[53]
miR-504	Tissue	55	OS	qRT-PCR	[52]
miR-7a, miR-24-3p	Tissue	25/50	PTT	ddPCR	[38,39]
miR-486-5p	Tissue	262	DB	qRT-PCR	[79]
miR-140-5p	Tissue	19	PTT	qRT-PCR	[58]
miR-103	Tissue	32	PTT	qRT-PCR	[56]
miR-219	Tissue	32	OS	qRT-PCR	[51]
miR-451	Tissue	72	OS	qRT-PCR	[50]
miR-375	Tissue	60	DB	qRT-PCR	[80]
miR-675	Tissue	92	OG	qRT-PCR	[42]
miR-34b, miR-34c	Tissue	52	DB	qRT-PCR	[81]
miR-588	Tissue	85	PTT	qRT-PCR	[55]
miR-200a-3p, miR-200a-5p, miR-200b-3p, miR-200b-5p, miR-429	Tissue	1341	DB	qRT-PCR	[82]
miR-663a	Tissue	62	DB	qRT-PCR	[83]
miR-218-5p	Tissue	NS	OS	qRT-PCR	[48]
miR-155	Tissue	1341	DB	qRT-PCR	[84]
miR-203	Tissue	125	DB	qRT-PCR	[85]
miR-34c, miR-183, miR-210	Tissue	103	OS, OG, OG	qRT-PCR	[47]
miR-23b	Tissue	NS	PTT	qRT-PCR	[63]
miR-34b-3p	Tissue	100	PTT	Microarray	[37]

This table summarizes studies focused on the connection between lung cancer and miRNA expression reported after the review by Feng et al. was published [31]. Abbreviations: DB—diagnostic biomarker, OS—onco-suppressor, OG—oncogene, PTT—possible therapeutic target, NS—not specified.

Wozniak et al. screened 754 miRNAs in 100 LC patients and a corresponding control group and developed a 24-plasma miRNA panel, which was capable of distinguishing these study groups based on differential miRNA expression [35]. A similar study was performed by Wang et al., where levels of five miRNAs were elevated after comparison of patients and healthy individuals [75]. Twenty miRNAs from plasma could be used as the diagnostic classifier for lung adenocarcinoma [36] and the combination of four miRNAs was validated out of 21 molecules as the microRNA expression signature for the LC patients [72]. Niu et al. (2018) detected ten differently expressed miRNAs when LC patients and healthy subjects were compared. Based on their results, some of these miRNAs were associated with adenocarcinoma or squamous cell carcinoma [67]. With more than 90% specificity and sensitivity, four plasma miRNAs combined together could serve as a reliable tool for LC diagnostics even in the early stage of the disease [65]. By microarray, 338 differently expressed miRNAs were detected in blood from LC patients and later, after evaluating in larger sample groups and using qRT-PCR, four of them were chosen as promising diagnostic instruments [33]. The most recent study focused on searching for the appropriate biomarkers for lung tumor detection was published in 2020. Thirty-five miRNAs were indicated as biomarkers with different expression in LC patients, and, after validation in three additional cohorts, a five miRNA panel was created [64].

As described in this review and shown previously [31], the miRNA-lung cancer link is well established. Studying this relationship has revealed, that production of miRNA is influenced by the lung tumor and the progression of the lung tumor is dependent on the miRNA levels as well. Some miRNAs serve as oncogenes, others as tumor suppressors. Some miRNA levels are upregulated and some downregulated, which influences the protein translation and tumor progression/suppression. In conclusion, several miRNAs could be used as an early diagnostic tool which might improve the lung cancer prognosis and because of their connection to protein production, some of them have been proposed as being a therapy target for individuals, who suffer from this disease.

3. Air Pollution and miRNA

In comparison with lung cancer, the link between miRNA expression and air pollution exposure has been less studied. The first reports focusing on this investigation were published in 2012. In this section we aim to summarize the current knowledge on deregulation of miRNA expression in human subjects exposed to various types of air pollutants. In contrast to the miRNA-lung cancer link discussed above, we present the topic in more detail, as the review literature on this topic is lacking. Although the latest review article on miRNAs as biomarkers of exposure to environmental pollutants was published in 2019, the authors focused specifically on the role of the environment without investigating the miRNA-air pollution-lung cancer relationship [86].

To identify studies that have focused on the investigation of air pollutants on the modulation of miRNA expression in humans, we searched the PubMed database for the string "miRNA air pollution" and limited the output to "Humans" as a species. This query yielded 97 results which were further checked to obtain the reports that analyzed miRNA expression in human subjects exposed to any type of air pollutant. Only studies that involved healthy subjects, or alternatively diseased participants not suffering from cancer were further considered. We also excluded review articles from our search. As a result, we identified 27 studies published between 2012 and 2020 focused on miRNA expression in humans exposed to various air pollutants (Table 2).

A total of 18 reports focused on the investigation of the effects of particulate matter (PM) of various aerodynamic diameter (PM10, PM2.5, ultrafine particles (UFP)), often along with other traffic- or combustion-related pollutants (NOx, CO, CO_2, black carbon (BC)). In 5 studies, the effects of tobacco/cigarette smoke were investigated, while other pollutants (e.g., liquid petroleum gas (LPG) and diesel exhaust, wood smoke, volatile organic compounds, ozone) were evaluated in 4 publications. The analytical methods included various variants of qRT-PCR (17 studies), microarrays and other hybridization-based approaches (8 studies) and NGS (2 reports). Most of the studies (21) investigated miRNA expression in blood-derived material (whole blood, serum, plasma, extracellular vesicles), other matrices included placenta (1×), saliva (1×), lung tissue (1×), spermatozoa (1×), bronchoalveolar lavage (1×) and sputum (1×). The data were obtained for 4940 subjects, that mostly included healthy participants of various age, but some suffered from heart disease, chronic obstructive pulmonary disease (COPD), or were atopic.

Table 2. An overview of studies focused on links between air pollution exposure and miRNA expression.

Pollutant	miRNA	Tissue	Subjects/Characteristics	Method	Reference
Effects of Environmental Air Pollutants					
PM2.5, UFP (PM0.1), black carbon, soot	miR-24-3p, miR-4454, miR-4763-3p, miR-425-5p, let-7d-5p, miR-502-5p, and miR-505-3p were associated with PM2.5 exposure	Blood	143, healthy	Microarray	[87]
PM10, PM2.5, PM0.1, HCHO, NO_2	miR-155 was associated with PM2.5 and HCHO exposure in the asthma group	Serum	180, healthy/180 asthmatic children	qRT-PCR	[88]
PM10, PM2.5, NO, NO_2, CO, CO_2, BC and UFP	miR-28-3p, miR-222-3p, miR-146-5p, miR-30b-5p/30c-5p, miR-320a-3p/320b/320c/320d/320e, miR-532-5p, miR-192-5p/215-5p, miR-144-3p, miR-425-5p were associated with exposure to a mixture of pollutants; no effect for PM10 or PM2.5 alone	Plasma	24, healthy	NGS	[89]
PM2.5	Negative link of miR-21, miR-146a and miR-222 expression with PM2.5 in 2nd trimester; positive link of miR-20a and miR-21 in 1st trimester exposure	Placenta	210 newborns	qRT-PCR	[90]
PM2.5	miR-199a/b and miR-223–3p modified links between PM2.5 and systolic blood pressure	Extracellular vesicles	22 healthy elderly	NanoStringnCounter® platform	[91]
PM10, PM2.5, black carbon, ultrafine particles and NO_2	54 miRNAs associated with exposure	Plasma	24 healthy/ischemic heart disease/COPD	NGS	[92]
PM10, PM2.5, NO, NO_2, CO, CO_2, BC and UFP	miR-197-3p, miR-29a-3p, miR-15a-5p, miR-16-5p and miR-92a-3p associated with exposure to pollutants	Blood	50 healthy, 20 COPD, 19 ischemic heart disease	Sureprint G3 Human V19 miRNA 8 × 60K (Agilent)	[93]
PM2.5	The expression of miR-21-5p, miR-187-3p, miR-146a-5p, miR-1-3p, miR-199a-5p was associated with the exposure	Blood	55 healthy	qRT-PCR	[94]
PM10	The expression of let-7c-5p; miR-106a-5p; miR-143-3p; miR-185-5p; miR-218-5p; miR-331-3p; miR-642-5p; miR-652-3p; miR-99b-5p was downregulated	Extracellular vesicles	1630 overweight/obese	QuantStudio™ 12 K Flex Real Time PCR	[95]
PM2.5, UFP	miR-222 expression affected by UFP, but not PM2.5; no effect was observed for miR-146a	Saliva	80 healthy children	qRT-PCR	[96]
PM2.5	Expression of miR-126-3p, miR-19b-3p, miR-93-5p, miR-223-3p, miR-142-3p, miR-23a-3p, miR-150-5p, miR-15a-5p, miR-191-5p, let-7a-5p affected by the exposure	Serum	22 healthy	NanoStringnCounter® platform	[97]
PM and associated metals	17 miRNAs affected by the exposure, including mir-196b, miR-302b, miR-200c, miR-30d	Extracellular vesicles	55 healthy steel plant workers	qRT-PCR	[98]

Table 2. Cont.

Pollutant	miRNA	Tissue	Subjects/Characteristics	Method	Reference
Effects of Environmental Air Pollutants					
PM10	miR-145, miR-197, miR-30b, miR-345, miR-26a, miR-425-5p, miR-331, miR-140-3p, miR-101 associated with the exposure	Blood	90 obese subjects	TaqMan Low-Density Array	[99]
PM10	Negative link with miR-21, miR-222, but not -miR-146a expression	Blood	50 healthy adults	qRT-PCR	[100]
PM2.5, metals	Positive link with miR-4516	Serum	120 healthy subjects	miRCURY LNA™	[101]
PM10, PM2.5, elemental carbon	No effect of PM2.5 exposure; PM10 affected 12 miRNAs; EC affected 28 miRNAs in the controls and 29 in truck drivers; miR-125a-5p, miR-1274a, miR-600, miR-1283, miR-10a were common in both groups	Blood	120 healthy subjects (truck drivers and controls)	NanoStringnCounter® platform	[102]
PM	Increased expression of miR-128 and miR-302c	Extracellular vesicles	63 healthy steel plant workers	qRT-PCR	[103]
PM2.5, black carbon, organic carbon, sulfates	Negative links with miR-1, miR-126, miR-135a, miR-146a, miR-155, miR-21, miR-222 and miR-9	Blood	153 elderly healthy men	qRT-PCR	[104]
Effects of Cigarette/Tobacco Smoke Exposure					
Biomass smoke (BS), tobacco smoke	miR-22-3p downregulated after BS exposure	Serum	50, COPD	qRT-PCR	[105]
Cigarette smoke	Expression of miR-29a, miR-93, let-7a, and let-7g affected	Serum	775, healthy, smokers/non-smokers	Low-density PCR array	[106]
Cigarette smoke	Modulation of miR-181c expression	Lung tissue	34 COPD	qRT-PCR	[107]
Tobacco smoke	Positive link with miR-223, but not with miR-155	Maternal and cord blood	441 mothers and newborns	qRT-PCR	[108]
Cigarette smoke	28 miRNAs differentially expressed in smokers when compared with non-smokers	Spermatozoa	13 healthy smokers and non-smokers	miRCURY LNA™	[109]
Effects of Other Pollutants					
Wood and LPG exhaust	miR-126 and miR-155 upregulated after wood smoke exposure	Plasma	52, healthy	qRT-PCR	[110]
Diesel exhaust, allergen	miR-183-5p, miR-324-5p and miR-132-3p induced by allergen; no modulatory effect of diesel exhaust	Bronchoalveolar lavage	15 atopic subjects	NanoStringnCounter® platform	[111]
VOC	Specific miRNAs for exposure to individual VOCs	Blood	50 healthy exposed workers	Microarray	[112]
Ozone	Increased expression of miR-132, miR-143, miR-145, miR-199a, miR-199b-5p, miR-222, miR-223, miR-25, miR-424, and miR-582-5p after the exposure	Sputum	20 healthy volunteers	Microarray	[113]

3.1. The Effect of Air Pollution on miRNA Expression in Healthy Adults

The majority of studies reported miRNA expression changes after exposure to air pollutants in general adult populations. Thus, the effects of PM2.5, UFP, black carbon and soot on miRNA expression were investigated in a multi-centric study among 143 healthy volunteers living in Switzerland, United Kingdom, Italy, and the Netherlands. The authors used the microarray technology to identify a total of seven microRNAs (miR-24-3p, miR-4454, miR-4763-3p, miR-425-5p, let-7d-5p, miR-502-5p, miR-505-3p) extracted from whole blood to be correlated with exposure to PM2.5. Interestingly, the effect of other pollutants was not significant [87]. Another study that involved 24 healthy subjects exposed to air pollutants during physical activity and the resting phase used NGS technology to correlate miRNA present in blood plasma with exposure to PM10, PM2.5, NO, NO_2, CO, CO_2, BC and UFP. Although the exposure to a mixture of the pollutants affected expression of nine miRNAs (miR-28-3p, miR-222-3p, miR-146-5p, miR-30b-5p/30c-5p and miR-320a-3p/320b/320c/320d/320e were positively associated; miR-532-5p, miR-192-5p/215-5p, miR-144-3p and miR-425-5p showed a negative relationship), no specific effects of PM2.5 and PM10 were detected. However, the effects of NO, NO_2, CO, CO_2, BC and UFP were observed [89]. In another report, a total of 24 non-smoking subjects (healthy, or suffering from ischemic heart disease (IHD), or COPD) were exposed to various levels of ambient air pollution and miRNA expression in blood plasma was assessed using NGS. The authors identified 54 circulating miRNAs associated with exposure to PM10, PM2.5, black carbon, UFP and NO_2 following only 2h exposure to air pollution. These molecules have been described as being related to negative consequences of traffic pollutants in the lung, heart, kidney and brain [92]. The effect of short (2h) PM10, PM2.5, NO, NO_2, CO, CO_2, BC and UFP exposure on miRNA expression in whole blood was further investigated using microarray technology among a total of 89 volunteers, including healthy subjects and those with COPD and IHD. The investigated populations originated from two cohorts with different levels of air pollution. The authors found miR-197-3p, miR-29a-3p, miR-15a-5p, miR-16-5p and miR-92a-3p linked with the exposure scenarios, although the expression of individual molecules was cohort-specific with little overlap between both sets of samples. These miRNAs play a role in cancers and Alzheimer's disease indicating a health risk associated with exposure to air pollutants. An effect of COPD and IHD on miRNA expression profiles was not found [93]. The potential role of PM2.5 on cytokines associated with systemic inflammation was assessed in 55 healthy volunteers exposed to different levels of the pollutant. A negative correlation of the exposure with miR-21-5p, miR-187-3p, miR-146a-5p, miR-1-3p and miR-199a-5p expression in whole blood confirmed the role of cytokines in response to exposure to air pollution [94]. Another study in 22 healthy subjects focused on the long-term effects of ambient PM2.5 exposure on miRNA expression in extracellular vesicles in serum involved in pathways related to cardiovascular diseases. The authors detected increased levels of miR-126-3p, miR-19b-3p, miR-93-5p, miR-223-3p, miR-142-3p, miR-23a-3p, miR-150-5p, miR-15a-5p and miR-191-5p let-7a-5p that are linked to oxidative stress, inflammation and atherosclerosis [97]. Targeted analysis of miR-21, miR-222 and miR-146a in the blood of 50 healthy subjects exposed to environmental levels of PM10 was performed using qRT-PCR in another study. An increase in PM10 concentrations was associated with a decrease of miR-21 and miR-222 expressions that are involved in inflammatory and oxidative stress pathways [100]. The specific role of metals in PM2.5 was studied in 120 healthy subjects exposed to moderate air pollution by measuring the expression of miR-4516 in serum. The expression of this miRNA was positively associated with Al, Pb and Cu levels suggesting an important role of miR-4516-autophagy pathway in response to PM2.5 and PM-associated metals. In a study involving 60 truck drivers and 60 office workers living in the highly polluted city of Beijing, the effect of PM2.5, PM10 and elemental carbon (EC) on miRNA expression in whole blood was analyzed using a hybridization technology. Interestingly, no consistent significant effects of either PM2.5, or PM10 exposure was observed. PM10 affected the expression of 12 miRNAs in office workers only, while short-term EC exposure had significant impacts on 28 miRNAs in office workers and 29 miRNAs in truck drivers, although only 5 miRNAs were common in both groups (miR-125a-5p, miR-1274a, miR-600, miR-1283, miR-10a). The deregulated miRNAs seem to play a role in the immune response [102].

3.2. The Effect of Air Pollution on miRNA Expression in Children

The effect of prenatal exposure to air pollutants on miRNA expression in placenta tissue was investigated by qRT-PCR by Tsamou et al. [90]. In a group of 210 newborns placenta tissue was collected upon delivery and mothers' exposure to PM2.5 in individual trimesters was correlated with expression levels of miRNA. The results showed an inverse relationship of PM2.5 levels in the 2nd trimester with miR-21, miR-146a and miR-222 expression, while miR-20a and miR-21 levels were positively associated with air pollution in the 1st trimester. The common putative target of these miRNAs is PTEN (tumor suppressor phosphatase and tensin homolog) that is involved in the pathways regulating cell survival, cell cycle, angiogenesis and metabolism suggesting the impact of PM2.5 exposure on these processes.

Research on environmental exposure to PM and other air pollutants in children was conducted by Liu et al. [88] and Vriens et al. [96]. The first study focused on a link between air pollution and childhood asthma. In a group of 180 asthmatic and 180 healthy children, the serum levels of miR-155 were analyzed by qRT-PCR and their correlation with HCHO, NO_2 and PM10, PM2.5 and PM1 was assessed. In asthmatic children the levels of miR-155 were significantly higher and were associated with indoor PM2.5 and HCHO concentrations. As this miRNA plays an important role in asthma progression, indoor air pollution seems to be involved in aggravation of the disease in this study group [88]. In a group of 80 healthy children, saliva was collected, expression of miR-222 and miR-146a assessed by qRT-PCR and link with recent exposure to PM2.2 and UFP investigated. While a positive correlation with UFP concentrations was detected for miR-222 levels, which was reported to participate in cell cycle regulation, no such effects were found for miR-146a [96].

3.3. The Effect of Air Pollution on miRNA Expression in Elderly Subjects

Two studies focused on miRNA expression associated with air pollution in elderly men originating from the Normative Aging Study [91,104]. In a small group of 22 subjects, exposure to PM2.5 was linked with increased blood pressure and positively associated with miR-199a/b and miR-223-3p expression in extracellular vesicles. The expression of miR-199a/b was further affected by DNA methylation near the enhancer region of the gene encoding this molecule. Both miRNAs seem to target proteins implicated in important cardiovascular functions [91]. The potential effect of PM2.5, black carbon, organic carbon, and sulphates on the expression of fourteen candidate miRNAs in blood leukocytes was investigated among 153 subjects. A negative correlation between pollutant levels and miR-1, miR-126, miR-135a, miR-146a, miR-155, miR-21, miR-222 and miR-9 was detected. The strongest link was found for 7-day moving averages of PM2.5 and black carbon, and 48-h moving averages for organic carbon. The deregulated miRNAs most likely participate in HMGB1/RAGE signaling pathway that is associated with the enhanced expression of proinflammatory cytokines [104].

3.4. The Effect of Air Pollution on miRNA Expression in Overweight/Obese Subjects

The role of miRNA expression in the risk of cardiovascular disease modified by exposure to PM10 in overweight/obese subjects was reported in two studies [95,99]. A larger investigation of 1630 subjects showed downregulation of let-7c-5p, miR-106a-5p, miR-143-3p, miR-185-5p, miR-218-5p, miR-331-3p, miR-642-5p, miR-652-3p and miR-99b-5p expression in extracellular vesicles after short-term exposure to PM10. These miRNAs exhibit a putative role in cardiovascular disease and mediate changes of fibrinogen levels associated with PM10 exposure suggesting a role of PM in increased coagulation [95]. In another study, decreased miRNA expression in the peripheral blood of 90 obese subjects was found after exposure to PM10 48 h before sample collection. These miRNAs included miR-145, miR-197, miR-30b, miR-345, miR-26a, miR-425-5p, miR-331, miR-140-3p and miR-101. PM10 exposure was associated with a blood pressure increase further modulated by miRNA-101 expression [99]. These reports indicate that miRNA expression represents a molecular mechanism underlying the effects of air pollution on blood pressure.

3.5. The Effect of Occupational Exposure to Polluted Air on miRNA Expression

miRNA expression was also assessed in occupationally exposed subjects. In extracellular vesicles of healthy steel plant workers miRNA levels were measured by qRT-PCR [98,103]. Among 55 subjects, 17 miRNAs were found to be affected, including mir-196b, miR-302b, miR-200c, miR-30d. The pathway analysis revealed the role of mir-196b in insulin biosynthesis; miR-302b, miR-200c, miR-30d were related to inflammatory and coagulation markers. Thus, inhalation exposure to PM with metallic components may have adverse cardiovascular and metabolic effects [98]. In a study of 63 workers, increased expression of miR-128 and miR-302c after 3 days exposure to PM was detected. Pathway analysis identified miR-128 as a part of coronary artery disease pathways, and miR-302c to be involved in coronary artery disease, cardiac hypertrophy and heart failure pathways [103]. Both studies thus highlight the role of PM exposure in negative impacts on the cardiovascular system.

3.6. The Effect of Tobacco Smoking on miRNA Expression

The effect of cigarette/tobacco smoke exposure on miRNA expression was studied among healthy subjects, those suffering from COPD, as well as in mothers and newborns. While COPD is a pulmonary disease linked with genetic and environmental factors, dysregulation of miRNAs has also been shown to play a role. The effect of tobacco smoke exposure in miRNA deregulation was investigated in serum and lung tissue of a total of 84 subjects [105,107]. Serum levels of miR-22-3p were upregulated in smoking COPD subjects when compared with COPD subjects exposed to biomass smoke. Non-exposed or healthy controls were not included in this study. miRNA-22-3p was suggested to activate antigen-presenting cells in lungs in relation to tobacco smoke exposure [105]. Another study revealed downregulation of miR-181c in lung tissues from smoking patients with COPD when compared with subjects who had never smoked. Overexpression of this miRNA decreases inflammatory response, neutrophil inflammation, ROS generation and inflammatory cytokines production [107]. In 775 healthy subjects, cigarette smoking was associated with expression of miR-29a, miR-93, let-7a, and let-7g using a machine learning approach suggesting these molecules as potential serum biomarkers of environmental tobacco smoke exposure [106]. In spermatozoa of 7 non-smokers and 6 smokers miRNA profiling revealed differences in the expression of 28 miRNAs that were shown to be involved in several pathways, including cellular proliferation, differentiation and death, as well as reproductive system disease [109]. The effect of prenatal cigarette smoke exposure on the expression of miR-155 and miR-223 was studied in the maternal and cord blood of 441 mothers/newborns pairs. A positive correlation was found between miR-223 expression and maternal urine cotinine levels, indoor concentrations of benzene and toluene. The effects were not observed for miR-155. The results indicate a role of miR-223 expression on regulatory T cell numbers in the cord blood with a subsequent allergy risk to children of mothers exposed to tobacco smoke [108].

3.7. miRNA Expression in Subjects Exposed to Other Sources of Air Pollution

The next paragraph summarizes the results from populations that do not fit to the above-reported groups. The effects of household air pollution on miRNAs associated with inflammatory response was studied among 52 healthy women who used wood and LPG for cooking. Specifically, the expression of miR-126 and miR-155 was assessed in plasma by qRT-PCR and the results correlated with 1-hydroxypyrene levels, as a marker of smoke exposure. The expression of both molecules was significantly higher in the subjects exposed to wood smoke. As the analyzed miRNAs are important modulators involved in vascular dysfunction and atherosclerosis, the results indicate a greater health risk associated with burning wood than using LPG [110]. In another study, fifteen atopic subjects were exposed for 2 h to filtered air or diesel exhaust followed by bronchial allergen challenge in a controlled study and the expression of miRNA was assessed in bronchoalveolar lavage. Diesel exhaust induced expression of a greater number of miRNAs when compared with the controls. The presence of allergen significantly modulated the expression of miR-183-5p, miR-324-5p and miR-132-3p, while diesel exhaust alone did not have this effect. Negative correlations were observed between miR-132-3p and CDKN1A, a regulator of cell cycle progression in G1, as well as miR-183-5p and HLA-A, human leukocyte antigens [111]. The impacts of exposure to volatile organic compounds (VOC), including toluene, xylene and ethylbenzene was investigated in 50 healthy occupationally exposed subjects and controls. miRNA expression was assessed in whole blood using microarray technique. Specific signature of exposure to individual compounds was found: expression of 467 miRNAs was associated with toluene exposure, 211 miRNAs with xylene exposure and 695 miRNAs with xylene inhalation. These signatures may serve as indicators of VOC exposure. However, identification of the potential mechanisms underlying the exposure was not performed in this study. The impacts of inhalation exposure to ozone on miRNA expression in human bronchial airways were investigated by Fry et al. [113]. Twenty healthy subjects were enrolled and exposed for 2 h. Sputum samples were collected 48 h pre-exposure and 6 h post-exposure and miRNA expression was assessed by microarrays. Ozone exposure increased the expression of 10 miRNAs (miR-132, miR-143, miR-145, miR-199a, miR-199b-5p, miR-222, miR-223, miR-25, miR-424, and miR-582-5p). Pathway analysis revealed, among other biological functions and properties, their link with inflammation and immune-related diseases.

3.8. miRNAs Commonly Deregulated by Various Types of Air Pollutants

Due to the diversity of the biological material used for the detection of miRNA expression, various analytical methods, characteristics of human subjects and exposure conditions, identification of commonly deregulated miRNA(s) that may serve as biomarker(s) of exposure to air pollutants is rather difficult. From the studies discussed in this review, miR-222 was found to be affected by air pollutant exposure in six articles, followed by miR-223 family (mir-223 and miR-223-3p), miR-21 family (miR-21 and miR-21-5p) and miR-155, each reported in four studies, and miR-126 family (miR-126 and miR-126–3p) and mir-425-5p, each described in three publications. Other miRNAs commonly appeared in two studies only or were unique for a single report.

4. miRNA Affected by Air Pollution Exposure and Implicated in Lung Cancer

In this section, we discuss the miRNAs that we identified to be commonly associated with air pollution exposure and lung cancer risk. Such miRNAs deserve the most attention as promising biomarkers that may inform of exposure to harmful pollutants potentially contributing to lung cancer development. An overview of the commonly deregulated miRNAs is provided in Table 3 and Figure 1; the most prominent molecules are discussed further in this section.

Table 3. A summary of miRNAs identified to be deregulated in lung cancer, as well as in air pollution-exposed subjects.

miRNA	Pollutant	References-Air Pollutants	References-Lung Cancer
miR-222	mixture of pollutants; PM2.5; UFP; PM10; black carbon, organic carbon, sulphates; ozone	[89,90,96,100,104,113]	[114]
let-7a-5p	PM2.5; Cigarette smoke	[87,97]	[64]
miR-21	PM2.5; PM10; black carbon, organic carbon, sulphates	[90,94,100,104]	[41,68,74,77]

Table 3. Cont.

miRNA	Pollutant	References-Air Pollutants	References-Lung Cancer
miR-29a family	Cigarette smoke	[93,106]	[44]
miR-93 family	PM2.5; Cigarette smoke	[97,106]	[36]
miR-126 family	PM2.5; black carbon, organic carbon, sulphates; wood smoke	[97,104,110]	[65,70]
miR-145	PM10; ozone	[99,113]	[65]
miR-155	PM2.5, HCHO; black carbon, organic carbon, sulphates; wood smoke	[88,104,108,110]	[35,84]
miR-223	PM2.5; tobacco smoke; ozone	[91,97,108,113]	[40]
miR-425 family	PM2.5; mixture of pollutants; PM10	[87,89,99]	[36,69]
miR-1-3p	PM2.5	[94]	[64]
miR-19bfamily	PM2.5	[97]	[36]
miR-22-3p	Biomass smoke (BS), tobacco smoke	[105]	[36]
miR-24-3p	PM2.5, UFP (PM0.1), black carbon, soot	[87]	[38,39]
miR-25	Ozone	[113]	[66,75]
miR-101	PM10	[99]	[61]
miR-142 family	PM2.5	[97]	[36]
miR-183 family	Diesel exhaust, allergen	[111]	[47]
miR-185	PM10	[95]	[36]
miR-196b family	PM and associated metals	[98]	[62]
miR-200c	PM and associated metals	[98]	[35,67]
miR-218-5p	PM10	[95]	[48]
miR-532	PM10, PM2.5, NO, NO_2, CO, CO_2, BC and UFP	[89]	[69]
miR-642 family	PM10		[35]
miR-1274a	PM10, PM2.5, elemental carbon	[102]	[36]

Text in bold red: miRNA commonly deregulated in six air pollution studies; text in bold: miRNAs commonly deregulated in 2–4 air pollution studies; regular font—miRNAs unique for a single air pollution study. See Figure 1 for graphical presentation. This overview reflects lung cancer studies reported since the Feng et al. review [31].

miR-222 appears to be deregulated in many cancers [115], including NSCLC [114] in which it targets tumor suppressors (PTEN, TIMP3) and enhances cellular migration by the activation of the AKT pathway. The molecule is involved in several steps of carcinogenesis, as e.g., tumor cell invasion and metastasis, regulation of apoptosis and drug resistance and the induction of tumor angiogenesis. Our literature review indicates that its expression was also associated with exposure to mixtures of air pollutants, specifically to PM10, PM2.5, UFP, black carbon, organic carbon, sulphates, and ozone. This link was described in six studies making miR-222 the molecule that is most commonly deregulated in the context of air pollution exposure.

let-7a-5p is involved in lung cancer development, most likely by targeting *BCL2L1*, *IGF1R*, *MAPK8*, and *FAS* genes thus affecting cell proliferation, growth arrest and apoptosis, as well as production and elimination of reactive oxygen species [116]. Its expression was found to be affected in subjects exposed to cigarette smoke and PM2.5. A variety of activities of **miR-21** have been described, including functions as an oncogene, that inhibits apoptosis, promotes cell differentiation and interstitial fibrosis. Its role in hypertension and lung cancer has also been reported [117,118]. In addition, its expression is affected by exposure to air pollutants (PM2.5 and PM10, black carbon, organic carbon, and sulphates) as reported in four studies. **miR-29a** was detected to be overexpressed in NSCLC tissues, where it was positively associated with malignancy of the disease and negatively associated with survival. The miRNA targets the *MTSS1* gene that encodes the protein inhibiting cell migration and proliferation [44]. Exposure to PM of various sizes, as well as to NOx, CO, CO_2, and cigarette smoke were factors involved in the deregulation of miR-29a expression in environmentally exposed subjects. **miR-93** plays a role in several human cancers, including lung cancer, although its effect can be inconsistent, as it may act both as an oncogene and tumor-suppressor. The target genes of this miRNA were reported to be closely related to transcription with *MAPK1*, *RBBP7* and *Smad7* being the hub genes [119]. The expression of miR-93-5p was affected in human subjects exposed to PM2.5 and cigarette smoke. Circulating **miR-126-3p** was associated with exposure to asbestos and with malignant mesothelioma [120], although in another study it suppressed the progression of NSCLC [121]. Low levels of miR-126-3p were associated with poor pathological stage, large tumor diameter and lymph node metastasis in lung adenocarcinoma. This miRNA was suggested to regulate the pathways involved in apoptosis and cancer [122]. PM2.5, black carbon or wood smoke were prominent pollutants affecting levels of this molecule. Expression of both strands of **miR-145** is downregulated in lung cancer where these molecules regulate cell cycle pathway genes and significantly reduce patient survival [123]. In human exposure studies, PM10 and ozone exposure were associated with expression of this molecule. **miR-155** is involved in a variety of processes linked to immunity, inflammation, and hematopoiesis. Its aberrant expression was observed in malignant and non-malignant diseases affecting the nervous, immune and cardiovascular system [124]. This molecule is also deregulated in lung disorders, including asthma and cystic fibrosis and lung cancer [125]. Similar to miR-126-3p, its expression was modified by PM2.5, black and organic carbon, as well as wood smoke exposure. These pollutants further affected the expression of **miR-425-5p** that appears to act as an oncogene in lung cancers, including squamous cell carcinoma [126] and NSCLC [127] in which the overexpression of the molecule was associated with poor prognosis.

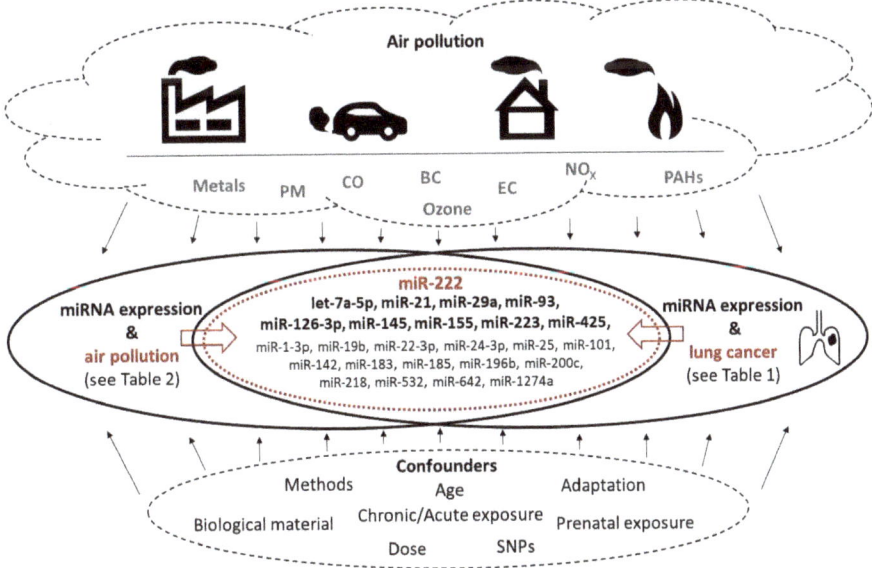

Figure 1. Graphical presentation of miRNAs commonly deregulated in lung cancer and human subjects exposed to various air pollutants. Factors affecting the results (types of air pollutants, methodological and other confounders) are also shown. See Table 3 for more details.

In contrast to previously mentioned miRNAs, **miR-223-3p** may have a function as a tumor-suppressor. The molecule is involved in inflammatory processes, it targets inflammasome components affecting the development of autoimmune diseases [128]. It also regulates the expression of GLUT4, a protein whose expression is altered in prediabetes and diabetes [129]. miR223-3p was further detected to be overexpressed in neutrophils of patients with asthma [130]. A recent study reported tumor-suppressing effects of this miRNA in lung squamous cell carcinoma [131]. Considering these results, deregulation of miR-223-3p following PM2.5 and ozone inhalation reflects the role of air pollutants in the development of immune system-related disorders rather than cancer.

5. Conclusions

In this review we aimed to summarize the current state of knowledge on miRNAs deregulated in lung cancer and miRNAs affected by exposure to air pollutants. As exposure to air pollution represents a dominant factor in the development of lung cancer and other respiratory system disorders, we further intended to identify the miRNAs commonly affected by both conditions. Such molecules could serve as biomarkers of choice for identification of human populations in greater risk of lung cancer resulting from exposure to air pollution. Our literature search identified a total of 25 miRNAs that meet such criteria. Among them, miR-222, miR-21, miR-126-3p, miR-155 and miR-425 may be considered the prominent molecules, as they were identified to be deregulated in multiple studies. PM2.5 is an air pollutant commonly affecting the expression of molecules. Thus, our observation is in agreement with the classification of air pollution as a human carcinogen [132]. It should however be noted that the number of studies investigating the link between air pollution and miRNA expression is limited when compared with the studies on cancer-miRNA relationship, and the methods used for detection of miRNA expression widely differ. Additionally, the effect of various confounders, including e.g., age of human subjects, lenght of exposure, genetic variability associated single nucleotide polymorphisms (SNPs) in genes encoding miRNAs, or the role of epigenetic adaptation should be considered. In particular, the process of epigenetic adaptation, previously reported by us and other authors (reviewed e.g., in [133–135]), significantly modifies the environment-organism interactions potentially resulting in a reduction of negative impacts of pollutants on the organism. These facts should be taken into account as they may potentially bias our conclusions.

Author Contributions: Conceptualization, A.R., P.R.J., M.S.; writing—original draft preparation, M.S., A.R., P.R.J., Z.S.; writing—review and editing, P.R.J., M.S., A.R., Z.S. All authors have read and agreed to the published version of the manuscript.

Funding: This research project was funded by the Ministry of Education, Youth and Sports of the Czech Republic project Healthy Aging in Industrial Environment HAIE (CZ.02.1.01/0.0/0.0/16_019/0000798), which is co-financed by the European Union (European Structural and Investment funds; Operation Programme Research, Development and Education). The study was further supported by the Ministry of Education, Youth and Sports of the Czech Republic (Research Infrastructures NanoEnviCZ, LM2018124; EATRIS-CZ, LM2018133), by the EU and the Ministry of Education, Youth and Sports of the Czech Republic as a JPND 2020 project ADAIR (8F20008) and by the Czech Science Foundation (18-02079S).

Institutional Review Board Statement: Not applicable.

Informed Consent Statement: Not applicable.

Data Availability Statement: Not applicable.

Conflicts of Interest: The authors declare no conflict of interest.

Abbreviations

CLL	Chronic lymphocytic leukemia
COPD	Chronic obstructive pulmonary disease
ddPCR	Droplet digital PCR
DNA	Deoxyribonucleic acid
EC	Elemental carbon
IHD	Ischemic heart disease
LC	Lung cancer
LPG	Liquid petroleum gas
miRNA	MicroRNA molecule
NGS	Next generation sequencing
NSCLC	Non-small cell lung cancer
PAH	Polycyclic aromatic hydrocarbon
PM	Particle matters
pre-miRNA	Precursor miRNA
pri-miRNA	Primary miRNA
qRT-PCR	Quantitative real-time polymerase chain reaction
RISC	RNA-induced silencing complex
RNA	Ribonucleic acid
SCLC	Small cell lung cancer
VOC	Volatile organic compound
WHO	World Health Organization

References

1. Lee, R.C.; Feinbaum, R.L.; Ambros, V.; The, C. Elegans Heterochronic Gene Lin-4 Encodes Small RNAs with Antisense Complementarity to Lin-14. *Cell* **1993**, *75*, 843–854. [CrossRef]
2. miRbase. Available online: http://mirbase.org/ (accessed on 1 December 2020).
3. Kozomara, A.; Birgaoanu, M.; Griffiths-Jones, S. MiRBase: From MicroRNA Sequences to Function. *Nucleic Acids Res.* **2019**, *47*, D155–D162. [CrossRef] [PubMed]
4. Alles, J.; Fehlmann, T.; Fischer, U.; Backes, C.; Galata, V.; Minet, M.; Hart, M.; Abu-Halima, M.; Grässer, F.A.; Lenhof, H.-P.; et al. An Estimate of the Total Number of True Human MiRNAs. *Nucleic Acids Res.* **2019**, *47*, 3353–3364. [CrossRef] [PubMed]
5. Tomari, Y.; Zamore, P.D. MicroRNA Biogenesis: Drosha Can't Cut It without a Partner. *Curr. Biol.* **2005**, *15*, R61–R64. [CrossRef]
6. Michlewski, G.; Cáceres, J.F. Post-Transcriptional Control of MiRNA Biogenesis. *RNA* **2019**, *25*, 1–16. [CrossRef]
7. Bernardo, B.C.; Charchar, F.J.; Lin, R.C.Y.; McMullen, J.R. A MicroRNA Guide for Clinicians and Basic Scientists: Background and Experimental Techniques. *Heart Lung Circ.* **2012**, *21*, 131–142. [CrossRef]
8. Tian, T.; Wang, J.; Zhou, X. A Review: MicroRNA Detection Methods. *Org. Biomol. Chem.* **2015**, *13*, 2226–2238. [CrossRef]
9. Bartošík, M.; Jiráková, L. Current Methods of MicroRNA Analysis. *Klin. Onkol.* **2018**, *31*. [CrossRef]
10. Krepelkova, I.; Mrackova, T.; Izakova, J.; Dvorakova, B.; Chalupova, L.; Mikulik, R.; Slaby, O.; Bartos, M.; Ruzicka, V. Evaluation of MiRNA Detection Methods for the Analytical Characteristic Necessary for Clinical Utilization. *Biotechniques* **2019**, *66*, 277–284. [CrossRef]
11. Tajadini, M.; Panjehpour, M.; Javanmard, S. Comparison of SYBR Green and TaqMan Methods in Quantitative Real-Time Polymerase Chain Reaction Analysis of Four Adenosine Receptor Subtypes. *Adv. Biomed. Res.* **2014**, *3*, 85. [CrossRef]
12. González-Bermúdez, L.; Anglada, T.; Genescà, A.; Martín, M.; Terradas, M. Identification of Reference Genes for RT-QPCR Data Normalisation in Aging Studies. *Sci. Rep.* **2019**, *9*, 13970. [CrossRef] [PubMed]
13. Backes, C.; Meese, E.; Keller, A. Specific MiRNA Disease Biomarkers in Blood, Serum and Plasma: Challenges and Prospects. *Mol. Diagn. Ther.* **2016**, *20*, 509–518. [CrossRef] [PubMed]
14. Vishnoi, A.; Rani, S. MiRNA Biogenesis and Regulation of Diseases: An Overview. In *MicroRNA Profiling*; Rani, S., Ed.; Methods in Molecular Biology; Springer: New York, NY, USA, 2017; Volume 1509, pp. 1–10. ISBN 978-1-4939-6522-9.
15. Wojciechowska, A.; Osiak, A.; Kozar-Kamińska, K. MicroRNA in Cardiovascular Biology and Disease. *Adv. Clin. Exp. Med.* **2017**, *26*, 868–874. [CrossRef] [PubMed]
16. Calin, G.A.; Dumitru, C.D.; Shimizu, M.; Bichi, R.; Zupo, S.; Noch, E.; Aldler, H.; Rattan, S.; Keating, M.; Rai, K.; et al. Frequent Deletions and Down-Regulation of Micro-RNA Genes MiR15 and MiR16 at 13q14 in Chronic Lymphocytic Leukemia. *Proc. Natl. Acad. Sci. USA* **2002**, *99*, 15524–15529. [CrossRef] [PubMed]
17. World Health Organization. Available online: https://www.who.int/ (accessed on 1 December 2020).
18. Pogribny, I.P. MicroRNA Dysregulation during Chemical Carcinogenesis. *Epigenomics* **2009**, *1*, 281–290. [CrossRef]
19. Chen, T. The Role of MicroRNA in Chemical Carcinogenesis. *J. Environ. Sci. Health Part C* **2010**, *28*, 89–124. [CrossRef]
20. Izzotti, A.; Pulliero, A. The Effects of Environmental Chemical Carcinogens on the MicroRNA Machinery. *Int. J. Hyg. Environ. Health* **2014**, *217*, 601–627. [CrossRef]

21. Ceccaroli, C.; Pulliero, A.; Geretto, M.; Izzotti, A. Molecular Fingerprints of Environmental Carcinogens in Human Cancer. *J. Environ. Sci. Health C Environ. Carcinog. Ecotoxicol. Rev.* **2015**, *33*, 188–228. [CrossRef]
22. Pogribny, I.P.; Beland, F.A.; Rusyn, I. The Role of MicroRNAs in the Development and Progression of Chemical-Associated Cancers. *Toxicol. Appl. Pharmacol.* **2016**, *312*, 3–10. [CrossRef]
23. Li, M.; Huo, X.; Davuljigari, C.B.; Dai, Q.; Xu, X. MicroRNAs and Their Role in Environmental Chemical Carcinogenesis. *Environ. Geochem. Health* **2019**, *41*, 225–247. [CrossRef]
24. Rzeszutek, I.; Singh, A. Small RNAs, Big Diseases. *Int. J. Mol. Sci.* **2020**, *21*, 5699. [CrossRef] [PubMed]
25. Peng, Y.; Croce, C.M. The Role of MicroRNAs in Human Cancer. *Signal Transduct. Target. Ther.* **2016**, *1*, 15004. [CrossRef] [PubMed]
26. Zhang, B.; Pan, X.; Cobb, G.P.; Anderson, T.A. MicroRNAs as Oncogenes and Tumor Suppressors. *Dev. Biol.* **2007**, *302*, 1–12. [CrossRef] [PubMed]
27. Celic, T.; Meuth, V.; Six, I.; Massy, Z.; Metzinger, L. The Mir-221/222 Cluster Is a Key Player in Vascular Biology via the Fine-Tuning of Endothelial Cell Physiology. *CVP* **2016**, *15*, 40–46. [CrossRef]
28. Takamizawa, J.; Konishi, H.; Yanagisawa, K.; Tomida, S.; Osada, H.; Endoh, H.; Harano, T.; Yatabe, Y.; Nagino, M.; Nimura, Y.; et al. Reduced Expression of the Let-7 MicroRNAs in Human Lung Cancers in Association with Shortened Postoperative Survival. *Cancer Res.* **2004**, *64*, 3753–3756. [CrossRef] [PubMed]
29. Travis, W.D.; Brambilla, E.; Burke, A.P.; Marx, A.; Nicholson, A.G. Introduction to The 2015 World Health Organization Classification of Tumors of the Lung, Pleura, Thymus, and Heart. *J. Thorac. Oncol.* **2015**, *10*, 1240–1242. [CrossRef]
30. Noone, A.-M.; Cronin, K.A.; Altekruse, S.F.; Howlader, N.; Lewis, D.R.; Petkov, V.I.; Penberthy, L. Cancer Incidence and Survival Trends by Subtype Using Data from the Surveillance Epidemiology and End Results Program, 1992–2013. *Cancer Epidemiol. Biomark. Prev.* **2017**, *26*, 632–641. [CrossRef]
31. Feng, B.; Zhang, K.; Wang, R.; Chen, L. Non-Small-Cell Lung Cancer and MiRNAs: Novel Biomarkers and Promising Tools for Treatment. *Clin. Sci.* **2015**, *128*, 619–634. [CrossRef]
32. Patnaik, S.K.; Kannisto, E.D.; Mallick, R.; Vachani, A.; Yendamuri, S. Whole Blood MicroRNA Expression May Not Be Useful for Screening Non-Small Cell Lung Cancer. *PLoS ONE* **2017**, *12*, e0181926. [CrossRef]
33. He, Q.; Fang, Y.; Lu, F.; Pan, J.; Wang, L.; Gong, W.; Fei, F.; Cui, J.; Zhong, J.; Hu, R.; et al. Analysis of Differential Expression Profile of MiRNA in Peripheral Blood of Patients with Lung Cancer. *J. Clin. Lab. Anal.* **2019**, *33*, e23003. [CrossRef]
34. Singh, A.; Kant, R.; Saluja, T.S.; Tripathi, T.; Srivastava, K.; Naithani, M.; Gupta, A.; Mirza, A.A.; Prakash, V.; Singh, S.K. Differential Diagnosis of Non-Small Cell Lung Carcinoma by Circulating MicroRNA. *J. Cancer Res. Ther.* **2020**, *16*, 127–131. [CrossRef]
35. Wozniak, M.B.; Scelo, G.; Muller, D.C.; Mukeria, A.; Zaridze, D.; Brennan, P. Circulating MicroRNAs as Non-Invasive Biomarkers for Early Detection of Non-Small-Cell Lung Cancer. *PLoS ONE* **2015**, *10*, e0125026. [CrossRef] [PubMed]
36. Tai, M.C.; Yanagisawa, K.; Nakatochi, M.; Hotta, N.; Hosono, Y.; Kawaguchi, K.; Naito, M.; Taniguchi, H.; Wakai, K.; Yokoi, K.; et al. Blood-Borne MiRNA Profile-Based Diagnostic Classifier for Lung Adenocarcinoma. *Sci. Rep.* **2016**, *6*, 31389. [CrossRef] [PubMed]
37. Feng, H.; Ge, F.; Du, L.; Zhang, Z.; Liu, D. MiR-34b-3p Represses Cell Proliferation, Cell Cycle Progression and Cell Apoptosis in Non-Small-Cell Lung Cancer (NSCLC) by Targeting CDK4. *J. Cell. Mol. Med.* **2019**, *23*, 5282–5291. [CrossRef] [PubMed]
38. Olbromski, M.; Grzegrzolka, J.; Jankowska-Konsur, A.; Witkiewicz, W.; Podhorska-Okolow, M.; Dziegiel, P. MicroRNAs Modulate the Expression of the SOX18 Transcript in Lung Squamous Cell Carcinoma. *Oncol. Rep.* **2016**, *36*, 2884–2892. [CrossRef]
39. Olbromski, M.; Rzechonek, A.; Grzegrzolka, J.; Glatzel-Plucinska, N.; Chachaj, A.; Werynska, B.; Podhorska-Okolow, M.; Dziegiel, P. Influence of MiR-7a and MiR-24-3p on the SOX18 Transcript in Lung Adenocarcinoma. *Oncol. Rep.* **2018**, *39*, 201–208. [CrossRef] [PubMed]
40. D'Antona, P.; Cattoni, M.; Dominioni, L.; Poli, A.; Moretti, F.; Cinquetti, R.; Gini, E.; Daffrè, E.; Noonan, D.M.; Imperatori, A.; et al. Serum MiR-223: A Validated Biomarker for Detection of Early-Stage Non-Small Cell Lung Cancer. *Cancer Epidemiol. Biomark. Prev.* **2019**, *28*, 1926–1933. [CrossRef] [PubMed]
41. Wen, Z.N.; Ling, Z.G.; Huang, Y.; Li, X. Expression and differential diagnostic value of serum microRNA for invasive pulmonary aspergillosis. *Zhonghua Jie He He Hu Xi Za Zhi* **2017**, *40*, 272–277. [CrossRef]
42. Feng, Y.; Yang, C.; Hu, D.; Wang, X.; Liu, X. MiR-675 Promotes Disease Progression of Non-Small Cell Lung Cancer via Activating NF-KB Signaling Pathway. *Cell. Mol. Biol.* **2017**, *63*, 7–10. [CrossRef]
43. Liang, Y.-Y.; Huang, J.-C.; Tang, R.-X.; Chen, W.-J.; Chen, P.; Cen, W.-L.; Shi, K.; Gao, L.; Gao, X.; Liu, A.-G.; et al. Clinical Value of MiR-198-5p in Lung Squamous Cell Carcinoma Assessed Using Microarray and RT-QPCR. *World J. Surg. Oncol.* **2018**, *16*, 22. [CrossRef]
44. Liu, M.; Zeng, X.; Lu, Y.-X.; Mo, Y.-J.; Liao, T.-H.; Gan, C.; Lu, X.-Q. Study on Molecular Mechanism of MiRNA-29a in Promoting Proliferation and Invasion of Non-Small-Cell Lung Cancer by Inhibiting MTSS1. *Eur. Rev. Med. Pharmacol. Sci.* **2018**, *22*, 5531–5538. [CrossRef] [PubMed]
45. He, J.; Yu, L.; Wang, C.-M.; Zhou, X.-F. MiR-1275 Promotes Non-Small Cell Lung Cancer Cell Proliferation and Metastasis by Regulating LZTS3 Expression. *Eur. Rev. Med. Pharmacol. Sci.* **2018**, *22*, 2680–2687. [CrossRef] [PubMed]

46. Maemura, K.; Watanabe, K.; Ando, T.; Hiyama, N.; Sakatani, T.; Amano, Y.; Kage, H.; Nakajima, J.; Yatomi, Y.; Nagase, T.; et al. Altered Editing Level of MicroRNAs Is a Potential Biomarker in Lung Adenocarcinoma. *Cancer Sci.* **2018**, *109*, 3326–3335. [CrossRef] [PubMed]
47. Pak, M.G.; Lee, C.-H.; Lee, W.-J.; Shin, D.-H.; Roh, M.-S. Unique MicroRNAs in Lung Adenocarcinoma Groups According to Major TKI Sensitive EGFR Mutation Status. *Diagn. Pathol.* **2015**, *10*, 99. [CrossRef] [PubMed]
48. Zhu, K.; Ding, H.; Wang, W.; Liao, Z.; Fu, Z.; Hong, Y.; Zhou, Y.; Zhang, C.-Y.; Chen, X. Tumor-Suppressive MiR-218-5p Inhibits Cancer Cell Proliferation and Migration via EGFR in Non-Small Cell Lung Cancer. *Oncotarget* **2016**, *7*, 28075–28085. [CrossRef] [PubMed]
49. Xia, Y.; Hu, C.; Lian, L.; Hui, K.; Wang, L.; Qiao, Y.; Liu, L.; Liang, L.; Jiang, X. MiR-497 Suppresses Malignant Phenotype in Non-small Cell Lung Cancer via Targeting KDR. *Oncol. Rep.* **2019**, *42*, 443–452. [CrossRef]
50. Goto, A.; Tanaka, M.; Yoshida, M.; Umakoshi, M.; Nanjo, H.; Shiraishi, K.; Saito, M.; Kohno, T.; Kuriyama, S.; Konno, H.; et al. The Low Expression of MiR-451 Predicts a Worse Prognosis in Non-Small Cell Lung Cancer Cases. *PLoS ONE* **2017**, *12*, e0181270. [CrossRef]
51. Sun, X.; Xu, M.; Liu, H.; Ming, K. MicroRNA-219 Is Downregulated in Non-Small Cell Lung Cancer and Inhibits Cell Growth and Metastasis by Targeting HMGA2. *Mol. Med. Rep.* **2017**, *16*, 3557–3564. [CrossRef]
52. Ye, M.-F.; Zhang, J.-G.; Guo, T.-X.; Pan, X.-J. MiR-504 Inhibits Cell Proliferation and Invasion by Targeting LOXL2 in Non Small Cell Lung Cancer. *Biomed. Pharmacother.* **2018**, *97*, 1289–1295. [CrossRef]
53. Liu, S.; Ge, X.; Su, L.; Zhang, A.; Mou, X. MicroRNA-454 Inhibits Non-small Cell Lung Cancer Cells Growth and Metastasis via Targeting Signal Transducer and Activator of Transcription-3. *Mol. Med. Rep.* **2018**, *17*, 3979–3986. [CrossRef]
54. Wu, Z.; Yuan, Q.; Yang, C.; Zhang, X.; Qi, P.; Huang, H.; Ma, Z. Downregulation of Oncogenic Gene TGFβR2 by MiRNA-107 Suppresses Non-Small Cell Lung Cancer. *Pathol. Res. Pract.* **2020**, *216*, 152690. [CrossRef] [PubMed]
55. Qian, L.; Lin, L.; Du, Y.; Hao, X.; Zhao, Y.; Liu, X. MicroRNA-588 Suppresses Tumor Cell Migration and Invasion by Targeting GRN in Lung Squamous Cell Carcinoma. *Mol. Med. Rep.* **2016**, *14*, 3021–3028. [CrossRef] [PubMed]
56. Yang, D.; Wang, J.-J.; Li, J.-S.; Xu, Q.-Y. MiR-103 Functions as a Tumor Suppressor by Directly Targeting Programmed Cell Death 10 in NSCLC. *Oncol. Res.* **2018**, *26*, 519–528. [CrossRef]
57. Pirooz, H.J.; Jafari, N.; Rastegari, M.; Fathi-Roudsari, M.; Tasharrofi, N.; Shokri, G.; Tamadon, M.; Sazegar, H.; Kouhkan, F. Functional SNP in MicroRNA-491-5p Binding Site of MMP9 3′-UTR Affects Cancer Susceptibility. *J. Cell. Biochem.* **2018**, *119*, 5126–5134. [CrossRef] [PubMed]
58. Flamini, V.; Jiang, W.G.; Cui, Y. Therapeutic Role of MiR-140-5p for the Treatment of Non-Small Cell Lung Cancer. *Anticancer Res.* **2017**, *37*, 4319–4327. [CrossRef]
59. Jeon, S.H.; Yoo, J.K.; Kim, C.M.; Lim, E.S.; Lee, S.J.; Lee, J.M.; Oh, S.-H.; Kim, J.K. The Novel Hsa-MiR-12528 Regulates Tumourigenesis and Metastasis through Hypo-Phosphorylation of AKT Cascade by Targeting IGF-1R in Human Lung Cancer. *Cell Death Dis.* **2018**, *9*, 493. [CrossRef]
60. Xu, L.; Xu, X.; Huang, H.; Ma, Z.; Zhang, S.; Niu, P.; Chen, Y.; Ping, J.; Lu, P.; Yu, C.; et al. MiR-1260b Promotes the Migration and Invasion in Non-Small Cell Lung Cancer via Targeting PTPRK. *Pathol. Res. Pract.* **2018**, *214*, 776–783. [CrossRef]
61. Fujiwara, Y.; Saito, M.; Robles, A.I.; Nishida, M.; Takeshita, F.; Watanabe, M.; Ochiya, T.; Yokota, J.; Kohno, T.; Harris, C.C.; et al. A Nucleolar Stress-Specific P53-MiR-101 Molecular Circuit Functions as an Intrinsic Tumor-Suppressor Network. *EBioMedicine* **2018**, *33*, 33–48. [CrossRef]
62. Liang, G.; Meng, W.; Huang, X.; Zhu, W.; Yin, C.; Wang, C.; Fassan, M.; Yu, Y.; Kudo, M.; Xiao, S.; et al. MiR-196b-5p-Mediated Downregulation of TSPAN12 and GATA6 Promotes Tumor Progression in Non-Small Cell Lung Cancer. *Proc. Natl. Acad. Sci. USA* **2020**, *117*, 4347–4357. [CrossRef]
63. Wang, H.X.; Wang, X.Y.; Fei, J.W.; Li, F.H.; Han, J.; Qin, X. MicroRNA-23B Inhibits Non-Small Cell Lung Cancer Proliferation, Invasion and Migration as Downregulation of RUNX2 and Inhibition of Wnt/B-Catenin Signaling Pathway. *J. Biol. Regul. Homeosl. Agents* **2020**, *34*, 825–835. [CrossRef]
64. Ying, L.; Du, L.; Zou, R.; Shi, L.; Zhang, N.; Jin, J.; Xu, C.; Zhang, F.; Zhu, C.; Wu, J.; et al. Development of a Serum MiRNA Panel for Detection of Early Stage Non-Small Cell Lung Cancer. *Proc. Natl. Acad. Sci. USA* **2020**, *117*, 25036–25042. [CrossRef]
65. Li, J.; Fang, H.; Jiang, F.; Ning, Y. External Validation of a Panel of Plasma MicroRNA Biomarkers for Lung Cancer. *Biomark. Med.* **2019**, *13*, 1557–1564. [CrossRef] [PubMed]
66. Zhang, Y.-L.; Zhang, Z.-L.; Zhu, X.-B.; Xu, L.; Lu, P.; Xu, M.; Liu, W.-J.; Zhang, X.-Y.; Yao, H.-M.; Ye, X.-W. Low Plasma MiR-25 Expression Is a Favorite Prognosis Factor in Non-Small Cell Lung Cancer. *Eur. Rev. Med. Pharmacol. Sci.* **2019**, *23*, 5251–5259. [CrossRef]
67. Niu, Y.; Su, M.; Wu, Y.; Fu, L.; Kang, K.; Li, Q.; Li, L.; Hui, G.; Li, F.; Gou, D. Circulating Plasma MiRNAs as Potential Biomarkers of Non-Small Cell Lung Cancer Obtained by High-Throughput Real-Time PCR Profiling. *Cancer Epidemiol. Biomark. Prev.* **2019**, *28*, 327–336. [CrossRef]
68. Sun, Y.; Mei, H.; Xu, C.; Tang, H.; Wei, W. Circulating MicroRNA-339-5p and -21 in Plasma as an Early Detection Predictors of Lung Adenocarcinoma. *Pathol. Res. Pract.* **2018**, *214*, 119–125. [CrossRef] [PubMed]
69. Wang, Y.; Zhao, H.; Gao, X.; Wei, F.; Zhang, X.; Su, Y.; Wang, C.; Li, H.; Ren, X. Identification of a Three-MiRNA Signature as a Blood-Borne Diagnostic Marker for Early Diagnosis of Lung Adenocarcinoma. *Oncotarget* **2016**, *7*, 26070–26086. [CrossRef] [PubMed]

70. Feng, M.; Zhao, J.; Wang, L.; Liu, J. Upregulated Expression of Serum Exosomal MicroRNAs as Diagnostic Biomarkers of Lung Adenocarcinoma. *Ann. Clin. Lab. Sci.* **2018**, *48*, 712–718. [PubMed]
71. Zhou, G.-H.; Yang, W.-H.; Sun, B. Clinical Impact of Serum MiR-661 in Diagnosis and Prognosis of Non-Small Cell Lung Cancer. *Eur. Rev. Med. Pharmacol. Sci.* **2017**, *21*, 5696–5701. [CrossRef] [PubMed]
72. Zhu, Y.; Li, T.; Chen, G.; Yan, G.; Zhang, X.; Wan, Y.; Li, Q.; Zhu, B.; Zhuo, W. Identification of a Serum MicroRNA Expression Signature for Detection of Lung Cancer, Involving MiR-23b, MiR-221, MiR-148b and MiR-423-3p. *Lung Cancer* **2017**, *114*, 6–11. [CrossRef] [PubMed]
73. Shang, A.Q.; Xie, Y.N.; Wang, J.; Sun, L.; Wei, J.; Lu, W.Y.; Lan, J.Y.; Wang, W.W.; Wang, L.; Wang, L.L. Predicative Values of Serum MicroRNA-22 and MicroRNA-126 Levels for Non-Small Cell Lung Cancer Development and Metastasis: A Case-Control Study. *Neoplasma* **2017**, *64*, 453–459. [CrossRef]
74. Sun, M.; Song, J.; Zhou, Z.; Zhu, R.; Jin, H.; Ji, Y.; Lu, Q.; Ju, H. Comparison of Serum MicroRNA21 and Tumor Markers in Diagnosis of Early Non-Small Cell Lung Cancer. *Dis. Markers* **2016**, *2016*, 3823121. [CrossRef] [PubMed]
75. Wang, C.; Ding, M.; Xia, M.; Chen, S.; Van Le, A.; Soto-Gil, R.; Shen, Y.; Wang, N.; Wang, J.; Gu, W.; et al. A Five-MiRNA Panel Identified From a Multicentric Case-Control Study Serves as a Novel Diagnostic Tool for Ethnically Diverse Non-Small-Cell Lung Cancer Patients. *EBioMedicine* **2015**, *2*, 1377–1385. [CrossRef] [PubMed]
76. Lu, J.; Gu, X.; Liu, F.; Rui, Z.; Liu, M.; Zhao, L. Antitumor Effects of Hsa-miR661-3p on Non-small Cell Lung Cancer in Vivo and in Vitro. *Oncol. Rep.* **2019**, *41*, 2987–2996. [CrossRef] [PubMed]
77. Kunita, A.; Morita, S.; Irisa, T.U.; Goto, A.; Niki, T.; Takai, D.; Nakajima, J.; Fukayama, M. MicroRNA-21 in Cancer-Associated Fibroblasts Supports Lung Adenocarcinoma Progression. *Sci. Rep.* **2018**, *8*, 8838. [CrossRef]
78. Luo, J.; Shi, K.; Yin, S.-Y.; Tang, R.-X.; Chen, W.-J.; Huang, L.-Z.; Gan, T.-Q.; Cai, Z.-W.; Chen, G. Clinical Value of MiR-182-5p in Lung Squamous Cell Carcinoma: A Study Combining Data from TCGA, GEO, and RT-QPCR Validation. *World J. Surg. Oncol.* **2018**, *16*, 76. [CrossRef] [PubMed]
79. Tessema, M.; Yingling, C.M.; Picchi, M.A.; Wu, G.; Ryba, T.; Lin, Y.; Bungum, A.O.; Edell, E.S.; Spira, A.; Belinsky, S.A. ANK1 Methylation Regulates Expression of MicroRNA-486-5p and Discriminates Lung Tumors by Histology and Smoking Status. *Cancer Lett.* **2017**, *410*, 191–200. [CrossRef]
80. Chen, L.-J.; Li, X.-Y.; Zhao, Y.-Q.; Liu, W.-J.; Wu, H.-J.; Liu, J.; Mu, X.-Q.; Wu, H.-B. Down-Regulated MicroRNA-375 Expression as a Predictive Biomarker in Non-Small Cell Lung Cancer Brain Metastasis and Its Prognostic Significance. *Pathol. Res. Pract.* **2017**, *213*, 882–888. [CrossRef]
81. Daugaard, I.; Knudsen, A.; Kjeldsen, T.E.; Hager, H.; Hansen, L.L. The Association between MiR-34 Dysregulation and Distant Metastases Formation in Lung Adenocarcinoma. *Exp. Mol. Pathol.* **2017**, *102*, 484–491. [CrossRef]
82. Xie, K.; Wang, C.; Qin, N.; Yang, J.; Zhu, M.; Dai, J.; Jin, G.; Shen, H.; Ma, H.; Hu, Z. Genetic Variants in Regulatory Regions of MicroRNAs Are Associated with Lung Cancer Risk. *Oncotarget* **2016**, *7*, 47966–47974. [CrossRef]
83. Zhang, Y.; Xu, X.; Zhang, M.; Wang, X.; Bai, X.; Li, H.; Kan, L.; Zhou, Y.; Niu, H.; He, P. MicroRNA-663a Is Downregulated in Non-Small Cell Lung Cancer and Inhibits Proliferation and Invasion by Targeting JunD. *BMC Cancer* **2016**, *16*, 315. [CrossRef]
84. Xie, K.; Ma, H.; Liang, C.; Wang, C.; Qin, N.; Shen, W.; Gu, Y.; Yan, C.; Zhang, K.; Dai, N.; et al. A Functional Variant in MiR-155 Regulation Region Contributes to Lung Cancer Risk and Survival. *Oncotarget* **2015**, *6*, 42781–42792. [CrossRef]
85. Tang, R.; Zhong, T.; Dang, Y.; Zhang, X.; Li, P.; Chen, G. Association between Downexpression of MiR-203 and Poor Prognosis in Non-Small Cell Lung Cancer Patients. *Clin. Transl. Oncol.* **2016**, *18*, 360–368. [CrossRef]
86. Kotsyfakis, M.; Patelarou, E. MicroRNAs as Biomarkers of Harmful Environmental and Occupational Exposures: A Systematic Review. *Biomarkers* **2019**, *24*, 623–630. [CrossRef]
87. Mancini, F.R.; Laine, J.E.; Tarallo, S.; Vlaanderen, J.; Vermeulen, R.; van Nunen, E.; Hoek, G.; Probst-Hensch, N.; Imboden, M.; Jeong, A.; et al. MicroRNA Expression Profiles and Personal Monitoring of Exposure to Particulate Matter. *Environ. Pollut.* **2020**, *263*, 114392. [CrossRef]
88. Liu, Q.; Wang, W.; Jing, W. Indoor Air Pollution Aggravates Asthma in Chinese Children and Induces the Changes in Serum Level of MiR-155. *Int. J. Environ. Health Res.* **2019**, *29*, 22–30. [CrossRef]
89. Krauskopf, J.; van Veldhoven, K.; Chadeau-Hyam, M.; Vermeulen, R.; Carrasco-Turigas, G.; Nieuwenhuijsen, M.; Vineis, P.; de Kok, T.M.; Kleinjans, J.C. Short-Term Exposure to Traffic-Related Air Pollution Reveals a Compound-Specific Circulating MiRNA Profile Indicating Multiple Disease Risks. *Environ. Int.* **2019**, *128*, 193–200. [CrossRef]
90. Tsamou, M.; Vrijens, K.; Madhloum, N.; Lefebvre, W.; Vanpoucke, C.; Nawrot, T.S. Air Pollution-Induced Placental Epigenetic Alterations in Early Life: A Candidate MiRNA Approach. *Epigenetics* **2018**, *13*, 135–146. [CrossRef]
91. Rodosthenous, R.S.; Kloog, I.; Colicino, E.; Zhong, J.; Herrera, L.A.; Vokonas, P.; Schwartz, J.; Baccarelli, A.A.; Prada, D. Extracellular Vesicle-Enriched MicroRNAs Interact in the Association between Long-Term Particulate Matter and Blood Pressure in Elderly Men. *Environ. Res.* **2018**, *167*, 640–649. [CrossRef] [PubMed]
92. Krauskopf, J.; Caiment, F.; van Veldhoven, K.; Chadeau-Hyam, M.; Sinharay, R.; Chung, K.F.; Cullinan, P.; Collins, P.; Barratt, B.; Kelly, F.J.; et al. The Human Circulating MiRNome Reflects Multiple Organ Disease Risks in Association with Short-Term Exposure to Traffic-Related Air Pollution. *Environ. Int.* **2018**, *113*, 26–34. [CrossRef] [PubMed]
93. Espín-Pérez, A.; Krauskopf, J.; Chadeau-Hyam, M.; van Veldhoven, K.; Chung, F.; Cullinan, P.; Piepers, J.; van Herwijnen, M.; Kubesch, N.; Carrasco-Turigas, G.; et al. Short-Term Transcriptome and MicroRNAs Responses to Exposure to Different Air Pollutants in Two Population Studies. *Environ. Pollut.* **2018**, *242*, 182–190. [CrossRef] [PubMed]

94. Chen, R.; Li, H.; Cai, J.; Wang, C.; Lin, Z.; Liu, C.; Niu, Y.; Zhao, Z.; Li, W.; Kan, H. Fine Particulate Air Pollution and the Expression of MicroRNAs and Circulating Cytokines Relevant to Inflammation, Coagulation, and Vasoconstriction. *Environ. Health Perspect.* **2018**, *126*, 017007. [CrossRef] [PubMed]
95. Pergoli, L.; Cantone, L.; Favero, C.; Angelici, L.; Iodice, S.; Pinatel, E.; Hoxha, M.; Dioni, L.; Letizia, M.; Albetti, B.; et al. Extracellular Vesicle-Packaged MiRNA Release after Short-Term Exposure to Particulate Matter Is Associated with Increased Coagulation. *Part. Fibre Toxicol.* **2017**, *14*, 32. [CrossRef]
96. Vriens, A.; Nawrot, T.S.; Saenen, N.D.; Provost, E.B.; Kicinski, M.; Lefebvre, W.; Vanpoucke, C.; Van Deun, J.; De Wever, O.; Vrijens, K.; et al. Recent Exposure to Ultrafine Particles in School Children Alters MiR-222 Expression in the Extracellular Fraction of Saliva. *Environ. Health* **2016**, *15*, 80. [CrossRef] [PubMed]
97. Rodosthenous, R.S.; Coull, B.A.; Lu, Q.; Vokonas, P.S.; Schwartz, J.D.; Baccarelli, A.A. Ambient Particulate Matter and MicroRNAs in Extracellular Vesicles: A Pilot Study of Older Individuals. *Part. Fibre Toxicol.* **2016**, *13*, 13. [CrossRef] [PubMed]
98. Pavanello, S.; Bonzini, M.; Angelici, L.; Motta, V.; Pergoli, L.; Hoxha, M.; Cantone, L.; Pesatori, A.C.; Apostoli, P.; Tripodi, A.; et al. Extracellular Vesicle-Driven Information Mediates the Long-Term Effects of Particulate Matter Exposure on Coagulation and Inflammation Pathways. *Toxicol. Lett.* **2016**, *259*, 143–150. [CrossRef]
99. Motta, V.; Favero, C.; Dioni, L.; Iodice, S.; Battaglia, C.; Angelici, L.; Vigna, L.; Pesatori, A.C.; Bollati, V. MicroRNAs Are Associated with Blood-Pressure Effects of Exposure to Particulate Matter: Results from a Mediated Moderation Analysis. *Environ. Res.* **2016**, *146*, 274–281. [CrossRef]
100. Louwies, T.; Vuegen, C.; Panis, L.I.; Cox, B.; Vrijens, K.; Nawrot, T.S.; De Boever, P. MiRNA Expression Profiles and Retinal Blood Vessel Calibers Are Associated with Short-Term Particulate Matter Air Pollution Exposure. *Environ. Res.* **2016**, *147*, 24–31. [CrossRef]
101. Li, X.; Lv, Y.; Hao, J.; Sun, H.; Gao, N.; Zhang, C.; Lu, R.; Wang, S.; Yin, L.; Pu, Y.; et al. Role of MicroRNA-4516 Involved Autophagy Associated with Exposure to Fine Particulate Matter. *Oncotarget* **2016**, *7*, 45385–45397. [CrossRef]
102. Hou, L.; Barupal, J.; Zhang, W.; Zheng, Y.; Liu, L.; Zhang, X.; Dou, C.; McCracken, J.P.; Díaz, A.; Motta, V.; et al. Particulate Air Pollution Exposure and Expression of Viral and Human MicroRNAs in Blood: The Beijing Truck Driver Air Pollution Study. *Environ. Health Perspect.* **2016**, *124*, 344–350. [CrossRef]
103. Bollati, V.; Angelici, L.; Rizzo, G.; Pergoli, L.; Rota, F.; Hoxha, M.; Nordio, F.; Bonzini, M.; Tarantini, L.; Cantone, L.; et al. Microvesicle-Associated MicroRNA Expression Is Altered upon Particulate Matter Exposure in Healthy Workers and in A549 Cells. *J. Appl. Toxicol.* **2014**, *35*, 59–67. [CrossRef]
104. Fossati, S.; Baccarelli, A.; Zanobetti, A.; Hoxha, M.; Vokonas, P.S.; Wright, R.O.; Schwartz, J. Ambient Particulate Air Pollution and MicroRNAs in Elderly Men. *Epidemiology* **2014**, *25*, 68–78. [CrossRef]
105. Velasco-Torres, Y.; Ruiz, V.; Montaño, M.; Pérez-Padilla, R.; Falfán-Valencia, R.; Pérez-Ramos, J.; Pérez-Bautista, O.; Ramos, C. Participation of the MiR-22-HDAC4-DLCO Axis in Patients with COPD by Tobacco and Biomass. *Biomolecules* **2019**, *9*, 837. [CrossRef]
106. Khan, A.; Thatcher, T.H.; Woeller, C.F.; Sime, P.J.; Phipps, R.P.; Hopke, P.K.; Utell, M.J.; Krahl, P.L.; Mallon, T.M.; Thakar, J. Machine Learning Approach for Predicting Past Environmental Exposures From Molecular Profiling of Post-Exposure Human Serum Samples. *J. Occup. Environ. Med.* **2019**, *61*, S55–S64. [CrossRef]
107. Du, Y.; Ding, Y.; Chen, X.; Mei, Z.; Ding, H.; Wu, Y.; Jie, Z. MicroRNA-181c Inhibits Cigarette Smoke–Induced Chronic Obstructive Pulmonary Disease by Regulating CCN1 Expression. *Respir. Res.* **2017**, *18*, 155. [CrossRef]
108. Herberth, G.; Bauer, M.; Gasch, M.; Hinz, D.; Röder, S.; Olek, S.; Kohajda, T.; Rolle-Kampczyk, U.; von Bergen, M.; Sack, U.; et al. Maternal and Cord Blood MiR-223 Expression Associates with Prenatal Tobacco Smoke Exposure and Low Regulatory T-Cell Numbers. *J. Allergy Clin. Immunol.* **2014**, *133*, 543–550. [CrossRef]
109. Marczylo, E.L.; Amoako, A.A.; Konje, J.C.; Gant, T.W.; Marczylo, T.H. Smoking Induces Differential MiRNA Expression in Human Spermatozoa: A Potential Transgenerational Epigenetic Concern? *Epigenetics* **2012**, *7*, 432–439. [CrossRef]
110. Ruiz-Vera, T.; Ochoa-Martínez, A.C.; Pruneda-Álvarez, L.G.; Zarazúa, S.; Pérez-Maldonado, I.N. Exposure to Biomass Smoke Is Associated with an Increased Expression of Circulating MiRNA-126 and MiRNA-155 in Mexican Women: A Pilot Study. *Drug Chem. Toxicol.* **2019**, *42*, 335–342. [CrossRef]
111. Rider, C.F.; Yamamoto, M.; Günther, O.P.; Hirota, J.A.; Singh, A.; Tebbutt, S.J.; Carlsten, C. Controlled Diesel Exhaust and Allergen Coexposure Modulates MicroRNA and Gene Expression in Humans: Effects on Inflammatory Lung Markers. *J. Allergy Clin. Immunol.* **2016**, *138*, 1690–1700. [CrossRef]
112. Song, M.-K.; Ryu, J.-C. Blood MiRNAs as Sensitive and Specific Biological Indicators of Environmental and Occupational Exposure to Volatile Organic Compound (VOC). *Int. J. Hyg. Environ. Health* **2015**, *218*, 590–602. [CrossRef]
113. Fry, R.C.; Rager, J.E.; Bauer, R.; Sebastian, E.; Peden, D.B.; Jaspers, I.; Alexis, N.E. Air Toxics and Epigenetic Effects: Ozone Altered MicroRNAs in the Sputum of Human Subjects. *Am. J. Physiol. Lung Cell. Mol. Physiol.* **2014**, *306*, L1129–L1137. [CrossRef]
114. Garofalo, M.; Di Leva, G.; Romano, G.; Nuovo, G.; Suh, S.-S.; Ngankeu, A.; Taccioli, C.; Pichiorri, F.; Alder, H.; Secchiero, P.; et al. MiR-221&222 Regulate TRAIL Resistance and Enhance Tumorigenicity through PTEN and TIMP3 Downregulation. *Cancer Cell* **2009**, *16*, 498–509. [CrossRef]
115. Amini, S.; Abak, A.; Sakhinia, E.; Abhari, A. MicroRNA-221 and MicroRNA-222 in Common Human Cancers: Expression, Function, and Triggering of Tumor Progression as a Key Modulator. *Lab. Med.* **2019**, *50*, 333–347. [CrossRef]

116. Zhang, L.; Hao, C.; Zhai, R.; Wang, D.; Zhang, J.; Bao, L.; Li, Y.; Yao, W. Downregulation of Exosomal Let-7a-5p in Dust Exposed-Workers Contributes to Lung Cancer Development. *Respir. Res.* **2018**, *19*, 235. [CrossRef]
117. Li, X.; Wei, Y.; Wang, Z. MicroRNA-21 and Hypertension. *Hypertens. Res.* **2018**, *41*, 649–661. [CrossRef]
118. Bica-Pop, C.; Cojocneanu-Petric, R.; Magdo, L.; Raduly, L.; Gulei, D.; Berindan-Neagoe, I. Overview upon MiR-21 in Lung Cancer: Focus on NSCLC. *Cell. Mol. Life Sci.* **2018**, *75*, 3539–3551. [CrossRef]
119. Gao, Y.; Deng, K.; Liu, X.; Dai, M.; Chen, X.; Chen, J.; Chen, J.; Huang, Y.; Dai, S.; Chen, J. Molecular Mechanism and Role of MicroRNA-93 in Human Cancers: A Study Based on Bioinformatics Analysis, Meta-analysis, and Quantitative Polymerase Chain Reaction Validation. *J. Cell. Biochem.* **2019**, *120*, 6370–6383. [CrossRef]
120. Micolucci, L.; Akhtar, M.M.; Olivieri, F.; Rippo, M.R.; Procopio, A.D. Diagnostic Value of MicroRNAs in Asbestos Exposure and Malignant Mesothelioma: Systematic Review and Qualitative Meta-Analysis. *Oncotarget* **2016**, *7*, 58606–58637. [CrossRef]
121. Liu, R.; Zhang, Y.S.; Zhang, S.; Cheng, Z.M.; Yu, J.L.; Zhou, S.; Song, J. MiR-126-3p Suppresses the Growth, Migration and Invasion of NSCLC via Targeting CCR1. *Eur. Rev. Med. Pharmacol. Sci.* **2019**, *23*, 679–689. [CrossRef]
122. Chen, Q.; Hu, H.; Jiao, D.; Yan, J.; Xu, W.; Tang, X.; Chen, J.; Wang, J. MiR-126-3p and MiR-451a Correlate with Clinicopathological Features of Lung Adenocarcinoma: The Underlying Molecular Mechanisms. *Oncol. Rep.* **2016**, *36*, 909–917. [CrossRef]
123. Mitra, R.; Adams, C.M.; Jiang, W.; Greenawalt, E.; Eischen, C.M. Pan-Cancer Analysis Reveals Cooperativity of Both Strands of MicroRNA That Regulate Tumorigenesis and Patient Survival. *Nat. Commun.* **2020**, *11*, 968. [CrossRef]
124. Gulei, D.; Raduly, L.; Broseghini, E.; Ferracin, M.; Berindan-Neagoe, I. The Extensive Role of MiR-155 in Malignant and Non-Malignant Diseases. *Mol. Asp. Med.* **2019**, *70*, 33–56. [CrossRef] [PubMed]
125. Mahesh, G.; Biswas, R. MicroRNA-155: A Master Regulator of Inflammation. *J. Interferon Cytokine Res.* **2019**, *39*, 321–330. [CrossRef] [PubMed]
126. Wang, J.; Li, Z.; Ge, Q.; Wu, W.; Zhu, Q.; Luo, J.; Chen, L. Characterization of MicroRNA Transcriptome in Tumor, Adjacent, and Normal Tissues of Lung Squamous Cell Carcinoma. *J. Thorac. Cardiovasc. Surg.* **2015**, *149*, 1404–1414.e4. [CrossRef]
127. Fu, Y.; Li, Y.; Wang, X.; Li, F.; Lu, Y. Overexpression of MiR-425-5p Is Associated with Poor Prognosis and Tumor Progression in Non-Small Cell Lung Cancer. *Cancer Biomark.* **2020**, *27*, 147–156. [CrossRef]
128. Boxberger, N.; Hecker, M.; Zettl, U.K. Dysregulation of Inflammasome Priming and Activation by MicroRNAs in Human Immune-Mediated Diseases. *J. Immunol.* **2019**, *202*, 2177–2187. [CrossRef]
129. Esteves, J.V.; Enguita, F.J.; Machado, U.F. MicroRNAs-Mediated Regulation of Skeletal Muscle GLUT4 Expression and Translocation in Insulin Resistance. *J. Diabetes Res.* **2017**, *2017*, 1–11. [CrossRef] [PubMed]
130. Gomez, J.L.; Chen, A.; Diaz, M.P.; Zirn, N.; Gupta, A.; Britto, C.; Sauler, M.; Yan, X.; Stewart, E.; Santerian, K.; et al. A Network of Sputum MicroRNAs Is Associated with Neutrophilic Airway Inflammation in Asthma. *Am. J. Respir. Crit. Care Med.* **2020**, *202*, 51–64. [CrossRef]
131. Luo, P.; Wang, Q.; Ye, Y.; Zhang, J.; Lu, D.; Cheng, L.; Zhou, H.; Xie, M.; Wang, B. MiR-223-3p Functions as a Tumor Suppressor in Lung Squamous Cell Carcinoma by MiR-223-3p-Mutant P53 Regulatory Feedback Loop. *J. Exp. Clin. Cancer Res.* **2019**, *38*, 74. [CrossRef]
132. IARC Working Group on the Evaluation of Carcinogenic Risks to Humans. In *Outdoor Air Pollution*; International Agency for Research on Cancer: Lyon, France, 2015; ISBN 978-92-832-0147-2.
133. Rossnerova, A.; Pokorna, M.; Svecova, V.; Sram, R.J.; Topinka, J.; Zölzer, F.; Rossner, P. Adaptation of the Human Population to the Environment: Current Knowledge, Clues from Czech Cytogenetic and "Omics" Biomonitoring Studies and Possible Mechanisms. *Mutat. Res. Rev. Mutat. Res.* **2017**, *773*, 188–203. [CrossRef]
134. Vineis, P.; Chatziioannou, A.; Cunliffe, V.T.; Flanagan, J.M.; Hanson, M.; Kirsch-Volders, M.; Kyrtopoulos, S. Epigenetic Memory in Response to Environmental Stressors. *FASEB J.* **2017**, *31*, 2241–2251. [CrossRef]
135. Rossnerova, A.; Izzotti, A.; Pulliero, A.; Bast, A.; Rattan, S.I.S.; Rossner, P. The Molecular Mechanisms of Adaptive Response Related to Environmental Stress. *Int. J. Mol. Sci.* **2020**, *21*, 7053. [CrossRef] [PubMed]

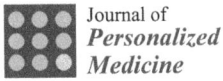

Article

miR-210 and miR-152 as Biomarkers by Liquid Biopsy in Invasive Ductal Carcinoma

Beatriz C. Lopes [1], Cristine Z. Braga [2], Fabrício V. Ventura [2], Jéssica G. de Oliveira [2], Edson M. Kato-Junior [2], Newton A. Bordin-Junior [3] and Debora A. P. C. Zuccari [1,2,4,*]

[1] Institute of Biosciences, Letters and Exact Sciences (IBILCE), Sao Jose do Rio Preto, Sao Paulo 15054-000, Brazil; beatrizclbio@gmail.com
[2] Faculdade de Medicina de Sao Jose do Rio Preto (FAMERP), Sao Jose do Rio Preto, Sao Paulo 15090-000, Brazil; cris_zamp@hotmail.com (C.Z.B.); ventura.bio.med@gmail.com (F.V.V.); jessicag.oliveira21@outlook.com (J.G.d.O.); edsonkato_jr@hotmail.com (E.M.K.-J.)
[3] Hospital de Base de Sao Jose do Rio Preto, Sao Jose do Rio Preto, Sao Paulo 15090-000, Brazil; bordinjunior@gmail.com
[4] Laboratory of Molecular Investigation of Cancer (LIMC), Avenue Brigadeiro Faria Lima, 5416, Vila Sao Pedro, Sao Jose do Rio Preto, Sao Paulo 15090-000, Brazil
* Correspondence: debora.zuccari@famerp.br; Fax: +55-17-3201-5885

Abstract: Detecting circulating microRNAs (miRNAs; miRs) by means of liquid biopsy is an important tool for the early diagnosis and prognosis of breast cancer (BC). We aimed to identify and validate miR-210 and miR-152 as non-invasive circulating biomarkers, for the diagnosis and staging of BC patients, confirming their involvement in tumor angiogenesis. Methods: RT-qPCR was performed and MiRNA expression analysis was obtained from plasma and fragments of BC and benign breast condition (BBC) women patients, plus healthy subjects. Additionally, the immunohistochemistry technique was carried out to analyze the expression of target proteins. Results: Tumor fragments showed increased expression of oncomiR-210 and decreased expression of miR-152 tumoral suppressor. Both miRNAs were increased in plasma samples from BC patients. The receiver operating characteristic (ROC) curve analysis revealed that only the expression of oncomiR-210 in tissue samples and only the expression of the miR-152 suppressor in plasma have the appropriate sensitivity and specificity for use as differential biomarkers between early/intermediate and advanced stages of BC patients. In addition, there was an increase in the expression of hypoxia-inducible factor 1-alpha (HIF-1α), insulin-like growth factor 1 receptor (IGF-1R), and vascular endothelial growth factor (VEGF) in BC patients. On the contrary, a decrease in Von Hippel–Lindau (VHL) protein expression was observed. Conclusions: This study showed that increased levels of miR-210 and decreased levels of miR152, in addition to the expressions of their target proteins, could indicate, respectively, the oncogenic and tumor suppressive role of these miRNAs in fragments. Both miRNAs are potential diagnostic biomarkers for BC by liquid biopsy. In addition, miR-152 proved to be a promising biomarker for disease staging.

Keywords: breast cancer; miRNAs; liquid biopsy; angiogenesis; biomarkers; early diagnosis

Citation: Lopes, B.C.; Braga, C.Z.; Ventura, F.V.; de Oliveira, J.G.; Kato-Junior, E.M.; Bordin-Junior, N.A.; Zuccari, D.A. P. C. miR-210 and miR-152 as Biomarkers by Liquid Biopsy in Invasive Ductal Carcinoma. *J. Pers. Med.* 2021, 11, 31. https://doi.org/10.3390/jpm11010031

Received: 12 November 2020
Accepted: 31 December 2020
Published: 6 January 2021

Publisher's Note: MDPI stays neutral with regard to jurisdictional claims in published maps and institutional affiliations.

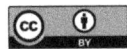

Copyright: © 2021 by the authors. Licensee MDPI, Basel, Switzerland. This article is an open access article distributed under the terms and conditions of the Creative Commons Attribution (CC BY) license (https://creativecommons.org/licenses/by/4.0/).

1. Introduction

The high mortality rate for breast cancer (BC) is mainly related to the development of metastasis, a process that depends on angiogenesis [1]. Data show that this malignant evolution is aggravated, in most cases, by the late diagnosis of the disease [2]. Therefore, the identification of biomarkers that can diagnose cancer in the early stage and predict the behavior of the tumor is of special interest to the patients.

As the tumor grows, there is a reduction in oxygen at the center of the tumor, creating adverse conditions of hypoxia, which induces increased expression of numerous pro-angiogenic factors, such as hypoxia-inducible factor 1-alpha (HIF-1α) and insulin-like growth factor type 1 receptor (IGF-1R) [3]. Increased levels of HIF-1α and IGF-1R stimulate vascular endothelial growth factor (VEGF) expression [4]. On the contrary, anti-angiogenic factors, such as Von Hippel–Lindau (VHL) protein act in the degradation of HIF-1α and, consequently, decrease the expression of VEGF [5].

Currently, liquid biopsy has been gaining ground as a promising tool for the detection of neoplasms, having the benefit of being less invasive and causing minimal discomfort and risk to patients. This procedure consists of the collection of any bodily fluid for the purpose of analyzing information from the tumor, including circulating nucleic acids—circulating tumor DNA (ctDNA) and circulating tumor RNA (ctRNA) [6].

These circulating biomarkers have advantages over tissue biomarkers as they are easily obtained and can also be monitored routinely, resulting in real-time detection, and consequently effective diagnosis and prognosis. With the advancement of this technique, a growing series of research studies have been developed for the purpose of discovering new circulating biomarkers that are more sensitive, characterizing specific subtypes of each tumor type [7].

Additionally, a class of small non-coding RNAs, called microRNAs (miRNAs; miRs), has been studied as potential biomarkers in cancer. MiRNAs are small, non-coding endogenous RNAs with approximately 22 nucleotides that control numerous cell pathways through the regulation of gene expression in the post-transcriptional phase [8,9].

A broad review showed the most significant miRNAs for BC and which regulators (hallmarks) they involved [10]. Among them, miR-210 is considered an oncogenic miRNA which exhibits regulation mediated by HIF-1α and VHL. HIF-1α promotes increased expression of miR-210 and this leads to stabilization of HIF-1α, suggesting that both miRNA and its target gene are involved in a positive feedback loop. HIF-1α, in turn, will stimulate the expression of genes that promote angiogenesis, such as VEGF [11–13]. In addition, studies have shown that miR-210 expression was significantly higher in patients with BC in the preoperative phase compared to women who underwent tumor removal surgery [14]. Moreover, a study showed that elevated levels of miR-210 lead to increased tumor progression and migration and reduced cell cycle arrest in MCF-7 breast tumor cells [15].

Another miRNA present in the review by Bertoli, Cava, and Castiglioni is miR-152, which belongs to the miR-148/152 family. This miRNA is involved in the regulation of angiogenesis, being considered a tumor suppressor in BC [10]. Studies investigated the regulation of the IGF-1R receptor by miR-152. The high expression of this miR inhibits the expression of IGF-1R through its binding to the 3′-UTR region, leading to the blocking of the expression of HIF-1α and VEGF [16,17]. In BC, miR-152 showed low levels of expression in tumor tissue compared to adjacent non-tumor tissue, as well as in a series of BC cell lines [18,19].

In summary, on tumor progression, the high expression of oncomiR-210 and the low expression of the miR-152 suppressor trigger the increase in VEGF. The mechanisms of action of both miRNAs in the angiogenic pathway are summarized in Figure 1.

In recent years, studies have shown that miRNAs are not only detected in tissues, but also in fluids [9]. The circulating miRNAs, that represent the miRNA population in the free portion of body fluids, have attracted interest in the field of biomarker discovery because they are involved in several gene regulation processes [20]. Therefore, it is of great importance for patients to validate tumor biomarkers that are capable of diagnosing and predicting the staging for BC and can still be detected by a non-invasive method such as liquid biopsy. The aim of this study was to validate two miRNAs involved in the angiogenic process, and to evaluate the potential of these as biomarkers of diagnosis and staging in BC.

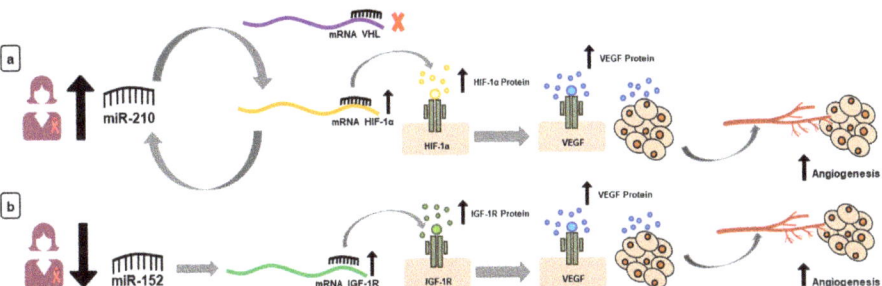

Figure 1. Candidate microRNAs (miRNAs) and their target proteins. (**a**) High levels of miR-210 in women with breast cancer (BC) leads to increased levels of hypoxia-inducible factor 1-alpha (HIF-1α) (activates a looping cascade) and, in addition, there is no blocking of HIF-1α by Von Hippel–Lindau (VHL) protein. Elevated levels of HIF-1α lead to an increase in vascular endothelial growth factor (VEGF). (**b**) With regard to miR-152, there is a low expression of this miRNA in women with BC, which leads to the increase of the IGF-1R protein and, later, of the VEGF protein.

2. Materials and Methods

This study was approved by the Research Ethics Committee (CEP) of the Faculty of Medicine of Sao Jose do Rio Preto (FAMERP), Sao Jose do Rio Preto, Brazil, #2.118.866/2017, and it was elaborated following the national and international rules of ethics in experiments with human samples.

2.1. Experimental Groups

The samples were collected from patients at their first medical appointment and selected by BI-RADS™ that indicated a higher probability of BC (4C and 5). Of the total samples, 30 women from the BC group and 5 from the benign breast condition (BBC) group were selected, based on the inclusion criteria pre-established in this study. The experimental groups of this study were as follows:

- Group Breast Cancer (BC): women with breast cancer (plasma/fragment: $n = 30$);
- Group Benign Breast Conditions (BBC): women with benign breast conditions (plasma/fragment: $n = 5$);
- Control: women with no atypical breast, and no history of BC in the family (plasma: $n = 15$; fragment: $n = 5$).

Inclusion criteria for BC: patients pathologically diagnosed with BC who had undergone surgical treatment; exclusion criteria for BC: patients who had received radiotherapy and chemotherapy before specimens were taken; exclusion criteria for all groups: women with other severe organ diseases; patients with any inflammatory process at the time of collection. All collections were performed at the Base Hospital, Sao Jose do Rio Preto, Brazil.

2.2. Collections

With respect to groups BC and BBC, the fragments were obtained by core biopsy performed. For the control group, the mammary fragments were obtained in mammoplasty reduction. Blood samples were collected by venipuncture (up to 5 mL per patient) and processed within one hour of collection.

2.3. Determination of Diagnosis and Pathological Prognosis Staging

All BC and BBC women included in this study had their diagnoses confirmed by the pathology team at the Base Hospital—Sao Jose do Rio Preto, SP/Brazil. To determine the staging of each patient, the most recent version (8th edition/2018) published by the American Joint Committee on Cancer (AJCC) was used.

The present study divided the women with staging Ia, Ib, IIa, and IIb and considered the respective patients to have an early/intermediatestage. Women with staging IIIa, IIIb, IIIc, and IV were considered to have an advanced stage.

2.4. Analysis of miRNA Expression by RT-qPCR

Plasma RNA extraction was performed with the miRNeasy Serum/Plasma Advanced kit (Qiagen, CA, USA) (200 µL plasma), and the Trizol™ reagent (Life Technologies, Carlsbad, CA, USA) was used for the fragments. The RNA concentration and purity was assessed using a spectrophotometer (NanoDrop™ 2000/2000c, Thermo Fisher Scientific, Waltham, MA, USA). The status purity was verified using A260/A280 ratios (range: 1.8–2.0). The complementary DNA (cDNA) was obtained by reverse transcriptase technique from the RNA extracted from the samples (50 ng). cDNA was synthesized from 50 ng of total RNA with the TaqMan™ MicroRNA Reverse Transcription kit (Applied Biosystems, Foster City, CA, USA).

The quantitative real-time polymerase chain reaction (qPCR) was performed using the StepOnePlus™ Real-Time PCR System (Applied Biosystems). Each sample were normalized against U6 levels. Reactions for miRNA expression analysis (and the reference gene, U6) were performed in triplicate (plasma) and duplicate (fragment) using 10 µL of 2 × TaqMan® Gene Expression Master Mix (Applied Biosystems), 1 µL of 20 × TaqMan Gene Expression Assay (Applied Biosystems), 3 µL cDNA by volume, and 6 µL of H2O DEPC, at a final volume of 20 µL.

The expression values of the miRNAs of interest were determined by the relative quantification (RQ) method in relation to normalizing of the gene used as reference ($2^{-\Delta\Delta Cq}$). Details of the sequences of miRNAs (miR-210 and miR-152) are available in Table S1, Supplementary Materials.

2.5. Analysis of Target Protein Expression by Immunohistochemistry

The protein expression of the target genes HIF-1α, IGF-IR, VHL, and VEGF was performed by immunohistochemistry assay, and their standardization followed the instructions provided by the manufacturer. Histological sections of 4 µm were obtained from paraffin-embedded material and adhered to silanized slides. The deparaffinization was performed on xylol followed by hydration, and subsequently incubated with hydrogen peroxide with the blocking of proteins (blocking non-specific reactions). The material was incubated with the primary antibody of each specific protein for 18 h at 4 °C. The Complement and HRP Conjugate (REVEAL™ Biotin-Free Polyvalent DAB - Spring Bioscience, Pleasanton, CA, USA) were applied, followed by the chromogenic substrate (DAB) and Harris hematoxylin.

All immunoreactions were accompanied by a positive control and a negative control (without primary antibody). The slides were observed under a 40× objective of the Olympus BX60 light equipment (Olympus, Shinjuku, Tokyo, Japan) and analyzed by optical densitometry. For each sample, 3 different fields were photographed only in the immunoreactive areas, in which 20 points were quantified with ImageJ software, totaling 60 quantified points for each slide. The values were obtained in arbitrary units (a.u.) and demonstrated the average optical density (DOM) for each sample. The details of the antibodies and the photomicrographs of the positive and negative controls are presented in Table S2 and Figure S1, respectively, Supplementary Materials.

2.6. Statistical Analysis

The results were submitted to descriptive analysis to determine normality. For each group, the Gaussian distribution test or D'Agostino and Pearson omnibus normality test was applied. The comparison of two parameters was performed using the Mann–Whitney test, and for three or more parameters the Kruskal–Wallis test (posteriorly Dunn post test) was performed. Data were presented as mean ± standard error of the mean (SEM). Values of $p < 0.05$ were considered significant and all analyses were performed using

GraphPad Prism 8 software (GraphPad Software, Inc., San Diego, CA, USA). In order to measure the diagnostic accuracy of each miRNA, the receiver operating characteristic (ROC) curve was used. In addition, the sensitivity and specificity of the optimum cutoff point were defined as those values that maximized the area under the curve (AUC).

3. Results
3.1. Characterization of Study Population

For the BC group, the demographic characteristics analyzed were age, distant metastasis, pathological prognosis staging, histological grade, and expression of hormonal receptors (ER, RP, HER2). Regarding age, among the 30 women included in this study, 25 (83.33%) had an age greater than or equal to 50 years, the mean age being 59 years (29–79 years). For the pathological prognosis staging, 14 samples (46.66%) were of the early/intermediate stages (Ia, Ib, IIa, and IIb), and 16 samples (53.34%) were of the advanced stage (IIIa, IIIb, IIIc, and IV). The histological grade of the tumor showed that 3 (10%), 20 (66.67%), and 7 (23.33%) samples were tumors that were low differentiated (Grade I), moderately differentiated (Grade II), and well differentiated (Grade III), respectively. Distant metastasis was found in 6 (20%) women with metastatic BC at the time of this study. For the expression of hormone receptors, the data show that 22 (73.33%), 19 (63.33%), and 14 (46.67%) samples were positive for ER, PR, and HER2, respectively. The mean age of the BBC group was 52 years (40–70 years), and the mean age of the control group was 49 years (23–70 years).

3.2. Expression Levels of miRNAs in Breast Cancer

Initially, we verified the expression of miR-210 and miR-152 in tumor fragments (BC), benign (BBC), and control to test the different levels of expression of these miRNAs in BC. MiR-210 showed increased expression in tumor fragments of BC compared to the BBC (* $p < 0.05$) (Figure 2a). However, there was no significant difference between BC fragments compared to the control group and between the BBC group and the control group. For miR-152, relative quantification showed decreased expression in tumor fragments of BC when compared to BBC fragments (** $p < 0.01$) and normal fragments (** $p < 0.01$) (Figure 2b).

Subsequently, we verified the expression levels of these miRNAs in plasma samples for the three different groups. With respect to miR-210, the relative quantification showed increased plasma expression for women with BC compared to the control group (** $p < 0.01$) (Figure 3a). However, there was no significant difference in plasma samples from the BC group compared to the BBC group or between the BBC group and the control group.

Surprisingly, we found that the tumor suppressor, miR-152, also had elevated levels in plasma samples from BC patients compared to the control group (* $p < 0.05$), different from the tumor fragments (Figure 3b). There was no significant difference in these miRs when compared to the BC group and women with BBC.

After finding the expression levels in the BC, BBC, and control groups, the miRNA expression levels were also analyzed in the staging groups. Our results show that miR-210 had increased expression in fragments of malignant neoplasms of advanced stage when compared to samples of early/intermediate stage BC fragments (** $p < 0.01$). In addition, there was increased expression in malignant neoplasms of advanced stage when compared to samples of BBC fragments (** $p < 0.01$) (Figure 4a). Regarding miR-152, relative quantification showed decreased expression in malignant neoplasm fragments of advanced stage in relation to the control group (* $p < 0.05$). The difference was also significant among women with early/intermediatestage malignant neoplasm vs. women with BBC (* $p < 0.05$) and control women (* $p < 0.05$) (Figure 4b). However, there was no difference between the different stages of BC for miR-152 in fragments.

For plasma samples, with respect to the miR-210, relative quantification showed increased expression in women with advanced stage of BC in relation to women controls (*** $p < 0.001$) (Figure 5a). However, there was no significant difference between the different stages of BC. Surprisingly, in addition to the increased expression level of the tumor suppressor, miR-152, in plasma of women with BC, this was also able to differentiate women with advanced stage from women with early/intermediate stage of BC and control women (* $p < 0.05$) (Figure 5b).

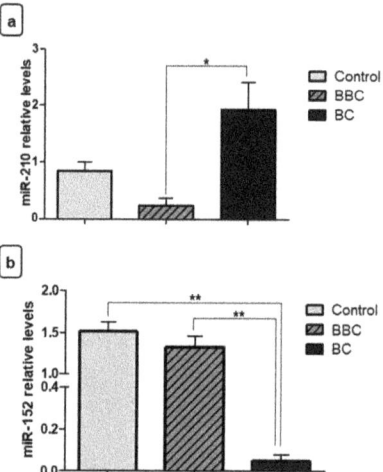

Figure 2. Evaluation of miRNA expression in fragments as diagnostic biomarkers. (**a**) Relative quantification showed that miR-210 exhibited increased expression in samples of tumor fragments from patients with breast cancer (BC) vs. those with benign breast conditions (BBC). (**b**) Contrastingly, miR-152 showed decreased expression in samples of BC fragments compared to the control group and to the BBC group. Significant value in Kruskal–Wallis and Dunn's post test (±SEM - standard error of the mean; * $p < 0.05$; ** $p < 0.01$).

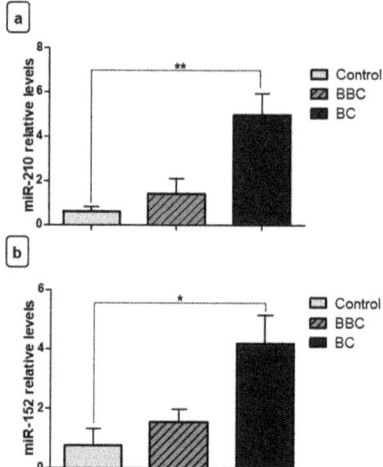

Figure 3. Evaluation of plasma miRNA expression as diagnostic biomarkers. (**a**) Relative quantification revealed that miR-210 showed increased expression in plasma samples from breast cancer (BC) patients vs. the control group. (**b**) The miR-152 also showed increased expression in plasma samples from women with BC vs. the control group. No significant difference was observed between the BC group and benign breast conditions (BBC) for any miRNA. Significant value in Kruskal–Wallis and Dunn's post test (±SEM - standard error of the mean; * $p < 0.05$, ** $p < 0.01$).

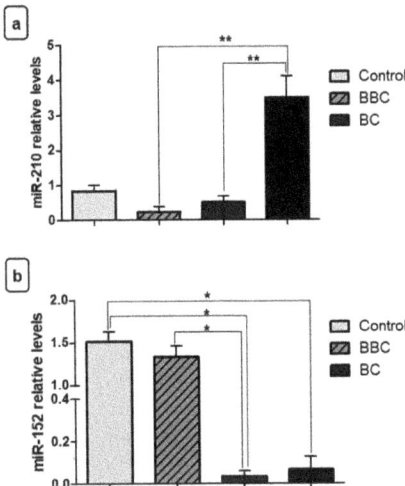

Figure 4. Evaluation of miRNA expression in fragments as staging biomarkers. (**a**) Relative quantification showed that there was increased expression of miR-210 in samples of breast cancer (BC) fragments with advanced stage when compared to women with early/intermediatestage of BC. Moreover, the increase was also significant with benign breast conditions (BBC). (**b**) miR-152 showed a significant decrease of expression in fragments from women with advanced stage of BC vs. the control group, and also decreased expression in early/intermediatestage malignant neoplasms when compared to women with BBC and the control group. There was no significant difference between the two stages' groups. Significant value in Kruskal–Wallis and Dunn's post test (±SEM - standard error of the mean; * $p < 0.05$; ** $p < 0.01$).

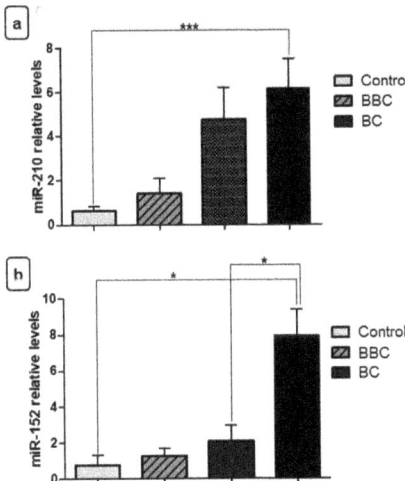

Figure 5. Evaluation of plasma miRNA expression as staging biomarkers. (**a**) Relative quantification showed that there was increased expression of miR-210 in plasma samples from women with breast cancer (BC) of advanced stage vs. controls. (**b**) With regard to miR-152, this showed increased expression in plasma samples from women with malignant neoplasms of advanced stage vs. women with early/intermediate stage and controls. Significant value in Kruskal–Wallis and Dunn's post test (±SEM - standard error of the mean; * $p < 0.05$; *** $p < 0.01$). BBC: benign breast conditions.

Finally, the miRNA expression levels were analyzed together to verify the strength of their combined use in plasma samples. Our results showed the combined amount of both miRNAs was able to differentiate patients with BC from control group (*** $p < 0.001$). However, there was no significant difference between the BC and BBC group (Figure 6a). In addition, the two miRNAs together were able to differentiate patients in advanced stage of BC from patients with early/intermediate stage of BC (** $p < 0.01$), advanced stage from BBC (* $p < 0.05$) and, lastly, advanced stage from control (*** $p < 0.001$). The other peer-compared groups showed no significant differences (Figure 6b).

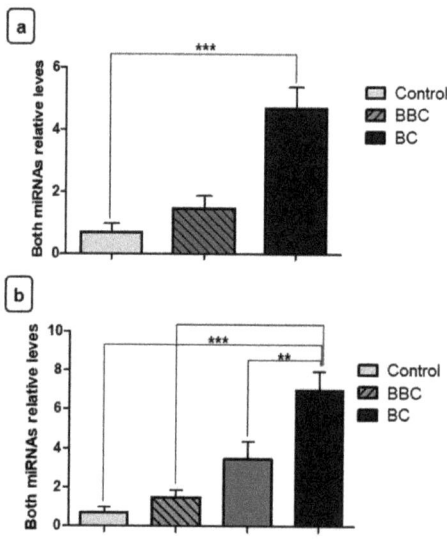

Figure 6. Evaluation of both miRNAs' plasma expression as staging biomarkers. (**a**) Relative quantification showed that there was increased expression of both miRNAs in plasma samples from women with breast cancer (BC) vs. the control group. (**b**) Relative quantification showed that there was increased expression of both miRNAs in plasma samples from women with advanced stage vs. early/intermediate, benign breast conditions (BBC) group and controls. Significant value in Kruskal–Wallis and Dunn's post test (±SEM - standard error of the mean; ** $p < 0.01$; *** $p < 0.01$).

3.3. miR-210 and miR-152 Are Stable in Bloodstream

Subsequently, the differences in the miRNA expression in fragments and plasma samples were analyzed for the BC group. The results reveal that miR-210 (** $p < 0.01$) (Figure 7a) and miR-152 (*** $p < 0.001$) (Figure 7b) presented increased expression in plasma samples compared to the fragments, indicating that oncomiR, and even the tumor suppressor, have stabilizing mechanisms in the bloodstream. Although both miRNAs were increased in plasma samples compared to the fragment, there was no significant difference in circulating levels between them (Figure 7c).

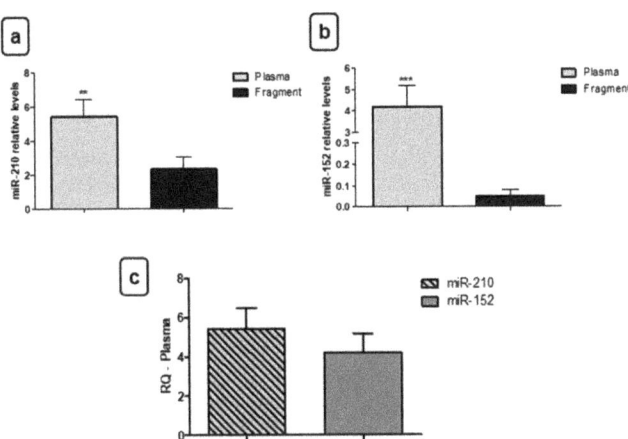

Figure 7. Both miR-210 and miR-152 are stable in blood. (**a**) For the breast cancer (BC) group, relative quantification showed that there was increased expression of miR-210 in plasma samples when compared with fragments. (**b**) The same occurred for miR-152; the relative quantification of this miRNA was higher in plasma samples compared to fragments. (**c**) There was no significant difference in circulating levels between miRNAs. Significant value in Kruskal–Wallis and Dunn's post test (±SEM - standard error of the mean; ** $p < 0.01$; *** $p < 0.01$).

3.4. Expression of miRNA Target Proteins by Immunohistochemistry

To confirm the action of miR-210 and miR-152 on the angiogenesis pathway, we verified the expression of the target proteins of both miRNAs by immunohistochemistry. All proteins showed cytoplasmic marking. Evaluation of protein expression by immunohistochemistry revealed increased levels of HIF-1α (*** $p < 0.0001$), IGF-1R (*** $p < 0.0001$), and VEGF (*** $p < 0.0001$) proteins in BC tissues compared to the control group. In addition, the proteins also showed increased expression in BC samples compared to the BBC group (HIF-1α *** $p < 0.0001$, IGF-1R *** $p < 0.0001$, and VEGF *** $p < 0.0001$). With respect to VHL, this protein showed decreased expression in BC samples when compared to the control group (*** $p < 0.0001$) and BBC group (*** $p < 0.0001$) (Figure 8).

3.5. Evaluation of miR-210 and miR-152 as Potential Diagnostic and Staging Biomarkers

Analysis of the ROC curve was used to determine miR-210 and miR-152 in plasma as a diagnostic biomarker to differentiate patients with BC from healthy individuals. The AUC for miR-210 for women with BC compared to the control group was 0.8427 (0.7174 to 0.9680) ($p = 0.0011$) with optimal sensitivity and specificity values of 76.9% and 90.9%, respectively, to the cut-off value of 1.690 as well as a positive predictive value of 95.24% and a negative predictive value of 62.44% (Figure 9a).

The AUC for miR-152 in plasma expression for women with BC compared to the control group was 0.7709 (0.6095 to 0.9324) ($p = 0.0105$) with optimal sensitivity and specificity values of 80% and 72.7%, respectively, to the cut-off value of 0.252 as well as a positive predictive value of 86.92% and a negative predictive value of 61.58%. (Figure 9b). Therefore, miR-210 and miR-152 expression in plasma samples have appropriate sensitivity and specificity to differentiate women without BC from women with BC (Figure 9).

ROC curve analysis was also performed to investigate the role of mir-152 in plasma as a staging biomarker for distinguishing advanced stage of BC patients from early/intermediate stage BC patient. On RT-qPCR, miR-210 did not show significantly different levels between women with early/intermediate stage of BC and women with advanced stage. The miR-152 showed good results in ROC analysis for women with advanced BC compared to women with early/intermediate stages of BC. The AUC was 0.8917 (0.7598 to 1.0000) ($p = 0.0019$) with optimal sensitivity and specificity values of 90% and 75%, respectively, to the cut-off value of 2.573 as well as a positive predictive value of 73.03% and a negative predictive value of 89.98% (Figure 9c).

Ultimately, the ROC curve was used with the combined amount of these two miRNAs to determine whether together they could be diagnostic and prognostic biomarkers for BC (Figure 10).

The AUC for both miRNAs in plasma expression for women with BC compared to the control group was 0.7542 (0.6345 to 0.8739) ($p = 0.0004$) with optimal sensitivity and specificity values of 83.33% and 68.0%, respectively, to the cut-off value of 0.9571 as well as a positive predictive value of 89.47% and a negative predictive value of 55.51% (Figure 10a). Thus, the combined amount expression in plasma samples has appropriate sensitivity and specificity to differentiate the control group to women with BC.

ROC curve analysis was also performed to investigate the role of miR-210 with miR-152 in plasma together as staging biomarkers for distinguishing advanced stage from early/intermediate stage of BC. The AUC was 0.7733 (0.6382 to 0.9084) ($p = 0.0016$) with optimal sensitivity and specificity values of 85.71% and 60%, respectively, to the cut-off value of 2.660 as well as a positive predictive value of 83.29% and a negative predictive value of 64.33% (Figure 10b). Therefore, miRNAs together showed good results in the analysis of the ROC curve as prognostic biomarkers. However, the AUC showed that miRNAs individually are better diagnostic and prognostic biomarkers for BC.

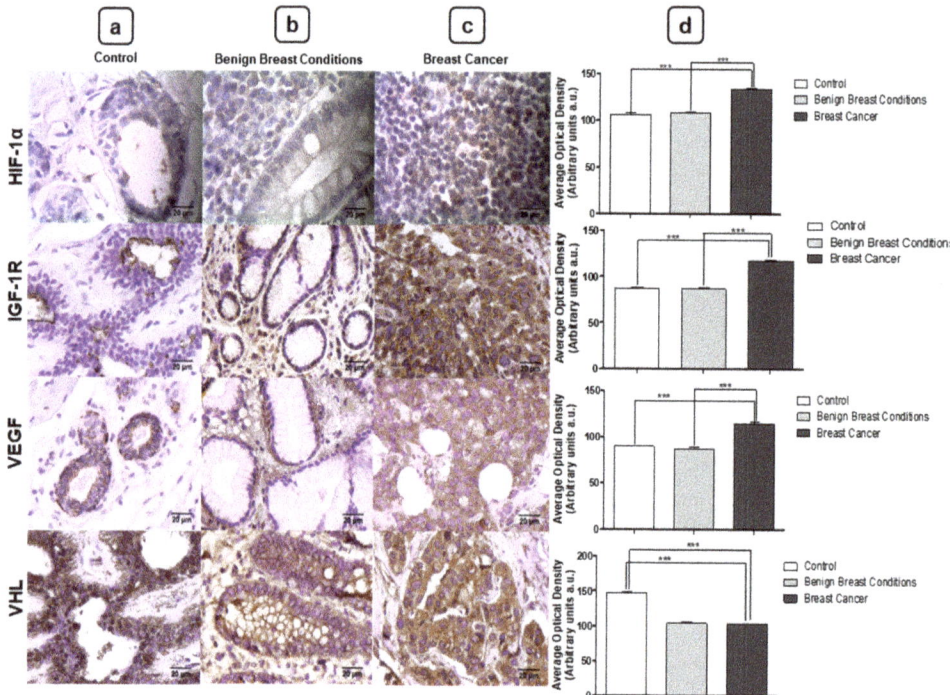

Figure 8. (a) Photomicrographs of (a) control, (b) benign breast conditions (BBC), and (c) breast cancer (BC). (d) Evaluation of protein expression in the three different groups. Hypoxia-inducible factor 1-alpha (HIF-1α), insulin-like growth factor 1 receptor (IGF-1R), and vascular endothelial growth factor (VEGF) showed a significant increase in the BC group compared to the group with BBC and the control group. Contrastingly, Von Hippel-Lindau (VHL) showed a significant decrease in the BC group compared to the group with BBC and the control group. Significant value in Kruskal–Wallis and Dunn's post test (±S.E.M - Standard Error of the Mean; *** $p < 0.001$ vs. the control group; *** $p < 0.001$ vs. the BBC group). Magnification of 40×. Bar: 20 μm.

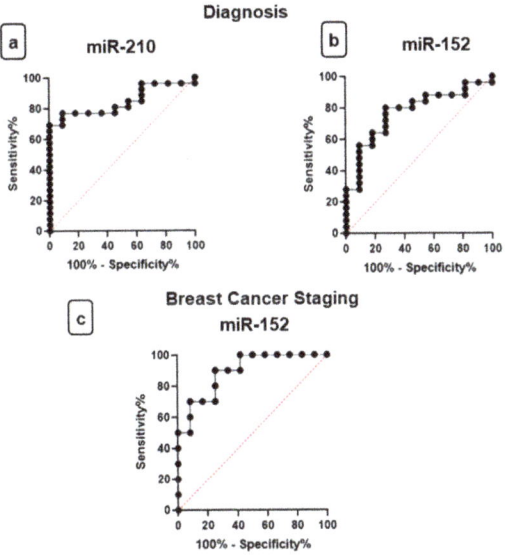

Figure 9. Receiver operating characteristic (ROC) curves investigate the diagnostic and staging power of miRNAs. (**a**) Plasma levels of miR-210 and (**b**) miR-152 discriminate breast cancer (BC) patients from healthy individuals—area under the curve (AUC) = 0.8427 and AUC = 0.709, respectively; cut-off value of 1.690 and of 0.252, respectively. Plasma levels of miR-152 (**c**) discriminate advanced stage of BC patients from early/intermediate stage of BC patients (AUC = 0.8917; cut-off value of 2.573).

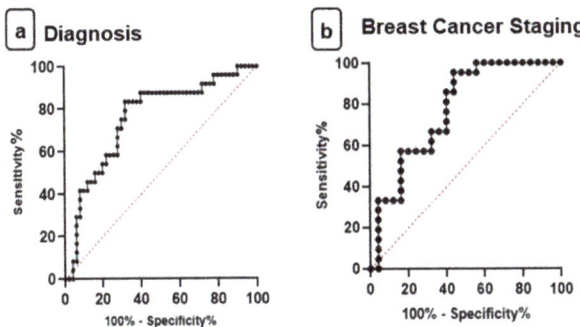

Figure 10. Receiver operating characteristic (ROC) curves investigate the diagnostic and staging power of amount combined of the miRNAs. (**a**) Plasma levels of miR-210 with miR-152 discriminate breast cancer (BC) patients from healthy individuals—area under the curve (AUC) = 0.7542; cut-off value of 0.9571. (**b**) Plasma levels of miR-210 with miR-152 discriminate advanced stage of BC patients from early/intermediate stage of BC patients (AUC = 0.7733; cut-off value of 2.660).

4. Discussion

This study aimed to identify and validate two promising circulating miRNAs as biomarkers for diagnosis and staging of BC. In the clinical routine, a useful biomarker is still not available that is able to detect early malignant breast tumors and also predict the clinical evolution of the disease, with the advantage of being minimally invasive and routinely quantified [21]. In addition to the benefits of liquid biopsy, studies show that miRNAs are stable in biological fluids, and therefore have been investigated as potential circulating biomarkers [9]. Thus, the well-consolidated miRNAs in BC were selected to verify if they have good potential as circulating biomarkers.

miR-210 has been reported as one of the most consistent miRNAs for this neoplasm [22]. In this study, the results showed increased expression levels of miR-210 in tumor fragment samples. Thakur et al. also observed increased expression of this miRNA in tissue and cell lines of BC (MDA-MB-231 and MCF-10) [23]. Subsequently, the oncomiR-210 target protein expressions involved in the angiogenesis pathway were validated. In BC samples, this study found increased levels of HIF-1α expression and decreased levels of VHL. In neuroblastoma tumors, Ognibene et al. also observed that most hypoxic tumors present high expression of HIF-1α, which is a prognostic indicator to stratify high-risk patients [24]. In renal carcinoma cells, densitometry analysis revealed that the protein expression of VHL in cancerous tissue was lower when compared to normal adjacent tissue of the patients [25].

Another miRNA addressed in this study was miR-152. This is considered a tumor miRNA suppressor well validated in several types of neoplasms, including BC [16,26]. In this study, decreased levels of miR-152 expression were observed in tumor fragments. In addition to these results, Wen et al. found that miR-152 expression levels were significantly lower in BC fragments than in non-cancerous tissues [27]. Furthermore, Ge et al. investigated the role of this miRNA in the initiation and progression of BC and found that miR-152 expression was significantly reduced in BC fragments and in cell lines [19]. MiR-152 acts on the angiogenesis pathway as a tumor suppressor, leading to IGF-1R blockade [16]. In agreement with our findings, studies have observed the overexpression of IGF-1R in BC samples, and this may influence the heterogeneity of molecular subtypes [28].

Both cascades of miR-210 and miR-152 have a final interference on the VEGF protein, which culminates in the development of new blood vessels for the tumor microenvironment [29]. In this study, the expression of VEGF in BC samples was validated. As with our results, previous studies have shown an increase of this protein in BC and also in other neoplasms [30,31].

After verifying the expression of these miRNAs and their target proteins in BC fragments, we questioned whether they could be potential circulating biomarkers for this neoplasm. According to Chen et al. [32], the source of circulating miRNAs in cancer patients is controlled by the following three mechanisms: (i) passive miRNA leakage from tumor cells, (ii) active secretion via microvesicles, and (iii) active secretion using an RNA-binding protein-dependent pathway, without microvesicles. Nonetheless, according to these authors, the miRNAs from sources (i) and (ii) have stability in the blood circulation, despite the presence of ribonucleases.

In the specific case of miR-210, this study found increased levels in the plasma of patients with BC, which coincides with the findings in the fragments. In agreement with these results, Madhavan et al. observed that miR 210 presented high levels in plasma samples from women with BC, and its expression was associated with the appearance of metastasis for up to two years after confirmation of the diagnosis [33]. Markou et al. also found significantly elevated plasma miR-210 levels in women with metastatic BC compared to healthy women [34]. Moreover, Qattan et al., comparing the expression levels of plasma miRNAs from women with BC and available RNASeq data from breast tumor tissue, also found that miR-210 showed increased levels of expression in both samples [35].

Cancer cells secrete various types of humoral factors in their tumor microenvironment and, among them, are extracellular vesicles (microvesicles and exosomes). Currently, evidence suggests the importance of communication between cancer cells and their microenvironment by releasing membrane exosomes that can fuse with nearby cells [36]. According to Adouh et al., circulating blood exosomes are the main contributing factors involved in the horizontal transfer of malignant characteristics to the target cells [37]. These horizontal molecular transfers can modulate cell-signaling pathways, such as the miR-210 pathway of angiogenesis. It is concluded, therefore, that the increased levels of miR-210 in plasma may reflect molecular changes in the cells from which they are derived [38].

Our results showed increased expression of circulating miR-152 in the plasma of women with BC. This was an interesting finding in this study because, as already described, miR-152 has a suppressive action on fragments of breast neoplasms. In the literature, there is only one study involving miR-152 and blood samples from patients with BC. The authors also observed increased plasma levels of miR-152 in patients with the disease and in patients with benign lesions compared to the control group. Furthermore, the increased expression of plasma miR-152 levels was also observed in patients with lung and colon cancer when compared to the control group [39]. Another study demonstrated that an increased level of circulating miR-152 was found in patients with bladder cancer, which was related to tumor recurrence of invasive bladder cancer [40]. In addition, Lin et al. showed that the tumor suppressor miR-34a was upregulated in esophageal cancer and concluded that this miRNA can serve as a potential biomarker in the detection of the early stages of this neoplasia [41]. Moreover, Qattan et al. observed an inverse pattern between plasma and tissue levels of patients with BC triple negative for let-7b, miR-29c, and miR-22. In all cases, plasma miRNA levels were higher than tissue levels [35].

According to Kosaka et al., negatively regulated miRNAs in cancer tissues are supplied during the initial stage of tumorigenesis by the surrounding cells that provide exosomes containing the decreased miRNAs. However, if the surrounding cells fail to meet demand, the cancer cells end up entering an advanced oncogenic stage. Thus, microRNAs secreted by exosomes can be useful for the maintenance and surveillance system against cancer progression [42].

In some cases, the exosomal mechanism can be used by metastatic cells to eliminate miRNAs with suppressive functions. For example, one study showed that miRNAs in the let-7 family, which preferentially act as a tumor suppressor, showed increased levels of expression in metastatic gastric cancer cells compared to non-metastatic parental cells. Therefore, the authors concluded that the let-7 miRNA family is rich in exosomes from a metastatic gastric cancer [43]. Yet, another study showed that tumor suppressor miR-23b, highly secreted by exosomes from metastatic cells, showed decreased levels in lymph node metastasis compared to primary tumors. Thus, the exosome-mediated secretion of tumor suppressor miRNA is selected during tumor progression as a mechanism to coordinate the activation of a metastatic cascade [44].

Therefore, exosomes play an important role in communicating with the tumor microenvironment, since cancer cells can modulate the stromal environment in their favor, or even surrounding cells can try to stop the evolution of malignancy by "delivering" protective miRNAs [45]. Many studies show that circulating miRNAs packaged by extracellular vesicles are protected from the degradation action of ribonucleases and, therefore, present high levels in the bloodstream. In this way, so as not to be degraded in the bloodstream, secretory vesicles carry circulating miRNAs [46,47].

In summary, we hypothesized that the discrepancies in the expected miR-152 expression in plasma and tissue fragments occur because circulating miRNAs packaged by extracellular vesicles are protected from the degradation action of ribonucleases and, thus, present high levels in the bloodstream. Despite the advances made regarding miR-152, further studies are needed to determine which regulatory mechanisms for miRNAs are secreted by exosomes, especially with regard to tumor suppressor miRNAs present in biological fluids. This will provide enormous opportunities for cancer-targeted therapies in the near future.

In order to establish the value of miRNAs as circulating biomarkers of diagnosis and staging, ROC curves were constructed and the AUC calculated. Hosmer and Lemeshow defined a rule that studies follow to identify good results in the ROC curves, based on respective AUC values: "0.5 = this suggests no discrimination, so we might as well flip a coin; 0.5–0.7 = we consider this poor discrimination, not much better than a coin toss;

0.7–0.8 = acceptable discrimination; 0.8–0.9 = excellent discrimination and >0.9 = outstanding discrimination" [48].

In the present study, results showed that miR-210 in plasma samples have excellent discrimination to be used as a biomarker of diagnosis, according to the AUC of the ROC curve comparing the control group and BC. With the same objective, other studies obtained similar results. Markou et al. evaluated miR-210 by ROC curve analysis and concluded that it was a valuable biomarker for discriminating patients from healthy individuals, with AUCs of 0.959 (95% Confidence Interval (CI) = 0.917–1.000, $p < 0.0001$) [34].

Despite the unexpected increased expression of miR-152 in women with BC, ROC curve analysis demonstrated that miR-152 expression in plasma samples has an acceptable discrimination to be used as a biomarker of diagnosis. Furthermore, miR-152 has shown greater sensitivity compared to miR-210, which demonstrated its greater capacity in the screening of BC. In contrast, miR-210 was shown to be the most specific in the analysis, which could indicate a greater capacity, compared to the miR-152, to confirm the diagnosis of BC, with lower false-positive results. In the same way, other authors obtained similar results. Chen et al. observed significant upregulated miR-152 expression with a 2.91-fold change in BC patients ($p = 0.00275$), when compared to normal controls. Furthermore, they evaluated miR-152 by ROC curve analysis and concluded that it was a valuable plasma biomarker for discriminating patients with BC and BBC from normal controls [39].

To investigate the role of miR-152 in plasma staging biomarkers, the values of AUC showed that miR-152 plasma expression has an outstanding discrimination to differentiate early/intermediate and advanced stage of BC patients. Furthermore, Dasari et al. evaluated that the level of miR-152 in peripheral blood was higher in patients with high-grade cervical intraepithelial neoplasia (CIN) compared with those with low-grade CIN, which demonstrates the prognostic importance of this miRNA in the carcinogenic process [49].

5. Conclusions

In conclusion, analysis of miRNA expression in the fragments showed increased miR-210 and decreased miR-152 in BC, also validated by the expression of their target proteins involved in angiogenesis. Among miRNAs, miR-210 had a potential as a diagnostic biomarker and miR-152 presented a potential as diagnostic and staging biomarkers. The combination of the two miRNAs has the potential to be used as diagnostic and prognostic biomarkers in BC, but not better than the miRNAs used individually. These results may contribute to the use of these miRNAs as promising circulating markers in addition to the benefit of being detected by liquid biopsy. In the future, it is also expected that the miRNAs may be potential therapeutic targets, contributing to advances in personalized medicine.

Supplementary Materials: The following are available online at https://www.mdpi.com/2075-4426/11/1/31/s1, Table S1: Description of microRNAs, Table S2: Primary antibodies used in immunohistochemical techniques and their respective specifications, Figure S1: Photomicrographs of the positive and negative controls of the target proteins during the immunohistochemistry reaction. Magnification of 40X. Bar: 20 μm.

Author Contributions: Conceptualization, B.C.L. and D.A.P.C.Z.; methodology, B.C.L., C.Z.B., F.V.V., J.G.d.O. and E.M.K.-J.; software, B.C.L., C.Z.B. and F.V.V.; validation, B.C.L., C.Z.B. and J.G.d.O.; formal analysis, B.C.L. and C.Z.B.; investigation, B.C.L. and C.Z.B.; resources, D.A.P.C.Z.; data curation, B.C.L. and D.A.P.C.Z.; writing—original draft preparation, B.C.L. and C.Z.B.; writing—review and editing, D.A.P.C.Z.; visualization, B.C.L. and D.A.P.C.Z.; supervision, D.A.P.C.Z. and N.A.B.-J.; project administration, D.A.P.C.Z.; funding acquisition, B.C.L. and D.A.P.C.Z. All authors have read and agreed to the published version of the manuscript.

Funding: Fundação de Amparo à Pesquisa do Estado de São Paulo (FAPESP) (2017/11807-3)/MSc. Beatriz Camargo Lopes. Fundação de Amparo à Pesquisa do Estado de São Paulo (FAPESP) (2017/15006-5)/PhD. Debora Aparecida Pires de Campos Zuccari. Fundação de Apoio à Pesquisa e Extensão de Sao Jose do Rio Preto (FAPERP) (028/2018)/MSc. Beatriz Camargo Lopes.

Institutional Review Board Statement: All procedures performed in studies involving human participants were in accordance with the ethical standards of the institutional and/or national research committee and with the 1964 Helsinki Declaration and its later amendments or comparable ethical standards. In addition, all procedures performed in studies were in accordance with the ethical standards of the institutional and/or national research committee (Research Ethics Committee (CEP) of the Faculty of Medicine of Sao Jose do Rio Preto (FAMERP), Sao Jose do Rio Preto, Brazil, #2.118.866/2017). This article does not contain any studies with animals performed by any of the authors.

Informed Consent Statement: Informed consent was obtained from all individual participants included in the study.

Data Availability Statement: The datasets used and/or analysed during the current study are available from the corresponding author on reasonable request.

Acknowledgments: The authors thank to the Laboratory of Morphology and Microanalysis (LMM) of the Institute of Biosciences, Letters and Exact Sciences (IBILCE), Sao Jose do Rio Preto, Brazil, for the support in obtaining the photomicrographs. Thanks to all patients and to the team of doctors, nurses and technicians at the Base Hospital, Sao Jose do Rio Preto, Brazil.

Conflicts of Interest: The authors declare no conflict of interest.

References

1. Crawford, Y.; Ferrara, N. VEGF inhibition: Insights from preclinical and clinical studies. *Cell Tissue Res.* **2009**, *335*, 261–269. [CrossRef] [PubMed]
2. Zhang, C.; Liu, K.; Li, T.; Fang, J.; Ding, Y.; Sun, L.; Tu, T.; Jiang, X.; Du, S.; Hu, J.; et al. miR-21: A gene of dual regulation in breast cancer. *Int. J. Oncol.* **2016**, *48*, 161–172. [CrossRef] [PubMed]
3. Boudreau, N.; Myers, C. Breast cancer-induced angiogenesis: Multiple mechanisms and the role of the microenvironment. *Breast Cancer Res.* **2003**, *5*, 140–146. [CrossRef] [PubMed]
4. Chiu, C.J.; Conley, Y.P.; Gorin, M.B.; Gensler, G.; Lai, C.Q.; Shang, F.; Taylor, A. Associations between Genetic Polymorphisms of Insulin-like Growth Factor Axis Genes and Risk for Age-related Macular Degeneration. *Investig. Ophthalmol. Vis. Sci.* **2011**, *52*, 9099–9107. [CrossRef]
5. Rahimi, N. The Ubiquitin-Proteasome System Meets Angiogenesis. *Mol. Cancer Ther.* **2012**, *11*, 538–548. [CrossRef]
6. Wu, F.T.; Lu, L.; Xu, W.; Li, J.Y. Circulating tumor DNA: Clinical roles in diffuse large B cell lymphoma. *Ann. Hematol.* **2018**, *98*, 255–269. [CrossRef]
7. Qi, Z.H.; Xu, H.X.; Zhang, S.R.; Xu, J.Z.; Li, S.; Gao, H.L.; Jin, W.; Wang, W.Q.; Wu, C.T.; Ni, Q.X.; et al. The Significance of Liquid Biopsy in Pancreatic Cance. *J. Cancer* **2018**, *9*, 3417–3426. [CrossRef]
8. Esquela-Kerscher, A.; Slack, F.J. Oncomirs-microRNAs with a role in cancer. *Nat. Rev. Cancer* **2006**, *6*, 259–269. [CrossRef]
9. Wei, J.; Gao, W.; Zhu, C.J.; Liu, Y.K.; Mei, Z.; Cheng, T.; Shu, Y.Q. Identification of plasma microRNA-21 as biomarker for early detection and chemosensity of non-small cell lung cancer. *Chin. J. Cancer* **2011**, *30*, 407–414. [CrossRef]
10. Bertoli, G.; Cava, C.; Castiglioni, I. MicroRNAs: New biomarkers for diagnosis, prognosis, therapy prediction and therapeutic tools for breast cancer. *Theranostics* **2015**, *5*, 1122–1143. [CrossRef]
11. Karakashev, S.V.; Reginato, M.J. Progress toward overcoming hypoxia-induced resistance to solid tumor therapy. *Cancer Manag. Res.* **2015**, *7*, 253–264. [CrossRef] [PubMed]
12. Agrawal, R.; Pandey, P.; Jha, P.; Dwivedi, V.; Sarkar, C.; Kulshreshtha, R. Hypoxic signature of microRNAs in glioblastoma: Insights from small RNA deep sequencing. *BMC Genom.* **2014**, *17*, 1–16. [CrossRef] [PubMed]
13. Jung, E.J.; Santarpia, L.; Kim, J.; Esteva, F.J.; Moretti, E.; Buzdar, A.U.; Di Leo, A.; Le, X.F.; Bast-Jr, R.C.; Park, S.T.; et al. Plasma microRNA 210 levels correlate with sensitivity to trastuzumab and tumor presence in breast cancer patients. *Cancer* **2012**, *118*, 2603–2614. [CrossRef] [PubMed]
14. Dang, K.; Myers, K.A. The role of Hypoxia-Induced miR-210 in Cancer Progression. *Int. J. Mol. Sci.* **2015**, *16*, 6353–6372. [CrossRef] [PubMed]
15. Liu, D.; Xia, H.; Wang, F.; Chen, C.; Long, J. MicroRNA-210 interacts with FBXO31 to regulate cancer proliferation cell cycle and migration in human breast cancer. *Onco Targets Ther.* **2016**, *9*, 5245–5255. [CrossRef]
16. Xu, Q.; Jiang, Y.; Yin, Y.; Li, Q.; He, J.; Jing, Y.; Qi, Y.-T.; Xu, Q.; Li, W.; Lu, B.; et al. A regulatory circuit of miR-148a/152 and DNMT1 in modulating cell transformation and tumor angiogenesis through IGF-IR and IRS1. *J. Mol. Cell Biol.* **2013**, *5*, 3–13. [CrossRef]
17. Sengupta, D.; Deb, M.; Rath, S.K.; Kar, S.; Parbin, S.; Pradhan, N.; Patra, S.K. DNA methylation and not H3K4 trimethylation dictates the expression status of miR-152 gene which inhibits migration of breast cancer cells via DNMT1/CDH1 loop. *Exp. Cell Res.* **2016**, *15*, 176–187. [CrossRef]
18. Liu, X.; Li, J.; Qin, F.; Dai, S. miR-152 as a tumor suppressor microRNA: Target recognition and regulation in cancer. *Oncol. Lett.* **2016**, *11*, 3911–3916. [CrossRef]

19. Ge, S.; Wang, D.; Kong, Q.; Gao, W.; Sun, J. Function of miR-152 as a Tumor Suppressor in Human Breast Cancer by Targeting PIK3CA. *Oncol. Res.* **2017**, *25*, 1363–1371. [CrossRef]
20. Roth, C.; Rack, B.; Müller, V.; Janni, W.; Pantel, K.; Schwarzenbach, H. Circulating microRNAs as blood-based markers for patients with primary and metastatic breast cancer. *Breast Cancer Res.* **2010**, *12*, R90. [CrossRef]
21. Duffy, M.J.; Harbeck, N.; Nap, M.; Molina, R.; Nicolini, A.; Senkus, E.; Cardoso, F. Clinical use of biomarkers in breast cancer: Updated guidelines from the European Group on Tumor Markers (EGTM). *Eur. J. Cancer* **2017**, *75*, 284–298. [CrossRef] [PubMed]
22. Qin, Q.; Furong, W.; Baosheng, L. Multiple functions of hypoxia-regulated miR-210 in cancer. *J. Exp. Clin. Cancer Res.* **2014**, *33*, 1–10. [CrossRef] [PubMed]
23. Thakur, S.; Grover, R.K.; Gupta, S.; Yadav, A.K.; Das, B.C. Identification of Specific miRNA Signature in Paired Sera and Tissue Samples of Indian Women with Triple Negative Breast Cancer. *PLoS ONE* **2016**, *11*, 1–21. [CrossRef] [PubMed]
24. Ognibene, M.; Cangelosi, D.; Morini, M.; Segalerba, D.; Bosco, M.C.; Sementa, A.R.; Eva, A.; Varesio, L. Immunohistochemical analysis of PDK1, PHD3 and HIF-1α expression defines the hypoxic status of neuroblastoma tumors. *PLoS ONE* **2017**, *12*, 1–19. [CrossRef] [PubMed]
25. Hogner, A.; Krause, H.; Jandrig, B.; Kasim, M.; Fuller, T.F.; Schostak, M.; Erbersdobler, A.; Patzak, A.; Kilic, E. PBRM1 and VHL expression correlate in human clear cell renal cell carcinoma with differential association with patient's overall survival. *Urol. Oncol. Semin. Orig. Investig.* **2018**, *36*, 94.e1–94.e14. [CrossRef]
26. Zhang, H.; Lu, Y.; Wang, S.; Sheng, X.; Zhang, S. MicroRNA-152 Acts as a Tumor Suppressor MicroRNA by Inhibiting Kruppel-Like Factor 5 in Human Cervical Cancer. *Oncol Res. Featur. Preclin. Clin. Cancer Ther.* **2019**, *27*, 335–340. [CrossRef] [PubMed]
27. Wen, Y.Y.; Liu, W.T.; Sun, H.R.; Ge, X.; Shi, Z.M.; Wang, M.; Ling-Zhi, L.; Zhang, J.Y.; Liu, L.Z.; Jiang, B.H. IGF-1-mediated PKM2/beta-catenin/miR-152 regulatory circuit in breast cancer. *Sci. Rep.* **2017**, *7*, 1–10. [CrossRef]
28. Sun, W.Y.; Yun, H.Y.; Song, Y.J.; Kim, H.; Lee, O.J.; Nam, S.J.; Koo, J.S. Insulin-like growth factor 1 receptor expression in breast cancer tissue and mammographic density. *Mol. Clin. Oncol.* **2015**, *3*, 572–580. [CrossRef]
29. Cebe-Suarez, S.; Zehnder-Fjallman, A.; Ballmer-Hofer, K. The role of VEGF receptors in angiogenesis; complex partnerships. *Cell Mol. Life Sci.* **2006**, *63*, 601–615. [CrossRef]
30. Maae, E.; Nielsen, M.; Steffensen, K.D.; Jakobsen, E.H.; Jakobsen, A.; Sorensen, F.B. Estimation of immunohistochemical expression of VEGF in ductal carcinomas of the breast. *J. Histochem. Cytochem.* **2011**, *59*, 750–760. [CrossRef]
31. Wen, S.; Shao, G.; Zheng, J.; Zeng, H.; Luo, J.; Gu, D. Apatinib regulates the cell proliferation and apoptosis of liver cancer by regulation of VEGFR2/STAT3 signaling. *Pathol. Res. Pract.* **2019**, *215*, 816–821. [CrossRef] [PubMed]
32. Chen, X.; Liang, H.; Zhang, J.; Zen, K.; Zhang, C.Y. Secreted microRNAs: A new form of intercellular communication. *Trends Cell Biolog.* **2012**, *22*, 125–132. [CrossRef] [PubMed]
33. Madhavan, D.; Peng, C.; Wallwiener, M.; Zucknick, M.; Nees, J.; Schott, S. Circulating miRNAs with prognostic value in metastatic breast cancer and for early detection of metastasis. *Carcinogenesis* **2016**, *37*, 461–470. [CrossRef] [PubMed]
34. Markou, A.; Zavridou, M.; Sourvinou, I.; Yousef, G.; Kounelis, S.; Malamos, N.; Georgoulias, V.; Lianidou, E. Direct Comparison of Metastasis-Related miRNAs Expression Levels in Circulating Tumor Cells, Corresponding Plasma, and Primary Tumors of Breast Cancer Patients. *Clin. Chem.* **2016**, *62*, 1002–1011. [CrossRef] [PubMed]
35. Qattan, A.M.; Intabli, H.; Alkhayal, W.; Eltabache, C.; Tweigieri, T.; Amer, S.B. Robust expression of tumor suppressor miRNA's let-7 and miR-195 detected in plasma of Saudi female breast cancer patients. *BMC Cancer* **2017**, *17*, 1–10. [CrossRef] [PubMed]
36. Yoshioka, Y.; Katsuda, T.; Ochiya, T. Extracellular vesicles and encapusulated miRNAs as emerging cancer biomarkers for novel liquid biopsy. *Jpn. J. Clin. Oncol.* **2018**, *48*, 1–8. [CrossRef] [PubMed]
37. Adouh, M.; Hamam, D.; Gao, Z.H.; Arena, V.; Arena, M.; Arena, G.O. Exosomes isolated from cancer patients sera transfer malignant traits and confer the same phenotype of primary tumors to oncosuppressor-mutated cells. *J. Exp. Clin. Cancer Res.* **2017**, *36*, 1–15. [CrossRef]
38. Dilsiz, N. Role of exosomes and exosomal microRNAs in cancer. *Future Sci.* **2020**, *6*, FSO465. [CrossRef]
39. Chen, H.; Liu, H.; Zou, H.; Chen, R.; Dou, Y.; Sheng, S.; Dai, S.; Ai, J.; Melson, J.; Kittles, R.A.; et al. Evaluation of Plasma miR-21 and miR-152 as Diagnostic Biomarkers for Common Types of Human Cancers. *J. Cancer* **2016**, *7*, 490–499. [CrossRef]
40. Jiang, X.; Du, L.; Wang, L.; Li, J.; Liu, Y.; Zheng, G.; Qu, A.; Zhang, X.; Pan, H.; Yang, Y.; et al. Serum microRNA expression signatures identified from genome-wide microRNA profiling serve as novel noninvasive biomarkers for diagnosis and recurrence of bladder cancer. *Int. J. Cancer* **2015**, *136*, 854–862. [CrossRef]
41. Lin, Y.; Lin, Z.; Fang, Z.; Li, H.; Zhi, X.; Zhang, Z. Plasma MicroRNA-34a as a Potential Biomarker for Early Diagnosis of Esophageal Cancer. *Clin. Lab.* **2019**, *65*. [CrossRef]
42. Kosaka, N.; Iguchi, H.; Yoshioka, Y.; Takeshita, F.; Matsuki, Y.; Ochiya, T. Secretory Mechanisms and Intercellular Transfer of MicroRNAs in Living Cells. *J. Biol. Chem.* **2010**, *285*, 17442–17452. [CrossRef]
43. Ohshima, K.; Inoue, K.; Fujiwara, A.; Hatakeyama, K.; Kanto, K.; Watanabe, Y.; Muramatsu, K.; Fukuda, Y.; Ogura, S.-I.; Yamaguchi, K.; et al. Let-7 microRNA family is selectively secreted into the extracellular environment via exosomes in a metastatic gastric cancer cell line. *PLoS ONE* **2010**, *8*, e13247. [CrossRef] [PubMed]
44. Ostenfeld, M.S.; Jeppesen, D.K.; Laurberg, J.R.; Boysen, A.T.; Bramsen, J.B.; Primdal-Bengtson, B.; Hendrix, A.; Lamy, P.; Dagnaes-Hansen, F.; Rasmussen, M.H.; et al. Cellular Disposal of miR23b by RAB27-Dependent Exosome Release Is Linked to Acquisition of Metastatic Properties. *Cancer Res.* **2014**, *74*, 5758–5771. [CrossRef]

45. Falcone, G.; Felsani, A.; D'Agnano, I. Signaling by exosomal microRNAs in cancer. *J. Exp. Clin. Cancer Res.* **2015**, *34*, 1–10. [CrossRef]
46. Wang, K.; Zhang, S.; Weber, J.; Baxter, D.; Galas, D.J. Export of microRNAs and microRNA-protective protein by mammalian cells. *Nucleic Acids Res.* **2010**, *38*, 7248–7259. [CrossRef] [PubMed]
47. Mitchell, P.S.; Parkin, R.K.; Kroh, E.M.; Fritz, B.R.; Wyman, S.K.; Pogosova-Agadjanyan, E.L.; Peterson, A.; Noteboom, J.; O'Briant, K.C.; Allen, A.; et al. Circulating microRNAs as stable blood-based markers for cancer detection. *Proc. Natl. Acad. Sci. USA* **2008**, *105*, 10513–10518. [CrossRef]
48. Hosmer, D.W., Jr.; Lemeshow, S.; Sturdivant, R.X. *Applied Logistic Regression*, 3rd ed.; Wiley: Hoboken, NJ, USA, 2013; p. 177.
49. Dasari, S.; Wudayagiri, R.; Valluru, L. Cervical Cancer: Biomarkers for Diagnosis and Treatment. *Clin. Chim. Acta* **2015**, *445*, 7–11. [CrossRef] [PubMed]

MDPI
St. Alban-Anlage 66
4052 Basel
Switzerland
Tel. +41 61 683 77 34
Fax +41 61 302 89 18
www.mdpi.com

Journal of Personalized Medicine Editorial Office
E-mail: jpm@mdpi.com
www.mdpi.com/journal/jpm

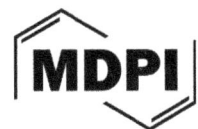

www.ingramcontent.com/pod-product-compliance
Lightning Source LLC
LaVergne TN
LVHW070139100526
838202LV00015B/1850

9 7 8 3 0 3 6 5 3 8 0 6 8